T0293665

Diagnosis and Treatment of Anemia

Diagnosis and Treatment of Anemia

Edited by Martha Pratt

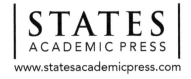
www.statesacademicpress.com

States Academic Press,
109 South 5th Street,
Brooklyn, NY 11249, USA

Visit us on the World Wide Web at:
www.statesacademicpress.com

ISBN: 978-1-63989-761-2

Cataloging-in-Publication Data

Diagnosis and treatment of anemia / edited by Martha Pratt.
     p. cm.
Includes bibliographical references and index.
ISBN 978-1-63989-761-2
1. Anemia. 2. Anemia--Pathophysiology. 3. Anemia--Diagnosis. 4. Anemia--Treatment.
5. Blood--Diseases. I. Pratt, Martha.
RC641 .A54 2023
616.152--dc23

Table of Contents

Preface

The purpose of the book is to provide a glimpse into the dynamics and to present opinions and studies of some of the scientists engaged in the development of new ideas in the field from very different standpoints. This book will prove useful to students and researchers owing to its high content quality.

Anemia is a blood disorder, where the capability of the blood to carry oxygen is decreased due to a low blood count, or due to low levels of hemoglobin. Chronic anemia has symptoms such as weakness, headaches, tiredness and short breath, while acute anemia shows symptoms like loss of consciousness, confusion, dizziness and increased thirst. The causes of anemia include loss of blood, fluid overload, impaired production of red blood cells, and increased reduction of red blood cells. Anemia is diagnosed on the basis of complete blood count. A blood test is utilized generally for determining the platelets and count of red blood cells and white blood cells. Tests such as serum ferritin, serum vitamin B12, and sample of bone marrow can help in determining the type of anemia and its cause. Treatment of anemia is dependent on its severity and cause, and includes iron supplementation in oral and injectable form, blood transfusions, intramuscular injections of vitamin B12, hyperbaric oxygen, and erythropoiesis-stimulating agents. This book aims to understand the diagnosis and treatment of anemia. It will serve as a reference to a broad spectrum of readers.

At the end, I would like to appreciate all the efforts made by the authors in completing their chapters professionally. I express my deepest gratitude to all of them for contributing to this book by sharing their valuable works. A special thanks to my family and friends for their constant support in this journey.

Editor

Red Blood Cell Homeostasis and Altered Vesicle Formation in Patients with Paroxysmal Nocturnal Hemoglobinuria

Joames K. Freitas Leal[1], Frank Preijers[2], Roland Brock[1], Merel Adjobo-Hermans[1] and Giel Bosman[1*]

[1]Department of Biochemistry, Radboud University Medical Center, Nijmegen, Netherlands, [2]Laboratory for Hematology, Department of Laboratory Medicine, Radboud University Medical Center, Nijmegen, Netherlands

*Correspondence:
Giel Bosman
giel.bosman@radboudumc.nl

A subset of the red blood cells (RBCs) of patients with paroxysmal nocturnal hemoglobinuria (PNH) lacks GPI-anchored proteins. Some of these proteins, such as CD59, inhibit complement activation and protect against complement-mediated lysis. This pathology thus provides the possibility to explore the involvement of complement in red blood cell homeostasis and the role of GPI-anchored proteins in the generation of microvesicles (MVs) *in vivo*. Detailed analysis of morphology, volume, and density of red blood cells with various CD59 expression levels from patients with PNH did not provide indications for a major aberration of the red blood cell aging process in patients with PNH. However, our data indicate that the absence of GPI-anchored membrane proteins affects the composition of red blood cell-derived microvesicles, as well as the composition and concentration of platelet-derived vesicles. These data open the way toward a better understanding on the pathophysiological mechanism of PNH and thereby to the development of new treatment strategies.

Keywords: red blood cells, paroxysmal nocturnal hemoglobinuria, aging, thrombosis, microvesicles

INTRODUCTION

Paroxysmal nocturnal hemoglobinuria (PNH) is a highly debilitating disease that is characterized by intravascular hemolysis, arterial, and venous thrombosis (Malato et al., 2012; Peacock-Young et al., 2018) and a variety of symptoms related to smooth muscle dystonia (DeZern and Brodsky, 2015). PNH is a rare disease with an incidence of 1–2 per 1,000,000 persons per year and is frequently associated with bone marrow failure such as aplastic anemia (Clemente et al., 2018). PNH is caused by clonal expansion of multipotent hematopoietic stem cells with somatic mutations in the *PIGA* gene. *PIGA* encodes for an enzyme that is critical in the synthesis of the first intermediate in the pathway of glycosylphosphatidylinositol (GPI) anchors. (Takeda et al., 1993; DeZern and Brodsky, 2015) As a consequence, the absence of *PIGA* activity results in hematopoietic cells that are deficient in GPI-anchored proteins. In RBCs, the absence of the GPI-anchored proteins decay-accelerating factor (DAF;

CD55) and membrane inhibitor of reactive lysis (MIRL; CD59) that protect against complement-mediated lysis renders red blood cells (RBCs) highly vulnerable to intravascular hemolysis (Risitano and Rotoli, 2008; Brodsky, 2014). This results not only in anemia but also in the release of free hemoglobin and iron, which catalyzes the generation of reactive oxygen species and subsequent NO depletion and vasoconstriction (Kahn et al., 2013; Rapido, 2017). For untreated patients, thrombosis is the most common cause of death (Hill et al., 2013; Griffin and Munir, 2017).

The monoclonal antibody eculizumab is the most effective drug used in PNH (Brodsky, 2009). Eculizumab blocks the cleavage of C5 by the C5 convertase into C5b and thereby inhibits the formation of the terminal membrane attack complex (MAC) C5b-9 and consequent hemolysis of abnormal RBCs. This reduces RBC destruction and transfusion requirements (Carroll and Sim, 2011; Risitano, 2012; Bayly-Jones et al., 2017). Nevertheless, the opsonizing effects of activated complement factors such as C3d may induce RBC phagocytosis (Risitano et al., 2009; DeZern and Brodsky, 2015).

At present, the mechanism(s) responsible for clonal expansion during hematopoiesis and the variable clinical manifestations of the disease have only partially been elucidated (Hill et al., 2017), but increased removal of RBC may contribute to the pathophysiology of PNH (Risitano and Rotoli, 2008). RBC homeostasis is dependent on the generation of young and removal of aged RBCs. The latter process is initiated by binding of senescent cell-specific IgG, the appearance of molecules that may trigger pathological reactions, such as immunoreactive epitopes on damaged membrane proteins, and exposure of phosphatidylserine (PS) in the outer leaflet of the lipid bilayer, all leading to phagocytosis (Bosman et al., 2008; Dinkla et al., 2014; Klei et al., 2017). From biophysical, immunochemical, proteomic, and metabolomic studies, a molecular picture of the pathways involved in the normal aging and removal process of RBCs has emerged: oxidative damage-induced, high-affinity binding of hemoglobin to the cytoplasmic domain of band 3, activation of Ca^{2+}-permeable channels, phosphorylation-controlled alterations in morphology and metabolism affecting ATP production and redox status, degradation of band 3 and/or aggregation of band 3 fragments, binding of IgG, and microvesicle (MV) generation (Ferru et al., 2011; Zolla and D'Alessandro, 2012; Bosman, 2016). Physiological anti-band 3 IgG has been reported to have a high affinity for dimeric C3b, thereby linking RBC phagocytosis to complement activation (Lutz and Bogdanova, 2013).

During physiological RBC aging, there is a small decrease in the content of GPI-anchored DAF and MIRL (Willekens et al., 2008), and in the content and activity of acetylcholinesterase (AChE), another GPI-anchored protein (Willekens et al., 2008; Freitas Leal et al., 2017). The latter observation suggests that the activities of DAF and/or MIRL might also decrease in healthy individuals and thereby contribute to complement-mediated opsonization and removal of old RBCs. AChE is increased in microvesicles, suggesting that changes in the distribution of GPI-anchored proteins in microdomains are associated with microvesicle (MV) generation (Salzer and Prohaska, 2001; Freitas Leal et al., 2017). As a consequence, the absence of GPI-anchored proteins may affect the microvesiculation process. Indeed, some data indicate that microvesiculation of RBCs and platelets may be impaired in PNH patients (Whitlow et al., 1993). Also, it has been shown that activated complement induces the massive formation of vesicles with a strong pro-coagulant activity (Ninomiya et al., 1999). Thus, the absence of GPI-anchored proteins may have a pronounced effect on RBC morphology, function, and survival (Whitlow et al., 1993). In addition, exposure of the pro-coagulant and removal signal PS, which is in general associated with abnormal membrane organization and vesiculation in damaged or stressed, but not in aged RBCs (Bosman et al., 2008), has been reported to be increased in RBCs of PNH patients (Sato et al., 2010).

Here, we have selected a number of aging-associated parameters from this current knowledge of the molecular mechanisms involved in physiological RBC homeostasis (Bosman et al., 2008, 2012; Lutz and Bogdanova, 2013; Bosman, 2016; Freitas Leal et al., 2018) that might be relevant for the pathophysiology of PNH, in order to explore the effect of the absence of GPI-linked proteins on RBC structure, function, aging, and removal in vivo. Our data, obtained from PNH patients with various clone sizes and following various treatment regimes, indicate no significant effects of the absence of GPI-linked proteins on RBC turnover but emphasize the heuristic value of more, detailed studies on the origin, composition, and activity of RBC-derived and platelet-derived microvesicles.

MATERIALS AND METHODS

Red Blood Cell Sampling

Blood was collected by venipuncture from healthy volunteers and 15 patients after obtaining written informed consent, and using EDTA as anticoagulant, following the guidelines of the local medical ethical committee (CMO regio Arnhem Nijmegen) and in accordance with the Declaration of Helsinki. Leukocytes and platelets were removed as described before using Ficoll-Paque (Freitas Leal et al., 2017). The time between blood collection, fractionation, and analysis was identical for all samples.

Red Blood Cell Fractionation and Microscopic Analysis

RBCs were fractionated according to cell density using discontinuous Percoll gradients ranging from 40% Percoll (1.060 g/ml) to 80% Percoll (1.096 g/ml) as described before (Willekens et al., 2008; Freitas Leal et al., 2017). The various RBC fractions were isolated and washed three times with Ringer's solution (Freitas Leal et al., 2017) by repeated centrifugation for 5 min at 400 g before analysis. RBC morphology was analyzed using a TCS SP5 confocal laser scanning microscope (Leica Microsystems, Mannheim, Germany) as described before (Cluitmans et al., 2015).

Isolation and Characterization of Microvesicles From Plasma

Microvesicles (MVs) were isolated from the platelet-rich plasma (PRP) obtained after differential centrifugation as described before (Dinkla et al., 2012, 2013, 2016).

Flow Cytometry Analysis

Classification of the RBCs according to PNH type was performed by flow cytometry using FITC-labeled CD235a (clone KC16, 1:100, Beckman Coulter, Fullerton, CA, USA) and PE-labeled CD59 (clone MEM43, 1:400, IQ products, Groningen, the Netherlands) as described before (Sutherland et al., 2015). PNH RBCs were classified based on CD59 content in type III (complete GPI-deficiency), type II (partial GPI-deficiency), and type I (normal expression) cells (Sutherland et al., 2015). APC-labeled CD71 (clone CY1G4, 1:200, Biolegend, San Diego, California, USA) was combined with PE-labeled CD59 to evaluate the percentage of reticulocytes per PNH type. FITC-labeled anti-C3c (1:200, Abcam, Cambridge, UK) and APC-labeled anti-C3d (1 μg/million cells, Assay Pro, St. Louis, Missouri, USA) were combined with PE-labeled CD59 to evaluate the degree of opsonization per PNH type. Staining of band 3 with eosin-5′ maleimide (EMA, Thermo Fisher Scientific, Landsmeer, the Netherlands) was performed by incubating 1 million RBCs with 25 μl of EMA (0.5 mg/ml in Ringer's solution) in the dark at RT for 15 min. (Cobb and Beth, 1990; Crisp et al., 2011). After staining, RBCs were washed three times with Ringer's solution and analyzed by flow cytometry [FACSCalibur instrument (BD Biosciences, Franklin Lakes NJ, USA)] using CELLQuest software (BD Biosciences). Data were analyzed with FlowJo cell analysis software v.10 (FlowJo, LLC, Ashland, OR) using 200,000 events. Microvesicle analysis was performed using mixtures of PE-labeled CD59 (1:400), FITC-labeled CD235a (1:100), and PE/Cy5-labeled CD41 (1:10) by flow cytometry as previously described (Dinkla et al., 2012, 2013). Sulfate latex microspheres (0.9 μm, Invitrogen, Carlsbad CA, USA) and washed Flow-Count calibration beads (Beckman Coulter, Brea CA, USA) were used for quantification (Dinkla et al., 2012). Microvesicles were classified based on CD59 positivity in CD59-negative (complete GPI-deficiency), low CD59 (partial GPI-deficiency), and wild type (normal expression).

Comparisons and Statistical Analyses

The exclusion criteria for the PNH patients were other hematological comorbidities besides aplastic anemia and having received a red blood cell transfusion within a period of 3 months before analysis. For most analyses, we compared PNH patients with control donors and PNH patients being treated with eculizumab with patients without eculizumab. Differences between groups were determined using a two-way ANOVA test. Non-parametric t-tests or one-way ANOVA tests were used to analyze differences between control and PNH samples. Wilcoxon matched pair tests were used to analyze differences between the various RBC fractions inside the groups, and the Fisher LSD test was used to compare controls and patient samples. Two-sided p'sless than 0.05 were used to determine statistical significance. Relations between the various parameters were estimated using the Pearson correlation coefficient.

RESULTS

RBC Morphology and Phenotype

During aging in vivo and in vitro, RBCs undergo a series of morphological changes that result in the appearance of deformed, mostly spherocytic cells. Semi-quantitative analysis of these changes has been shown to be informative on RBC hemostasis and on the relationship between morphology, deformability, and survival (Cluitmans et al., 2015). Microscopic analysis of RBCs from patients with PNH showed a tendency to a decrease in the numbers of cells with the regular discocyte form and a concomitant increase in the numbers of echinocyte-like and otherwise misshapen cells, especially in the densest cell fractions (Figure 1A). The majority of the patients' RBCs were type I according to CD59 expression levels (Figure 1B), and we found no differences in the percentages of type II and type III cells between the various Percoll layers (Figure 1C). Treatment with eculizumab did not result in significant differences in CD59-deficient cells (Figure 1D).

Membrane/Band 3 Content (Eosine 5′-Maleimide)

RBC aging is accompanied by changes in membrane organization that are associated with the appearance of removal signals and with the loss of cell membrane. Especially, changes in the integral membrane protein band 3 play a pivotal role in the generation of senescence-specific antigens, in the interaction between lipid bilayer and cytoskeleton, and in the generation of microvesicles (Willekens et al., 2008; Bosman et al., 2012; Lutz and Bogdanova, 2013; Freitas Leal et al., 2018). The amount of binding of the band 3 probe eosine 5′-maleimide (EMA) is mostly a sensitive marker of band 3 content, but also of Rh, Rh glycoprotein, and CD47, and/or of the loss of membrane (Cobb and Beth, 1990; Huisjes et al., 2018). Flow cytometric analysis of the binding of EMA showed a higher EMA signal in all RBC fractions from two different PNH patients tested, independent of cell density and treatment (Figure 2). There was no significant difference in the density-associated decrease between control donors or any of the PNH patients. Also, there was no statistically significant correlation between EMA fluorescence and the RBC size (forward scatter) in the RBC fractions of controls and PNH patients taken together ($r = 0.31$, $p = 0.18$, $N = 20$).

Complement Deposition (C3c and C3d)

Activation of complement may lead to deposition of complement fragments on RBC through the CR1 receptor, and the presence of C3b fragments induces phagocytosis of eculizumab-treated, CD59-negative RBCs in vitro (Lin et al., 2015). We therefore also probed for the presence of C3c and C3d

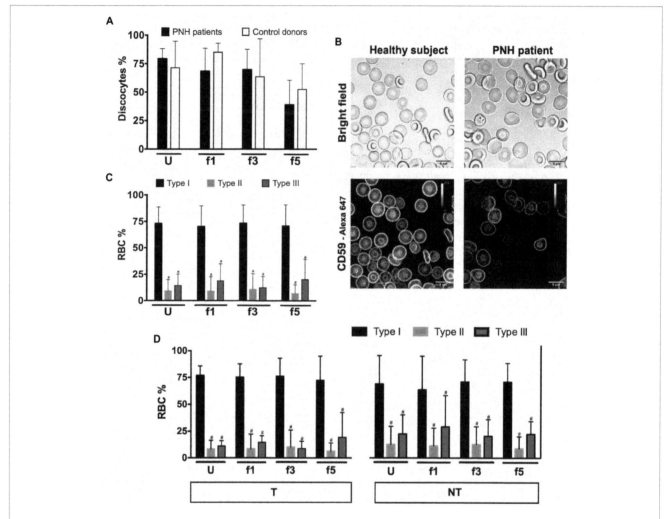

FIGURE 1 | RBCs morphology and phenotype of PNH patients. **(A)** Percentage of discocytes per Percoll fraction in PNH patients ($N = 5$) and healthy control donors ($N = 5$); **(B)** bright field and fluorescence images of anti-CD59-Alexa 647 stained RBCs from a healthy subject and a PNH patient, showing CD59 density; **(C)** RBCs of PNH patients ($N = 9$) were separated according to density and analyzed by flow cytometry regarding their CD59 content (type I, II, and III); **(D)** RBCs of PNH patients being treated with eculizumab (T; $N = 5$) and non-treated PNH patients (NT; $N = 4$) separated according to density and analyzed by flow cytometry according to their CD59 content (type I, II, and III). #Significantly different from type I in the same Percoll fraction ($p < 0.05$). U, unseparated; f1, f3, f5, fractions of increasing density isolated by Percoll density separation (Materials and Methods).

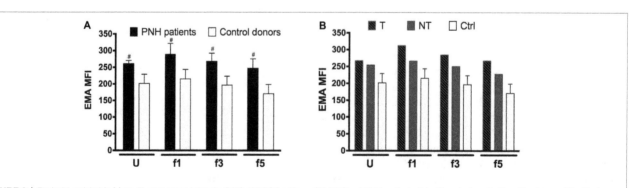

FIGURE 2 | Eosin 5′-maleimide Mean Fluorescence Intensity (MFI) of RBC fractions. **(A)** RBCs of PNH patients ($N = 2$) and of control healthy donors ($N = 7$) of various Percoll fractions were stained with eosin 5′-maleimide (EMA). The degree of staining is expressed as the mean fluorescence intensity (MFI). **(B)** EMA MFI of RBCs of a PNH patient being treated with (T) and without (NT) eculizumab, separated according to density. Ctrl, healthy donors ($N = 7$). The samples were analyzed as described before (see Materials and Methods). #Significantly different from control ($p < 0.05$). U, unseparated; f1, f3, f5, fractions of increasing density isolated by Percoll density separation (Materials and Methods).

in density-separated RBCs. For both proteins, we observed a tendency to an increase in the percentage of positive cells with cell density (**Figure 3**). Thus, the content of RBC-bound C3c as well as C3d may increase with cell age, also on type I RBCs with a normal content of CD59 (**Figure 3**). These findings are in agreement with previous indications for the involvement of complement in phagocytosis *in vitro* (Lutz, 2004; Arese et al., 2005). We found no significant correlations between these parameters and treatment with eculizumab (data not shown).

Reticulocytes

Aberrant RBC structure resulting in a decreased mean life and leading to anemia is, in many cases, compensated by increased erythropoiesis, as indicated by changes in the size of the reticulocyte fraction. The hematological data show a large variability in the size of the reticulocyte fractions of our patients, without any significant correlation with other patient variables, although most eculizumab-treated patients had higher reticulocyte numbers than the patients without eculizumab (**Supplementary Table 1**). Flow cytometric analysis of the RBCs of a few PNH patients showed similar data, also without significant differences between donors or RBC fractions (**Figures 4A,B**). In general, most reticulocytes were

found in the lightest density fractions upon Percoll separation, i.e., fraction 1 (**Figure 4A**), as shown before for healthy individuals (Willekens et al., 2008). The fraction of type III, CD59-lacking reticulocytes was considerably higher than the other types (**Figure 4C**), which may reflect a disturbed differentiation and/or maturation process in the absence of GPI-linked proteins (Sato et al., 2010).

Microvesicles

Microvesicle generation is an integral part of the physiological RBC aging process, and changes in microvesicle concentration as well as composition occur in patients with disturbed RBC homeostasis (Freitas Leal et al., 2018). We found no significant differences in the concentrations of RBC-derived microvesicles between PNH patients and controls (**Figure 5A**). However, the concentration of PS-negative microvesicles in the plasma of PNH patients was higher than in the plasma of control donors (**Figure 5B**). The concentration of CD59-high RBC-derived microvesicles was higher than that of the other types in the plasma of control donors but not in the plasma of PNH patients (**Figure 5C**). Platelet-derived microvesicle concentrations were much higher in the plasma of PNH patients than in controls (**Figure 5D**), both the PS-positive and the PS-negative microvesicles (**Figure 5E**). Remarkably, almost all platelet-derived

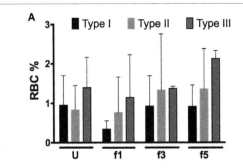
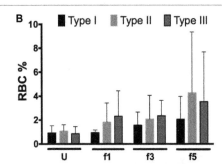

FIGURE 3 | Complement deposition on density-separated RBCs. **(A)** Percentage of C3c-positive RBCs in the PNH RBC population divided per CD59 content (type I, II, and III) per density (Percoll fraction; N = 2); **(B)** percentage of C3d-positive RBCs in the PNH RBC population according to CD59 content (type I, II, and III) per Percoll fraction (type I, II, and III; N = 3). The samples were analyzed as described before (see Materials and Methods). U, unseparated; f1, f3, f5, fractions of increasing density isolated by Percoll density separation (Materials and Methods).

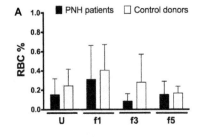
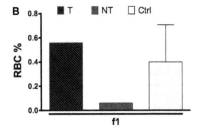
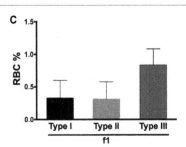

FIGURE 4 | Reticulocytes in patients with PNH. **(A)** Percentage of CD71-expressing RBCs from the blood of PNH patients (N = 2) and healthy control donors RBCs (N = 4) of various Percoll fractions after staining with APC-labeled CD71; **(B)** percentage of APC-CD71-positive RBCs of a PNH patient being treated with eculizumab (T), a non-treated PNH patient (NT), and healthy control donors in the reticulocyte-enriched Percoll fraction 1 (Ctrl; N = 4); **(C)** percentage of APC-CD71-positive RBCs in the PNH RBC population per CD59 content (type I, II, and III) in fraction 1 (N = 2). The samples were analyzed as described before (see Materials and Methods). U, unseparated; f1, f3, f5, fractions of increasing density isolated by Percoll density separation (Materials and Methods).

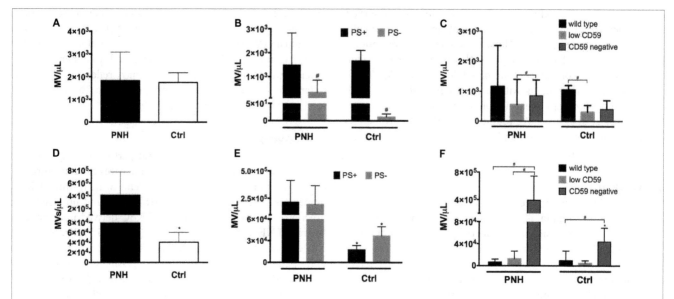

FIGURE 5 | Microvesicle numbers and composition in the blood of patients with PNH. **(A)** Concentration per microliter (MV/µl) of RBC-derived, CD235a-positive microvesicles in the blood of PNH patients (N = 9) and control healthy donors (N = 6); **(B)** concentration of RBC-derived microvesicles in the blood of PNH patients (N = 9) and control healthy donors (N = 3), distinguished according to their reactivity to Annexin V (phosphatidylserine-positive (PS+) or negative (PS–); **(C)** RBC-derived microvesicles were categorized into wild type, CD59-low and CD59-negative PNH, N = 9; Ctrl, N = 3, as described for RBCs (Materials and Methods); **(D)** concentration of CD41-positive, platelet-derived microvesicles in the blood of PNH patients (N = 9) and control healthy donors (N = 6); **(E)** concentration of platelet-derived microvesicles according their reactivity to Annexin V (PS+ or PS–; PNH, N = 9; Ctrl, N = 3); **(F)** platelet-derived microvesicles were categorized into wild type, CD59-low and CD59-negative as described for RBCs and quantified and analyzed by flow cytometry as described before (PNH, N = 9; Ctrl, N = 3). #Significantly different from the other parameter (p < 0.05); *Significantly different from the patients' samples (p < 0.05).

microvesicles were devoid of CD59, including those from the plasma of control donors (**Figure 5F**). We observed no statistically significant correlations between the numbers of RBC-derived and platelet-derived vesicles (r = −0.40, p = 0.28, N = 9).

DISCUSSION

RBC Aging and Generation of Microvesicles

Red blood cells of PNH patients lack the key GPI-anchored membrane proteins that protect against activated complement. We postulated that this change in membrane composition has a more wide-spread effect on membrane organization and thereby on various aspects of RBC homeostasis. The most obvious aspects derive from the role of complement in removal of senescent RBCs and the involvement of GPI-linked proteins in microdomain-associated generation of microvesicles (Lutz, 2004; Lutz and Bogdanova, 2013; de Back et al., 2014; Saha et al., 2016; Pollet et al., 2018). In this exploratory study, we did not find significant indications for a pronounced alteration of RBC homeostasis in patients with PNH, as based on cell volume, cell density, and morphology or on clinical hematology parameters, including LDH values (**Supplementary Table 1**). Thus, in most of our patients, the lack of GPI-anchored proteins does not seem to cause a major disturbance of the physiological RBC aging mechanisms.

Nevertheless, there were clear differences related to membrane composition and microvesicle formation. The EMA

measurements showed significant differences between the RBCs of PNH patients and of control donors (**Figure 2**). The tendency to a density-associated decrease in EMA staining might be due to loss of band 3 and/or membrane with aging by vesiculation, both in RBCs from control donors and from PNH patients. This has been postulated before for physiological aging *in vivo* (Willekens et al., 2008). However, the absence of a statistically significant correlation between EMA fluorescence and the RBC size, based on the cytometer parameter forward scatter, suggests that in the RBCs from PNH patients, the band 3 protein content is not a direct function of cell size. EMA staining is affected by changes in band 3 conformation and membrane organization as well (e.g., Cobb and Beth, 1990; Huisjes et al., 2018). Combined with the considerable fractions of PS-negative and CD59-lacking microvesicles in the blood of PNH patients (**Figure 5**), these data indicate that the organization of the RBC membrane, as well as the mechanism of microvesicle generation, are altered by the absence of GPI-linked proteins. This may be a direct effect, but also the consequence of the deposition of C3b. The latter not only affects lateral mobility of CD59 and band 3 molecules but also membrane viscosity and deformability (Karnchanaphanurach et al., 2009; Glodek et al., 2010). Our *in vivo* data support the involvement of GPI-linked proteins in microvesicle formation during RBC aging *in vitro* (Salzer et al., 2008; Freitas Leal et al., 2017). The differences in mechanisms leading to the generation of microvesicles with and without PS at their outside remain to be established, as well as the effect on biological activity.

Since PS exposure contributes to recognition and removal of microvesicles by macrophages (Willekens et al., 2005), its absence may not only affect their pro-coagulant activity but also their lifespan. Fusion between microvesicles and RBCs may underlie the reported transfer between CD55 and CD59 from normal RBCs to RBCs without these proteins (Sloand et al., 2004). Thus, microvesicles generated by PNH RBCs may also fuse with normal RBCs, thereby affecting their membrane organization as well. Furthermore, increased levels of RBC-derived microvesicles may affect NO bioavailability (Said et al., 2018) and induce activation of endothelial cells and tissue factor expression (Collier et al., 2013), thereby contributing to the wide-spread thrombosis in patients with PNH.

Platelet Microvesicles and Thrombosis

Platelets without CD59 have been described to catalyze the rate of prothrombin conversion upon treatment with complement C5b-9 in vitro, and this was associated with an increase in microvesicle formation (Wiedmer et al., 1993). RBC-derived and platelet-derived, phosphatidylserine-positive microvesicles have been reported to be increased approximately two-fold in the blood of PNH patients (Hugel et al., 1999). We found equal concentrations of RBC-derived microvesicles in the plasma of PNH patients and healthy donors, but much larger RBC-derived, phosphatidylserine-negative microvesicle concentrations in the blood of PNH patients (**Figure 5B**), and larger concentrations of platelet-derived vesicles (**Figure 5D**). In the plasma of eculizumab-treated PNH patients, the numbers of RBC-derived vesicles were lower than in patients who had not been treated with eculizumab (**Supplementary Figure S1**). The absence of a statistically significant correlation between the concentrations of RBC-derived and platelet-derived microvesicles indicates that the absence of GPI-linked proteins affects microvesicle generation from RBCs and platelets through different mechanisms. Although in control donors, most platelets are CD59-positive (Jin et al., 1997), almost all platelet-derived microvesicles were CD59-negative (**Figure 5**). There were approximately equal concentrations of platelet-derived vesicles with and without PS at their surface (**Figure 5E**). These data strongly suggest that the absence of GPI-linked proteins does not only have a pronounced stimulatory effect on the generation of microvesicles but also on their composition. The latter may be related to the presence of tissue factor and is likely to affect their function (Devalet et al., 2014). Our recent finding that platelet-derived microvesicles can prevent differentiation of regulatory T-cells through P-selectin (Dinkla et al., 2016) emphasizes their pivotal role in the pathophysiology of many diseases that may include PNH (Devalet et al., 2014). Although the name suggests otherwise, most platelet-derived microvesicles originate not from platelets, but from megakaryocytes in the bone marrow (Flaumenhaft et al., 2009; Rank et al., 2010). It is not known how the absence of GPI-linked proteins affects megakaryocyte biology and/or platelet

activation. These data support the importance of an extensive characterization of origin, composition, and biological activity of CD41-positive microvesicles. Such studies may help in establishing an urgently needed, robust marker of platelet activation.

CONCLUSION

The heterogeneity of the patient population and the concomitant small numbers available for statistical comparisons of all parameters preclude a robust answer on the question whether RBC aging is altered in patients with PNH. However, the combined results of the selected aging-associated parameters (Bosman et al., 2008, 2012; Lutz and Bogdanova, 2013) do not reveal a major aberration of the physiological RBC aging process in patients with PNH. Remarkably, formation of microvesicles by RBCs is altered in patients with PNH. This is likely due to PNH-related differences in membrane organization that is associated with the absence of GPI-linked proteins. The conspicuous lack of phosphatidylserine exposure on many RBC-derived microvesicles in PNH patients may affect their time in the circulation as well as their contribution to hemostasis and thrombosis. In platelets, PNH-related processes seem not only to induce the appearance of large numbers of phosphatidylserine-negative microvesicles but also to cause excessive formation of microvesicles. Future investigations leading to a better understanding of the mechanisms underlying vesiculation, effect of vesiculation on RBC function and survival, and effect of the various microvesicles on thrombosis in patients with PNH may be instrumental in developing new treatment strategies (Kulasekararaj et al., 2019).

AUTHOR CONTRIBUTIONS

JF performed all measurements, the analyses, and wrote the first version of the manuscript. FP provided the samples, some protocols, and assisted in writing the manuscript. RB, MA-H, and GB contributed to the setup of the study, the interpretation of the data, and the writing of the manuscript.

SUPPLEMENTARY MATERIAL

SUPPLEMENTARY FIGURE S1 | Microvesicle numbers and composition in the blood of patients with PNH CD59 level and treatment. **(A)** Concentration (MV/µl) of CD235a-positive, RBC-derived microvesicles (MVs) in the blood of PNH patients who did not receive treatment (NT; $N = 3$), PNH patients who were treated with eculizumab (T; $N = 6$), and control healthy donors ($N = 6$); **(B)** concentration of RBC-derived microvesicles in the blood of PNH patients who did not receive treatment (NT; $N = 3$), PNH patients who were being treated with eculizumab (T; $N = 6$) and control donors ($N = 6$) according their reactivity to Annexin V (phosphatidylserine positive (PS+) or negative (PS–); **(C)** RBC-derived microvesicles in the blood of PNH patients who did not receive treatment (NT; $N = 3$), PNH patients who were being treated with eculizumab (T; $N = 6$) categorized in wild type, CD59-low and CD59-negative as described for

RBCs (Materials and Methods); **(D)** concentration of platelet-derived microvesicles (CD41-positive) from the blood of PNH patients who did not receive treatment with eculizumab (NT; $N = 3$), PNH patients who were being treated with eculizumab (T; $N = 6$) and control healthy donors ($N = 6$); **(E)** concentration of platelet-derived microvesicles in the blood of PNH patients who did not receive treatment with eculizumab (NT; $N = 3$), PNH patients who were being treated with eculizumab (T; $N = 6$) and control healthy donors ($N = 6$), according their reactivity to Annexin V (PS+ or PS–); **(F)** platelet-derived microvesicles from the blood of PNH patients who did not receive treatment with eculizumab (NT; $N = 3$), PNH patients who were being treated with eculizumab (T; $N = 6$) were categorized in wild type, low CD59, and CD59-negative as described for RBCs and quantified and analyzed by flow cytometry as described before (see Materials and Methods). #Significantly different from the other parameter in the same group ($p < 0.05$). *Significantly different between groups ($p < 0.05$).

SUPPLEMENTARY TABLE 1 | Clinical data of PNH patients. AA, PNH patient with aplastic anemia; N, PNH patient without hematological comorbidities; T, in treatment; NT, not in treatment; RBC, red blood cells ($\times 10^{12}$/L); RBC CS (II/III), red blood cell clone size (type II and III); Hb, hemoglobin (g/dl); Ht, hematocrit (%); MCV, mean corpuscular volume (fl); MCH, mean corpuscular hemoglobin (pg); MCHC, mean corpuscular hemoglobin concentration (g/dl); RDW, red blood cell distribution width (%); Retic, reticulocytes (promille); RBC Tr, red blood cell transfusion in the last 3 months; Leuk, Leukocytes ($\times 10^9$/L); Gran CS., granulocytes clone size; Plt, platelet ($\times 10^9$/L); LDH, lactate dehydrogenase (U/L); –, not available. Reference values for healthy adults: RBC: for men, 4.7–6.1 $\times 10^{12}$/L and for women, 4.2–5.4 $\times 10^{12}$/L; Hb: for men, 8.5–11 mmol/L and for women, 7.5–10 mmol/dl; Ht: for men, 0.4–0.54 and for women, 0.36–0.46; MCV: 80–96 fl; MCH: 1.7–2.1 fmol; MCHC: 19.3–22.5 mmol/L; RDW: 11.5–14.5%; Retic: 8–26 promille; Leuk: 4.5–11 $\times 10^9$/L; Plt: 150–400 $\times 10^9$/L; LDH: 135–225 U/L.

REFERENCES

Arese, P., Turrini, F., and Schwarzer, E. (2005). Band 3/complement-mediated recognition and removal of normally senescent and pathological human erythrocytes. *Cell. Physiol. Biochem.* 16, 133–146. doi: 10.1159/000089839

Bayly-Jones, C., Bubeck, D., and Dunstone, M. A. (2017). The mystery behind membrane insertion: a review of the complement membrane attack complex. *Philos. Trans. R. Soc. Lond. Ser. B Biol. Sci.* 372:20160221. doi: 10.1098/rstb.2016.0221

Bosman, G. (2016). The proteome of the red blood cell: an auspicious source of new insights into membrane-centered regulation of homeostasis. *Proteome* 4:35. doi: 10.3390/proteomes4040035

Bosman, G. J. C. G. M., Lasonder, E., Groenen-Döpp, Y. A. M., Willekens, F. L. A., and Werre, J. M. (2012). The proteome of erythrocyte-derived microparticles from plasma: new clues for erythrocyte aging and vesiculation. *J. Proteome* 76, 203–210. doi: 10.1016/j.jprot.2012.05.031

Bosman, G. J. C. G. M., Werre, J. M., Willekens, F. L. A., and Novotný, V. M. J. (2008). Erythrocyte ageing *in vivo* and *in vitro*: structural aspects and implications for transfusion. *Transfus. Med.* 18, 335–347. doi: 10.1111/j.1365-3148.2008.00892.x

Brodsky, R. A. (2009). How I treat paroxysmal nocturnal hemoglobinuria. *Blood* 113, 6522–6527. doi: 10.1182/blood-2009-03-195966

Brodsky, R. A. (2014). Paroxysmal nocturnal hemoglobinuria. *Blood* 124, 2804–2811. doi: 10.1182/blood-2014-02-522128

Carroll, M. V., and Sim, R. B. (2011). Complement in health and disease. *Adv. Drug Deliv. Rev.* 63, 965–975. doi: 10.1016/j.addr.2011.06.005

Clemente, M. J., Przychodzen, B., Hirsch, C. M., Nagata, Y., Bat, T., Wlodarski, M. W., et al. (2018). Clonal PIGA mosaicism and dynamics in paroxysmal nocturnal hemoglobinuria. *Leukemia* 32, 2507–2511. doi: 10.1038/s41375-018-0138-5

Cluitmans, J. C. A., Tomelleri, C., Yapici, Z., Dinkla, S., Bovee-Geurts, P., Chokkalingam, V., et al. (2015). Abnormal red cell structure and function in neuroacanthocytosis. *PLoS One* 10:e0125580. doi: 10.1371/journal.pone.0125580

Cobb, C. E., and Beth, A. H. (1990). Identification of the Eosinyl-5-maleimide reaction site on the human erythrocyte anion-exchange protein: overlap with the reaction sites of other chemical probes. *Biochemistry* 29, 8283–8290. doi: 10.1021/bi00488a012

Collier, M. E. W., Mah, P. M., Xiao, Y., Maraveyas, A., and Ettelaie, C. (2013). Microparticle-associated tissue factor is recycled by endothelial cells resulting in enhanced surface tissue factor activity. *Thromb. Haemost.* 110, 966–976. doi: 10.1160/TH13-01-0055

Crisp, R. L., Solari, L., Vota, D., García, E., Miguez, G., Chamorro, M. E., et al. (2011). A prospective study to assess the predictive value for hereditary spherocytosis using five laboratory tests (cryohemolysis test, eosin-5′-maleimide flow cytometry, osmotic fragility test, autohemolysis test, and SDS-PAGE) on 50 hereditary spherocytosis fa. *Ann. Hematol.* 90, 625–634. doi: 10.1007/s00277-010-1112-0

de Back, D. Z., Kostova, E. B., van Kraaij, M., van den Berg, T. K., and van Bruggen, R. (2014). Of macrophages and red blood cells; a complex love story. *Front. Physiol.* 5:9. doi: 10.3389/fphys.2014.00009

Devalet, B., Mullier, F., Chatelain, B., Dogne, J.-M., and Chatelain, C. (2014). The central role of extracellular vesicles in the mechanisms of thrombosis in paroxysmal nocturnal haemoglobinuria: a review. *J. Extracell. Vesicles* 3, 1–8. doi: 10.3402/jev.v3.23304

DeZern, A. E., and Brodsky, R. A. (2015). Paroxysmal nocturnal hemoglobinuria. A complement-mediated hemolytic anemia. *Hematol. Oncol. Clin. North Am.* 29, 479–494. doi: 10.1016/j.hoc.2015.01.005

Dinkla, S., Brock, R., Joosten, I., and Bosman, G. J. C. G. M. (2013). Gateway to understanding microparticles: standardized isolation and identification of plasma membrane-derived vesicles. *Nanomedicine* 8, 1657–1668. doi: 10.2217/nnm.13.149

Dinkla, S., Peppelman, M., Der Raadt, J., Atsma, F., Novotný, V. M. J., Van Kraaij, M. G. J., et al. (2014). Phosphatidylserine exposure on stored red blood cells as a parameter for donor-dependent variation in product quality. *Blood Transfus.* 12, 204–209. doi: 10.2450/2013.0106-13

Dinkla, S., Van Cranenbroek, B., Van Der Heijden, W. A., He, X., Wallbrecher, R., Dumitriu, I. E., et al. (2016). Platelet microparticles inhibit IL-17 production by regulatory T cells through P-selectin. *Blood* 127, 1976–1986. doi: 10.1182/blood-2015-04-640300

Dinkla, S., Wessels, K., Verdurmen, W. P. R., Tomelleri, C., Cluitmans, J. C. A., Fransen, J., et al. (2012). Functional consequences of sphingomyelinase-induced changes in erythrocyte membrane structure. *Cell Death Dis.* 3:e410. doi: 10.1038/cddis.2012.143

Ferru, E., Giger, K., Pantaleo, A., Campanella, E., Grey, J., Ritchie, K., et al. (2011). Regulation of membrane-cytoskeletal interactions by tyrosine phosphorylation of erythrocyte band 3. *Blood* 117, 5998–6006. doi: 10.1182/blood-2010-11-317024

Flaumenhaft, R., Dilks, J. R., Richardson, J., Alden, E., Patel-Hett, S. R., Battinelli, E., et al. (2009). Megakaryocyte-derived microparticles: direct visualization and distinction from platelet-derived microparticles. *Blood* 113, 1112–1121. doi: 10.1182/blood-2008-06-163832

Freitas Leal, J. K., Adjobo-Hermans, M. J. W., and Bosman, G. J. C. G. M. (2018). Red blood cell homeostasis: mechanisms and effects of microvesicle generation in health and disease. *Front. Physiol.* 9:703. doi: 10.3389/fphys.2018.00703

Freitas Leal, J. K., Adjobo-Hermans, M. J. W., Brock, R., and Bosman, G. J. C. G. M. (2017). Acetylcholinesterase provides new insights into red blood cell ageing *in vivo* and *in vitro*. *Blood Transfus.* 15, 232–238. doi: 10.2450/2017.0370-16

Glodek, A. M., Mirchev, R., Golan, D. E., Khoory, J. A., Burns, J. M., Shevkoplyas, S. S., et al. (2010). Ligation of complement receptor 1 increases erythrocyte membrane deformability. *Blood* 116, 6063–6071. doi: 10.1182/blood-2010-04-273904

Griffin, M., and Munir, T. (2017). Management of thrombosis in paroxysmal nocturnal hemoglobinuria: a clinician's guide. *Ther. Adv. Hematol.* 8, 119–126. doi: 10.1177/2040620716681748

Hill, A., DeZern, A. E., Kinoshita, T., and Brodsky, R. A. (2017). Paroxysmal nocturnal haemoglobinuria. *Nat. Rev. Dis. Primers.* 3:17028. doi: 10.1038/nrdp.2017.28

Hill, A., Kelly, R. J., and Hillmen, P. (2013). Thrombosis in paroxysmal nocturnal hemoglobinuria. *Blood* 121, 4985–4996. doi: 10.1182/blood-2012-09-311381

Hugel, B., Socié, G., Vu, T., Toti, F., Gluckman, E., Freyssinet, J. M., et al. (1999). Elevated levels of circulating procoagulant microparticles in patients with paroxysmal nocturnal hemoglobinuria and aplastic anemia. *Blood* 93, 3451–3456.

Huisjes, R., Satchwell, T. J., Verhagen, L. P., Schiffelers, R. M., van Solinge, W. W., Toye, A. M., et al. (2018). Quantitative measurement of red cell surface protein expression reveals new biomarkers for hereditary spherocytosis. *Int. J. Lab. Hematol.* 40, e74–e77. doi: 10.1111/ijlh.12841

Jin, J. Y., Tooze, J. A., Marsh, J. C. W., and Gordon-Smith, E. C. (1997). Glycosylphosphatidyl-inositol (GPI)-linked protein deficiency on the platelets of patients with aplastic anaemia and paroxysmal nocturnal haemoglobinuria: two distinct patterns correlating with expression on neutrophils. *Br. J. Haematol.* 96, 493–496. doi: 10.1046/j.1365-2141.1997. d01-2047.x

Kahn, M., Maley, J., Lasker, G., and Kadowitz, P. (2013). Updated role of nitric oxide in disorders of erythrocyte function. *Cardiovasc. Hematol. Disord. Drug Targets* 13, 83–87. doi: 10.2174/1871529X11313010009

Karnchanaphanurach, P., Mirchev, R., Ghiran, I., Asara, J. M., Papahadjopoulos-Sternberg, B., Nicholson-Weller, A., et al. (2009). C3b deposition on human erythrocytes induces the formation of a membrane skeleton-linked protein complex. *J. Clin. Invest.* 119, 788–801. doi: 10.1172/JCI36088

Klei, T. R. L., Meinderts, S. M., van den Berg, T. K., and van Bruggen, R. (2017). From the cradle to the grave: the role of macrophages in erythropoiesis and erythrophagocytosis. *Front. Immunol.* 8. doi: 10.3389/fimmu.2017.00073

Kulasekararaj, A. G., Hill, A., Rottinghaus, S. T., Langemeijer, S., Wells, R., Gonzalez-Fernandez, F. A., et al. (2019). Ravulizumab (ALXN1210) vs eculizumab in C5-inhibitor-experienced adult patients with PNH: the 302 study. *Blood* 133, 540–549. doi: 10.1182/blood-2018-09-876805

Lin, Z., Schmidt, C. Q., Koutsogiannaki, S., Ricci, P., Risitano, A. M., Lambris, J. D., et al. (2015). Complement C3dg-mediated erythrophagocytosis: implications for paroxysmal nocturnal hemoglobinuria. *Blood* 126, 891–894. doi: 10.1182/blood-2015-02-625871

Lutz, H. U. (2004). Innate immune and non-immune mediators of erythrocyte clearance. *Cell. Mol. Biol.* (*Noisy-le-Grand*) 50, 107–116.

Lutz, H. U., and Bogdanova, A. (2013). Mechanisms tagging senescent red blood cells for clearance in healthy humans. *Front. Physiol.* 4:387. doi: 10.3389/fphys.2013.00387

Malato, A., Saccullo, G., Lo Coco, L., Mancuso, S., Santoro, M., Martino, S., et al. (2012). Thrombotic complications in paroxysmal nocturnal haemoglobinuria: a literature review. *Blood Transfus.* 10, 428–435. doi: 10.2450/2012.0161-11

Ninomiya, H., Kawashima, Y., Hasegawa, Y., and Nagasawa, T. (1999). Complement-induced procoagulant alteration of red blood cell membranes with microvesicle formation in paroxysmal nocturnal haemoglobinuria (PNH): implication for thrombogenesis in PNH. *Br. J. Haematol.* 106, 224–231. doi: 10.1046/j.1365-2141.1999.01483.x

Peacock-Young, B., Macrae, F. L., Newton, D. J., and Ariëns, R. A. S. (2018). The prothrombotic state in paroxysmal nocturnal hemoglobinuria: a multifaceted source. *Haematologica* 103, 9–17. doi: 10.3324/haematol.2017.177618

Pollet, H., Conrard, L., Cloos, A.-S., and Tyteca, D. (2018). Plasma membrane lipid domains as platforms for vesicle biogenesis and shedding? *Biomol. Ther.* 8:94. doi: 10.3390/biom8030094

Rank, A., Nieuwland, R., Delker, R., Köhler, A., Toth, B., Pihusch, V., et al. (2010). Cellular origin of platelet-derived microparticles *in vivo. Thromb. Res.* 126, e255–e259. doi: 10.1016/j.thromres.2010.07.012

Rapido, F. (2017). The potential adverse effects of haemolysis. *Blood Transfus.* 15, 218–221. doi: 10.2450/2017.0311-16

Risitano, A. M. (2012). Paroxysmal nocturnal hemoglobinuria and other complement-mediated hematological disorders. *Immunobiology* 217, 1080–1087. doi: 10.1016/j.imbio.2012.07.014

Risitano, A. M., Notaro, R., Marando, L., Serio, B., Ranaldi, D., Seneca, E., et al. (2009). Complement fraction 3 binding on erythrocytes as additional mechanism of disease in paroxysmal nocturnal hemoglobinuria patients treated by eculizumab. *Blood* 113, 4094–4100. doi: 10.1182/blood-2008-11-189944

Risitano, A. M., and Rotoli, B. (2008). Paroxysmal nocturnal hemoglobinuria: pathophysiology, natural history and treatment options in the era of biological agents. *Biologics* 2, 205–222.

Saha, S., Anilkumar, A. A., and Mayor, S. (2016). GPI-anchored protein organization and dynamics at the cell surface. *J. Lipid Res.* 57, 159–175. doi: 10.1194/jlr.R062885

Said, A. S., Rogers, S. C., and Doctor, A. (2018). Physiologic impact of circulating RBC microparticles upon blood-vascular interactions. *Front. Physiol.* 8, 1–14. doi: 10.3389/fphys.2017.01120

Salzer, U., and Prohaska, R. (2001). Stomatin, flotillin-1, and flotillin-2 are major integral proteins of erythrocyte lipid rafts. *Blood* 97, 1141–1143. doi: 10.1182/blood.V97.4.1141

Salzer, U., Zhu, R., Luten, M., Isobe, H., Pastushenko, V., Perkmann, T., et al. (2008). Vesicles generated during storage of red cells are rich in the lipid raft marker stomatin. *Transfusion* 48, 451–462. doi: 10.1111/j.1537-2995.2007.01549.x

Sato, S., Kozuma, Y., Hasegawa, Y., Kojima, H., Chiba, S., and Ninomiya, H. (2010). Enhanced expression of CD71, transferrin receptor, on immature reticulocytes in patients with paroxysmal nocturnal hemoglobinuria. *Int. J. Lab. Hematol.* 32, e137–e143. doi: 10.1111/j.1751-553X.2009.01148.x

Sloand, E. M., Mainwaring, L., Keyvanfar, K., Chen, J., Maciejewski, J., Klein, H. G., et al. (2004). Transfer of glycosylphosphatidylinositol-anchored proteins to deficient cells after erythrocyte transfusion in paroxysmal nocturnal hemoglobinuria. *Blood* 104, 3782–3788. doi: 10.1182/blood-2004-02-0645

Sutherland, D. R., Illingworth, A., Keeney, M., and Richards, S. J. (2015). "High-sensitivity detection of PNH red blood cells, red cell precursors, and white blood cells" in *Current protocols in cytometry* (Hoboken, NJ, USA: John Wiley & Sons, Inc.), 6.37.1–6.37.29.

Takeda, J., Miyata, T., Kawagoe, K., Iida, Y., Endo, Y., Fujita, T., et al. (1993). Deficiency of the GPI anchor caused by a somatic mutation of the PIG-A gene in paroxysmal nocturnal hemoglobinuria. *Cell* 73, 703–711. doi: 10.1016/0092-8674(93)90250-T

Whitlow, M., Iida, K., Marshall, P., Silber, R., and Nussenzweig, V. (1993). Cells lacking glycan phosphatidylinositol-linked proteins have impaired ability to vesiculate. *Blood* 81, 510–516.

Wiedmer, T., Hall, S. E., Ortel, T. L., Kane, W. H., Rosse, W. F., and Sims, P. J. (1993). Complement-induced vesiculation and exposure of membrane prothrombinase sites in platelets of paroxysmal nocturnal hemoglobinuria. *Blood* 82, 1192–1196.

Willekens, F. L. A., Werre, J. M., Groenen-Döpp, Y. A. M., Roerdinkholder-Stoelwinder, B., De Pauw, B., and Bosman, G. J. C. G. M. (2008). Erythrocyte vesiculation: a self-protective mechanism? *Br. J. Haematol.* 141, 549–556. doi: 10.1111/j.1365-2141.2008.07055.x

Willekens, F. L. A., Werre, J. M., Kruijt, J. K., Roerdinkholder-Stoelwinder, B., Groenen-Döpp, Y. A. M., Van Den Bos, A. G., et al. (2005). Liver Kupffer cells rapidly remove red blood cell-derived vesicles from the circulation by scavenger receptors. *Blood* 105, 2141–2145. doi: 10.1182/blood-2004-04-1578

Zolla, L., and D'Alessandro, A. (2012). Shaking hands with the future through omics application in transfusion medicine and clinical biochemistry. *Blood Transfus.* 10, 10–12. doi: 10.2450/2012.001S

2

The Spectrum of *SPTA1*-Associated Hereditary Spherocytosis

Satheesh Chonat[1,2], Mary Risinger[3], Haripriya Sakthivel[4], Omar Niss[4,5], Jennifer A. Rothman[6], Loan Hsieh[7], Stella T. Chou[8,9], Janet L. Kwiatkowski[8,9], Eugene Khandros[8,9], Matthew F. Gorman[10], Donald T. Wells[11], Tamara Maghathe[4], Neha Dagaonkar[12], Katie G. Seu[4], Kejian Zhang[13], Wenying Zhang[5,14] and Theodosia A. Kalfa[4,5]*

[1] Department of Pediatrics, Emory University School of Medicine, Atlanta, GA, United States, [2] Aflac Cancer and Blood Disorders Center, Children's Healthcare of Atlanta, Atlanta, GA, United States, [3] College of Nursing, University of Cincinnati, Cincinnati, OH, United States, [4] Cancer and Blood Diseases Institute, Cincinnati Children's Hospital Medical Center, Cincinnati, OH, United States, [5] Department of Pediatrics, University of Cincinnati College of Medicine, Cincinnati, OH, United States, [6] Duke University Medical Center, Durham, NC, United States, [7] Division of Hematology, CHOC Children's Hospital and UC Irvine Medical Center, Orange, CA, United States, [8] Division of Hematology, Children's Hospital of Philadelphia, Philadelphia, PA, United States, [9] Department of Pediatrics, Perelman School of Medicine, University of Pennsylvania, Philadelphia, PA, United States, [10] Kaiser Permanente Santa Clara Medical Center, Santa Clara, CA, United States, [11] Dell Children's Medical Center, Austin, TX, United States, [12] Genomics Analysis Facility, Institute for Genomic Medicine, Columbia University, New York, NY, United States, [13] Coyote Bioscience Co., Ltd., San Jose, CA, United States, [14] Laboratory of Genetics and Genomics, Division of Human Genetics, Cincinnati Children's Hospital Medical Center, Cincinnati, OH, United States

*Correspondence:
Theodosia A. Kalfa
theodosia.kalfa@cchmc.org

Hereditary spherocytosis (HS) is the most common red blood cell (RBC) membrane disorder causing hereditary hemolytic anemia. Patients with HS have defects in the genes coding for ankyrin (*ANK1*), band 3 (*SLC4A1*), protein 4.2 (*EPB42*), and α (*SPTA1*) or β-spectrin (*SPTB*). Severe recessive HS is most commonly due to biallelic *SPTA1* mutations. α-spectrin is produced in excess in normal erythroid cells, therefore *SPTA1*-associated HS ensues with mutations causing significant decrease of normal protein expression from both alleles. In this study, we systematically compared genetic, rheological, and protein expression data to the varying clinical presentation in eleven patients with *SPTA1*-associated HS. The phenotype of HS in this group of patients ranged from moderately severe to severe transfusion-dependent anemia and up to *hydrops fetalis* which is typically fatal if transfusions are not initiated before term delivery. The pathogenicity of the mutations could be corroborated by reduced *SPTA1* mRNA expression in the patients' reticulocytes. The disease severity correlated to the level of α-spectrin protein in their RBC cytoskeleton but was also affected by other factors. Patients carrying the low expression α^{LEPRA} allele *in trans* to a null *SPTA1* mutation were not all transfusion dependent and their anemia improved or resolved with partial or total splenectomy, respectively. In contrast, patients with near-complete or complete α-spectrin deficiency have a history of having been salvaged from fatal *hydrops fetalis*, either because they were born prematurely and started transfusions early or because they had intrauterine transfusions. They have suboptimal reticulocytosis or reticulocytopenia and remain transfusion dependent even after splenectomy; these patients require either lifetime transfusions and iron chelation or stem cell transplant. Comprehensive genetic and phenotypic evaluation is critical to provide accurate diagnosis in patients with *SPTA1*-associated HS and guide toward appropriate management.

Keywords: *SPTA1*, α-spectrin, α^LEPRA, hereditary spherocytosis, next generation sequencing, hemolytic anemia, hydrops fetalis

INTRODUCTION

Hereditary spherocytosis (HS) is the most common red blood cell (RBC) cytoskeleton disorder causing hereditary hemolytic anemia (HHA), characterized by sphere-shaped erythrocytes (spherocytes) with increased osmotic fragility. HS can affect all ethnic groups but is more common in people of northern European ancestry where the prevalence is 1 in 1000–2500 (Gallagher, 2005). Spherocytes are formed because of loss of membrane due to quantitative defects in proteins that link the cytoskeleton to the lipid bilayer ("vertical" linkages) (Eber and Lux, 2004). The scaffolding network of the RBC cytoskeleton is assembled by α- and β-spectrin heterodimers self-associating in a head-to-head fashion to form tetramers, bound to the lipid membrane via the anchoring complex of ankyrin, protein 4.2, and band 3 (Salomao et al., 2008). In autosomal dominant HS, which accounts for approximately 75% of cases, mutations of ankyrin (*ANK1*), band 3 (*SLC4A1*), and β-spectrin (*SPTB*) genes predominate. Recessive HS is most often due to compound heterozygosity for defects in the genes encoding ankyrin, α-spectrin (*SPTA1*), or protein 4.2 (*EPB42*) (Eber and Lux, 2004; Gallagher, 2005; Mohandas, 2018).

Two normal *SPTA1* alleles allow for overproduction of α-spectrin chains (Hanspal and Palek, 1987). Therefore, HS due to α-spectrin deficiency manifests when both of the *SPTA1* alleles are affected by mutations causing significant quantitative defect. Two *SPTA1* low expression alleles were identified early-on to be associated with RBC membrane disorders and their study helped to determine the quantitative requirements of the RBC cytoskeleton for α-spectrin (Wilmotte et al., 1993; Wichterle et al., 1996). α^LELY (Low Expression LYon) has a minor allele frequency (MAF) of 25.5% (gnomad.broadinstitute.org) and consists of the mutation c.6531-12C>T in intron 45, causing partial skipping of exon 46 in half of the transcripts and consequently a 50% decrease in the amount of α-spectrin (Wilmotte et al., 1993; Marechal et al., 1995). α^LELY *in trans* to an *SPTA1* allele with a hereditary elliptocytosis (HE)-associated mutation modifies the phenotype from HE to hereditary pyropoikilocytosis (Niss et al., 2016). In contrast, α^LELY *in trans* to a null *SPTA1* allele causes no disease, indicating that production of ~25% of normal α-spectrin is enough for normal RBC cytoskeleton assembly (Delaunay et al., 2004). α^LEPRA (Low Expression PRAgue) is a deep intronic *SPTA1* mutation (c.4339-99C > T). Positioned at -99 of intron 30, it activates an alternative acceptor splice site at position -70 of the same intron. The alternative splicing results in frameshift and premature termination of translation, leading to decreased α-spectrin production. This allele (MAF

of 0.5% per gnomad.broadinstitute.org) produces only about 16% of full-length spectrin as compared to the normal *SPTA1* allele, based on studies with metabolic labeling of erythroblasts *in vitro* (Wichterle et al., 1996). α^LEPRA *in trans* to a null *SPTA1* allele (leading to a total α-spectrin production of about 8%) has been shown to cause severe autosomal recessive HS, with anemia and jaundice that resolve with splenectomy (Wichterle et al., 1996; Delaunay et al., 2004). Complete α-spectrin deficiency has been shown to cause lethal anemia *in utero* (Whitfield et al., 1991).

We present here eleven patients with HS due to α-spectrin deficiency and discuss their phenotype/genotype correlation (**Table 1**).

MATERIALS AND METHODS

Next Generation Sequencing (NGS) of Genes Associated With HHA

Patients with the clinical diagnosis of HHA and their parents were enrolled in an Institutional Review Board-approved research protocol based at Cincinnati Children's Hospital Medical Center. DNA was isolated from peripheral blood (in the case of patient 9 from liver tissue preserved in paraffin after autopsy), and analyzed on an NGS HHA panel; the regions of interest for enrichment and DNA sequencing included the coding exons plus 20 bases of intronic boundaries for 32 genes known to be associated with RBC membrane and enzyme disorders and with congenital dyserythropoietic anemias: *ABCG5, ABCG8, AK1, ALDOA, ANK1, C15orf41, CDAN1, EPB41, EPB42, G6PD, GATA1, GCLC, GPI, GPX1, GSR, GSS, HK1, KIF23, KLF1, NT5C3A, PFKM, PGK1, PIEZO1, PKLR, RHAG, SEC23B, SLC2A1(GLUT1), SLC4A1, SPTA1, SPTB, TPI1,* and *XK*. Regulatory regions and deep intronic areas of these genes with published disease-causing mutations were included in the HHA panel design. Sanger sequencing was used to confirm all mutations found in patients and in parental samples (except for parents of patients #7 and #11) to establish the phase.

Osmotic Gradient Ektacytometry

Whole blood samples were collected in K2-EDTA-containing vials from study subjects at least 3 months after last transfusion to avoid misinterpretation from the presence of donor RBCs. Samples from healthy volunteers were collected at same time and shipped as travel controls. Specimens were stored or shipped at 4°C and were analyzed within 24 h of sample collection using

TABLE 1 | Genetic mutations and associated phenotype in HS due to *SPTA1* mutations.

Phenotype	Patient	Allele 1	Allele 2	Age at time of report and comments	Ektacytometry	α-spectrin in RBC ghosts (% of control)
GROUP I (patients 1–4) Severe, recessive HS (transfusion-dependent, responding to splenectomy)	1	c.4339-99C > T	c.4295del (p.L1432*)	11 year-old, chronic transfusion requirement with partial response to partial splenectomy, resolved after total splenectomy		54%
	2	c.4339-99C > T	c.5102A > T (p.L1701*)	7 year-old, chronic transfusion requirement, improved with partial splenectomy		64%
	3	c.4339-99C > T	c.3267A > T (p.Y1089*)	11 year-old, not splenectomized due to family preference, continues to require frequent transfusions	Not evaluable in a transfused sample	
	4	Mutation not identified	Gross deletion of *SPTA1*	3.5 year-old, RT-PCR demonstrated significantly decreased α-spectrin expression; hemoglobin has normalized after recent splenectomy	Not evaluable in a transfused sample	
GROUP II (patients 5–8) Severe to moderately severe, recessive HS	5	c.4339-99C > T	c.1120C > T (p.R374*)	4 year-old, chronic transfusion requirement for first three years with improved pattern since.	Sample not provided after age 3, when transfusion-independent	
	6	c.4339-99C > T	c.1351-1G > T	7 year-old, occasional transfusion requirement, resolved after splenectomy at 5 years of age		59%
	7	c.4339-99C>T	c.2671C > T (p.R891*)	4 year-old, has not been transfused so far, Hgb 7.1-8.9 g/dL, ARC 420-572 x $10^3/\mu l$.		61%
	8	c.4339-99C > T	c.3257delT	8 year-old, transfused once as neonate, Hgb 10.6–11.8 g/dL, ARC 354–535 × $10^3/\mu l$; now Hgb 15–16 g/dL with normal ARC after splenectomy at 6 years of age (splenectomy performed because of chronic abdominal pain due to co-morbidities)		Not performed.
GROUP III (patients 9-11) Life-threatening anemia in utero leading to fatal *hydrops fetalis* if untreated (transfusion-dependent, not responding to splenectomy)	9	c.4206delG (fs)	c.4180delT (fs) in haplotype with c.6631C > T (p.R2211C)	Died at birth. Post-mortem diagnosis from parental studies and DNA extracted from liver tissue saved in paraffin block	N/A	
	10	c.6788+11C > T	c.6788+11C > T	11 year-old, born prematurely at EGA of 33 weeks with *hydrops fetalis*, remained transfusion-dependent even after splenectomy; now doing well after matched sibling transplant	Not evaluable in a transfused sample (required chronic transfusions up until bone marrow transplant)	26% (performed in CD71+ cells)
	11	c.6154del (p.Ala2052fs)	c.6154del (p.Ala2052fs)	2 year-old, severe in-utero anemia requiring five *in-utero* transfusions. Born with severe neonatal hyperbilirubinemia requiring exchange transfusion. Remains transfusion-dependent	Not evaluable in a transfused sample	

Of note, all the SPTA1 variants reported here except c.4339-99C > T (α^{LEPRA}) and c.2671C > T; p.R891 (Bogardus et al., 2014) have not been previously described.*

LoRRca® MaxSis (Mechatronics, United States LLC, Warwick, RI, United States). RBC deformation was recorded while the cells were exposed to a constant shear stress of 30 Pa and an increasing osmotic gradient (0–600 mOsm/kg) in order to generate the ektacytometry curve (Da Costa et al., 2016; Zaninoni et al., 2018).

Capillary Electrophoresis and Immunodetection

Red blood cell membrane "ghosts" were prepared from patients #1, #6, and #7, at least 3 months after last transfusion, by hypotonic lysis (Bennett, 1983) and cytoskeletal proteins were evaluated by immunodetection using the size-based capillary electrophoresis instrument Wes (ProteinSimple, San Jose, CA, United States). Capillary immuno-electrophoresis was also performed on lysates prepared from isolated CD71+ cells from patient #10 (with a similarly prepared healthy volunteer sample as control).

Quantitative Real-Time PCR (qPCR) of Reticulocyte mRNA

Reticulocytes were magnetically isolated from whole blood collected in K2-EDTA-containing vials from patients #4 and #10, in order to validate the pathogenicity of their genotype findings, using anti-CD71 microbeads and positive selection through an AutoMACS separator (Miltenyi Biotec). A reticulocyte sample from patient 1 was prepared similarly, to be used as positive control. RNA was isolated using the QiaAmp RNA Blood Mini kit (QIAGEN) and reverse transcription was performed using the High-Capacity cDNA Reverse Transcription Kit (Applied Biosystems). *SPTA1* mRNA expression level was determined by qPCR using a StepOnePlus Real-Time PCR System (Applied Biosystems) and FAM-labeled Taqman probes (Thermo Fisher Scientific) for *SPTA1* spanning exons 48–49 (Assay ID Hs01005878_m1) and *ACTB* (Assay ID Hs01060665_g1) as a reference gene.

RESULTS AND DISCUSSION

We observed three different phenotypes in patients with recessive HS due to biallelic *SPTA1* mutations, verified to be *in trans* by parental targeted sequencing (**Table 1**). The heterozygous parents did not have any evidence of hemolytic anemia as expected, since even α^{LELY} *in trans* to a null *SPTA1* allele, producing a total of ~25% of normal α-spectrin, causes no disease (Delaunay et al., 2004).

The first four patients listed in **Table 1** (within Group I) had the well-known phenotype of *SPTA1*-associated HS, i.e., severe, transfusion-dependent HHA with brisk reticulocytosis (Agre et al., 1982; Wichterle et al., 1996). These patients presented with hyperbilirubinemia and non-immune hemolytic anemia soon after birth, requiring their first transfusion as neonates, before any meaningful RBC phenotypical testing could be obtained. They continued to require frequent transfusions, precluding any further erythrocyte phenotype work-up until splenectomy. Patients 1–3 had a *SPTA1* nonsense mutation (expected to lead to nonsense-mediated decay of the transcript)

in trans to the low expression α^{LEPRA} mutation (c.4339-99C > T). Patient 1 required monthly transfusions for hemoglobin (Hgb) in the range of 6.4–7.5 g/dL with absolute reticulocyte count (ARC) of $130–360 \times 10^9$/L for the first four years of life, with consequent iron overload, requiring chelation treatment with deferasirox. After molecular diagnosis of *SPTA1*-associated HS utilizing NGS of the HHA panel, he underwent partial splenectomy at 4 years of age. He was able to remain transfusion-free for 18 months with Hgb 8.7–11 g/dL, but then his anemia gradually worsened with increasing transfusion requirement. He had a follow-up total splenectomy at 7 years of age; at that time the remaining splenic tissue had been impressively regrown to 435 g, based on the pathology report. The patient has had no further transfusion requirement for the past 4 years, with Hgb now in 12.7–15.8 g/dL range. Blood smear from a non-transfused blood sample after splenectomy shows many spherocytes and moderate poikilocytosis, as expected with α-spectrin deficiency (Eber and Lux, 2004), and ektacytometry reveals the typical HS curve (Da Costa et al., 2016; **Figure 1A**). Patient 2 had a similar course for the first 2.5 years. After molecular diagnosis of *SPTA1*-associated HS, he underwent partial splenectomy and he remains transfusion-free since then with Hgb in the range of 9–10.8 g/dL and minimal regrowth of the remaining splenic tissue based on ultrasound (108–123 ml). Patient 3 has not yet had splenectomy due to parental preference and continues to require frequent transfusions.

Patient 4 had a similar clinical presentation but NGS for the HHA-panel was negative. Deletion/duplication assay by Comparative Genomic Hybridization was performed and identified a heterozygous deletion at 1q23.1 involving the *SPTA1* gene. No mutation was identified *in trans*. Since the patient remained transfusion dependent precluding phenotypical evaluation of his RBCs, α-spectrin mRNA expression in his reticulocytes was evaluated by qPCR and was found decreased at levels comparable to patient 1, confirming *SPTA1*-associated recessive HS (**Figure 1B**). Hgb normalized at ~13 g/dL with no need for further transfusions post total splenectomy at 3 years of age.

Regrowth of the splenic remnant after partial splenectomy is a possibility, occasionally requiring a second surgery. Nevertheless, in both patients 1 and 2 who had splenectomy before 5 years of age in order to limit the transfusional iron overload, partial splenectomy was a reasonable choice with the goal to preserve splenic immune function (Englum et al., 2016). The different response of these two patients to partial splenectomy was most likely due to difference in splenic regrowth, rather than a difference in phenotypic severity. α-spectrin in the erythrocyte ghosts of patient 1 was determined by immunoelectrophoresis to be 54% vs. 64% for patient 2 in comparison to normal control (**Figure 1C**).

Surprisingly, we identified four patients (patients 5–8 in **Table 1**, comprising Group II) who, despite having equivalent genotype with the first four patients of a null *SPTA1* mutation *in trans* to α^{LEPRA}, appeared to have a milder phenotype, ranging from improvement in transfusion requirement after frequent transfusions in the first 2–3 years of life (patients 5 and 6)

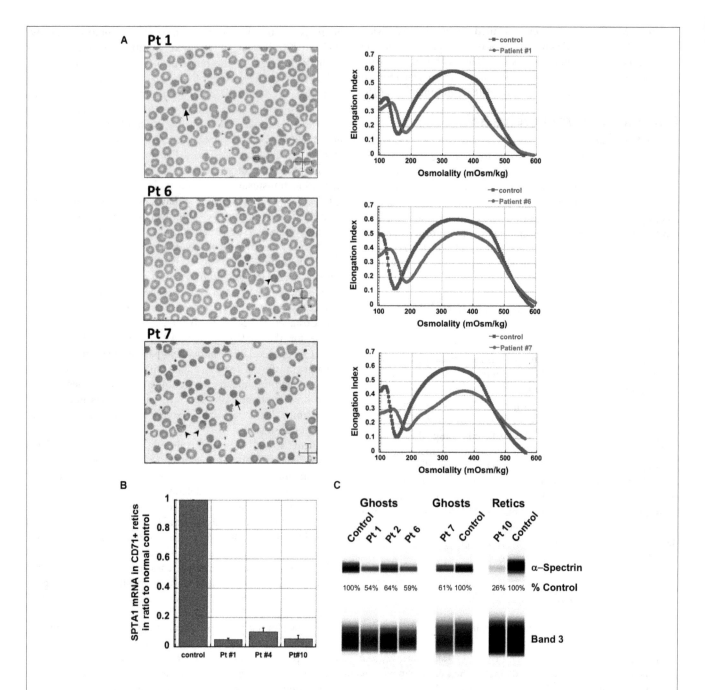

FIGURE 1 | Studies in peripheral blood of patients with *SPTA1*-associated HS. **(A)** Peripheral blood smears on the left from patients 1, 6 and 7 showing multiple spherocytes (arrows) lacking central pallor due to decreased surface area to volume ratio and aniso-poikilocytosis. Patient 7 also has polychromasia with increased reticulocytes (arrowheads) indicating significant hemolysis prior to splenectomy. Ektacytometry, on the right, demonstrates the typical HS curve for the patients (red) vs. control (blue). HS is characterized by increased Omin indicating decreased RBC surface to volume ratio and decreased Elmax (maximum Elongation Index) which depends mostly on the cytoskeleton mechanics. Frequently, the declining portion of the curve (represented by Ohyp, the osmolality value where the cells are at half of the maximum elongation) is also decreased (as in patient 1) indicating increased intracellular viscosity, however, it may also be normal as in patients 6 and 7 (Clark et al., 1983; Zaninoni et al., 2018). **(B)** qPCR in RNA isolated from patients' reticulocytes demonstrated severely decreased α-spectrin expression. Patient 1 who has α^{LEPRA} *in trans* to a null *SPTA1* mutation was found to express α-spectrin at about 5% in comparison to normal control at levels similar to the original calculations for α^{LEPRA} (about 16% of full-length spectrin as compared to the normal *SPTA1* allele based on studies with metabolic labeling of erythroblasts *in vitro* (Wichterle et al., 1996), and therefore a total of 8% α-spectrin when α^{LEPRA} is *in trans* to a null allele). qPCR appears to be a useful diagnostic assay when an unknown low-expression allele is suspected *in trans* to a null *SPTA1* mutation or deletion in a disease suspected to be severe HS, such as the case of patient 4.
(C) Quantitation of α-spectrin/band 3 ratio in RBC ghosts (Patients 1, 2, 6, and 7) and reticulocytes (Patient 10) expressed as percent of α-spectrin/band 3 ratio in corresponding normal control samples by immunodetection using size-based capillary electrophoresis. Agre et al. (1985) in one of the first descriptions of HS due to α-spectrin deficiency noted that the clinical severity of anemia was proportional to a degree of spectrin deficiency, ranging from 53% of normal spectrin content in severely anemic patients to 31% of normal in nearly lethal cases.

to well compensated hemolysis (patient 8). The milder severity of the disease did not seem to correlate with RBC osmotic fragility or deformability based on ektacytometry (**Figure 1A**) or the α-spectrin quantitation in RBC ghosts which was only slightly lower compared to the α-spectrin level in patient 2 (**Figure 1C**). Additional gene polymorphisms and mutations found in the HHA panel (**Supplementary Table S1**) did not explain the milder phenotype noted in the patients of Group II versus Group I. Heterogeneity in the level of normal α-spectrin expression from the α-LEPRA allele (c.4339-99C > T), variability in HIF-pathway, and erythropoietin response, and sometimes a different tolerance to anemia by patients and/or parents may be contributing to differences in the phenotype between Group I and Group II patients.

The third phenotype (Group III in **Table 1**) associated with HS due to near-complete or complete α-spectrin deficiency is less well known since it has been typically embryonal lethal causing fatal *hydrops fetalis* in the third trimester of pregnancy or perinatally, such as the case of patient 9. His parents requested genetic counseling after having a fetus and a newborn child die with the clinical picture of *hydrops fetalis*. Both parents were found to carry a frameshift *SPTA1* mutation. DNA isolated from the patient's liver tissue, preserved in paraffin after autopsy, was sequenced and revealed that the patient was compound heterozygous for these *SPTA1* mutations, predicting absence of normal α-spectrin production. With the progress of fetal medicine allowing prenatal diagnosis of severe anemia and *in utero* transfusions, more of these patients are now surviving to term and the disease is increasingly recognized.

Patient 10 was born prematurely at 33 weeks of gestation with severe non-immune hemolytic anemia requiring transfusion soon after birth. He remained transfusion dependent and total splenectomy did not significantly improve his hemolytic anemia. NGS for the HHA-panel revealed homozygosity for an intronic *SPTA1* variant, likely causing alternative splicing and severely decreased expression of α-spectrin, as verified by qPCR (**Figure 1B**) and immunoelectrophoresis performed in lysates prepared from isolated reticulocytes. The patient is now doing well after bone marrow transplant. Patient 11, an infant of Amish-Mennonite origin required five in-utero transfusions for severe anemia and had significant neonatal hyperbilirubinemia at birth requiring exchange transfusion. HHA gene panel revealed homozygosity for a *SPTA1* frameshift mutation, explaining her severe reticulocytopenia since her reticulocytes with complete

α-spectrin deficiency are extremely fragile, failing to survive the shear stress in circulation.

The genetic and phenotypic information gathered from our patient cohort demonstrates that patients with recessive *SPTA1*-associated HS due to the low expression *SPTA1* variant α^{LEPRA} *in trans* to a null *SPTA1* mutation respond to either partial or total splenectomy by significant improvement or resolution of anemia, respectively. In contrast, patients with near complete or complete α-spectrin deficiency because of biallelic null or rare intronic *SPTA1* mutations that result in severely decreased expression of the protein, are unlikely to have a measurable response to splenectomy and require either lifetime transfusions and iron chelation or stem cell transplant. This group of patients have typically reticulocytopenia and history of having been salvaged from fatal *hydrops fetalis*, either because they were born prematurely and started transfusions early or because they had intrauterine transfusions.

Next generation sequencing panels are robust and rapid diagnostic tools for HHA, especially when frequent transfusions preclude phenotypic evaluation of the patients' RBCs. Specialized assays such as qPCR of reticulocyte mRNA can be used for verification of the diagnosis. Comprehensive genetic and phenotypic evaluation is critical to provide insights into the variable phenotypes of patients with HHA and guide toward appropriate management.

AUTHOR CONTRIBUTIONS

SC, MR, KZ, WZ, and TK contributed to the conception and design of the study. SC, MR, HS, TM, ND, and KS performed the experiments. SC, ON, JR, LH, STC, JK, EK, MG, DW, and TK provided the clinical information. TK organized the database. SC and TK wrote the first draft of the manuscript. MR, HS, and KS wrote sections of the manuscript. All authors revised, read, and approved the submitted version of the manuscript.

ACKNOWLEDGMENTS

We are grateful to the CCHMC hematology clinical research support team, patients, and families for their enthusiastic participation in this study.

REFERENCES

Agre, P., Casella, J. F., Zinkham, W. H., McMillan, C., and Bennett, V. (1985). Partial deficiency of erythrocyte spectrin in hereditary spherocytosis. *Nature* 314, 380–383. doi: 10.1038/314380a0

Agre, P., Orringer, E. P., and Bennett, V. (1982). Deficient red-cell spectrin in severe, recessively inherited spherocytosis. *N. Engl. J. Med.* 306, 1155–1161. doi: 10.1056/NEJM198205133061906

Bennett, V. (1983). Proteins involved in membrane–cytoskeleton association in human erythrocytes: spectrin, ankyrin, and band 3. *Meth. Enzymol.* 96, 313–324. doi: 10.1016/s0076-6879(83)96029-9

Bogardus, H., Schulz, V. P., Maksimova, Y., Miller, B. A., Li, P., Forget, B. G., et al. (2014). Severe nondominant hereditary spherocytosis due to uniparental

isodisomy at the SPTA1 locus. *Haematologica* 99, e168–e170. doi: 10.3324/haematol.2014.110312

Clark, M. R., Mohandas, N., and Shohet, S. B. (1983). Osmotic gradient ektacytometry: comprehensive characterization of red cell volume and surface maintenance. *Blood* 61, 899–910.

Da Costa, L., Suner, L., Galimand, J., Bonnel, A., Pascreau, T., Couque, N., et al. (2016). Diagnostic tool for red blood cell membrane disorders: assessment of a new generation ektacytometer. *Blood Cells Mol. Dis.* 56, 9–22. doi: 10.1016/j.bcmd.2015.09.001

Delaunay, J., Nouyrigat, V., Proust, A., Schischmanoff, P. O., Cynober, T., Yvart, J., et al. (2004). Different impacts of alleles alphaLEPRA and alphaLELY as assessed versus a novel, virtually null allele of the SPTA1 gene in trans. *Br. J. Haematol.* 127, 118–122. doi: 10.1111/j.1365-2141.2004.05160.x

Eber, S., and Lux, S. E. (2004). Hereditary spherocytosis–defects in proteins that connect the membrane skeleton to the lipid bilayer. *Semin Hematol.* 41, 118–141. doi: 10.1053/j.seminhematol.2004.01.002

Englum, B. R., Rothman, J., Leonard, S., Reiter, A., Thornburg, C., Brindle, M., et al. (2016). Hematologic outcomes after total splenectomy and partial splenectomy for congenital hemolytic anemia. *J. Pediatr. Surg.* 51, 122–127. doi: 10.1016/j.jpedsurg.2015.10.028

Gallagher, P. G. (2005). Red cell membrane disorders. *Hematology Am. Soc. Hematol. Educ. Program* 2005, 13–18. doi: 10.1182/asheducation-2005.1.13

Hanspal, M., and Palek, J. (1987). Synthesis and assembly of membrane skeletal proteins in mammalian red cell precursors. *J. Cell Biol.* 105, 1417–1424. doi: 10.1083/jcb.105.3.1417

Marechal, J., Wilmotte, R., Kanzaki, A., Dhermy, D., Garbarz, M., Galand, C., et al. (1995). Ethnic distribution of allele alpha LELY, a low-expression allele of red-cell spectrin alpha-gene. *Br. J. Haematol.* 90, 553–556. doi: 10.1111/j.1365-2141.1995.tb05583.x

Mohandas, N. (2018). Inherited hemolytic anemia: a possessive beginner's guide. *Hematology Am. Soc. Hematol. Educ. Program* 2018, 377–381. doi: 10.1182/asheducation-2018.1.377

Niss, O., Chonat, S., Dagaonkar, N., Almansoori, M. O., Kerr, K., Rogers, Z. R., et al. (2016). Genotype-phenotype correlations in hereditary elliptocytosis and hereditary pyropoikilocytosis. *Blood Cells Mol. Dis.* 61, 4–9. doi: 10.1016/j.bcmd.2016.07.003

Salomao, M., Zhang, X., Yang, Y., Lee, S., Hartwig, J. H., Chasis, J. A., et al. (2008). Protein 4.1R-dependent multiprotein complex: new insights into the structural organization of the red blood cell membrane. *Proc. Natl. Acad. Sci. U.S.A.* 105, 8026–8031. doi: 10.1073/pnas.0803225105

Whitfield, C. F., Follweiler, J. B., Lopresti-Morrow, L., and Miller, B. A. (1991). Deficiency of alpha-spectrin synthesis in burst-forming units-erythroid in lethal hereditary spherocytosis. *Blood* 78, 3043–3051.

Wichterle, H., Hanspal, M., Palek, J., and Jarolim, P. (1996). Combination of two mutant alpha spectrin alleles underlies a severe spherocytic hemolytic anemia. *J. Clin. Invest.* 98, 2300–2307. doi: 10.1172/JCI119041

Wilmotte, R., Marechal, J., Morle, L., Baklouti, F., Philippe, N., Kastally, R., et al. (1993). Low expression allele alpha LELY of red cell spectrin is associated with mutations in exon 40 (alpha V/41 polymorphism) and intron 45 and with partial skipping of exon 46. *J. Clin. Invest.* 91, 2091–2096. doi: 10.1172/JCI116432

Zaninoni, A., Fermo, E., Vercellati, C., Consonni, D., Marcello, A. P., Zanella, A., et al. (2018). Use of laser assisted optical rotational cell analyzer (lorrca maxsis) in the diagnosis of rbc membrane disorders, enzyme defects, and congenital dyserythropoietic anemias: a monocentric study on 202 patients. *Front. Physiol.* 9:451. doi: 10.3389/fphys.2018.00451

3

Clinical Diagnosis of Red Cell Membrane Disorders: Comparison of Osmotic Gradient Ektacytometry and Eosin Maleimide (EMA) Fluorescence Test for Red Cell Band 3 (AE1, SLC4A1) Content for Clinical Diagnosis

Ahmar Urooj Zaidi[1]*, Steven Buck[1,2], Manisha Gadgeel[2], Miguel Herrera-Martinez[2], Araathi Mohan[2], Kenya Johnson[2], Shruti Bagla[2], Robert M. Johnson[2] and Yaddanapudi Ravindranath[1,2]

[1] Children's Hospital of Michigan, Detroit, MI, United States, [2] Wayne State University School of Medicine, Detroit, MI, United States

*Correspondence:
Ahmar Urooj Zaidi
ahmar@wayne.edu

The measurement of band 3 (AE1, SLC4A1, CD233) content of red cells by eosin-5- maleimide (EMA) staining is swiftly replacing conventional osmotic fragility (OF) test as a tool for laboratory confirmation of hereditary spherocytosis across the globe. Our group has systematically evaluated the EMA test as a method to screen for a variety of anemias in the last 10 years, and compared these results to those obtained with the osmotic gradient ektacytometry (osmoscans) which we have used over three decades. Our overall experience allowed us to characterize the distinctive patterns with the two tests in several congenital erythrocyte membrane disorders, such as hereditary spherocytosis (HS), hereditary elliptocytosis (HE), Southeast Asian Ovalocytosis (SAO), hereditary pyropoikilocytosis (HPP) variants, erythrocyte volume disorders, various red cell enzymopathies, and hemoglobinopathies. A crucial difference between the two methodologies is that osmoscans measure red blood cell deformability of the entire sample of RBCs, while the EMA test examines the band 3 content of individual RBCs. EMA content is influenced by cell size as smaller red cells have lower amount of total membrane than larger cells. The SAO mutation alters the EMA binding site resulting in a lower EMA MCF even as the band 3 content itself is unchanged. Thus, EMA scan results should be interpreted with caution and both the histograms and dot plots should be analyzed in the context of the clinical picture and morphology.

Keywords: red blood cell, anemia, membrane, Hematology, erythrocyte

INTRODUCTION

Our ability to accurately recognize the mechanistic basis of red cell disorders is continuing to evolve, none more so than the erythrocyte membrane disorders and enzymopathies. The human erythrocyte is the most abundant cell in the human body (Bianconi et al., 2013) and perhaps the most studied cell. There are approximately 20 major proteins and over 800 minor proteins in the red blood cell membrane. Integral membrane proteins are organized around band 3, an anion-exchange channel. The membrane skeleton, primarily composed of spectrin, actin and its associated proteins complete the composition of the phospholipid bilayer enabling it to maintain its shape (Lux, 2016). There are several other proteins that manage the regulation of volume and hydration that are implicated in rare, but important, disorders of the red blood cell membrane (Andolfo et al., 2016).

There have been many important contributions to red blood cell membrane science since the original osmotic fragility (OF) test (Hunter, 1940). One such contribution came almost four decades ago, the ektacytometer (Bessis et al., 1980). The ektacytometer is a laser diffractometer that measures the deformability potential of a population of red blood cells over an osmotic gradient, and allows the characterization of many of the common red blood cell membranopathies. Red cells undergo shape change from discoid to elliptocyte configuration as they traverse through the capillaries and the micropores in the splenic sinusoids. This *in vivo* phenomenon is mimicked in the ektacytometer. The cells are exposed to an increasing osmotic gradient, and cell deformability (shift from discoid to elliptical shape) is gauged by how light scatters as the cell responds to shear forces. The result of this test, is a characteristic graph (the Osmoscan), that shows the amount of deformability on the y-axis, and osmolality on the x-axis (**Figure 1**; Mohandas et al., 1980).

The major components of the red cells that determine deformability are the biconcave shape of the red cells, the membrane fluidity and the internal viscosity of the cell. There are several key features of the osmoscan that allow us to understand the deformability properties of the red blood cells being tested (Clark et al., 1983). The most significant measures, are the O_{min} , DI_{max} (y axis the value of the index at isotonicity or the ellipticity/deformability index maximum, EI/DI_{max}), and O_{hyper}. The O_{min} is the point at which red blood cells have attained their critical hemolytic value, due to osmotic shifting of water into the cell in a hypotonic environment; beyond this point, the now spherocytic red blood cells would lyse with a further decrease in osmolality. Thus, the EI at O_{min} measures the changes in surface to volume (S/V) ratio. The deformability index maximum is the index value at isotonicity, and the point at which red blood cells have attained the maximum ellipticity (DI_{max}, EI_{max}). Deformability index reflects the membrane integrity and elasticity. The O_{hyper} is the osmolality at which the index is midway between the maximal deformability and O_{min}. O_{hyper} is increased in states of cellular hydration either because of decreased mean corpuscular hemoglobin concentration or net increase of water content (such as stomatocytosis/cryohydrocytosis). These values, when compared to normal red blood cells provide unique signatures in cells with membrane pathologies. However, despite the ability of the ektacytometer to aid in the clinical diagnosis of red blood cell membrane disorders (Groner et al., 1980; Johnson and Ravindranath, 1996), its use was limited until recently because of the non-availability of the original Technicon made instruments. A newer clinical grade version with digitized osmoscans, LoRRca Maxsis®, has become available and its usage will expand. Even with the new-generation ektacytometer gaining

increasing popularity, the ability of centers to perform this test remains limited and yet approved by US FDA for clinical testing (Da Costa et al., 2016).

Almost 20 years after the introduction of ektacytometry, King et al. (2000) devised a simple alternative to standard OF test for laboratory confirmation of HS by using eosin maleimide fluorescence to measure band 3 content (AE1, SLC4A1). HS cells lose membrane through vesiculation, and along with it band-3 protein. The test uses the functional property of the fluorochrome, eosin-5-maleimide (EMA), which covalently binds to the 430th residue (lysine) on the first extracellular loop of band 3 (Cobb and Beth, 1990). This test provides investigators with insight on the amount of band 3, or functional loss of membrane, that exists in pathologic red blood cell. The results of the EMA test are reported as mean channel fluorescence (MCF) compared to a control sample- MCF ratio (patient's MCF/control MCF). However, as described below, the slope of the EMA curve on both sides indicates valuable information on the variation in cell size; trailing shoulders on the right side is prominent in patients with high reticulocyte count and the leading shoulder on the left indicates presence of fragmented red cells. Thus, EMA test should be interpreted not solely on the MCF, but also on the overall pattern of EMA intensity. The measurement of band 3 content by flow cytometry has enabled for rapid diagnosis of spherocytosis in intact red blood cells and is fast replacing the OF test.

A crucial difference between the ektacytometry and EMA test is that osmoscans measure red blood cell deformability of the entire sample of RBCs, while the EMA test examines the band 3 content of individual RBCs. One is a measure of deformability under shear stress (function) and the other an estimate of a critical membrane protein (structure). Further, the ektacytometer is a test that simulates flow of red blood cells through the vasculature, and is able to capture the spirit of the dynamic red blood cell; the test is a measure of RBC geometry, cytoplasmic viscosity, cell volume regulation and fluidity of the membrane (Mohandas et al., 1980). The testing is limited by the availability of the instrument, the need for specialized staff and the need to delay analysis after transfusion (Da Costa et al., 2016). The EMA is user-friendly, with quick turnaround time of testing, and flow cytometers are readily available in most institutions. Though the EMA only describes reduction in band 3 protein and does not interact with other integral proteins, it can serve as a reliable indirect measure of cytoskeletal health (King et al., 2004) but mild defects may result in indeterminate results (Bolton-Maggs et al., 2012).

Our group has systematically evaluated both the EMA test and osmoscans obtained as a method to screen for a variety of anemias over the past 10 years and compared these results. Our experience allowed us to characterize distinctive patterns in a variety of congenital hemolytic anemias (red cell membrane disorders, erythrocyte volume disorders, enzymopathies/hemoglobinopathies) and as well in some acquired disorders. We have not systematically evaluated the OF test by flow cytometry (Won and Suh, 2009; Crisp et al., 2012). In this review, we will describe both the ektacytometry-osmoscans and EMA tests from patients and the lessons we have learned from practical experience.

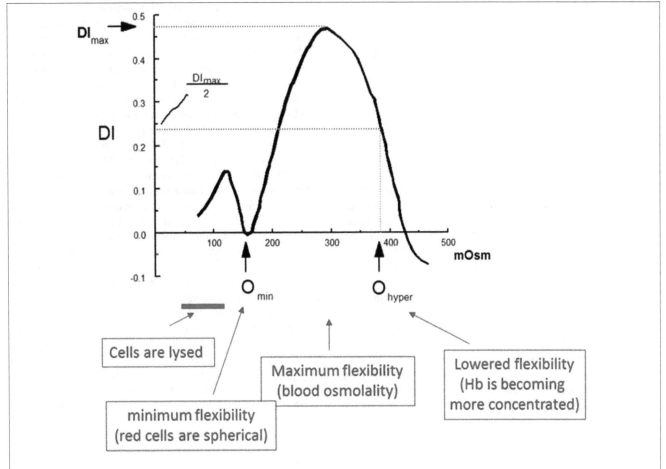

FIGURE 1 | Several key features of the osmoscan allow us to understand the deformability properties of the red blood cells being tested. The most significant measures, are the O_{min}, DI_{max} (y-axis the value of the index at isotonicity (or the deformability index maximum, DI_{max}) and O_{hyper}. The O_{min} is the point at which red blood cells have attained their critical hemolytic value, due to osmotic shifting of water into the cell in a hypotonic environment; beyond this point, the now spherocytic red blood cells would lyse with a further decrease in osmolality adapted with permission from Johnson and Ravindranath (1996).

MATERIALS AND METHODS

All individuals studied were patients at the Children's Hospital of Michigan/Wayne State University School of Medicine, and the data has been collected from routine clinical testing. This review was approved by the Wayne State University Human Investigation Committee. We reviewed records of children with suspected red blood cell membranopathies or anemias who underwent both osmotic gradient ektacytometry and flow cytometry studies using eosin-5-maleimide from 2007 to 2017. In all cases, the peripheral blood smears were reviewed by members of the division of Pediatric Hematology/Oncology. Osmotic gradient ektacytometry was performed on an ektacytometer manufactured by Technicon Instruments (Miles Diagnostics, Tarrytown, NY, United States). This instrument includes two pumps to generate buffer gradients, a microprocessor that controls the viscometer motor and gradient pumps, an image analyzer and a keyboard with a display. For standard clinical testing, the rotor speed was set at 150 RPM, operating at a shear stress of 159.3 dynes/cm^3 (all of the tests were done by Gerard Goyette until 2015 and following his untimely death by MG). The

analog curves were digitized (done by MHM and KJ) and O_{min} and O_{max} values were used to compare diagnostic reliability in dominant HS and general characteristics of the curves relative to normal were used to describe changes in other membrane disorders. For EMA flow cytometry, cells were stained in the dark for 30 min at room temperature with agitation, washed with 1 ml cold PBS, and re-suspended in 0.5 ml PBS plus fixative (PBS plus 0.5% formaldehyde). Acquisition was performed on a Coulter XL Flow Cytometer (Coulter Corp., Miami, FL, United States) equipped with a 488 nm Argon laser. Results were analyzed using EXPO-32 software (by SB and MG). We reviewed complete blood counts on the days of the sampling and entered them into a database without patient identifiers.

Cases

Table 1. Number of patients for each disorder.

Hereditary Spherocytosis (HS)

Hereditary spherocytosis (HS) is the most commonly inherited red blood cell membranopathy with significant clinical heterogeneity. Features like anemia, jaundice and splenomegaly

TABLE 1 | Number of cases.

43	Hereditary Spherocytosis
8	Hereditary Elliptocytosis
3	Hereditary Pyropoikilocytosis
3	ABO Incompatibility
4	AIHA
3	Southeast Asian Ovalocytosis
3	Erythrocyte Volume Disorders

are common, and jaundice may be the only sign in neonates (Ribeiro et al., 2000; Delaunay, 2007; An and Mohandas, 2008; Nussenzveig et al., 2014; Andolfo et al., 2016; Da Costa et al., 2016). Hydrops fetalis is an exceedingly rare complication in HS (Gallagher et al., 1995; Ribeiro et al., 2000). While the molecular defects are protean, in general, it is the weakened vertical linkages between the membrane skeleton and the lipid bilayer's integral proteins that drive this disease process (Palek and Lux, 1983; Perrotta et al., 2008). This disruption of linkage between the lipid bilayer and the cytoskeleton via ankyrin (band 2.1) results in echinocyte formation. More specifically defects in ankyrin, band 3, beta spectrin, alpha spectrin or protein 4.2 cause spherocytosis through loss of membrane surface area. As erythrocytes age they begin to exhibit a variety of membrane abnormalities including the loss of potassium and water, leading to cell dehydration and increased cell density, and the loss of surface area, likely owing

to gradual release of membrane microvesicles (Lux, 2014). The spherocyte generates characteristic results on osmoscans with the entire curve being inside of the control-O_{min} is increased, EI/DI_{Max} is lower and O_{hyper} is reduced. The three aspects of HS cells driving these changes are the loss of surface area, reduced S/V ratio and the high internal viscosity (Clark et al., 1983). The loss of band 3 content results in decreased EMA binding. The MCF (mean channel of fluorescence) is reduced variably with the histogram shifted to left (see **Figure 2**).

In 43 patients with HS, the EMA MCF was 395.69 ± 53.48, whereas in 76 normal controls the value is 514.50 ± 15.25 (Zaidi et al., 2015; **Table 2**). Thus compared to controls HS is easily diagnosable disease by either EMA or osmoscan. The severity of spherocytic defect, can be depicted in an osmoscan based on the degree of reduction in the y-coordinate of the elongation index's maximum point (Johnson and Ravindranath, 1996). **Figure 2A** shows a typical osmoscan of three samples: control (black line), mild HS (blue line), and severe HS (red line). In patients with low MCF and this typical osmoscan tracing, a diagnosis of HS is certain. There is good correlation between values for O_{min}, S/V ratio and MCF in dominant HS (Zaidi et al., 2015). However, in our cohort of patients, we were unable to find any replicable association or relationship with clinical indicators of severity-hemoglobin/hematocrit, reticulocyte counts, bilirubin and other red blood cell parameters (MCHC, MCH, MCV, RDW) with either O_{min} or MCF values. This suggests that phagocytosis of damaged red cells and the extent of compensatory erythropoeitic

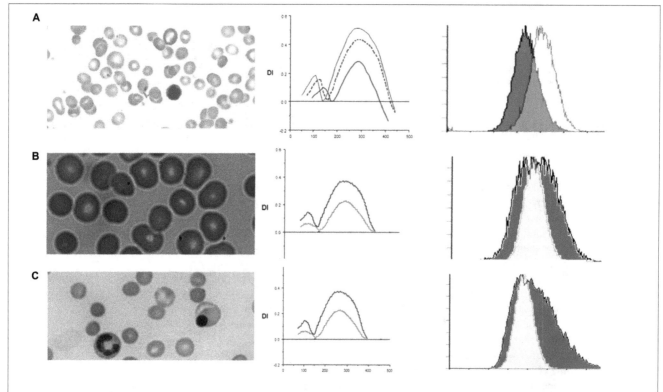

FIGURE 2 | (A) Depiction of smear in left panel, Osmoscan (blue line: mild HS, red line: severe HS) in middle panel, and EMA histogram in right panel in cases of hereditary spherocytosis. **(B)** Depiction of smear in left panel, Osmoscan in middle panel, EMA histogram in right panel in cases of ABO Hemolytic Anemia.
(C) Depiction of smear in left panel, Osmoscan in middle panel, and EMA histogram in right panel in cases of autoimmune hemolytic anemia.

TABLE 2 | Hereditary spherocytosis.

	HS (*n* = 43)			Normal controls (*n* = 76)	
	Mean	SD		Mean	SD
MCF	395.69	53.48	MCF	514.50	15.25
O_{min} (*X*-axis)	166.11	14.65	O_{min} (*X*-axis)	147.67	6.90
DI_{MAX} (*Y*-axis)	0.34	0.08	DI_{MAX} (*Y*-axis)	0.49	0.05

TABLE 3 | ABO hemolytic disease.

	ABO (*n* = 3)			Normal controls (*n* = 76)	
	Mean	SD		Mean	SD
MCF	554.40	42.97	MCF	514.50	15.25
O_{min} (*x*-axis)	175.39	25.34	O_{min} (*x*-axis)	147.67	6.90
DI_{MAX} (*y*-axis)	0.31	0.02	DI_{MAX} (*y*-axis)	0.49	0.05

TABLE 4 | Autoimmune hemolytic anemia.

	AIHA (*n* = 4)			Normal controls (*n* = 76)	
	Mean	SD		Mean	SD
MCF	497.63	66.84	MCF	514.50	15.25
O_{min} (*x*-axis)	169.24	6.53	O_{min} (*x*-axis)	147.67	6.90
DI_{MAX} (*y*-axis)	0.35	0.06	DI_{MAX} (*y*-axis)	0.49	0.05

response are critical additive determinants of clinical severity. Molecular testing was done only in a few cases and thus we cannot make sweeping comments, but the reader is referred to a recent publication by the Dutch group (Huisjes et al., 2019). Lowest MCF values in HS cases were seen in a teenager with band 3 mutation (SLC4A1; NM_000342.3; c.2423G > T, pArg808Leu) and in a child with ankyrin mutation (ANK1 NM-000037.3; c.2023dup;pVal675Glyfs*118). Arginine mutations appear to cause severe band 3 deficiency because of decreased incorporation of band 3 protein in to the lipid bilayer (Palek and Lux, 1983; Gallagher, 2013). However, the teenager (status post splenectomy) with SLC4A1 Arg808Leu had a hemoglobin of 17.8 g/dL, MCF 301.1 (ratio 59% when compared to mean control values) when tested at age 15.5 years. A young girl with ANK1 mutation had hemoglobin 6.5 g/dL at age 6 weeks and 8.5 g/dL at age 12 months with no interventions. Her brother had a hemoglobin of 10.3 g/dL at 18 months, and their father at age 26 had a hemoglobin of 13.6 g/dL; neither were transfused nor had splenectomy, and had the same mutation as the index patient. The EI_{Max} on the osmoscan was reduced to an equal degree in all three patients (51, 55, 56% of control).

Neither the osmoscans nor the EMA histograms can distinguish dominant HS from recessive HS. In the only child with recessive HS we have evaluated, the EMA MCF was 348 with MCF ratio of 0.87; the child had two alpha spectrin mutations (SPTA1 c.3267A > T, p.Y1089X and alpha-LEPRA [c.4339-99C > T]), in trans; the case was included in two recent publications on recessive HS (Chonat et al., 2015; Gallagher et al., 2019).

Heterozygotes with EPB42 mutations exhibit milder changes from our limited experience (2 cases) consistent with published data (Kalfa et al., 1993). Thus, in general, our findings are in agreement with the detailed structure-function correlations reported by the von Wijk laboratory (Huisjes et al., 2019).

Spherocytes in Immune (Allo/Auto) Hemolytic Anemias

Immune hemolytic anemia is the result of antibody mediated destruction of red cells. It can be caused by maternally transferred alloantibodies as in neonates with Rh sensitization and A/B blood group infants born to type O mothers. In older children and adults acquired autoantibodies can cause hemolytic anemia. Variable numbers of spherocytes are present on smears. The osmoscan by itself cannot distinguish acquired from congenital spherocytosis, as is evident from the patterns shown in **Figure 2**. In ABO hemolytic disease, on the ektacytometer, the O_{min} and DI_{max} (*Y*-axis) may appear similar to normal adult controls;

neonatal red cells typically have high osmoscans (Johnson et al., 1999) and age matched neonatal controls usually are not available concurrently and thus a "normal" scan may actually indicate underlying spherocytosis (congenital or caused by antibody due to blood group incompatibility). An additional confounding variable is the high reticulocyte count. Evaluation of the slope of the curve on EMA test is frequently informative with leftward leaning curve indicating a gradual loss of membrane due to the antibody as opposed to the rapid loss caused by structural defects in HS where the whole curve is shifted left. This is consistent with the reported data on this topic (Johnson et al., 1999). Diagnosis of neonatal HS and distinction from spherocytosis associated with ABO incompatibility remains a challenge; family history is helpful and repeat testing 8–10 weeks postnatally should clarify the diagnosis in *de novo* congenital HS cases (see **Figures 2B,C** and **Tables 3, 4**).

Hereditary Elliptocytosis (HE) and Hereditary Pyropoikilocytosis (HPP)

Hereditary elliptocytosis (HE) is clinically heterogeneous disorder. The presence of elliptically shaped red cells on the peripheral blood smear is the characteristic feature of HE. HE patients can have a diverse spectrum of clinical findings ranging from life threatening anemias to asymptomatic carrier state (Lazarova et al., 2017). The inheritance of HE is autosomal dominant, with rare reports of recessive mutations. Homozygous and compound heterozygous HE variants present with moderate anemia and hemolysis (Delaunay, 2007; An and Mohandas, 2008). Weakened lateral linkages in membrane skeletons due to either defective spectrin dimer-dimer interaction or weakened spectrin-actin-protein 4.1R junctional complex results in the decrease of mechanical stability in these patients (Gallagher, 2004). Significant fragmentation of red blood cells in addition to the classic elliptocytes are a feature of the disease (see **Figure 3**). Newborn infants may show high level of red cell fragmentation, so called hemolytic HE (as seen in **Figure 3A**), which improves by age 1–2 years (as seen in **Figure 3B**; Palek and Lux, 1983; Mentzer et al., 1987; An and Mohandas, 2008). In the family

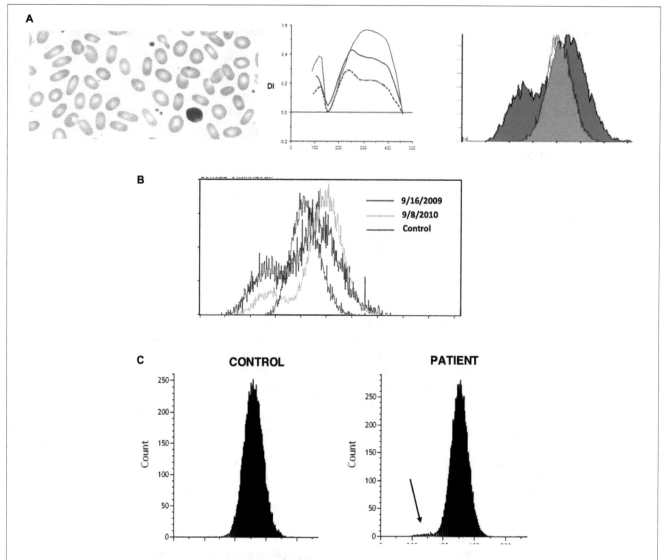

FIGURE 3 | (A) Depiction of smear in left panel, Osmoscan in middle panel (blue line depicts a mild case, red line depicts a severe case), and EMA histogram in right panel in cases of hereditary elliptocytosis with severe fragmentation. **(B)** Changes in the EMA histogram in a HE patient with severe fragmentation at birth, and improvement 1 year later. **(C)** EMA in an older child showing a prominent left shoulder, but mostly resolved fragmentation.

with 4.1 deficiency, homozygotes had more severe disease than heterozygotes.

Hereditary elliptocytosis cases show distinctive indented plateau on osmoscans pattern (Tchernia et al., 1981; Johnson and Ravindranath, 1996; Silveira et al., 1997). HE cells generate a trapezoidal profile in an osmoscan, with a normally positioned O_{min} and O_{hyper} but diminished EI_{Max}. The truncated curve reflects the inability of the already elliptical cells to deform further under shear stress. These findings were conformed in more recent work (Suemori et al., 2015) and has been re-appraised with the use of the new generation ektacytometers (Da Costa et al., 2016).

On EMA scans a bimodal pattern comprised of distinct population of cells with decreased MCF (representing fragmented cells) and a population with normal to high MCF may be present, especially in neonates. The EMA histograms reflect the level of fragmentation seen on smears. In infants who show

high numbers of fragmented cells ("hemolytic HE") two distinct populations one with low MCF and another with high MCF) can be identified (**Figure 3A**). Often in such cases the level of fragmentation decreases as the infant gets older and the EMA histograms reflect this with a decrease in the size of the red cell population with low MCF (**Figure 3B**). This feature also distinguishes hemolytic HE cases from cases of HPP where the extreme fragmentation gives a single population of cells with low MCF (**Figure 4**). In older children and adults the curve may overlap the control or shifted slightly to right but a trailing population of fragment cells can identified on the left shoulder of the curve (**Figure 3C**). This is an important finding as, it expands the value of the EMA test beyond the diagnosis of HS. In a recently reported work, heterogeneity in the ovalization of the HE patients had no association with EMA binding (Suemori et al., 2015).

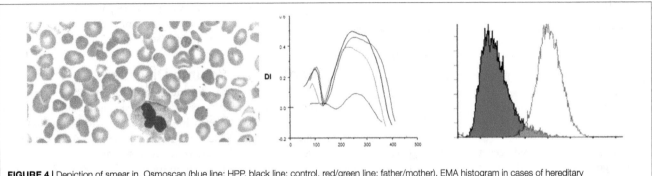

FIGURE 4 | Depiction of smear in, Osmoscan (blue line: HPP, black line: control, red/green line: father/mother), EMA histogram in cases of hereditary pyropoikilocytosis.

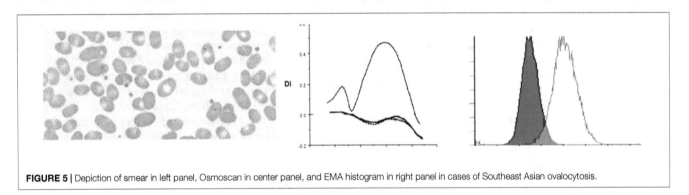

FIGURE 5 | Depiction of smear in left panel, Osmoscan in center panel, and EMA histogram in right panel in cases of Southeast Asian ovalocytosis.

Hereditary pyropoikilocytosis (HPP), originally thought to be a unique and separate disease process, has been reclassified as a subset of HE due to double heterozygosity of mutations in the alpha-spectrin gene (Gallagher, 2004). This severe subset of HE-type disorders, in which red blood cells appear like those seen in thermal burn patients (Zarkowsky et al., 1975), is characterized by neonatal jaundice and transfusion dependent hemolytic anemia that persists through life. A peripheral smear shows microspherocytosis or micropoikilocytes more than elliptocytes. A protein analysis of the phospholipid bilayer of HPP reveals a mild spectrin reduction but a greater increase in spectrin dimer content than in common HE (Zarkowsky et al., 1975). We have seen 3 families with HPP phenotype. In one family despite the name of the disorder we were unable to show heat instability by morphology or circular dichroism studies in purified spectrin (Ravindranath and Johnson, 1985). Molecular studies (courtesy of Bernard Forget, Yale University) showed double heterozygosity for mutations near the dimer-dimer association site in alpha spectrin (Alpha1 74 c.28 CGT to CAT p.Arg > His and Alpha1 50a at c209 CTG > CCG, Leu to Pro). There was significant reduction in alpha spectrin. In these patients (n = 3) there was extreme cellular fragmentation and transfusion requirements abated only after splenectomy. We noted the lowest MCF values, with MCF 213.9 ± 52 in these cases, consistent with the MCV values of <50 fl. There is also a very clear change in the O_{min} and the deformability index was severely decreased (see **Figure 5**). The red cells in HPP appear to have a significantly decreased ability to maintain deformability in the face of hypotonicity, evidenced by their critical hemolytic value occurring at an osmolality much higher than normal controls and

TABLE 5 | Hereditary elliptocytosis.

Hereditary elliptocytosis (n = 8)			Normal controls (n = 76)		
	Mean	SD		Mean	SD
MCF	478.69	28.42	MCF	514.50	15.25
O_{min} (x-axis)	147.59	21.06	O_{min} (x-axis)	147.67	6.90
DI_{MAX} (y-axis)	0.22	0.05	DI_{MAX} (y-axis)	0.49	0.05

TABLE 6 | Hereditary pyropoikilocytosis.

Hereditary pyropoikilocytosis (n = 3)			Normal controls (n = 76)		
	Mean	SD		Mean	SD
MCF	213.85	52.26	MCF	514.50	15.25
O_{min} (x-axis)	175.75	13.44	O_{min} (x-axis)	147.67	6.90
DI_{MAX} (y-axis)	0.11	0.14	DI_{MAX} (y-axis)	0.49	0.05

HS cases. These parameters distinguish HPP cases from common hemolytic HE especially in infants where the fragmentation could be mistaken for HPP. Both osmoscans and EMA test separate the two entities (see **Tables 5, 6**).

Southeast Asian Ovalocytosis (SAO)

The first report of Southeast Asian Ovalocytosis (SAO) was over five decades ago (Eng, 1965) in malaria endemic regions of Papua New Guinea and Laos. It has now been described in other South East Asian populations and in African Americans (Ravindranath et al., 1994). The condition is inherited in

TABLE 7 | Southeast Asian ovalocytosis.

Southeast Asian ovalocytosis ($n = 3$)			Normal controls (n = 76)		
	Mean	SD		Mean	SD
MCF	334.13	22.01	MCF	514.50	15.25
O_{min} (x-axis)	NA	NA	O_{min} (x-axis)	147.67	6.90
DI_{MAX} (y-axis)	−7.33	6.43	DI_{MAX} (y-axis)	0.49	0.05

a dominant fashion and genetic studies generally reveal heterozygotes. Subsequently, the genetic lesion has been found to be related to a mutation in band 3 (anion exchanger 1; SLC4A1) (Tse and Lux, 1999). The mutation results in the deletion of eight amino acid residues in band 3, that result in misfolding of the first transmembrane domain (Tanner et al., 1991). Most patients present with minimal hemolysis, though neonatal hyperbilirubinemia is described. Patients will have stomatocytic elliptocytes, that are pathognomonic to SAO (Liu et al., 1990; Tanner et al., 1991; Cheung et al., 2005). Ektacytometry studies show completely non-deformable red blood cells, with no discernable deformability across a wide osmotic gradient, resulting in a characteristic near flat curve (Mohandas et al., 1984; Ravindranath et al., 1994). EMA testing presents a unique signature as the 8 amino acid deletion in the first *trans* membrane loop of AE1 renders lysine 430 inaccessible to binding with EMA, band 3 content itself is not decreased (Moriyama et al., 1992). The reduction of MCF in our three patients (one Philippino, two African Americans) with SAO from normal controls was approximately 35% of control MCF value,

and approximately 16% lower from HS patients. This indicates the EMA can be used as a screening method for SAO, although ektacytometry is more specific (see **Figure 5** and **Table 7**).

Erythrocyte Volume Disorders

Erythrocyte volume disorders include hereditary xerocytosis (now referred to as dehydrated stomatocytosis) and stomatocytosis (overhydrated stomatocytosis) (Mohandas and Gallagher, 2008; Andolfo et al., 2016). A recent major discovery is the linkage of xerocytosis cases with mutation in the mechanosensitive calcium transporter PIEZO1 (Zarychanski et al., 2012). Other genes implicated in EVDs are the Gardos channel KCNN4 and potassium channel ABCB6. Anemia may be mild or in some cases mild erythrocytosis has been reported. The morphology is not always distinct with a variable mixture of xerocytes and stomatocytes. In three patients with erythrocyte volume disorders associated with PIEZO1 mutations we observed mixed patterns on osmoscans, similar to mild HS or a right shift of the curve suggesting increased cellular hydration (Knight et al., 2019). Classical xerocytosis with cellular dehydration results in a left shifted curve. In our experience the most common cause for a left shifted curve on osmoscans is in patients with hemoglobin C by itself or in combination with sickle hemoglobin (HbSC), consistent with the known effect of hemoglobin C on the Gardos channel (Hannemann et al., 2015). In our three patients with PIEZO1 mutations (c.4766 C > T p.Thr1589Ile, c.5182 C > T p.Arg1728Cys, c.6835C > T p.Arg2279Cys) EMA MCF scans were not diagnostic while Osmoscans were abnormal (Johnson and Ravindranath, 1996;

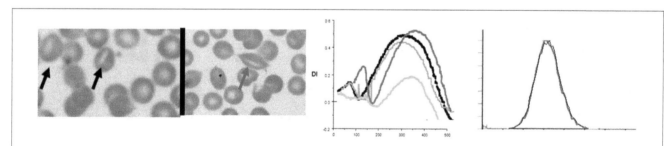

FIGURE 6 | Depiction of smear (black arrows point to classical stomatocytes and red arrow to a "lipstick" stomatocyte, Osmoscans in middle panel- black line: control; yellow line: hereditary spherocytosis, red line: overhydrated stomatocytosis [PIEZO1 (p.Arg1728Cys)], and blue line: dehydrated stomatocytosis [PIEZO1 (p.Thr1589Ile)], EMA histograms in right panel in cases of stomatocytosis overlap control histograms.

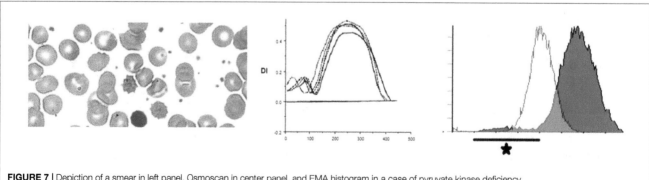

FIGURE 7 | Depiction of a smear in left panel, Osmoscan in center panel, and EMA histogram in a case of pyruvate kinase deficiency.

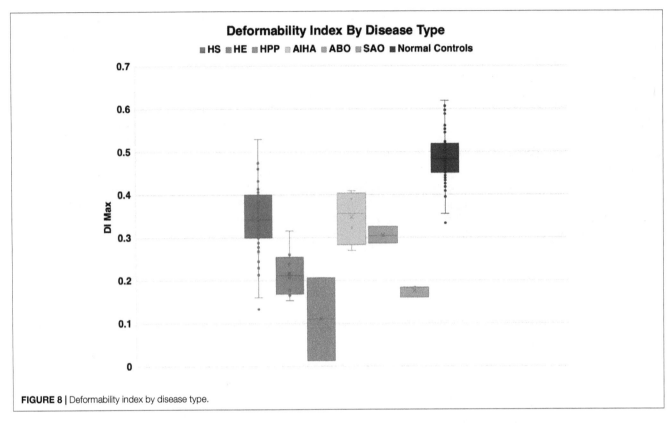

FIGURE 8 | Deformability index by disease type.

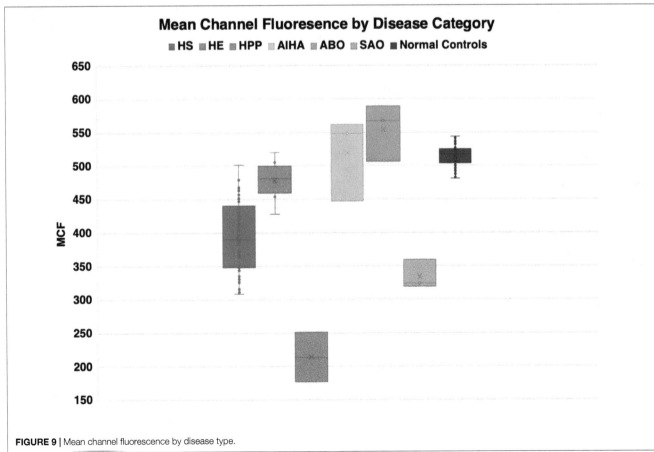

FIGURE 9 | Mean channel fluorescence by disease type.

Da Costa et al., 2013; Andolfo et al., 2016; Knight et al., 2019). The clinical findings of xerocytes (dense spherocytes) and stomatocytes coupled with left or right shifted osmoscan curves should raise the suspicion of erythrocyte volume disorders; mutation testing is necessary for confirmation. The variable Osmoscan pattern may reflect the diverse mutations in PIEZO1 and their impact on the calcium and cation fluxes (Knight et al., 2019; see **Figure 6**).

Other Disorders With Low MCF Values on EMA Test

Red cells from individuals with iron deficiency anemia and thalassemias show low MCF values on EMA scan but can be distinguished from HS cases because of a left shoulder of smaller cells indicating the anisopoikilocytosis in these disorders. A left shoulder may also be seen in cases with hemolytic uremic syndrome and other thrombotic microangiopathies indicating the level of circulating fragmented red cells.

RBC Enzyme Deficiency

In G6PD deficiency and glycolytic enzyme disorders ektacytometry shows high osmoscans indicating greater deformability of red cells (Johnson and Ravindranath, 1996). EMA test in patients with glycolytic enzyme deficiencies, in this case phosphoglycerate kinase 1, show higher MCF with right shifted curves reflecting the high MCV noted in these cases (low mean cell age) (Zaidi et al., 2019). In addition our review of patients with glycolytic enzyme deficiency (in 3 cases of pyruvate kinase (PK) deficiency (post splenectomy) and a new case of phosphoglycerate kinase (PGK1) deficiency) revealed a previously unsuspected signature -on scatter plots and histograms there is a distinctive tail of small cells – presumably the ATP depleted dense spiculated cells (Zaidi et al., 2019; see **Figure 7**).

CONCLUSION

Eosin-5-maleimide testing and osmoscans are complementary

and the combined information can lead to better diagnosis of red cell membrane disorders. There are very salient and key differences in the diagnostic ability of the EMA test and ektacytometry. The EMA provides a static, quantifiable measurement of the amount of band 3 protein, while the ektacytometer provides a fluid, physiologically simulated test that assesses red blood cell deformability in an active fashion (**Figures 8, 9**). In interpreting the EMA test, attention should be paid to not only the MCF value, but also the slope of the curve on either side, which together reflect the heterogeneity of cell size (**Figure 2**). The lowest MCF values were seen in HPP cases; SAO cases had MCF values intermediate between HPP and HS cases (**Figure 9**). In erythrocyte volume disorders EMA tests may be normal, but changes in cell hydration can be suspected better on the osmoscan. At present, the use of the Osmoscan is limited by the availability of the instrument, and the need for specialized staff. The EMA is user-friendly, with quick turnaround time of testing, and flow cytometers are readily available in most institutions. These tests can provide very different results, and should be used in combination with morphology on blood smears and blood counts including the red cell indices. Molecular testing is needed for confirmation of erythrocyte volume disorders.

AUTHOR CONTRIBUTIONS

AM set up the EMA test. MH-M, SBa, and KJ digitized the osmoscans and determined the O_{min}, DI_{max}, and O_{hyper} values. Ektacytometry testing was done under supervision of RJ. AZ wrote the manuscript. RJ gifted the ektacytometer to YR. YR supervises the red cell and flow cytometry laboratories. All authors contributed to the article and approved the submitted version.

ACKNOWLEDGMENTS

Gerard Goyette, now deceased, performed the osmoscans for several decades and we gratefully acknowledge his many contributions to our work over the past 3 decades.

REFERENCES

An, X., and Mohandas, N. (2008). Disorders of red cell membrane. *Br. J. Haematol.* 141, 367–375. doi: 10.1111/j.1365-2141.2008.07091.x

Andolfo, I., Russo, R., Gambale, A., and Iolascon, A. (2016). New insights on hereditary erythrocyte membrane defects. *Haematologica* 101, 1284–1294. doi: 10.3324/haematol.2016.142463

Bessis, M., Mohandas, N., and Feo, C. (1980). Automated ektacytometry: a new method of measuring red cell deformability and red cell indices. *Blood Cells* 6, 315–327.

Bianconi, E., Piovesan, A., Facchin, F., Beraudi, A., Casadei, R., Frabetti, F., et al. (2013). An estimation of the number of cells in the human body. *Ann. Hum. Biol.* 40, 463–471. doi: 10.3109/03014460.2013.807878

Bolton-Maggs, P. H. B., Langer, J. C., Iolascon, A., Tittensor, P., and King, M. J. (2012). Guidelines for the diagnosis and management of hereditary spherocytosis - 2011 update. *Br. J. Haematol.* 156, 37–49. doi: 10.1111/j.1365-2141.2011.08921.x

Cheung, J. C., Cordat, E., and Reithmeier, R. A. F. (2005). Trafficking defects of the Southeast Asian ovalocytosis deletion mutant of anion exchanger 1 membrane proteins. *Biochem. J.* 392, 425–434. doi: 10.1042/BJ20051076

Chonat, S., Risinger, M., Dagaonkar, N., Maghathe, T., Rothman, J., Connor, J., et al. (2015). The spectrum of alpha-spectrin associated hereditary spherocytosis. *Blood* 126:941. doi: 10.1182/blood.v126.23.941.941

Clark, M. R., Mohandas, N., and Shohet, S. B. (1983). Osmotic gradient ektacytometry: comprehensive characterization of red cell volume and surface maintenance. *Blood* 61, 899–910. doi: 10.1182/blood.v61.5.899.bloodjournal615899

Cobb, C. E., and Beth, A. H. (1990). Identification of the eosinyl-5-maleimide reaction site on the human erythrocyte anion-exchange protein: overlap with the reaction sites of other chemical probes. *Biochemistry* 29, 8283–8290. doi: 10.1021/bi00488a012

Crisp, R. L., Solari, L., Gammella, D., Schvartzman, G. A., Rapetti, M. C., and Donato, H. (2012). Use of capillary blood to diagnose hereditary spherocytosis. *Pediatr. Blood Cancer* 59, 1299–1301. doi: 10.1002/pbc.24157

Da Costa, L., Galimand, J., Fenneteau, O., and Mohandas, N. (2013). Hereditary spherocytosis, elliptocytosis, and other red cell membrane disorders. *Blood Rev.* 27, 16–178. doi: 10.1016/j.blre.2013.04.003

Da Costa, L., Suner, L., Galimand, J., Bonnel, A., Pascreau, T., Couque, N., et al. (2016). Diagnostic tool for red blood cell membrane disorders: assessment of a new generation ektacytometer. *Blood Cells, Mol. Dis.* 56, 9–22. doi: 10.1016/j.bcmd.2015.09.001

Delaunay, J. (2007). The molecular basis of hereditary red cell membrane disorders. *Blood Rev.* 21, 1–20. doi: 10.1016/j.blre.2006.03.005

Eng, L. I. (1965). Hereditary ovalocytosis and haemoglobin E-ovalocytosis in Malayan aborigines. *Nature* 208:1329. doi: 10.1038/2081329a0

Gallagher, P. G. (2004). Hereditary Elliptocytosis: spectrin and Protein 4.1R. *Semin. Hematol.* 41, 142–164. doi: 10.1053/j.seminhematol.2004.01.003

Gallagher, P. G. (2013). Abnormalities of the erythrocyte membrane. *Pediatr. Clin. North Am.* 60, 1349–1362. doi: 10.1016/j.pcl.2013.09.001

Gallagher, P. G., Maksimova, Y., Lezon-Geyda, K., Newburger, P. E., Medeiros, D., Hanson, R. D., et al. (2019). Aberrant splicing contributes to severe α-spectrin–linked congenital hemolytic anemia. *J. Clin. Invest.* 129, 2878–2887. doi: 10.1172/JCI127195

Gallagher, P. G., Weed, S. A., Tse, W. T., Benoit, L., Morrow, J. S., Marchesi, S. L., et al. (1995). Recurrent fatal hydrops fetalis associated with a nucleotide substitution in the erythrocyte β-spectrin gene. *J. Clin. Invest.* 95, 1174–1182. doi: 10.1172/JCI117766

Groner, W., Mohandas, N., and Bessis, M. (1980). New optical technique for measuring erythrocyte deformability with the ektacytometer. *Clin. Chem.* 26, 1435–1442. doi: 10.1093/clinchem/26.10.1435

Hannemann, A., Rees, D. C., Tewari, S., and Gibson, J. S. (2015). Cation homeostasis in red cells from patients with sickle cell disease heterologous for HbS and HbC (HbSC Genotype). *EBiomedicine* 2, 1669–1676. doi: 10.1016/j.ebiom.2015.09.026

Huisjes, R., Makhro, A., Llaudet-Planas, E., Hertz, L., Petkova-Kirova, P., Verhagen, L. P., et al. (2019). Density, heterogeneity and deformability of red cells as markers of clinical severity in hereditary spherocytosis. *Haematologica* 2018:188151. doi: 10.3324/haematol.2018.188151

Hunter, F. T. (1940). A photoelectric method for the quantitative determination of erythrocyte fragility. *J. Clin. Invest.* 19, 691–694. doi: 10.1172/JCI101172

Johnson, R. M., Panchoosingh, H., Goyette, G., and Ravindranath, Y. (1999). Increased erythrocyte deformability in fetal erythropoiesis and in erythrocytes deficient in glucose-6-phosphate dehydrogenase and other glycolytic enzymes. *Pediatr. Res.* 45, 106–113. doi: 10.1203/00006450-199901000-00018

Johnson, R. M., and Ravindranath, Y. (1996). Osmotic scan ektacytometry in clinical diagnosis. *J. Pediatr. Hematol. Oncol.* 18, 122–129. doi: 10.1097/00043426-199605000-00005

Kalfa, T. A., Connor, J. A., and Begtrup, A. H. (1993). *EPB42-Related Hereditary Spherocytosis.* Available online at: http://www.ncbi.nlm.nih.gov/pubmed/24624460 (accessed January 7, 2019).

King, M. J., Behrens, J., Rogers, C., Flynn, C., Greenwood, D., and Chambers, K. (2000). Rapid flow cytometric test for the diagnosis of membrane cytoskeleton-associated haemolytic anaemia. *Br. J. Haematol.* 111, 924–933. doi: 10.1111/j.1365-2141.2000.02416.x

King, M.-J., Smythe, J. S., and Mushens, R. (2004). Eosin-5-maleimide binding to band 3 and Rh-related proteins forms the basis of a screening test for hereditary spherocytosis. *Br. J. Haematol.* 124, 106–113. doi: 10.1046/j.1365-2141.2003.04730.x

Knight, T., Zaidi, A. U., Wu, S., Gadgeel, M., Buck, S., and Ravindranath, Y. (2019). Mild erythrocytosis as a presenting manifestation of PIEZO1 associated erythrocyte volume disorders. *Pediatr. Hematol. Oncol.* 36, 317–326. doi: 10.1080/08880018.2019.1637984

Lazarova, E., Gulbis, B., van Oirschot, B., and van Wijk, R. (2017). Next-generation osmotic gradient ektacytometry for the diagnosis of hereditary spherocytosis: interlaboratory method validation and experience. *Clin. Chem. Lab. Med.* 55, 394–402. doi: 10.1515/cclm-2016-0290

Liu, S.-C., Zhai, S., Palek, J., Golan, D. E., Amato, D., Hassan, K., et al. (1990). Molecular defect of the band 3 protein in southeast asian ovalocytosis. *N. Engl. J. Med.* 323, 1530–1538. doi: 10.1056/NEJM199011293232205

Lux, S. E. (2014). *Chapter 15 - Red Cell Membrane*, 8th Edn. Amsterdam: Elsevier, doi: 10.1016/B978-1-4557-5414-4.00015-2

Lux, S. E. (2016). Anatomy of the red cell membrane skeleton: unanswered questions. *Blood* 127, 187–199. doi: 10.1182/blood-2014-12

Mentzer, W. C., Iarocci, T. A., Mohandas, N., Lane, P. A., Smith, B., Lazerson, J., et al. (1987). Modulation of erythrocyte membrane mechanical stability by 2,3-diphosphoglycerate in the neonatal poikilocytosis/elliptocytosis syndrome. *J. Clin. Invest.* 79, 943–949. doi: 10.1172/JCI112905

Mohandas, N., Clark, M. R., Jacobs, M. S., and Shohet, S. B. (1980). Analysis of factors regulating erythrocyte deformability. *J. Clin. Invest.* 66, 563–573. doi: 10.1172/JCI109888

Mohandas, N., and Gallagher, P. G. (2008). Red cell membrane: past, present, and future. *Blood* 112, 3939–3948. doi: 10.1182/blood-2008-07-161166

Mohandas, N., Lie-Injo, L. E., Friedman, M., and Mak, J. W. (1984). Rigid membranes of Malayan ovalocytes: a likely genetic barrier against malaria. *Blood* 63, 1385–1392. doi: 10.1182/blood.v63.6.1385.bloodjournal6361385

Moriyama, R., Ideguchi, H., Lombardo, C. R., Van Dort, H. M., and Low, P. S. (1992). Structural and functional characterization of band 3 from Southeast Asian ovalocytes. *J. Biol. Chem.* 267, 25792–25797.

Nussenzveig, R. H., Christensen, R. D., Prchal, J. T., Yaish, H. M., and Agarwal, A. M. (2014). Novel α-spectrin mutation in trans with α-spectrin causing severe neonatal jaundice from hereditary spherocytosis. *Neonatology* 106, 355–357. doi: 10.1159/000365586

Palek, J., and Lux, S. E. (1983). Red cell membrane skeletal defects in hereditary and acquired hemolytic anemias. *Semin. Hematol.* 20, 189–224.

Perrotta, S., Gallagher, P. G., and Mohandas, N. (2008). Hereditary spherocytosis. *Lancet* 372, 1411–1426. doi: 10.1016/S0140-6736(08)61588-3

Ravindranath, Y., Goyette, G., and Johnson, R. M. (1994). Southeast Asian ovalocytosis in an African-American family. *Blood* 84, 2823–2824. doi: 10.1182/blood.v84.8.2823.bloodjournal8482823

Ravindranath, Y., and Johnson, R. M. (1985). Altered spectrin association and membrane fragility without abnormal spectrin heat sensitivity in a case of congenital hemolytic anemia. *Am. J. Hematol.* 20, 53–65. doi: 10.1002/ajh.2830200108

Ribeiro, M. L., Alloisio, N., Almeida, H., Gomes, C., Texier, P., Lemos, C., et al. (2000). Severe hereditary spherocytosis and distal renal tubular acidosis associated with the total absence of band 3. *Blood* 96, 1602–1604.

Silveira, P., Cynober, T., Dhermy, D., Mohandas, N., and Tchernia, G. (1997). Red Blood cell abnormalities in hereditary elliptocytosis and their relevance to variable clinical expression. *Am. J. Clin. Pathol.* 108, 391–399. doi: 10.1093/ajcp/108.4.391

Suemori, S. I., Wada, H., Nakanishi, H., Tsujioka, T., Sugihara, T., and Tohyama, K. (2015). Analysis of hereditary elliptocytosis with decreased binding of eosin-5-maleimide to red blood cells. *Biomed Res. Int.* 2015:451861. doi: 10.1155/2015/451861

Tanner, M. J., Bruce, L., Martin, P. G., Rearden, D. M., and Jones, G. L. (1991). Melanesian hereditary ovalocytes have a deletion in red cell band 3. *Blood* 78, 2785–2786. doi: 10.1182/blood.v78.10.2785.bloodjournal78102785

Tchernia, G., Mohandas, N., and Shohet, S. B. (1981). Deficiency of skeletal membrane protein band 4.1 in homozygous hereditary elliptocytosis. Implications for erythrocyte membrane stability. *J. Clin. Invest.* 68, 454–460. doi: 10.1172/jci110275

Tse, W. T., and Lux, S. E. (1999). Red blood cell membrane disorders. *Br. J. Haematol.* 104, 2–13. doi: 10.1111/j.1365-2141.1999.01130.x

Won, D., and Suh, J. S. (2009). Flow cytometric detection of erythrocyte osmotic fragility. *Cytom. Part B Clin. Cytom.* 76B, 135–141. doi: 10.1002/cyto.b.20448

Zaidi, A. U., Bagla, S., and Ravindranath, Y. (2019). Identification of a novel variant in phosphoglycerate kinase-1 (PGK1) in an African-American child (PGK1 Detroit). *Pediatr. Hematol. Oncol.* 36, 302–308. doi: 10.1080/08880018.2019.1639863

Zaidi, A. U., Herrera-Martinez, M., Goyette, G. W., Buck, S., Gadgeel, M., Mohan, A., et al. (2015). Red Cell Band 3 Content Evaluation By Eosin Maleimide (EMA) Fluorescence: Beyond Diagnosis of Dominant Hereditary Spherocytosis (HS). *Blood* 126:3343. doi: 10.1182/blood.v126.23.3343.3343

Zarkowsky, H. S., Mohandas, N., Speaker, C. B., and Shohet, S. B. (1975). A congenital haemolytic anaemia with thermal sensitivity of the erythrocyte membrane. *Br. J. Haematol.* 29, 537–543. doi: 10.1111/j.1365-2141.1975.tb02740.x

Zarychanski, R., Schulz, V. P., Houston, B. L., Maksimova, Y., Houston, D. S., Smith, B., et al. (2012). Mutations in the mechanotransduction protein PIEZO1 are associated with hereditary xerocytosis. *Blood* 120, 1908–1915. doi: 10.1182/blood-2012-04-422253

4

The Pleiotropic Effects of GATA1 and KLF1 in Physiological Erythropoiesis and in Dyserythropoietic Disorders

Gloria Barbarani[1], Cristina Fugazza[1], John Strouboulis[2] and Antonella E. Ronchi[1]*

[1] Dipartimento di Biotecnologie e Bioscienze, Università degli Studi Milano-Bicocca, Milan, Italy, [2] School of Cancer & Pharmaceutical Sciences, Faculty of Life Sciences & Medicine, King's College London, London, United Kingdom

*Correspondence:
Antonella E. Ronchi
antonella.ronchi@unimib.it

In the last few years, the advent of new technological approaches has led to a better knowledge of the ontogeny of erythropoiesis during development and of the journey leading from hematopoietic stem cells (HSCs) to mature red blood cells (RBCs). Our view of a well-defined hierarchical model of hematopoiesis with a near-homogeneous HSC population residing at the apex has been progressively challenged in favor of a landscape where HSCs themselves are highly heterogeneous and lineages separate earlier than previously thought. The coordination of these events is orchestrated by transcription factors (TFs) that work in a combinatorial manner to activate and/or repress their target genes. The development of next generation sequencing (NGS) has facilitated the identification of pathological mutations involving TFs underlying hematological defects. The examples of GATA1 and KLF1 presented in this review suggest that in the next few years the number of TF mutations associated with dyserythropoietic disorders will further increase.

Keywords: erythropoiesis, dyserythropoiesis, transcription factors, GATA1, KLF1

INTRODUCTION

Erythropoiesis leads to the production of the proper number of RBCs required by the body under homeostatic and stress conditions. In healthy adults, erythropoiesis ensures the release in the blood stream of 2×10^6 RBCs/second, but this number dramatically increases to respond to inadequate tissue oxygenation (Tsiftsoglou et al., 2009; Dzierzak and Philipsen, 2013; Nandakumar et al., 2016).

Insufficient quantitative or qualitative production of fully functional RBCs, whether acquired or inherited, results in a wide spectrum of diseases generally defined as anemias.

The causes of anemias are variable and reflect the complexity of the differentiation and maturation of erythrocytes. In some cases, the number of RBCs is extremely low because of the failure to produce erythroid progenitors, as in Diamond-Blackfan Anemia (DBA) (Da Costa et al., 2018). In other cases, impaired differentiation leads to the accumulation of erythroid precursors in the bone marrow [β-thalassemia (Rivella, 2015), congenital dyserythropoietic anemia, CDA (Iolascon et al., 2011)] or to the unbalanced production of different blood cell types [myelodysplastic syndromes, MDS (Levine et al., 2007; Lefevre et al., 2017)], resulting in insufficient RBC numbers in the bloodstream.

In other forms of anemias, RBCs are produced but defects in some crucial gene products [typically specific enzymes (Koralkova et al., 2014; Grace et al., 2018), membrane proteins or cytoskeletal components (Mohandas and Gallagher, 2008; Perrotta et al., 2008), sickle globin chains (Rees et al., 2010), channel proteins (Glogowska and Gallagher, 2015), specific pathways (Bianchi et al., 2009; Schwarz et al., 2009)] result in RBCs with decreased oxygen delivery capacity and/or shortened lifespan. Very often, different diseases share common features: for example imbalanced globin chains in β-thalassemia is accompanied by the accumulation of defective precursors in the bone marrow and by ineffective erythropoiesis (IE), as is also observed in CDA (Libani et al., 2008; Iolascon et al., 2011; Ribeil et al., 2013; Rivella, 2015).

Recently, thanks to the advent of new technologies, including NGS using small pools of cells or single cells (Nestorowa et al., 2016; Paul et al., 2016; Ye et al., 2017; Giladi et al., 2018), the development of improved panels of surface markers (Guo et al., 2013; Notta et al., 2016) and the design of *in vivo* cell tracing systems (Dykstra and Bystrykh, 2014; Perie et al., 2014; Pei et al., 2017; Rodriguez-Fraticelli et al., 2018; Upadhaya et al., 2018), our understanding of hematopoiesis -and erythropoiesis- has greatly expanded. In parallel, genome wide association approaches (GWAS) (Menzel et al., 2007; Sankaran et al., 2008; Uda et al., 2008; Soranzo et al., 2009; van der Harst et al., 2012), massive genome and exome sequencing (Chami et al., 2016) led to the identification of new variant/modifier alleles influencing erythropoiesis associated with TFs.

In this scenario, TFs not only control lineage commitment transitions but are emerging as key-players underpinning, so far unexplained erythroid diseases. Here, we consider GATA1 and KLF1 as paradigmatic TFs. By focusing on these examples, we aim to provide evidence of their pleiotropic effects rather than to give a complete list of GATA1 or KLF1 mutations identified so far.

ERYTHROPOIESIS

Erythropoiesis During Development

The first wave of erythropoiesis originates in the yolk sac, where Primitive Erythroid Cells (EryPs) sustain the oxygenation demand of the growing embryo (Dzierzak and Philipsen, 2013). EryPs are large in size and still nucleated when released in the circulation, where they later enucleate (Isern et al., 2011; Dzierzak and Philipsen, 2013; Palis, 2014). In mouse, at E8.25 a second wave of erythro-myelo-precursors (EMPs) originates in the yolk sac and colonizes the fetal liver, generating the first definitive RBCs (Palis, 2016). Finally, around E10.5, hematopoietic stem cells (HSCs) from aorta-gonad-mesonephros (AGM), placenta and possibly other yet unknown sites, colonize the fetal liver. These cells will sustain definitive hematopoiesis for the remainder of gestation and, around birth, will migrate to the bone marrow, the site of adult hematopoiesis (Dzierzak and Philipsen, 2013).

From HSC to RBC

Until recently, the "classical model" of hematopoiesis was considered a paradigm of a stepwise, hierarchical cellular specification system, whereby HSCs generated multipotent progenitors with progressively restricted lineage potential through a sequence of binary choices. The grand entrance of new single-cell separation technologies, *in vivo* lineage tracing systems and single-cell analysis, provided novel and surprising insights, prompting the idea that early transcriptional priming develops into the acquisition of specific lineage programs (Cabezas-Wallscheid et al., 2014; Haas et al., 2018). In this context, erythroid cells would originate early in the hematopoietic hierarchy, i.e., from stem/multipotential progenitor stages (Guo et al., 2013; Notta et al., 2016; Tusi et al., 2018), soon after the emergence of the megakaryocytic lineage (Upadhaya et al., 2018).

The first clearly recognizable unipotent erythroid progenitor, identified decades ago in *in vitro* clonogenic assays, is the BFU-E (burst-forming unit-erythroid), that differentiate into rapidly dividing colony-forming-unit erythroid (CFU-E) (Hattangadi et al., 2011; Koury, 2016; Dulmovits et al., 2017). The entry of CFU-Es into erythroid terminal differentiation marks the transition into final maturation (Hwang et al., 2017; Tusi et al., 2018).

EXTRACELLULAR AND INTRACELLULAR SIGNALS

Red blood cell differentiation, their production in homeostatic and stress condition, is governed by an integrated complex interplay of extracellular and cell-cell signals within the microenvironment that activate the appropriate downstream intracellular signals, ultimately converging on key TFs. Although these aspects are beyond the scope of this review, we give a glimpse of the major players in these regulatory networks in **Figure 1**.

THE ROLE OF TRANSCRIPTION FACTORS

Transcription factors, together with cofactors and chromatin modifiers, dictate the lineage-specific, stage-specific transcriptional programs by coordinately activating and/or repressing their targets through their binding to DNA (Portela and Esteller, 2010; Dore and Crispino, 2011; Love et al., 2014). The advent of NGS has rapidly expanded our understanding of TFs functions in physiological erythropoiesis, discovering TF mutations as cause of yet unexplained hematological -and dyserythropoietic- defects. Here, we focus on the key examples of GATA1 and KLF1 and their mutations to provide a glimpse of the complexity of their actions (**Figure 2**).

The Example of the "Master Regulator" GATA1

The X-linked *GATA1* gene encodes a zinc finger TF expressed in the hematopoietic system in erythroid, megakaryocytic and, at lower levels, in eosinophilic, dendritic, and mast cells (Yu et al., 2002a; Ferreira et al., 2005; Gutierrez et al., 2007; Kozma et al., 2010).

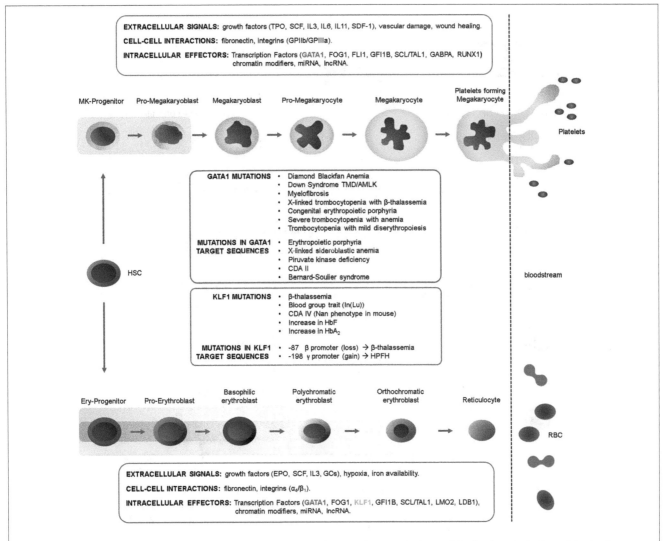

FIGURE 1 | Erythropoiesis and megakaryopoiesis are regulated at multiple levels. A complex network of extracellular signals -activating intracellular signaling pathways-, cell–cell interactions within the niche and intracellular effectors regulate cell differentiation in homeostatic conditions and in response to stress stimuli (Ferreira et al., 2005; Hattangadi et al., 2011; Songdej and Rao, 2017). These signals converge on TFs and chromatin modifiers which ultimately define the transcriptome at each given stage. The main growth factors, integrins and transcription factors involved in these processes are indicated. The GATA1 (red rectangles) and KLF1 (green rectangles) windows of expression are indicated (see also **Figure 2B**). HSC, Hematopoietic Stem cell; TPO, thrombopoietin; SCF, Stem cell Factor; IL, interleukin; SDF-1, stromal-derived factor-1; GPIIb/IIIa, integrins α_{IIb}/β_3 (CD41/CD61); EPO, erythropoietin; GCs, glucocorticoids. α_4/β_1, integrins α_4/β_1 (CD49d/CD29).

GATA1 has three main functional domains: an N-terminal activation domain (N-TAD) and two homologous zinc (Zn) finger domains in the C-terminal half of the protein. The N-terminal Zn finger binds to the GATA1 main cofactor FOG1 (Friend-of-GATA) and modulates the affinity of GATA1 for binding to complex sites *in vitro* (Trainor et al., 1996; Newton et al., 2001; Yu et al., 2002b). The C-terminal Zn finger (C-ZnF) binds to DNA (WGATAR motif).

GATA1 produces two isoforms: the full length protein (GATA1-FL, 47 kDa) and a shorter variant (GATA1s, 40 kDa), translated from codon 84 within the third exon. GATA1s lacks the N-TAD and results in a protein with a reduced transactivation activity (Calligaris et al., 1995). *Gata1* knockout in mice (Pevny et al., 1991) results in embryonic lethality around E10.5–E11.5

due to severe anemia, with GATA1-null cells undergoing massive apoptosis at the proerythroblastic stage (Pevny et al., 1995; Fujiwara et al., 1996). The conditional erythroid knockout in adult mice causes aplastic anemia, revealing its essential role in both steady-state and stress erythropoiesis (Gutierrez et al., 2008).

By contrast, megakaryoblasts lacking GATA1 proliferate abnormally but fail to undergo terminal differentiation (Shivdasani et al., 1997; Vyas et al., 1999). Since these first studies, many other reports revealed the many roles of GATA1 in the erythro/megakaryocytic differentiation (Ferreira et al., 2005). *GATA1* mutations identified in patients underscore this pleiotropy: mutations altering the quantity or quality of GATA1 can lead to a variety of phenotypes. Depending on the type of mutation and whether germline or somatic, the severity

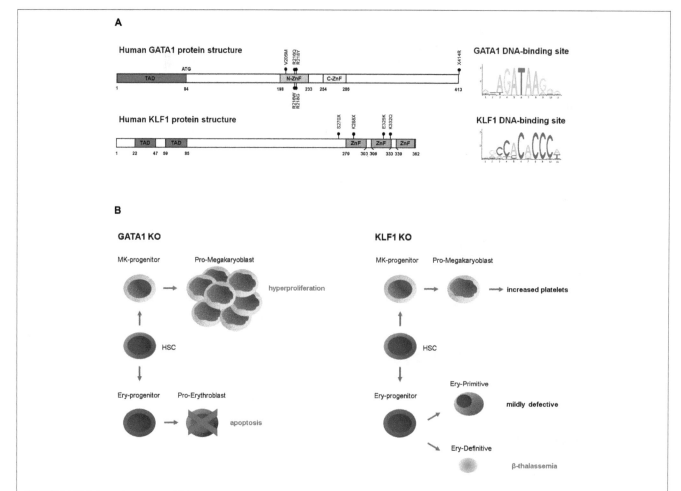

FIGURE 2 | (A) Schematic structure of GATA1 and KLF1 proteins and of their DNA-binding motifs. The position of the mutations discussed in this review are indicated. ZnF, zinc fingers; TAD, transactivation domains. The DNA consensus are from the JASPAR database (http://jaspar2016.genereg.net/). **(B)** Phenotype of *GATA1* (Pevny et al., 1991, 1995; Fujiwara et al., 1996; Shivdasani et al., 1997; Gutierrez et al., 2008) and *KLF1* (Nuez et al., 1995; Perkins et al., 1995; Hodge et al., 2006; Nilson et al., 2006; Frontelo et al., 2007; Tallack and Perkins, 2010) gene knockouts in mouse.

of the disease and the involvement of the erythroid and/or megakaryocytic compartments greatly varies.

"QUANTITATIVE MUTATIONS": GENE DOSAGE AND BACKGROUND EFFECTS AT WORK

Mutations Causing GATA1-FL Loss: Inherited

Diamond-Blackfan anemia (DBA) is an inherited bone marrow failure syndrome characterized by severe anemia due to a great reduction in BFU-Es, without involvement of other hematopoietic lineages. Heterozygous mutations in ribosomal proteins account for about 65% of DBA cases. In 2012 an exome sequencing approach discovered the first *GATA1* mutation in a DBA patient (Sankaran et al., 2012). This mutation (c.220G > C transversion) causes the skipping of exon 2, determining GATA1-FL loss, while retaining GATA1s. Unrelated

DBA patients were reported to carry the same mutation (Klar et al., 2014), or mutations in the ATG of GATA1-FL (Ludwig et al., 2014; Parrella et al., 2014). Of interest, in a family reported by Hollanda et al. (2006) the inherited loss of GATA1-FL results in macrocytic anemia of various severity in the different patients (with variable involvement of megakaryocytes and neutrophils).

Mutations Causing GATA1-FL Loss: Acquired

Somatic mutations in *GATA1*, preventing the synthesis of GATA1-FL, predispose newborn Down Syndrome (DS) patients to develop (in 10–20% of cases) transient myeloproliferative disease (TMD) (Wechsler et al., 2002; Xu et al., 2003; Hitzler and Zipursky, 2005). This pre-leukemic condition often spontaneously resolves. However, in about 30% of TMD cases, it develops into acute pediatric megakaryoblastic leukemia (AMKL) (Wechsler et al., 2002; Magalhaes et al., 2006). All the DS-TMD *GATA1* mutations identified so far, map in exon 2 and either introduce a STOP codon or alter splicing such that only GATA1s is translated (Mundschau et al., 2003; Rainis et al., 2003). The loss of GATA1-FL in premalignant cells characterizes virtually all cases of DS-TMD. The detection of clone-specific *GATA1* mutations in DS-TMD and AMKL proves that AMKL derive from the TMD clone (Rainis et al., 2003; Ahmed et al., 2004; Hitzler and Zipursky, 2005). Moreover, *GATA1* mutations are extremely rare in AMKL blasts of non-DS patients, clearly indicating a specific cooperation of *GATA1* mutations with trisomy 21 (Gruber and Downing, 2015). The restoration of GATA1-FL expression in DS-AMKL-derived cells partially restores erythroid differentiation, further supporting the notion that the loss of GATA1-FL is essential for leukemogenesis (Xu et al., 2003). Importantly, DS-AMKL *GATA1* mutations have very little effect on erythropoiesis, suggesting that the co-occurrence trisomy 21 confers the property of specific targeting megakaryoblasts in DS patients.

Various evidences suggest that TMD likely emerges in a yolk sac/fetal liver progenitor *in utero* (Shimada et al., 2004). In agreement with this hypothesis, in mouse, a knockin allele abolishing GATA1-FL (and leaving GATA1s intact) results in a transient reduction of erythroid cells accompanied by increased megakaryopoiesis that resolves around E14.5 (Li et al., 2005). Despite these observations, the fetal cell type originating TMD and molecular mechanisms by which *GATA1* mutations specifically synergizes with trisomy 21 are still unclear (Crispino, 2005).

GATA1 Low Levels and Disease

The notion that low levels of GATA1 lead to the development of myelofibrosis comes from studies in the GATA1-low mouse model, that also develops anemia with age (Vannucchi et al., 2002). In line with this first observation, the majority of patients with primary myelofibrosis (PMF) have GATA1-deficient megakaryocytes (Migliaccio et al., 2005). Of interest, in PMF patients, the reduced level of GATA1 is due to its impaired translation secondary to RPS14 deficiency (Gilles et al., 2017). The connection between GATA1 levels and RP proteins hinges on additional observations: indeed, in cells from DBA patients who are haploinsufficient for RPS19, GATA1 translation is greatly reduced (Ludwig et al., 2014; O'Brien et al., 2017; Khajuria et al., 2018).

Together, these examples again point toward the importance of the correct GATA1 protein dosage and indicates *GATA1* post-transcriptional regulation as an important determinant of GATA1 protein level.

"QUALITATIVE MUTATIONS": THE IMPORTANCE OF PROTEIN-PROTEIN INTERACTIONS AND MORE

Mutations Abolishing the Interaction With FOG1

In Tsang et al. (1997) identified by yeast two-hybrid a novel zinc finger protein, named FOG1, binding to the

N-ZnF of GATA1. GATA1 mutants unable to bind FOG1 (but still retaining DNA binding) do not rescue the severe block in terminal erythroid maturation of GATA1-deficient cells (Tsang et al., 1997). Instead, a compensatory FOG1 mutation restoring the interaction, rescues the GATA1$^-$ phenotype, demonstrating that the interaction between the two proteins is essential for erythroid and megakaryocytic differentiation (Crispino et al., 1999; Chang et al., 2002). In Nichols et al. (2000) described a family with dyserythropoietic anemia and thrombocytopenia caused by a GATA1 (V205M) mutation abolishing the GATA1:FOG1 interaction.

Other Allelic Variants, Other Interactions, Other Phenotypes

Remarkably, distinct substitutions at a single residue lead to very different outcomes, underlying the complexity of the GATA1 networks. The R216Q substitution causes X-linked thrombocytopenia with β-Thalassemia (Yu et al., 2002b; Balduini et al., 2004), whereas R216W patients also show features of congenital erythropoietic porphyria (CEP) (Phillips et al., 2007; Di Pierro et al., 2015). The D218Y mutation causes severe thrombocytopenia with anemia (Freson et al., 2002), whereas the D218G substitution causes macrothrombocytopenia with mild dyserythropoiesis and no anemia (Freson et al., 2001; Mehaffey et al., 2001).

Notably, whereas the D218Y diminishes the FOG1:GATA1 interaction, the D218G and R216Q do not, but they rather impair GATA1 ability to recruit the TAL1 cofactor complex (Campbell et al., 2013).

MUTATIONS IN THE GATA1 DNA TARGET SEQUENCES AS A CAUSE OF HUMAN ERYTHROID DISORDERS

Ultimately, TFs elicit their function by binding to DNA motifs on their target genes. Thus, it is expected that mutations creating new -or disrupting- specific binding sites could have phenotypic consequences. Although these mutations remain very elusive, over the years an increasing number of cases has accumulated, implicating these polymorphisms as a source of disease. Such mutations have been associated with congenital erythropoietic porphyria (Solis et al., 2001), X-linked sideroblastic anemia (Campagna et al., 2014; Kaneko et al., 2014), pyruvate kinase deficiency (Manco et al., 2000), CDAII (Russo et al., 2017), Bernard–Soulier syndrome (Ludlow et al., 1996) or linked to erythroid trait variants such as δ-thalassemia (Matsuda et al., 1992) and blood groups (Tournamille et al., 1995; Nakajima et al., 2013; Oda et al., 2015; Moller et al., 2018). Interestingly, a mutation abolishing a GATA1 consensus in the *KLF1* promoter (see below), causes a reduction of KLF1, which in turn results in reduced transcription of the KLF1 target genes more sensitive to KLF1 levels, such as *BCAM*, encoding for the Lutheran (Lu) antigen (Singleton et al., 2008).

E/KLF1: An Unsuspected Key-Player in Various Types of Dyserythropoiesis

KLF1 gene, located on chromosome 19, encodes for a proline-rich protein containing three zinc fingers (Bieker, 1996; Mas et al., 2011; **Figure 1B**), expressed in the bone marrow and in the erythroid lineage. KLF1 mainly acts by recruiting coactivators and chromatin remodelers, thus contributing to the large epigenetics changes which shape erythroid maturation (Shyu et al., 2014).

As for GATA1, the first evidence for an essential role in erythropoiesis came from the observation that *KLF1* knockout mice die *in utero* around E15 due to fatal anemia (Nuez et al., 1995; Perkins et al., 1995). Given that KLF1 is an important activator of β-globin, lethality was first attributed to β-thalassemia. However, this is not the sole explanation for the defect: the rescue of the α/β imbalance obtained by the transgenic expression of γ-globin is not sufficient to rescue hemolysis, thus pointing to additional roles for KLF1 (Perkins et al., 2000). In 2015, the first case of severe neonatal anemia with kernicterus due to *KLF1* compound heterozygosis was described in man (Magor et al., 2015), with an erythroid phenotype largely mirroring that observed in mice: hydrops fetalis, hemolytic anemia, jaundice, hepatosplenomegaly, marked erythroblastosis and high levels of HbF. Another report confirms that in humans, although compatible with life, the loss of KLF1 severely impairs erythropoiesis (Lee et al., 2016).

QUANTITATIVE MUTATIONS OF KLF1: HAPLOINSUFFICIENCY/HYPOMORPHIC ALLELES

KLF1 is haplosufficient. The loss of one allele is asymptomatic and only genes particularly sensitive to *KLF1* gene dosage are affected. This is observed in the Lutheran In(Lu) Blood group, where either frameshift mutations, introducing premature termination, or amino acids substitutions in the zinc binding domain, lead to reduced or ineffective KLF1 production (Singleton et al., 2008; Helias et al., 2013). Interestingly, the search for possible mutations in an erythroid TF -that turned out to be KLF1- as a cause of the In(Lu) phenotype came from transcriptomic analyses showing that In(Lu) cells express reduced levels of many erythroid-specific genes associated with red cell maturation, including *BCAM* (encoding for the Lu antigen), *ALAS2*, *HBB*, *SLC4A1*, and *CD44* (Singleton et al., 2008). More recently, extended serological and FACS analysis of In(Lu) samples also revealed a reduced expression of *CD35*, *ICAM4*, and *CD147* (Fraser et al., 2018). Interestingly, in one single case the In(Lu) phenotype has been associated with a GATA1 mutation (X414R) (Singleton et al., 2013).

It is now clear that different KLF1 target genes are differentially sensitive not only to KLF1 levels (when one allele carries an inactivating mutation), but also to the type of KLF1 mutation, making it difficult to clearly separate "quantitative" from "qualitative" effects of KLF1 mutations.

Indeed, KLF1 coordinately regulates the expression of a multitude of red cell specific genes including heme biosynthesis genes [*ALAS2*, *HMBS*, *TFR2* (Singleton et al., 2008)], red cell enzymes [such as pyruvate kinase genes -*PKLR* (Viprakasit et al., 2014)], globins (see below) or cell cycle proteins (Hodge et al., 2006; Pilon et al., 2008; Tallack et al., 2009; Gnanapragasam et al., 2016). Thus, depending on the type of mutation, a specific subset of targets can be affected, leading to a broad spectrum of phenotypes (Perkins et al., 2016).

The Semi-Dominant Phenotype in Nan (Neonatal Anemia) Mouse and in Human CDAIV

This is particularly evident in the case of the neonatal anemia (Nan) semi-dominant (Nan/+) mouse phenotype (Heruth et al., 2010; Siatecka et al., 2010) and in the phenotype observed in human Congenital dyserythropoietic anemia type IV (CDA IV) (Wickramasinghe et al., 1991; Arnaud et al., 2010; Jaffray et al., 2013; Ravindranath et al., 2018). In the Nan mouse model, the E339D substitution in the second ZnF within the Nan allele, alters Nan-KLF1 binding specificity, resulting in an aberrant transcriptome (Gillinder et al., 2017). The homologous E325K heterozygous mutation in CDA IV patients causes the reduced expression of a subset of KLF1 targets (such as *AQP1* and *CD44*), whereas other targets are normally expressed (such as *BCAM*) (Singleton et al., 2011). In analogy with the Nan mouse mutation, it is likely that also in man the E325K mutation could alter the mutant-KLF1 DNA-binding specificity, resulting in detrimental gain of function effects. On the basis of the different charge of the variant residues (Aspartic Acid or Lysine) it is possible to speculate that subsets of targets can be differentially affected by the different mutant proteins, likely explaining the distinct human and mice pathologies (Arnaud et al., 2010; Siatecka et al., 2010). On the other hand, traits common to mouse and human phenotypes could likely result from the reduced (50%) WT-KLF1.

The Intricate Link Between KLF1, Globin Expression and the Hemoglobin Switching: Direct and Indirect Effects

KLF1 was originally identified by its ability to bind to the β-globin promoter (Miller and Bieker, 1993) and the connection between KLF1 and β-thalassemia is demonstrated by the paradigmatic −87 mutation in the β-globin promoter CACC box (Feng et al., 1994).

Accordingly, the more evident phenotype of *KLF1* knockout mice is a marked β-thalassemia associated with increased *HBG1/HBG2*, suggesting that KLF1 interferes at different levels with globin genes expression. Indeed, the ablation of KLF1 perturbs the 3-dimensional conformation of the β-globin locus (Noordermeer and de Laat, 2008; Schoenfelder et al., 2010). Moreover, mutations creating *de novo* KLF1 motifs can also alter the relative expression within the β-locus: this is the case of the −198 mutation in the γ-promoter that introduces a new KLF1 binding site, generating the British type HFPH (Wienert et al., 2017). Besides these direct effects of loss or gain of KLF1 binding, an intricate network of indirect effects downstream to KLF1 haploinsufficiency/mutations must be considered. Borg et al. (2010) reported a Maltese family with HPFH and mild hypochromatic microcytic RBCs, caused by the KLF1 K288X non-sense mutation, ablating the DNA binding domain. Transcription profiling and functional studies in cells from these subjects revealed low levels of BCL11a, the most important known *HBG1/HBG2* repressor, suggesting that failure to properly activate BCL11a is the major cause of the observed HPFH (Borg et al., 2011). This was proven true also in the KLF1-deficient mouse model (Zhou et al., 2010). However, the situation is far more complicated: in another family described shortly thereafter, KLF1 haploinsufficiency did not result in HPFH (Satta et al., 2011). Instead, in this family, HPFH was observed only in compound heterozygotes (non-sense S270X and K332Q missense mutations) together with increased red cell protoporphyrin, a trait observed in the Nan mouse phenotype. Large-scale screening of patients with hemoglobinopathies of different ethnic origin supported the association of *KLF1* mutations with elevated HbF, thus confirming that KLF1 variants are an important source of HbF variation (Gallienne et al., 2012). Finally, more subtle effects of *KLF1* polymorphisms also account for an appreciable proportion of cases with borderline elevated HbA_2 (Perseu et al., 2011). Thus, again, the pleiotropic effects of KLF1 are the sum of quantitative and qualitative effects, possibly in combination with other genetic modifiers.

CONCLUSION AND PERSPECTIVES

The recent identification of mutations/variants alleles associated with RBC traits involving TFs has greatly increased thanks to new technologies and is expected to further increase in the next few years. This will help not only to explain so far unexplained diseases -and possibly to envisage new therapeutic strategies-, but also to better understand the structure and function of TFs themselves and their involvement in the different gene regulatory networks. This, in turn, will shed light on the contribution of TFs and their target sequences as a source of genetic variability underlying the wide spectrum of the observed erythroid phenotypes.

AUTHOR CONTRIBUTIONS

AR conceived and wrote the manuscript. GB, CF, and JS contributed with ideas and discussion. CF created figures.

ACKNOWLEDGMENTS

We thank Dr. Stephan Menzel for critical reading of the manuscript.

REFERENCES

Ahmed, M., Sternberg, A., Hall, G., Thomas, A., Smith, O., O'Marcaigh, A., et al. (2004). Natural history of GATA1 mutations in Down syndrome. *Blood* 103, 2480–2489. doi: 10.1182/blood-2003-10-3383

Arnaud, L., Saison, C., Helias, V., Lucien, N., Steschenko, D., Giarratana, M. C., et al. (2010). A dominant mutation in the gene encoding the erythroid transcription factor KLF1 causes a congenital dyserythropoietic anemia. *Am. J. Hum. Genet.* 87, 721–727. doi: 10.1016/j.ajhg.2010.10.010

Balduini, C. L., Pecci, A., Loffredo, G., Izzo, P., Noris, P., Grosso, M., et al. (2004). Effects of the R216Q mutation of GATA-1 on erythropoiesis and megakaryocytopoiesis. *Thromb. Haemost.* 91, 129–140. doi: 10.1160/TH03-05-0290

Bianchi, P., Fermo, E., Vercellati, C., Boschetti, C., Barcellini, W., Iurlo, A., et al. (2009). Congenital dyserythropoietic anemia type II (CDAII) is caused by mutations in the SEC23B gene. *Hum. Mutat.* 30, 1292–1298. doi: 10.1002/humu.21077

Bieker, J. J. (1996). Isolation, genomic structure, and expression of human erythroid Kruppel-like factor (EKLF). *DNA Cell Biol.* 15, 347–352. doi: 10.1089/dna.1996.15.347

Borg, J., Papadopoulos, P., Georgitsi, M., Gutierrez, L., Grech, G., Fanis, P., et al. (2010). Haploinsufficiency for the erythroid transcription factor KLF1 causes hereditary persistence of fetal hemoglobin. *Nat. Genet.* 42, 801–805. doi: 10.1038/ng.630

Borg, J., Patrinos, G. P., Felice, A. E., and Philipsen, S. (2011). Erythroid phenotypes associated with KLF1 mutations. *Haematologica* 96, 635–638. doi: 10.3324/haematol.2011.043265

Cabezas-Wallscheid, N., Klimmeck, D., Hansson, J., Lipka, D. B., Reyes, A., Wang, Q., et al. (2014). Identification of regulatory networks in HSCs and their immediate progeny via integrated proteome, transcriptome, and DNA methylome analysis. *Cell Stem Cell* 15, 507–522. doi: 10.1016/j.stem.2014.07.005

Calligaris, R., Bottardi, S., Cogoi, S., Apezteguia, I., and Santoro, C. (1995). Alternative translation initiation site usage results in two functionally distinct forms of the GATA-1 transcription factor. *Proc. Natl. Acad. Sci. U.S.A.* 92, 11598–11602. doi: 10.1073/pnas.92.25.11598

Campagna, D. R., de Bie, C. I., Schmitz-Abe, K., Sweeney, M., Sendamarai, A. K., Schmidt, P. J., et al. (2014). X-linked sideroblastic anemia due to ALAS2 intron 1 enhancer element GATA-binding site mutations. *Am. J. Hematol.* 89, 315–319. doi: 10.1002/ajh.23616

Campbell, A. E., Wilkinson-White, L., Mackay, J. P., Matthews, J. M., and Blobel, G. A. (2013). Analysis of disease-causing GATA1 mutations in murine gene complementation systems. *Blood* 121, 5218–5227. doi: 10.1182/blood-2013-03-488080

Chami, N., Chen, M. H., Slater, A. J., Eicher, J. D., Evangelou, E., Tajuddin, S. M., et al. (2016). Exome genotyping identifies pleiotropic variants associated with red blood cell traits. *Am. J. Hum. Genet.* 99, 8–21. doi: 10.1016/j.ajhg.2016.05.007

Chang, A. N., Cantor, A. B., Fujiwara, Y., Lodish, M. B., Droho, S., Crispino, J. D., et al. (2002). GATA-factor dependence of the multitype zinc-finger protein FOG-1 for its essential role in megakaryopoiesis. *Proc. Natl. Acad. Sci. U.S.A.* 99, 9237–9242. doi: 10.1073/pnas.142302099

Crispino, J. D. (2005). GATA1 mutations in Down syndrome: implications for biology and diagnosis of children with transient myeloproliferative disorder and acute megakaryoblastic leukemia. *Pediatr. Blood Cancer* 44, 40–44. doi: 10.1002/pbc.20066

Crispino, J. D., Lodish, M. B., MacKay, J. P., and Orkin, S. H. (1999). Use of altered specificity mutants to probe a specific protein-protein interaction in differentiation: the GATA-1:FOG complex. *Mol. Cell* 3, 219–228. doi: 10.1016/S1097-2765(00)80312-3

Da Costa, L., Narla, A., and Mohandas, N. (2018). An update on the pathogenesis and diagnosis of Diamond-Blackfan anemia. *F1000Res.* 7:F1000 Faculty Rev-1350. doi: 10.12688/f1000research.15542.1

Di Pierro, E., Russo, R., Karakas, Z., Brancaleoni, V., Gambale, A., Kurt, I., et al. (2015). Congenital erythropoietic porphyria linked to GATA1-R216W mutation: challenges for diagnosis. *Eur. J. Haematol.* 94, 491–497. doi: 10.1111/ejh.12452

Dore, L. C., and Crispino, J. D. (2011). Transcription factor networks in erythroid cell and megakaryocyte development. *Blood* 118, 231–239. doi: 10.1182/blood-2011-04-285981

Dulmovits, B. M., Hom, J., Narla, A., Mohandas, N., and Blanc, L. (2017). Characterization, regulation, and targeting of erythroid progenitors in normal and disordered human erythropoiesis. *Curr. Opin. Hematol.* 24, 159–166. doi: 10.1097/MOH.0000000000000328

Dykstra, B., and Bystrykh, L. V. (2014). No monkeying around: clonal tracking of stem cells and progenitors in the macaque. *Cell Stem Cell* 14, 419–420. doi: 10.1016/j.stem.2014.03.006

Dzierzak, E., and Philipsen, S. (2013). Erythropoiesis: development and differentiation. *Cold Spring Harb. Perspect. Med.* 3:a011601. doi: 10.1101/cshperspect.a011601

Feng, W. C., Southwood, C. M., and Bieker, J. J. (1994). Analyses of beta-thalassemia mutant DNA interactions with erythroid Kruppel-like factor (EKLF), an erythroid cell-specific transcription factor. *J. Biol. Chem.* 269, 1493–1500.

Ferreira, R., Ohneda, K., Yamamoto, M., and Philipsen, S. (2005). GATA1 function, a paradigm for transcription factors in hematopoiesis. *Mol. Cell Biol.* 25, 1215–1227. doi: 10.1128/MCB.25.4.1215-1227.2005

Fraser, N. S., Knauth, C. M., Schoeman, E. M., Moussa, A., Perkins, A. C., Walsh, T., et al. (2018). Investigation of the variable In(Lu) phenotype caused by KLF1 variants. *Transfusion* 58, 2414–2420. doi: 10.1111/trf.14926

Freson, K., Devriendt, K., Matthijs, G., Van Hoof, A., De Vos, R., Thys, C., et al. (2001). Platelet characteristics in patients with X-linked macrothrombocytopenia because of a novel GATA1 mutation. *Blood* 98, 85–92. doi: 10.1182/blood.V98.1.85

Freson, K., Matthijs, G., Thys, C., Marien, P., Hoylaerts, M. F., Vermylen, J., et al. (2002). Different substitutions at residue D218 of the X-linked transcription factor GATA1 lead to altered clinical severity of macrothrombocytopenia and anemia and are associated with variable skewed X inactivation. *Hum. Mol. Genet.* 11, 147–152. doi: 10.1093/hmg/11.2.147

Frontelo, P., Manwani, D., Galdass, M., Karsunky, H., Lohmann, F., Gallagher, P. G., et al. (2007). Novel role for EKLF in megakaryocyte lineage commitment. *Blood* 110, 3871–3880. doi: 10.1182/blood-2007-03-082065

Fujiwara, Y., Browne, C. P., Cunniff, K., Goff, S. C., and Orkin, S. H. (1996). Arrested development of embryonic red cell precursors in mouse embryos lacking transcription factor GATA-1. *Proc. Natl. Acad. Sci. U.S.A.* 93, 12355–12358. doi: 10.1073/pnas.93.22.12355

Gallienne, A. E., Dreau, H. M., Schuh, A., Old, J. M., and Henderson, S. (2012). Ten novel mutations in the erythroid transcription factor KLF1 gene associated with increased fetal hemoglobin levels in adults. *Haematologica* 97, 340–343. doi: 10.3324/haematol.2011.055442

Giladi, A., Paul, F., Herzog, Y., Lubling, Y., Weiner, A., Yofe, I., et al. (2018). Single-cell characterization of haematopoietic progenitors and their trajectories in homeostasis and perturbed haematopoiesis. *Nat. Cell Biol.* 20, 836–846. doi: 10.1038/s41556-018-0121-4

Gilles, L., Arslan, A. D., Marinaccio, C., Wen, Q. J., Arya, P., McNulty, M., et al. (2017). Downregulation of GATA1 drives impaired hematopoiesis in primary myelofibrosis. *J. Clin. Invest.* 127, 1316–1320. doi: 10.1172/JCI82905

Gillinder, K. R., Ilsley, M. D., Nebor, D., Sachidanandam, R., Lajoie, M., Magor, G. W., et al. (2017). Promiscuous DNA-binding of a mutant zinc finger protein corrupts the transcriptome and diminishes cell viability. *Nucleic Acids Res.* 45, 1130–1143. doi: 10.1093/nar/gkw1014

Glogowska, E., and Gallagher, P. G. (2015). Disorders of erythrocyte volume homeostasis. *Int. J. Lab. Hematol.* 37(Suppl. 1), 85–91. doi: 10.1111/ijlh.12357

Gnanapragasam, M. N., McGrath, K. E., Catherman, S., Xue, L., Palis, J., and Bieker, J. J. (2016). EKLF/KLF1-regulated cell cycle exit is essential for erythroblast enucleation. *Blood* 128, 1631–1641. doi: 10.1182/blood-2016-03-706671

Grace, R. F., Bianchi, P., van Beers, E. J., Eber, S. W., Glader, B., Yaish, H. M., et al. (2018). Clinical spectrum of pyruvate kinase deficiency: data from the Pyruvate Kinase Deficiency Natural History Study. *Blood* 131, 2183–2192. doi: 10.1182/blood-2017-10-810796

Gruber, T. A., and Downing, J. R. (2015). The biology of pediatric acute megakaryoblastic leukemia. *Blood* 126, 943–949. doi: 10.1182/blood-2015-05-567859

Guo, G., Luc, S., Marco, E., Lin, T. W., Peng, C., Kerenyi, M. A., et al. (2013). Mapping cellular hierarchy by single-cell analysis of the cell surface repertoire. *Cell Stem Cell* 13, 492–505. doi: 10.1016/j.stem.2013.07.017

Gutierrez, L., Nikolic, T., van Dijk, T. B., Hammad, H., Vos, N., Willart, M., et al. (2007). Gata1 regulates dendritic-cell development and survival. *Blood* 110, 1933–1941. doi: 10.1182/blood-2006-09-048322

Gutierrez, L., Tsukamoto, S., Suzuki, M., Yamamoto-Mukai, H., Yamamoto, M., Philipsen, S., et al. (2008). Ablation of Gata1 in adult mice results in aplastic crisis, revealing its essential role in steady-state and stress erythropoiesis. *Blood* 111, 4375–4385. doi: 10.1182/blood-2007-09-115121

Haas, S., Trumpp, A., and Milsom, M. D. (2018). Causes and consequences of hematopoietic stem cell heterogeneity. *Cell Stem Cell* 22, 627–638. doi: 10.1016/j.stem.2018.04.003

Hattangadi, S. M., Wong, P., Zhang, L., Flygare, J., and Lodish, H. F. (2011). From stem cell to red cell: regulation of erythropoiesis at multiple levels by multiple proteins, RNAs, and chromatin modifications. *Blood* 118, 6258–6268. doi: 10.1182/blood-2011-07-356006

Helias, V., Saison, C., Peyrard, T., Vera, E., Prehu, C., Cartron, J. P., et al. (2013). Molecular analysis of the rare in(Lu) blood type: toward decoding the phenotypic outcome of haploinsufficiency for the transcription factor KLF1. *Hum. Mutat.* 34, 221–228. doi: 10.1002/humu.22218

Heruth, D. P., Hawkins, T., Logsdon, D. P., Gibson, M. I., Sokolovsky, I. V., Nsumu, N. N., et al. (2010). Mutation in erythroid specific transcription factor KLF1 causes Hereditary Spherocytosis in the Nan hemolytic anemia mouse model. *Genomics* 96, 303–307. doi: 10.1016/j.ygeno.2010.07.009

Hitzler, J. K., and Zipursky, A. (2005). Origins of leukaemia in children with Down syndrome. *Nat. Rev. Cancer* 5, 11–20. doi: 10.1038/nrc1525

Hodge, D., Coghill, E., Keys, J., Maguire, T., Hartmann, B., McDowall, A., et al. (2006). A global role for EKLF in definitive and primitive erythropoiesis. *Blood* 107, 3359–3370. doi: 10.1182/blood-2005-07-2888

Hollanda, L. M., Lima, C. S., Cunha, A. F., Albuquerque, D. M., Vassallo, J., Ozelo, M. C., et al. (2006). An inherited mutation leading to production of only the short isoform of GATA-1 is associated with impaired erythropoiesis. *Nat. Genet.* 38, 807–812. doi: 10.1038/ng1825

Hwang, Y., Futran, M., Hidalgo, D., Pop, R., Iyer, D. R., Scully, R., et al. (2017). Global increase in replication fork speed during a p57(KIP2)-regulated erythroid cell fate switch. *Sci. Adv.* 3:e1700298. doi: 10.1126/sciadv.1700298

Iolascon, A., Russo, R., and Delaunay, J. (2011). Congenital dyserythropoietic anemias. *Curr. Opin. Hematol.* 18, 146–151. doi: 10.1097/MOH.0b013e32834521b0

Isern, J., He, Z., Fraser, S. T., Nowotschin, S., Ferrer-Vaquer, A., Moore, R., et al. (2011). Single-lineage transcriptome analysis reveals key regulatory pathways in primitive erythroid progenitors in the mouse embryo. *Blood* 117, 4924–4934. doi: 10.1182/blood-2010-10-313676

Jaffray, J. A., Mitchell, W. B., Gnanapragasam, M. N., Seshan, S. V., Guo, X., Westhoff, C. M., et al. (2013). Erythroid transcription factor EKLF/KLF1 mutation causing congenital dyserythropoietic anemia type IV in a patient of Taiwanese origin: review of all reported cases and development of a clinical diagnostic paradigm. *Blood Cells Mol. Dis.* 51, 71–75. doi: 10.1016/j.bcmd.2013.02.006

Kaneko, K., Furuyama, K., Fujiwara, T., Kobayashi, R., Ishida, H., Harigae, H., et al. (2014). Identification of a novel erythroid-specific enhancer for the ALAS2 gene and its loss-of-function mutation which is associated with congenital sideroblastic anemia. *Haematologica* 99, 252–261. doi: 10.3324/haematol.2013.085449

Khajuria, R. K., Munschauer, M., Ulirsch, J. C., Fiorini, C., Ludwig, L. S., McFarland, S. K., et al. (2018). Ribosome levels selectively regulate translation and lineage commitment in human hematopoiesis. *Cell* 173, 90–103.e19. doi: 10.1016/j.cell.2018.02.036

Klar, J., Khalfallah, A., Arzoo, P. S., Gazda, H. T., and Dahl, N. (2014). Recurrent GATA1 mutations in Diamond-Blackfan anaemia. *Br. J. Haematol.* 166, 949–951. doi: 10.1111/bjh.12919

Koralkova, P., van Solinge, W. W., and van Wijk, R. (2014). Rare hereditary red blood cell enzymopathies associated with hemolytic anemia - pathophysiology, clinical aspects, and laboratory diagnosis. *Int. J. Lab. Hematol.* 36, 388–397. doi: 10.1111/ijlh.12223

Koury, M. J. (2016). Tracking erythroid progenitor cells in times of need and times of plenty. *Exp. Hematol.* 44, 653–663. doi: 10.1016/j.exphem.2015.10.007

Kozma, G. T., Martelli, F., Verrucci, M., Gutierrez, L., Migliaccio, G., Sanchez, M., et al. (2010). Dynamic regulation of Gata1 expression during the maturation of conventional dendritic cells. *Exp. Hematol.* 38, 489–503.e1. doi: 10.1016/j.exphem.2010.03.006

Lee, H. H., Mak, A. S., Kou, K. O., Poon, C. F., Wong, W. S., Chiu, K. H., et al. (2016). An unusual hydrops fetalis associated with compound heterozygosity for kruppel-like factor 1 mutations. *Hemoglobin* 40, 431–434. doi: 10.1080/03630269.2016.1267017

Lefevre, C., Bondu, S., Le Goff, S., Kosmider, O., and Fontenay, M. (2017). Dyserythropoiesis of myelodysplastic syndromes. *Curr. Opin. Hematol.* 24, 191–197. doi: 10.1097/MOH.0000000000000325

Levine, R. L., Pardanani, A., Tefferi, A., and Gilliland, D. G. (2007). Role of JAK2 in the pathogenesis and therapy of myeloproliferative disorders. *Nat. Rev. Cancer* 7, 673–683. doi: 10.1038/nrc2210

Li, Z., Godinho, F. J., Klusmann, J. H., Garriga-Canut, M., Yu, C., and Orkin, S. H. (2005). Developmental stage-selective effect of somatically mutated leukemogenic transcription factor GATA1. *Nat. Genet.* 37, 613–619. doi: 10.1038/ng1566

Libani, I. V., Guy, E. C., Melchiori, L., Schiro, R., Ramos, P., Breda, L., et al. (2008). Decreased differentiation of erythroid cells exacerbates ineffective erythropoiesis in beta-thalassemia. *Blood* 112, 875–885. doi: 10.1182/blood-2007-12-126938

Love, P. E., Warzecha, C., and Li, L. (2014). Ldb1 complexes: the new master regulators of erythroid gene transcription. *Trends Genet.* 30, 1–9. doi: 10.1016/j.tig.2013.10.001

Ludlow, L. B., Schick, B. P., Budarf, M. L., Driscoll, D. A., Zackai, E. H., Cohen, A., et al. (1996). Identification of a mutation in a GATA binding site of the platelet glycoprotein Ibbeta promoter resulting in the Bernard-Soulier syndrome. *J. Biol. Chem.* 271, 22076–22080. doi: 10.1074/jbc.271.36.22076

Ludwig, L. S., Gazda, H. T., Eng, J. C., Eichhorn, S. W., Thiru, P., Ghazvinian, R., et al. (2014). Altered translation of GATA1 in diamond-Blackfan anemia. *Nat. Med.* 20, 748–753. doi: 10.1038/nm.3557

Magalhaes, I. Q., Splendore, A., Emerenciano, M., Figueiredo, A., Ferrari, I., and Pombo-de-Oliveira, M. S. (2006). GATA1 mutations in acute leukemia in children with Down syndrome. *Cancer Genet. Cytogenet.* 166, 112–116. doi: 10.1016/j.cancergencyto.2005.10.008

Magor, G. W., Tallack, M. R., Gillinder, K. R., Bell, C. C., McCallum, N., Williams, B., et al. (2015). KLF1-null neonates display hydrops fetalis and a deranged erythroid transcriptome. *Blood* 125, 2405–2417. doi: 10.1182/blood-2014-08-590968

Manco, L., Ribeiro, M. L., Maximo, V., Almeida, H., Costa, A., Freitas, O., et al. (2000). A new PKLR gene mutation in the R-type promoter region affects the gene transcription causing pyruvate kinase deficiency. *Br. J. Haematol.* 110, 993–997. doi: 10.1046/j.1365-2141.2000.02283.x

Mas, C., Lussier-Price, M., Soni, S., Morse, T., Arseneault, G., Di Lello, P., et al. (2011). Structural and functional characterization of an atypical activation domain in erythroid Kruppel-like factor (EKLF). *Proc. Natl. Acad. Sci. U.S.A.* 108, 10484–10489. doi: 10.1073/pnas.1017029108

Matsuda, M., Sakamoto, N., and Fukumaki, Y. (1992). Delta-thalassemia caused by disruption of the site for an erythroid-specific transcription factor, GATA-1, in the delta-globin gene promoter. *Blood* 80, 1347–1351.

Mehaffey, M. G., Newton, A. L., Gandhi, M. J., Crossley, M., and Drachman, J. G. (2001). X-linked thrombocytopenia caused by a novel mutation of GATA-1. *Blood* 98, 2681–2688. doi: 10.1182/blood.V98.9.2681

Menzel, S., Garner, C., Gut, I., Matsuda, F., Yamaguchi, M., Heath, S., et al. (2007). A QTL influencing F cell production maps to a gene encoding a zinc-finger protein on chromosome 2p15. *Nat. Genet.* 39, 1197–1199. doi: 10.1038/ng2108

Migliaccio, A. R., Rana, R. A., Vannucchi, A. M., and Manzoli, F. A. (2005). Role of GATA-1 in normal and neoplastic hemopoiesis. *Ann. N. Y. Acad. Sci.* 1044, 142–158. doi: 10.1196/annals.1349.019

Miller, I. J., and Bieker, J. J. (1993). A novel, erythroid cell-specific murine transcription factor that binds to the CACCC element and is related to the Kruppel family of nuclear proteins. *Mol. Cell Biol.* 13, 2776–2786. doi: 10.1128/MCB.13.5.2776

Mohandas, N., and Gallagher, P. G. (2008). Red cell membrane: past, present, and future. *Blood* 112, 3939–3948. doi: 10.1182/blood-2008-07-161166

Moller, M., Lee, Y. Q., Vidovic, K., Kjellstrom, S., Bjorkman, L., Storry, J. R., et al. (2018). Disruption of a GATA1-binding motif upstream of XG/PBDX abolishes Xg(a) expression and resolves the Xg blood group system. *Blood* 132, 334–338. doi: 10.1182/blood-2018-03-842542

Mundschau, G., Gurbuxani, S., Gamis, A. S., Greene, M. E., Arceci, R. J., and Crispino, J. D. (2003). Mutagenesis of GATA1 is an initiating event in Down syndrome leukemogenesis. *Blood* 101, 4298–4300. doi: 10.1182/blood-2002-12-3904

Nakajima, T., Sano, R., Takahashi, Y., Kubo, R., Takahashi, K., Kominato, Y., et al. (2013). Mutation of the GATA site in the erythroid cell-specific regulatory element of the ABO gene in a Bm subgroup individual. *Transfusion* 53(11 Suppl. 2), 2917–2927. doi: 10.1111/trf.12181

Nandakumar, S. K., Ulirsch, J. C., and Sankaran, V. G. (2016). Advances in understanding erythropoiesis: evolving perspectives. *Br. J. Haematol.* 173, 206–218. doi: 10.1111/bjh.13938

Nestorowa, S., Hamey, F. K., Pijuan Sala, B., Diamanti, E., Shepherd, M., Laurenti, E., et al. (2016). A single-cell resolution map of mouse hematopoietic stem and progenitor cell differentiation. *Blood* 128, e20–e31. doi: 10.1182/blood-2016-05-716480

Newton, A., Mackay, J., and Crossley, M. (2001). The N-terminal zinc finger of the erythroid transcription factor GATA-1 binds GATC motifs in DNA. *J. Biol. Chem.* 276, 35794–35801. doi: 10.1074/jbc.M106256200

Nichols, K. E., Crispino, J. D., Poncz, M., White, J. G., Orkin, S. H., Maris, J. M., et al. (2000). Familial dyserythropoietic anaemia and thrombocytopenia due to an inherited mutation in GATA1. *Nat. Genet.* 24, 266–270. doi: 10.1038/73480

Nilson, D. G., Sabatino, D. E., Bodine, D. M., and Gallagher, P. G. (2006). Major erythrocyte membrane protein genes in EKLF-deficient mice. *Exp. Hematol.* 34, 705–712. doi: 10.1016/j.exphem.2006.02.018

Noordermeer, D., and de Laat, W. (2008). Joining the loops: beta-globin gene regulation. *IUBMB Life* 60, 824–833. doi: 10.1002/iub.129

Notta, F., Zandi, S., Takayama, N., Dobson, S., Gan, O. I., Wilson, G., et al. (2016). Distinct routes of lineage development reshape the human blood hierarchy across ontogeny. *Science* 351:aab2116. doi: 10.1126/science.aab2116

Nuez, B., Michalovich, D., Bygrave, A., Ploemacher, R., and Grosveld, F. (1995). Defective haematopoiesis in fetal liver resulting from inactivation of the EKLF gene. *Nature* 375, 316–318. doi: 10.1038/375316a0

O'Brien, K. A., Farrar, J. E., Vlachos, A., Anderson, S. M., Tsujiura, C. A., Lichtenberg, J., et al. (2017). Molecular convergence in ex vivo models of Diamond-Blackfan anemia. *Blood* 129, 3111–3120. doi: 10.1182/blood-2017-01-760462

Oda, A., Isa, K., Ogasawara, K., Kameyama, K., Okuda, K., Hirashima, M., et al. (2015). A novel mutation of the GATA site in the erythroid cell-specific regulatory element of the ABO gene in a blood donor with the Am B phenotype. *Vox Sang.* 108, 425–427. doi: 10.1111/vox.12229

Palis, J. (2014). Primitive and definitive erythropoiesis in mammals. *Front. Physiol.* 5:3. doi: 10.3389/fphys.2014.00003

Palis, J. (2016). Hematopoietic stem cell-independent hematopoiesis: emergence of erythroid, megakaryocyte, and myeloid potential in the mammalian embryo. *FEBS Lett.* 590, 3965–3974. doi: 10.1002/1873-3468.12459

Parrella, S., Aspesi, A., Quarello, P., Garelli, E., Pavesi, E., Carando, A., et al. (2014). Loss of GATA-1 full length as a cause of Diamond-Blackfan anemia phenotype. *Pediatr. Blood Cancer* 61, 1319–1321. doi: 10.1002/pbc.24944

Paul, F., Arkin, Y., Giladi, A., Jaitin, D. A., Kenigsberg, E., Keren-Shaul, H., et al. (2016). Transcriptional heterogeneity and lineage commitment in myeloid progenitors. *Cell* 164, 325. doi: 10.1016/j.cell.2015.12.046

Pei, W., Feyerabend, T. B., Rossler, J., Wang, X., Postrach, D., Busch, K., et al. (2017). Polylox barcoding reveals haematopoietic stem cell fates realized in vivo. *Nature* 548, 456–460. doi: 10.1038/nature23653

Perie, L., Hodgkin, P. D., Naik, S. H., Schumacher, T. N., de Boer, R. J., and Duffy, K. R. (2014). Determining lineage pathways from cellular barcoding experiments. *Cell Rep.* 6, 617–624. doi: 10.1016/j.celrep.2014.01.016

Perkins, A., Xu, X., Higgs, D. R., Patrinos, G. P., Arnaud, L., Bieker, J. J., et al. (2016). Kruppeling erythropoiesis: an unexpected broad spectrum of human red blood cell disorders due to KLF1 variants. *Blood* 127, 1856–1862. doi: 10.1182/blood-2016-01-694331

Perkins, A. C., Peterson, K. R., Stamatoyannopoulos, G., Witkowska, H. E., and Orkin, S. H. (2000). Fetal expression of a human Agamma globin transgene rescues globin chain imbalance but not hemolysis in EKLF null mouse embryos. *Blood* 95, 1827–1833.

Perkins, A. C., Sharpe, A. H., and Orkin, S. H. (1995). Lethal beta-thalassaemia in mice lacking the erythroid CACCC-transcription factor EKLF. *Nature* 375, 318–322. doi: 10.1038/375318a0

Perrotta, S., Gallagher, P. G., and Mohandas, N. (2008). Hereditary spherocytosis. *Lancet* 372, 1411–1426. doi: 10.1016/S0140-6736(08)61588-3

Perseu, L., Satta, S., Moi, P., Demartis, F. R., Manunza, L., Sollaino, M. C., et al. (2011). KLF1 gene mutations cause borderline HbA(2). *Blood* 118, 4454–4458. doi: 10.1182/blood-2011-04-345736

Pevny, L., Lin, C. S., D'Agati, V., Simon, M. C., Orkin, S. H., and Costantini, F. (1995). Development of hematopoietic cells lacking transcription factor GATA-1. *Development* 121, 163–172.

Pevny, L., Simon, M. C., Robertson, E., Klein, W. H., Tsai, S. F., D'Agati, V., et al. (1991). Erythroid differentiation in chimaeric mice blocked by a targeted mutation in the gene for transcription factor GATA-1. *Nature* 349, 257–260. doi: 10.1038/349257a0

Phillips, J. D., Steensma, D. P., Pulsipher, M. A., Spangrude, G. J., and Kushner, J. P. (2007). Congenital erythropoietic porphyria due to a mutation in GATA1: the first trans-acting mutation causative for a human porphyria. *Blood* 109, 2618–2621. doi: 10.1182/blood-2006-06-022848

Pilon, A. M., Arcasoy, M. O., Dressman, H. K., Vayda, S. E., Maksimova, Y. D., Sangerman, J. I., et al. (2008). Failure of terminal erythroid differentiation in EKLF-deficient mice is associated with cell cycle perturbation and reduced expression of E2F2. *Mol. Cell Biol.* 28, 7394–7401. doi: 10.1128/MCB.01087-08

Portela, A., and Esteller, M. (2010). Epigenetic modifications and human disease. *Nat. Biotechnol.* 28, 1057–1068. doi: 10.1038/nbt.1685

Rainis, L., Bercovich, D., Strehl, S., Teigler-Schlegel, A., Stark, B., Trka, J., et al. (2003). Mutations in exon 2 of GATA1 are early events in megakaryocytic malignancies associated with trisomy 21. *Blood* 102, 981–986. doi: 10.1182/blood-2002-11-3599

Ravindranath, Y., Johnson, R. M., Goyette, G., Buck, S., Gadgeel, M., and Gallagher, P. G. (2018). KLF1 E325K-associated congenital dyserythropoietic anemia type IV: insights into the variable clinical severity. *J. Pediatr. Hematol. Oncol.* 40, e405–e409. doi: 10.1097/MPH.0000000000001056

Rees, D. C., Williams, T. N., and Gladwin, M. T. (2010). Sickle-cell disease. *Lancet* 376, 2018–2031. doi: 10.1016/S0140-6736(10)61029-X

Ribeil, J. A., Arlet, J. B., Dussiot, M., Moura, I. C., Courtois, G., and Hermine, O. (2013). Ineffective erythropoiesis in beta -thalassemia. *ScientificWorldJournal.* 2013:394295. doi: 10.1155/2013/394295

Rivella, S. (2015). beta-thalassemias: paradigmatic diseases for scientific discoveries and development of innovative therapies. *Haematologica* 100, 418–430. doi: 10.3324/haematol.2014.114827

Rodriguez-Fraticelli, A. E., Wolock, S. L., Weinreb, C. S., Panero, R., Patel, S. H., Jankovic, M., et al. (2018). Clonal analysis of lineage fate in native haematopoiesis. *Nature* 553, 212–216. doi: 10.1038/nature25168

Russo, R., Andolfo, I., Gambale, A., De Rosa, G., Manna, F., Arillo, A., et al. (2017). GATA1 erythroid-specific regulation of SEC23B expression and its implication in the pathogenesis of congenital dyserythropoietic anemia type II. *Haematologica* 102, e371–e374. doi: 10.3324/haematol.2016.162966

Sankaran, V. G., Ghazvinian, R., Do, R., Thiru, P., Vergilio, J. A., Beggs, A. H., et al. (2012). Exome sequencing identifies GATA1 mutations resulting in Diamond-Blackfan anemia. *J. Clin. Invest.* 122, 2439–2443. doi: 10.1172/JCI63597

Sankaran, V. G., Menne, T. F., Xu, J., Akie, T. E., Lettre, G., Van Handel, B., et al. (2008). Human fetal hemoglobin expression is regulated by the developmental stage-specific repressor BCL11A. *Science* 322, 1839–1842. doi: 10.1126/science.1165409

Satta, S., Perseu, L., Moi, P., Asunis, I., Cabriolu, A., Maccioni, L., et al. (2011). Compound heterozygosity for KLF1 mutations associated with remarkable

increase of fetal hemoglobin and red cell protoporphyrin. *Haematologica* 96, 767–770. doi: 10.3324/haematol.2010.037333

Schoenfelder, S., Sexton, T., Chakalova, L., Cope, N. F., Horton, A., Andrews, S., et al. (2010). Preferential associations between co-regulated genes reveal a transcriptional interactome in erythroid cells. *Nat. Genet.* 42, 53–61. doi: 10.1038/ng.496

Schwarz, K., Iolascon, A., Verissimo, F., Trede, N. S., Horsley, W., Chen, W., et al. (2009). Mutations affecting the secretory COPII coat component SEC23B cause congenital dyserythropoietic anemia type II. *Nat. Genet.* 41, 936–940. doi: 10.1038/ng.405

Shimada, A., Xu, G., Toki, T., Kimura, H., Hayashi, Y., and Ito, E. (2004). Fetal origin of the GATA1 mutation in identical twins with transient myeloproliferative disorder and acute megakaryoblastic leukemia accompanying Down syndrome. *Blood* 103:366. doi: 10.1182/blood-2003-09-3219

Shivdasani, R. A., Fujiwara, Y., McDevitt, M. A., and Orkin, S. H. (1997). A lineage-selective knockout establishes the critical role of transcription factor GATA-1 in megakaryocyte growth and platelet development. *EMBO J.* 16, 3965–3973. doi: 10.1093/emboj/16.13.3965

Shyu, Y. C., Lee, T. L., Chen, X., Hsu, P. H., Wen, S. C., Liaw, Y. W., et al. (2014). Tight regulation of a timed nuclear import wave of EKLF by PKCtheta and FOE during Pro-E to Baso-E transition. *Dev. Cell* 28, 409–422. doi: 10.1016/j.devcel.2014.01.007

Siatecka, M., Sahr, K. E., Andersen, S. G., Mezei, M., Bieker, J. J., and Peters, L. L. (2010). Severe anemia in the Nan mutant mouse caused by sequence-selective disruption of erythroid Kruppel-like factor. *Proc. Natl. Acad. Sci. U.S.A.* 107, 15151–15156. doi: 10.1073/pnas.1004996107

Singleton, B. K., Burton, N. M., Green, C., Brady, R. L., and Anstee, D. J. (2008). Mutations in EKLF/KLF1 form the molecular basis of the rare blood group In(Lu) phenotype. *Blood* 112, 2081–2088. doi: 10.1182/blood-2008-03-145672

Singleton, B. K., Lau, W., Fairweather, V. S., Burton, N. M., Wilson, M. C., Parsons, S. F., et al. (2011). Mutations in the second zinc finger of human EKLF reduce promoter affinity but give rise to benign and disease phenotypes. *Blood* 118, 3137–3145. doi: 10.1182/blood-2011-04-349985

Singleton, B. K., Roxby, D. J., Stirling, J. W., Spring, F. A., Wilson, C., Poole, J., et al. (2013). A novel GATA1 mutation (Stop414Arg) in a family with the rare X-linked blood group Lu(a-b-) phenotype and mild macrothrombocytic thrombocytopenia. *Br. J. Haematol.* 161, 139–142. doi: 10.1111/bjh.12184

Solis, C., Aizencang, G. I., Astrin, K. H., Bishop, D. F., and Desnick, R. J. (2001). Uroporphyrinogen III synthase erythroid promoter mutations in adjacent GATA1 and CP2 elements cause congenital erythropoietic porphyria. *J. Clin. Invest.* 107, 753–762. doi: 10.1172/JCI10642

Songdej, N., and Rao, A. K. (2017). Hematopoietic transcription factor mutations: important players in inherited platelet defects. *Blood* 129, 2873–2881. doi: 10.1182/blood-2016-11-709881

Soranzo, N., Spector, T. D., Mangino, M., Kuhnel, B., Rendon, A., Teumer, A., et al. (2009). A genome-wide meta-analysis identifies 22 loci associated with eight hematological parameters in the HaemGen consortium. *Nat. Genet.* 41, 1182–1190. doi: 10.1038/ng.467

Tallack, M. R., Keys, J. R., Humbert, P. O., and Perkins, A. C. (2009). EKLF/KLF1 controls cell cycle entry via direct regulation of E2f2. *J. Biol. Chem.* 284, 20966–20974. doi: 10.1074/jbc.M109.006346

Tallack, M. R., and Perkins, A. C. (2010). Megakaryocyte-erythroid lineage promiscuity in EKLF null mouse blood. *Haematologica* 95, 144–147. doi: 10.3324/haematol.2009.010017

Tournamille, C., Colin, Y., Cartron, J. P., and Le Van Kim, C. (1995). Disruption of a GATA motif in the Duffy gene promoter abolishes erythroid gene expression in Duffy–negative individuals. *Nat. Genet.* 10, 224–228. doi: 10.1038/ng0695-224

Trainor, C. D., Omichinski, J. G., Vandergon, T. L., Gronenborn, A. M., Clore, G. M., and Felsenfeld, G. (1996). A palindromic regulatory site within vertebrate GATA-1 promoters requires both zinc fingers of the GATA-1 DNA-binding domain for high-affinity interaction. *Mol. Cell Biol.* 16, 2238–2247. doi: 10.1128/MCB.16.5.2238

Tsang, A. P., Visvader, J. E., Turner, C. A., Fujiwara, Y., Yu, C., Weiss, M. J., et al. (1997). FOG, a multitype zinc finger protein, acts as a cofactor for transcription factor GATA-1 in erythroid and megakaryocytic differentiation. *Cell* 90, 109–119. doi: 10.1016/S0092-8674(00)80318-9

Tsiftsoglou, A. S., Vizirianakis, I. S., and Strouboulis, J. (2009). Erythropoiesis: model systems, molecular regulators, and developmental programs. *IUBMB Life* 61, 800–830. doi: 10.1002/iub.226

Tusi, B. K., Wolock, S. L., Weinreb, C., Hwang, Y., Hidalgo, D., Zilionis, R., et al. (2018). Population snapshots predict early haematopoietic and erythroid hierarchies. *Nature* 555, 54–60. doi: 10.1038/nature25741

Uda, M., Galanello, R., Sanna, S., Lettre, G., Sankaran, V. G., Chen, W., et al. (2008). Genome-wide association study shows BCL11A associated with persistent fetal hemoglobin and amelioration of the phenotype of beta-thalassemia. *Proc. Natl. Acad. Sci. U.S.A.* 105, 1620–1625. doi: 10.1073/pnas.0711566105

Upadhaya, S., Sawai, C. M., Papalexi, E., Rashidfarrokhi, A., Jang, G., Chattopadhyay, P., et al. (2018). Kinetics of adult hematopoietic stem cell differentiation in vivo. *J. Exp. Med.* 215:2815. doi: 10.1084/jem.20180136

van der Harst, P., Zhang, W., Mateo Leach, I., Rendon, A., Verweij, N., Sehmi, J., et al. (2012). Seventy-five genetic loci influencing the human red blood cell. *Nature* 492, 369–375. doi: 10.1038/nature11677

Vannucchi, A. M., Bianchi, L., Cellai, C., Paoletti, F., Rana, R. A., Lorenzini, R., et al. (2002). Development of myelofibrosis in mice genetically impaired for GATA-1 expression (GATA-1(low) mice). *Blood* 100, 1123–1132. doi: 10.1182/blood-2002-06-1913

Viprakasit, V., Ekwattanakit, S., Riolueang, S., Chalaow, N., Fisher, C., Lower, K., et al. (2014). Mutations in Kruppel-like factor 1 cause transfusion-dependent hemolytic anemia and persistence of embryonic globin gene expression. *Blood* 123, 1586–1595. doi: 10.1182/blood-2013-09-526087

Vyas, P., Ault, K., Jackson, C. W., Orkin, S. H., and Shivdasani, R. A. (1999). Consequences of GATA-1 deficiency in megakaryocytes and platelets. *Blood* 93, 2867–2875.

Wechsler, J., Greene, M., McDevitt, M. A., Anastasi, J., Karp, J. E., Le Beau, M. M., et al. (2002). Acquired mutations in GATA1 in the megakaryoblastic leukemia of Down syndrome. *Nat. Genet.* 32, 148–152. doi: 10.1038/ng955

Wickramasinghe, S. N., Illum, N., and Wimberley, P. D. (1991). Congenital dyserythropoietic anaemia with novel intra-erythroblastic and intra-erythrocytic inclusions. *Br. J. Haematol.* 79, 322–330. doi: 10.1111/j.1365-2141.1991.tb04541.x

Wienert, B., Martyn, G. E., Kurita, R., Nakamura, Y., Quinlan, K. G. R., and Crossley, M. (2017). KLF1 drives the expression of fetal hemoglobin in British HPFH. *Blood* 130, 803–807. doi: 10.1182/blood-2017-02-767400

Xu, G., Nagano, M., Kanezaki, R., Toki, T., Hayashi, Y., Taketani, T., et al. (2003). Frequent mutations in the GATA-1 gene in the transient myeloproliferative disorder of Down syndrome. *Blood* 102, 2960–2968. doi: 10.1182/blood-2003-02-0390

Ye, F., Huang, W., and Guo, G. (2017). Studying hematopoiesis using single-cell technologies. *J. Hematol. Oncol.* 10:27. doi: 10.1186/s13045-017-0401-7

Yu, C., Cantor, A. B., Yang, H., Browne, C., Wells, R. A., Fujiwara, Y., et al. (2002a). Targeted deletion of a high-affinity GATA-binding site in the GATA-1 promoter leads to selective loss of the eosinophil lineage in vivo. *J. Exp. Med.* 195, 1387–1395.

Yu, C., Niakan, K. K., Matsushita, M., Stamatoyannopoulos, G., Orkin, S. H., and Raskind, W. H. (2002b). X-linked thrombocytopenia with thalassemia from a mutation in the amino finger of GATA-1 affecting DNA binding rather than FOG-1 interaction. *Blood* 100, 2040–2045.

Zhou, D., Liu, K., Sun, C. W., Pawlik, K. M., and Townes, T. M. (2010). KLF1 regulates BCL11A expression and gamma- to beta-globin gene switching. *Nat. Genet.* 42, 742–744. doi: 10.1038/ng.637

5

Characterization of Two Cases of Congenital Dyserythropoietic Anemia Type I Shed Light on the Uncharacterized C15orf41 Protein

Roberta Russo[1,2*†], Roberta Marra[1,2†], Immacolata Andolfo[1,2], Gianluca De Rosa[1,2], Barbara Eleni Rosato[1,2], Francesco Manna[2], Antonella Gambale[1,2], Maddalena Raia[2], Sule Unal[3], Susanna Barella[4] and Achille Iolascon[1,2]

[1] Dipartimento di Medicina Molecolare e Biotecnologie Mediche, Università degli Studi di Napoli Federico II, Naples, Italy,
[2] CEINGE Biotecnologie Avanzate, Naples, Italy, [3] Division of Pediatric Hematology, Hacettepe University, Ankara, Turkey,
[4] SSD Talassemie, Anemie Rare e Dismetabolismi del Ferro, Ospedale Pediatrico Microcitemico Antonio Cao, Azienda
Ospedaliera Brotzu, Cagliari, Italy

*Correspondence:
Roberta Russo
roberta.russo@unina.it

[†] These authors have contributed
equally to this work

CDA type I is a rare hereditary anemia, characterized by relative reticulocytopenia, and congenital anomalies. It is caused by biallelic mutations in one of the two genes: (i) CDAN1, encoding Codanin-1, which is implicated in nucleosome assembly and disassembly; (ii) C15orf41, which is predicted to encode a divalent metal ion-dependent restriction endonuclease with a yet unknown function. We described two cases of CDA type I, identifying the novel variant, Y94S, in the DNA binding domain of C15orf41, and the H230P mutation in the nuclease domain of the protein. We first analyzed the gene expression and the localization of C15orf41. We demonstrated that C15orf41 and CDAN1 gene expression is tightly correlated, suggesting a shared mechanism of regulation between the two genes. Moreover, we functionally characterized the two variants, establishing that the H230P leads to reduced gene expression and protein level, while Y94S induces a slight decrease of expression. We demonstrated that C15orf41 endogenous protein exhibits nuclear and cytosolic localization, being mostly in the nucleus. However, no altered nuclear-cytosolic compartmentalization of mutated C15orf41 was observed. Both mutants accounted for impaired erythroid differentiation in K562 cells, and H230P mutant also exhibits an increased S-phase of the cell cycle in these cells. Our functional characterization demonstrated that the two variants have different effects on the stability of the mutated mRNA, but both resulted in impaired erythroid maturation, suggesting the block of cell cycle dynamics as a putative pathogenic mechanism for C15orf41-related CDA I.

Keywords: CDA (I–III), C15ORF41, functional characterization of proteins, genetic testing, anemia

INTRODUCTION

Congenital dyserythropoietic anemias (CDAs) are hereditary diseases, belonging to the bone marrow (BM) failure syndromes, which embrace a heterogeneous set of rare hereditary anemias that result from impaired erythropoiesis and various kinds of abnormalities during late stages of erythropoiesis (Gambale et al., 2016). Among them, CDA type I (CDA I) is characterized by anemia of variable degree, generally macrocytic, relative reticulocytopenia, and congenital anomalies, such as syndactyly, chest deformity, and short stature. The original classification system for CDAs was based on specific erythroblasts morphological abnormalities on BM light microscopy (Roy and Babbs, 2019). The morphological pathognomonic feature of CDA I is the presence of thin chromatin bridges between the nuclei pairs of erythroblasts. On electron microscopy, heterochromatin is denser than normal, and forms demarcated clumps with small translucent vacuoles, giving rise to the metaphor of "Swiss cheese appearance" (Kellermann et al., 2010; Roy and Babbs, 2019).

CDA I is inherited as an autosomal recessive disorder caused by mutations in two different loci, *CDAN1* and *C15orf41*, which account for the 90% of CDA I cases. *CDAN1* (chr15q15.2) was the first gene in which pathogenic variants causative of CDA type I (OMIM # 224120) were identified (Dgany et al., 2002). It encodes a ubiquitously expressed and cell-cycle regulated protein, Codanin-1 (Noy-Lotan et al., 2009), which acts in nucleosome assembly and disassembly through the formation of the cytosolic Asf1-H3-H4-importin-4 complex. Codanin-1 binds directly to Asf1 via a conserved B-domain, implying a mutually exclusive interaction with the chromatin assembly factor 1 (CAF-1) and HIRA. Previous studies on osteosarcoma U-2-OS cells silenced for Codanin-1 showed accelerated DNA replication rate and increased levels of chromatin-bound Asf1, suggesting that Codanin-1 guards a limiting step in chromatin replication (Ask et al., 2012). More recently, *C15orf41* (chr15q14) was discovered as the second locus associated with CDA I (OMIM # 615631). It is an uncharacterized gene that is predicted to encode a divalent metal-ion dependent restriction endonuclease with homology to the Holliday junction resolvases (Babbs et al., 2013). It was suggested that C15orf41-encoded protein, similarly to Codanin-1, interacts with Asf1b (Ewing et al., 2007), supporting the hypothesis that both C15orf41 and Codanin-1 could interplay during DNA replication and chromatin assembly (Gambale et al., 2016).

To date, only five *C15orf41* variants have been reported (Babbs et al., 2013; Palmblad et al., 2018; Russo et al., 2018). We herein described two cases of *C15orf41*-CDA I carrying the aminoacidic substitutions p.Tyr94Ser and p.His230Pro that are located in the two different domains of the C15orf41 protein. Our functional characterization demonstrated that the two variants have different effects on the stability of the mutated mRNA. However, both mutations account for impaired erythroid maturation. This study improves the current understanding of the role of this uncharacterized protein in both the physiological conditions and the pathogenic mechanism of the disease.

MATERIALS AND METHODS

Patients and Genetic Testing

The diagnosis of CDA I was based on history, clinical findings, laboratory data, morphological analysis of both peripheral blood and marrow smears, and genetic testing.

Local university ethical committees approved both the DNA sampling and the collection of patients' data from Medical Genetics Ambulatory in Naples (University Federico II, DAIMedLab).

Written informed consent was obtained from the patients for the participation in the study and the publication of the case report.

Genomic DNA preparation and mutational screening for *CDAN1*, *SEC23B*, and *C15orf41* genes by direct sequencing were performed as previously described (Russo et al., 2013). High-throughput sequencing by the custom multi-gene panel for hereditary anemias was performed as described (Russo et al., 2018).

The pathogenicity of the novel exonic variants has been evaluated by InterVar, a bioinformatics software tool for clinical interpretation of genetic variants based on the ACMG/AMP 2015 guideline[1]. Mainly, the pathogenicity of each variant was assessed by gathering evidence from various sources: population data, computational and predictive data, functional data, localization of the variant in a mutational hotspot and critical and well-established functional domain, and segregation data (Richards et al., 2015; Russo et al., 2018).

Cloning and Site Direct Mutagenesis

cDNA encoding full-length wild-type (WT) *C15orf41* sequence was cloned in the pCMV-Tag1 vector for mammalian cell expression (Invitrogen) in the BglII and XhoI sites, to obtain an N-terminal tagged protein with FLAG. The point mutations c.281A > C, p.Tyr94Ser (Y94S) and c.689A > C, p.His230Pro (H230P) were introduced into the pCMV-Tag1 vector by using a QuikChange site-directed mutagenesis kit (Stratagene) (Russo et al., 2017). The coding sequence was sequenced after mutagenesis.

Cell Cultures, Transfections, and Stable Clones Production

Hek-293, HepG2, HuH7, MG-63, HEL, and K562 cells were obtained from American Type Culture Collection (ATCC, Manassas, VA, United States). Cells were maintained in Dulbecco's modified Eagle medium (DMEM) (Invitrogen) or RPMI 1640 medium (Invitrogen) supplemented with 10% fetal bovine serum (Invitrogen), 100 U/mL penicillin (Invitrogen), and 100 mg/mL streptomycin (Invitrogen) in a humidified 5% CO_2 atmosphere at 37°C, according to the manufacturer's instructions. Hek-293 cells (400×10^3) were transfected with pCMV-Tag1-C15orf41 plasmids (2.5 µg/well) using the DNA Transfection Reagent (TransFectin Lipid Reagent, Bio-Rad) according to the manufacturer's procedures. Cells were collected 16, 24, and 48 h after the transfection to perform RNA and protein extractions. For generating K562 stably over-expressing *C15ORF41* gene, 10^6 cells were transfected with pCMV-Tag1-C15orf41 plasmids using Hily Max DNA Transfection Reagent (Dojindo Laboratories). After 48 h, G418 (0.6 mg/mL) was added as a selection marker. Clones were generated according to the limiting dilution method (see **Supplementary Material** for further details).

---

[1] http://wintervar.wglab.org/

Erythroid Differentiation and Flow Cytometry

Erythroid differentiation of K562-C15orf41 stable clones (2×10^5/mL) was performed adding 50 μM hemin (Sigma) to the culture medium, after 24 h of starvation (Andolfo et al., 2010). Cells were collected before hemin addition (0 days) and two days after hemin addition (2 days). For cell cycle analysis, K562 stable clones were harvested by centrifugation, resuspended in PBS containing 3.75% Nonidet P-40, 100 μg/ml RNase A and 40 μg/ml propidium iodide, and incubated at room temperature for 3 h in the dark. The cell antigen profile was analyzed by flow cytometry through evaluation of CD71 (proerythroblasts) and CD235a (proerythroblasts and orthochromatic erythroblasts). Samples were analyzed on a FACS flow cytometer (Becton Dickinson Immunocytometry Systems, BDIS).

Gene Expression Analysis

Total RNA was extracted either from peripheral blood leukocytes (PBLs), reticulocytes and from cell lines using TRIzol reagent (Life Technologies). Synthesis of cDNA from total RNA (2 μg) was performed using SensiFAST™ cDNA Synthesis Kit (Bioline). Quantitative RT-PCR (qRT-PCR) using Power SYBR Green PCR Master Mix (Applied Biosystems) was performed on Applied Biosystems 7900HT Sequence Detection System using standard cycling conditions. β-actin was used as internal control, while the Neomycin resistance gene was used as a control of transfection efficiency for K562 stable clones. Relative gene expression was calculated by using the $2^{-\Delta Ct}$ method, as described (Russo et al., 2013).

Subcellular Fractionation and Western Blotting

Proteins were extracted from cell lines using RIPA lysis buffer containing protease inhibitor cocktail (1×). Subcellular fractionation in nuclear and cytoplasmic proteins was performed using NE-PER™ Nuclear and Cytoplasmic Extraction Reagents (Thermo Fisher Scientific™). Equal amounts of protein from each lysate, as determined by a Bradford assay, were subjected to 12% sodium dodecyl sulfate-polyacrylamide gel electrophoresis (SDS-PAGE), and blotted onto polyvinylidene difluoride membranes (Biorad). Detection was performed with mouse anti-FLAG antibody (1:1000) (Sigma-Aldrich) and rabbit anti-C15orf41 (1:500) (Atlas Antibodies HPA061023). Since this antibody was recommended for immunofluorescence (IF) we tested its specificity for western blotting (WB) by using C15orf41 over-expression cells as a positive control (Bordeaux et al., 2010) (**Supplementary Figure S1**).

Mouse anti-TBP (TATA Binding Protein) (1:1000) (Sigma-Aldrich) and mouse anti-α-TUBULIN (1:5000) (Abcam) were used as a control for equal loading for cytosolic and nuclear proteins' extracts, respectively. Mouse anti-β-actin (1:12000) (Sigma-Aldrich) was used as a loading control for total proteins' extracts. Labeled bands were visualized and densitometric analysis performed with the BioRad Chemidoc using Quantity One software (BioRad) to obtain an integrated optical density (OD) value.

Immunofluorescence Analysis

For IF analysis 3×10^5 cells were fixed for 10 min in 4% Paraformaldehyde (PFA, Sigma) and washed in 50 mM PBS/NH4Cl (Sigma-Aldrich, Milan, Italy). After washing in PBS 1×, cells were allowed on 35 mm IBIDI μ-Dishes (Ibidi GmbH, Martinsried, Germany) coated with 0.05% poly-L-lysine (Sigma-Aldrich, Milan, Italy) to adhere. Permeabilization was performed with 0.2% Triton/PBS, followed by blocking with 1% BSA/PBS. The seeded cells were immunologically stained with rabbit anti-C15orf41 antibody (1:25) (Atlas Antibodies HPA061023), mouse anti-NUCLEOPHOSMIN (1:200), and secondary antibodies (1:200) (Alexa Fluor 546 anti-rabbit, Life Technologies and Alexa Fluor 488 anti-mouse). Nuclei were stained with 1 μg/ml DRAQ5 in PBS for 15 min at room temperature. Cells were preserved in PBS 1× and imaged using a LEICA TCS SP8 meta confocal microscope, equipped with an oil immersion plan Apochromat 63× objective 1.4 NA. The following settings were used: Green channel excitation of Alexa488 by the argon laser 488 nm line was detected with the 505–550 nm emission bandpass filter. Red channel excitation of Alexa546 by the Helium/Neon laser 543 nm line was detected with the 560–700 nm emission bandpass filter (using the Meta monochromator). Blue channel excitation of DRAQ5 by the blue diode laser 647 nm and emission bandpass filter.

Statistical Analysis

Statistical significance of differences in protein and gene expression was determined using the Mann–Whitney test or Student's t-test. Correlation analysis of C15orf41 with CDAN1 gene expression was performed by Pearson correlation test. A two-sided p-value < 0.05 was considered statistically significant.

For the in silico correlation analysis between C15orf41 and CDAN1 gene expression in normal hematopoietic cell subpopulations we used the dataset "Normal Hematopoietic Subgroups – (GEO ID: gse19599)," stored in the R2: Genomics Analysis and Visualization Platform[2], a biologist-friendly, web-based genomics analysis, and visualization application.

RESULTS

Clinical Cases and Genetic Testing

Clinical features and genetic data of the two probands are summarized in **Table 1**. Case 1 (A-II.2) was a 7-years-old female, second child from healthy non-consanguineous parents of Italian origin (Sardinia). At birth, cholestatic hepatopathy, dysmorphic features (bilateral syndactyly of the IV–V toes), and severe anemia (Hb 5.5 gr/dl) were observed. Family history was not indicative of anemia. At diagnosis, the proband presented transfusion-dependent normocytic anemia with a blood transfusion frequency every 15–20 days, and low reticulocyte count (**Table 1**). BM analysis showed: erythroid hyperplasia with 6% of cells showing megaloblastic features, nuclear abnormalities, and nuclear/cytoplasmic maturation

---

[2]http://r2.amc.nl

TABLE 1 | Clinical features of the two patients enrolled in the study.

	Case 1 (A-II.2)	Case 2 (B-II.1)*	Reference range[‡]
Age at diagnosis	7 years	2.4 years	–
Distal limb anomalies/ other features	Toes syndactyly	Thoracic dysplasia; short limbs	–
Complete blood count			
RBC ($\times 10^6/\mu$L)	2.72	3.67	3.9–5.6
Hb (g/dL)	7.8	10.6	11.0–16.0
Hct (%)	22.2	31.4	33.0–45.0
MCV (fL)	81.6	85.4	70.0–91.0
MCH (pg)	20.2	28.8	23.0–33.0
MCHC (g/dL)	24.8	33.8	23.0–33.0
Retics %	5.8	1.0	0.5–2.0
Retics count ($\times 10^3/\mu$L)	158000	36700	–
PLT ($\times 10^3/\mu$L)	–	518.0	150.0–450.0
Biochemical, laboratory data and iron balance			
Total bilirubin (mg/dL)	1.90	1.46	0.2–1.2
LDH (U/L)	779	511	125.0–243.0
Ferritin (ng/mL)	825	1512	22.0–275.0
TSAT (%)	75	89	15.0–45.0
C15ORF41 variants			
HGVS (Coding)[a]	c.281A > C	c.689A > C	–
HGVS (Protein)[b]	p.Tyr94Ser	p.His230Pro	–
RefSeq ID	rs587777101	–	–
MAF	C = 0.00001	–	–
InterVar (evidence codes)[§]	Pathogenic (PS1, PS3, PM2, PP4)	Likely pathogenic (PS3, PM2, PP4)	–

*Patient RP0_39 described in Russo et al. (2018); [‡]Reference ranges from AOU Federico II, University of Naples, Italy; [a]NM_001130010; [b]NP_001123482; [§] InterVar evidence scores by the website http://wintervar.wglab.org/evds.php; PS1, same amino acid change as an established pathogenic variant; PS3, well-established functional studies show a deleterious effect; PM2, absent (or at an extremely low frequency if recessive) in population databases; PP4, patient's phenotype is highly specific for a single gene etiology; TSAT, transferrin saturation; MAF, minor allele frequency.

asynchrony; 4% of erythroblasts were bi- and tri-nucleated; the granulopoietic/erythropoietic ratio (G:E) = 0.53. A substantial percentage of erythroblasts showed inter-nuclear bridges (5%), a typical feature of CDA I. Accordingly, genetic testing for *CDAN1* was performed, but no causative variants were identified. Conversely, when we analyzed *C15orf41* gene, we observed the presence of the transversion c.281A > C in the homozygous state, resulting in a novel aminoacidic substitution p.Tyr94Ser (Y94S). It is an ultra-rare variant (rs587777101) with a minor allele frequency (MAF) C = 0.00001 in the ExAC database. In agreement with the recessive inheritance pattern, both parents were heterozygous (**Figure 1A**).

Case 2 was a 2.4-years-old male, born from 3rd degree consanguineous parents of Turkish origin. At birth, recurrent pneumonia, thoracic dysplasia, and short limbs were observed. Family history was negative for anemia or jaundice. The proband presented transfusion-dependent normocytic anemia (12 transfusions/year), low reticulocyte count, growth retardation, and increased ferritin level, suggesting an iron loading condition (**Table 1**). No splenomegaly was observed at physical examination and abdominal echography. BM analysis showed severe megaloblastic changes and normoblasts with double or multiple nuclei, a morphological feature suggestive of CDA II. Accordingly, we firstly performed Sanger sequencing analysis for CDA II-disease gene *SEC23B*, finding no causative variants. Then, as a second-step analysis, we enrolled the patient

in our multi-gene panel for hereditary anemias, identifying the transversion c.689A > C in *C15orf41* in the homozygous state, resulting in the amino acid substitution p.His230Pro (H230P), as reported (Russo et al., 2018). In agreement with the recessive inheritance pattern, both parents were heterozygous (**Figure 1B**).

C15orf41 and *CDAN1* Gene Expression Are Directly Correlated

To evaluate the effect of the two identified mutations on C15orf41 gene expression, we initially analyzed *C15orf41* expression in PBLs isolated from the two probands and healthy controls (HCs). To note, *C15orf41* is a ubiquitous gene, showing a comparable level of expression in both PBLs and reticulocytes (**Supplementary Figure S2**). No difference in gene expression levels of the proband A-II.2 compared to those detected in HCs was observed, suggesting that Y94S variant does not affect gene expression. Conversely, we found a marked down-regulation of *C15orf41*-H230P in the second proband B-II.1 (**Figure 2A**). Likewise, we saw a similar trend of *CDAN1* expression in the two patients. Notably, the proband A-II.2 did not show any alterations of *CDAN1* expression compared to those seen in HCs, while the B-II.1 proband revealed a decrease of *CDAN1* expression level, although not statistically significant (**Figure 2B**). Of note, a direct correlation between *C15orf41* and *CDAN1* expression genes in healthy subjects was observed ($r = 0.62$, $p = 0.0006$) (**Figure 2C**). We confirmed

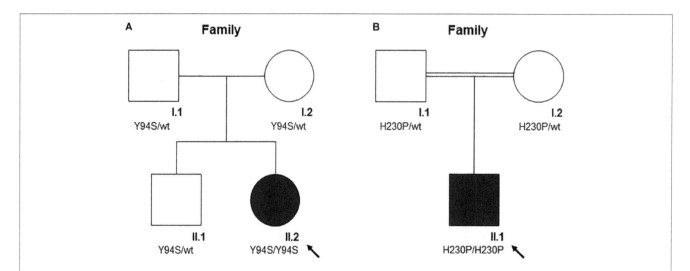

FIGURE 1 | The pedigree of the two families (**A** and **B**). Square denote males, circle females, solid symbols affected persons. The black arrow indicates probands. **(A)** The pedigree of family A is shown. According to the autosomal recessive inheritance pattern, the parents of A-II.2 are heterozygous for the variant c.281A > C, p.Tyr94Ser. **(B)** The pedigree of family B is shown. According to the autosomal recessive inheritance pattern, consanguineous parents of B-II.1 are heterozygous for the variant c.689A > C, p.His230Pro.

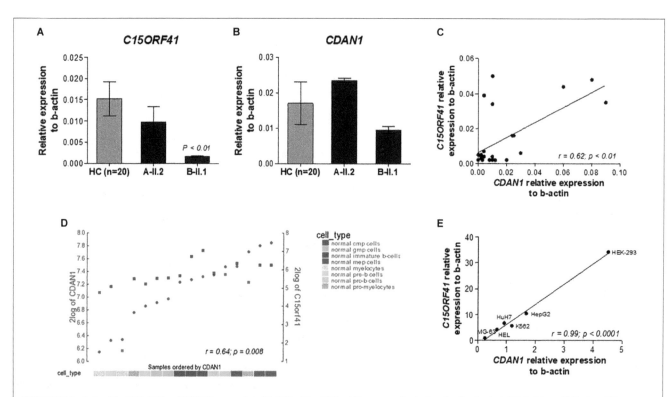

FIGURE 2 | Analysis of the *C15orf41* and *CDAN1* expression. **(A)** *C15orf41* mRNA relative expression to β-*actin* of patients A-II.2, B-II.1, and HCs (*n* = 20) are shown. Data are presented as mean ± SE. *P* value by Student's *t*-test. **(B)** *CDAN1* mRNA relative expression to β-*actin* of patients A-II.2, B-II.1 and HCs (*n* = 20) is shown. Data are presented as mean ± SE. **(C)** Correlation analysis between *C15orf41* and *CDAN1* gene expression, performed on 20 HCs and two probands, showed a direct correlation between the two genes (Pearson correlation *r* = 0.62, *p* = 0.01). **(D)** YY-plot of correlation analysis performed by R2 database to investigate the expression level of *C15orf41* and *CDAN1* genes in the expression dataset for normal flow sorted hematopoietic cell subpopulation (GEO ID: gse19599); CMP, common myeloid progenitor; GMP, granulocyte-macrophage progenitor. Pearson correlation *r* = 0.64, *p* = 0.008. **(E)** Correlation analysis between *C15orf41* and *CDAN1* expression, performed in MG-63, HEL, K562, HuH7, HepG2, and Hek-293 cell lines. MG-63, bone osteosarcoma cells; HEL, human erythroblasts; HuH7, hepatocellular carcinoma cells; HepG2, hepatocellular carcinoma cells (Pearson correlation *r* = 0.99, *p* < 0.0001).

the *ex vivo* data on *C15orf41-CDAN1* correlation by *in silico* analysis of the expression dataset for normal hematopoietic cell subpopulations, obtained by R2 database (**Figure 2D**). Additionally, we achieved comparable results by gene expression profiling of different human cell lines (Hek-293, HepG2, HuH7, MG-63, HEL, and K562 cells), where a significant direct correlation between *C15orf41* and *CDAN1* expression was observed (**Figure 2E**).

C15orf41 Localization Into Nuclear and Cytosolic Compartments

We first assessed the turnover and localization of the C15orf41 protein in Hek293 cells transiently transfected with pCMV-tag1-C15orf41. Time-course analysis showed a gradual increase of *C15orf41* gene expression in cells transfected with WT clone at 16, 24, and 48 h compared to those transfected with empty vector (EV) (**Figure 3A**). Conversely, WB analysis on the same harvested cells revealed a marked increase of C15orf41 protein level at 16 h after transfection, with a progressive decrease of the C15orf41-FLAG signal, which resulted highly down-regulated at 48 h after the transfection (**Figure 3B**).

To investigate C15orf41 localization, we assessed the endogenous protein levels and localization of the protein by both WB and IF on a nuclear and a cytosolic fraction of Hek-293 cells (**Figures 3C,D**). Both analyses confirmed that the protein was mainly expressed in the nucleus, but also in the cytosol compartment, even if in a smaller amount, suggesting a role of the protein in these two cellular compartments (**Figure 3D** and **Supplementary Figure S3**). No co-localization of C15orf41 with nucleoli was observed (**Supplementary Figure S3**).

Characterization of C15orf41-H230P and -Y94S Mutants

To study *in vitro* the pathogenetic effect of the two variants, we evaluated gene expression and protein level of both C15orf41-H230P and C15orf41-Y94S mutants at 16 h after transfection in Hek-293. In agreement with the *ex vivo* data on both patients, we observed a sharp decrease of both gene expression and protein levels in cells over-expressing C15orf41-H230P mutant compared to C15orf41-WT ones (**Figures 4A,B** and **Supplementary Figure S1**). Conversely, only a slight reduction in gene expression and protein level in cells over-expressing C15orf41-Y94S was observed (**Figures 4A,B** and **Supplementary Figure S1**).

To obtain a reliable cellular model, able to be induced to erythroid differentiation, we developed K562 cells stably over-expressing C15orf41-WT and both mutants. Over-expressing clones were selected by measuring *Neomycin* relative gene expression in each K562 clone and comparing the digestion pattern of mutant vs. WT clones (**Supplementary Figure S4**). K562 selected clones WT#3 and Y94S#5 showed strong over-expression of *C15orf41* compared to those observed in K562 EV#3 clone. Instead, H230P#10 cells showed a marked gene down-regulation respect to WT#3 cells (**Figure 5A**). WB analysis confirmed the same trend for all the clones (**Figure 5B**).

To investigate if both mutants could affect erythroid differentiation, we treated K562 cells with hemin. Evaluation of CD71 and CD235 differentiation markers showed a statistically significant decreased percentage of $CD71^+/CD235^+$ cells in both Y94S and H230P clones compared to the WT one (**Figure 5C**). Moreover, we observed a slight increase of the rate of S-phase at cell cycle analysis in K562 cells over-expressing Y94S and H230P mutants compared to WT, although not statistically significant (**Figure 5D** and **Supplementary Figure S5**). To note, immunolocalization analysis of C15orf41 protein in K562 stable clones highlighted a preferential localization of the mutated proteins within nuclear compartment compared to WT one, similarly to those observed in Hek-293 cells transiently over-expressing C15orf41 mutants (**Figure 5E**).

DISCUSSION

CDA type I is an autosomal recessive disorder that belongs to the heterogeneous group of inherited BM failure syndromes. To date, two causative genes have been associated to this condition: *CDAN1* that is the most frequently mutated; *C15orf41* that has been found mutated in five unrelated patients, so far (Babbs et al., 2013; Palmblad et al., 2018; Russo et al., 2018). Most of the CDA I patients exhibit lifelong macrocytic anemia with variable values of Hb. *C15orf41* patients show clinical features like *CDAN1* ones. Anyhow, a slight difference in Hb level and MCV value has been observed between the two subgroups of patients (Gambale et al., 2016).

We herein described two unrelated cases of C15orf41-related CDA I. Both patients presented clinical characteristics, hematological status, and morphological features of erythroblasts compatible with a suspicion of CDA I. Particularly, the presence of a substantial amount of inter-nuclear bridges between erythroblasts, a typical feature of CDA I, at the BM analysis of the case 1 (A-II.2), prompted us to perform the molecular screening of both CDA I causative genes. No causative variants in *CDAN1* were identified, while genetic testing of *C15orf41* highlighted the presence of the homozygous missense mutation Y94S. This variant resulted annotated on public databases as ultra-rare single nucleotide variant. Of note, it is a novel missense change at an amino acid residue where a different pathogenic missense change, Y94C, has been previously described (Babbs et al., 2013). Case 2 (B-II.1) was initially suspected of suffering from CDA type II, since he presented normocytic anemia and non-specific morphological erythroblast features, such as the presence of bi- and multi-nuclearity, megaloblastic changes, but no inter-nuclear bridges. Of note, among syndromes showing dyserythropoiesis, there is not a full concordance between experienced hematologists in recognition of these features (Goasguen et al., 2018). Indeed, accurate molecular screening remains the most reliable diagnosis for these patients. First genetic testing for *SEC23B* revealed no mutations in this gene. Thus, the patient was analyzed by a t-NGS panel for red blood cell disorders, that allowed us the identification of the homozygous missense variant H230P in the *C15orf41* gene (Russo et al., 2018).

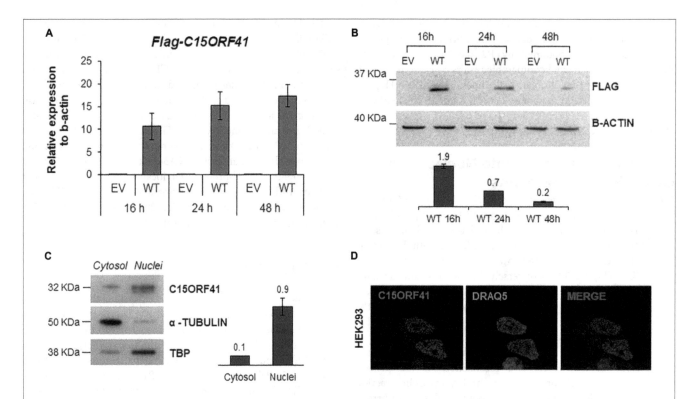

FIGURE 3 | C15orf41-WT expression and subcellular localization. **(A)** The panel shows *FLAG-C15orf41* mRNA relative expression to β-actin of Hek-293 cells over-expressing pCMV-tag1-C15orf41 WT compared to those transfected with empty vector (EV) at 16, 24, and 48 after the transfection. Data from two different transfections are presented as mean ± SD. **(B)** The panel shows WB analysis of Hek-293 cells over-expressing pCMV-tag1-C15orf41 WT compared to those transfected with EV at 16, 24, and 48 h after the transfection. β-actin is loading control. Sizes (in kDa) are on the left. The histogram shows the densitometric quantification based on β-actin amount. Data derived from two experiments are presented as mean ± SD. **(C)** WB on cytosolic and nuclear fractions of Hek-293 cells showing C15orf41 expression. TBP and α- TUBULIN are shown as a loading control of nuclear and cytosolic compartments, respectively. The histogram shows the densitometric quantification based on TBP and α- TUBULIN amounts. Data derived from three experiments are presented as mean ± SD. Sizes (in kDa) are on the left. **(D)** Immunofluorescence analysis of Hek-293 cells is shown. Rabbit anti-C15orf41 antibody was used to stain C15orf41 protein. DRAQ5 was used as a nuclear marker. Overlapping of both signals (MERGE) is shown on the right.

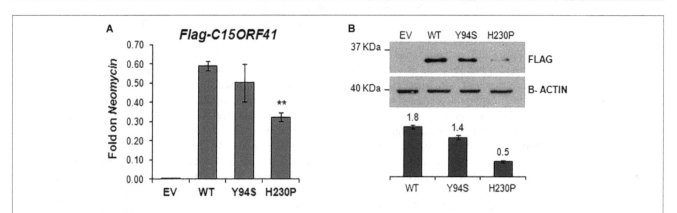

FIGURE 4 | *In vitro* characterization of C15orf41 mutants. **(A)** The panel shows *FLAG-C15orf41* mRNA expression normalized on *Neomycin* of Hek-293 cells over-expressing pCMV-tag1-C15orf41-WT, -Y94S, and -H230P compared to those transfected with EV at 16 h after the transfection. *P* value by Student's *t*-test. *******P* < 0.01. **(B)** The panel shows WB analysis of Hek-293 cells over-expressing pCMV-tag1-C15orf41-WT, -Y94S, and -H230P compared to those transfected with EV at 16 h after the transfection. The histogram shows the densitometric quantification based on the β-actin as a loading control. Data derived from three experiments are presented as mean ± SD. Sizes (in kDa) are on the left.

To investigate the expression and subcellular localization of C15orf41, we expressed the full-length WT protein fused to a FLAG-tag. Time-course analysis evidenced an indirect correlation between gene expression and protein levels, suggesting a rapid turnover of the protein. It was recently found that C15orf41 has at least three post-translational modification sites, such as K50 (Acetylation), T114 (Phosphorylation) and K176 (Ubiquitination) (Ahmed et al., 2018). Since

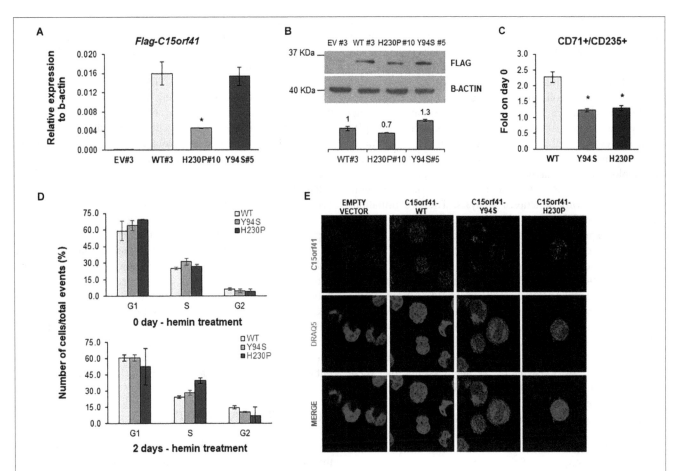

FIGURE 5 | Analysis of K562-C15orf41 over-expressing clones during hemin-induced erythroid differentiation. **(A)** *FLAG-C15orf41* mRNA relative expression to β-actin of K562 cells stably over-expressing C15orf41-WT, -Y94S, and -H230P compared to the EV. Data derived from two experiments are presented as mean ± SD. *P* value by Student's *t*-test. *P < 0.05. **(B)** WB analysis of K562 cells stably over-expressing C15orf41-WT, -H230P, and -Y94S compared to the EV. The histogram shows the densitometric quantification based on the β-actin. Data derived from two experiments are presented as mean ± SD. Sizes (in kDa) are on the left. **(C)** Erythroid differentiation markers of C15orf41-K562 stable clones. The histogram shows the percentage of CD71$^+$/CD125$^+$ cells at two days of hemin treatment normalized on untreated cells (0 days). Data derived from two experiments are presented as mean ± SD. *P* value by Student's *t*-test. *P < 0.05. **(D)** The histograms show the number of K562 over-expressing pCMV-tag1-C15orf41-WT, -Y94S, and -H230P cells on total events (%) in G1, S, and G2 phases of the cell cycle. Data derived from two experiments are presented as mean ± SD. **(E)** Immunofluorescence analysis of K562 stable clones is shown. Rabbit anti-C15orf41 antibody was used to stain C15orf41 protein. DRAQ5 was used as a nuclear marker. Overlapping of both signals (MERGE) is shown at the bottom.

that ubiquitination is one of the most common signals for proteasome-mediated degradation (Hershko and Ciechanover, 1998), we speculated that C15orf41 is degraded via proteasome during the cell cycle. Moreover, this data is corroborated by the fact that it could be a cell cycle-regulated protein, as well as Codanin-1 (Noy-Lotan et al., 2009), and that the two proteins could interact. Our *ex vivo* and *in vitro* analyses demonstrated that *C15orf41* and *CDAN1* gene expression levels were directly correlated in patients, healthy controls, and different cell lines. Of note, Codanin-1 was proved to be part of the cytosolic Asf1-H3-H4-importin-4 complex, which is implicated in nucleosome assembly and disassembly (Ask et al., 2012).

Similarly, C15orf41 was predicted to interact with Asf1b (Ewing et al., 2007). These data suggested that both proteins are needed together to accomplish their function, thus could be regulated by the same mechanism, could control each other

in a positive feedback loop, or could interact with each other. To note, *CDAN1* and *C15orf41* are ubiquitously expressed genes, but their alterations mainly affect the erythroid lineage. One possible explanation may be that erythroid progenitors have a uniquely fast cell cycle, although CDA patients do not manifest abnormalities of other tissues containing fast-dividing cell types, such as gut epithelium or hair follicles. Other hypotheses include nuclear extrusion in erythroblasts, which requires the eviction of histones, such as H3 and H4, and C15orf41 and Codanin-1 may play a role in this process (Roy and Babbs, 2019).

The analysis of cytosolic and nuclear fractions demonstrated that C15orf41 endogenous protein exhibits mainly nuclear localization. Accordingly, nuclear localization signals and nuclear export signals were predicted in the amino acid sequence, confirming that the protein is exported from the nucleus to the cytoplasm and vice-versa. Once again, changes in C15orf41 nuclear-cytoplasmic localization could represent a mechanism, or the effect, of its regulation. According to the predicted Holliday junction resolvase function of C15ORF41 and its potential role in DNA repair machinery as guardians of genome integrity and viability, we initially hypothesized that C15orf41 could localize in the nucleoli. Indeed, it was recently demonstrated that the nucleolus, long regarded as a mere ribosome producing factory, plays a crucial role in monitoring and responding to cellular stress, as well as in DNA repair mechanisms (Mayer and Grummt, 2005; Ogawa and Baserga, 2017). However, our immunolocalization data did not support this hypothesis.

We further characterized the identified variants by both *ex vivo* and *in vitro* functional analyses. The two mutations showed different behavior. Indeed, the Y94S variation did not affect gene expression, and only slightly decreased the protein level. On the contrary, the H230P mutation induced a sharp decrease in gene expression and protein level.

Of note, Y94S variant is located in the two turn-helix-turn DNA binding domains (DBD) of the protein, together with the previously identified Y94C and P20R mutations (Babbs et al., 2013; Palmblad et al., 2018). On the contrary, H230P variant is located in the PD-(D/E) XK nuclease domain, as well as the two causative mutations L178Q and Y238C (Babbs et al., 2013; Palmblad et al., 2018). Therefore, we might assume that these variants could have a different effect on both the protein function and the pathogenetic mechanism of the disease.

Since no impaired expression of C15orf41-Y94S was observed, we speculate that this mutation could affect the three-dimensional structure of the protein and, thus, undermine the binding to the DNA.

Since CDA I mutated proteins affect mainly the erythroid lineage, we developed K562 cells stably over-expressing C15orf41 WT and mutants to induce erythroid differentiation. This cellular model allowed us to demonstrate that both mutant clones showed impaired erythroid differentiation, exhibiting a decreased percentage of CD71$^+$/CD235$^+$ cells at two days of hemin treatment. Moreover, both Y94S and H230P clones were retained in the S phase of the cell cycle during differentiation, although with a different degree. It has been already demonstrated that

there is an interdependence between S-phase progression and an essential commitment step during erythroid differentiation in which, within few hours, cells become dependent on the hormone erythropoietin, undergo activating changes in chromatin of red cell genes, and activate GATA-1, the erythroid master transcriptional regulator. Arresting S-phase progression at this time prevents the execution of this commitment step and subsequent induction of red cell genes (Pop et al., 2010). Of note, *CDAN1*-CDA Ia cultured erythroblasts showed an increase in S-phase cells, suggesting a cell cycle arrest (Tamary et al., 1996). Nevertheless, based on the present data, we are not able to establish if the increased number of cells in S-phase represents faster cycling cells or a block in S-phase.

This study represents the first investigation of both the expression and the localization of C15orf41. Our *ex vivo* and *in vitro* analyses demonstrated that C15orf41 and CDAN1 are tightly correlated, suggesting a shared mechanism of regulation between the two genes and related proteins. The different behavior of both Y94S-DBD-mutation and H230P-PD-(D/E) XK-mutation could be related to the dual function of the C15orf41 protein within separate subcellular compartments. Nevertheless, both variants resulted in impaired erythroid maturation, suggesting the block of cell cycle dynamics as a putative pathogenic mechanism for C15orf41-related CDA I.

AUTHOR CONTRIBUTIONS

RR, RM, and IA designed and conducted the study, and prepared the manuscript. AI critically reviewed the study. GDR and BR collaborated to the generation of cellular models. FM performed Sanger sequencing and t-NGS. MR performed flow cytometry analyses. SU, SB, and AG cared for the patients.

ACKNOWLEDGMENTS

We thank Alessia Romano of the CEINGE Advanced Light Microscopy Facility for expert help in data acquisition.

REFERENCES

Ahmed, M. S., Shahjaman, M., Kabir, E., and Kamruzzaman, M. (2018). Structure modeling to function prediction of uncharacterized human protein C15orf41. *Bioinformation* 14, 206–212. doi: 10.6026/97320630014206

Andolfo, I., De Falco, L., Asci, R., Russo, R., Colucci, S., Gorrese, M., et al. (2010). Regulation of divalent metal transporter 1 (DMT1) non-IRE isoform by the microRNA Let-7d in erythroid cells. *Haematologica* 95, 1244–1252. doi: 10.3324/haematol.2009.020685

Ask, K., Jasencakova, Z., Menard, P., Feng, Y., Almouzni, G., Groth, A., et al. (2012). Codanin-1, mutated in the anaemic disease CDAI, regulates Asf1 function in S-phase histone supply. *EMBO J.* 31, 2013–2023. doi: 10.1038/emboj.2012.55

Babbs, C., Roberts, N. A., Sanchez-Pulido, L., McGowan, S. J., Ahmed, M. R., Brown, J. M., et al. (2013). Homozygous mutations in a predicted endonuclease are a novel cause of congenital dyserythropoietic anemia type I. *Haematologica* 98, 1383–1387. doi: 10.3324/haematol.2013.089490

Bordeaux, J., Welsh, A., Agarwal, S., Killiam, E., Baquero, M., Hanna, J., et al. (2010). Antibody validation. *Biotechniques* 48, 197–209. doi: 10.2144/000113382

Dgany, O., Avidan, N., Delaunay, J., Krasnov, T., Shalmon, L., Shalev, H., et al. (2002). Congenital dyserythropoietic anemia type I is caused by mutations in codanin-1. *Am. J. Hum. Genet.* 71, 1467–1474. doi: 10.1086/344781

Ewing, R. M., Chu, P., Elisma, F., Li, H., Taylor, P., Climie, S., et al. (2007). Large-scale mapping of human protein-protein interactions by mass spectrometry. *Mol. Syst. Biol.* 3:89. doi: 10.1038/msb4100134

Gambale, A., Iolascon, A., Andolfo, I., and Russo, R. (2016). Diagnosis and management of congenital dyserythropoietic anemias. *Expert Rev. Hematol.* 9, 283–296. doi: 10.1586/17474086.2016.1131608

Goasguen, J. E., Bennett, J. M., Bain, B. J., Brunning, R., Vallespi, M. T., Tomonaga, M., et al. (2018). Dyserythropoiesis in the diagnosis of the myelodysplastic syndromes and other myeloid neoplasms: problem areas. *Br. J. Haematol.* 182, 526–533. doi: 10.1111/bjh.15435

Hershko, A., and Ciechanover, A. (1998). The ubiquitin system. *Annu. Rev. Biochem.* 67, 425–479. doi: 10.1146/annurev.biochem.67.1.425

Kellermann, K., Neuschwander, N., Högel, J., and Schwarz, K. (2010). The morphological diagnosis of congenital dyserythropoietic anemia: results of a quantitative analysis of peripheral blood and bone marrow cells. *Haematologica* 95, 1034–1036. doi: 10.3324/haematol.2009.014563

Mayer, C., and Grummt, I. (2005). Cellular stress and nucleolar function. *Cell Cycle* 4, 1036–1038. doi: 10.4161/cc.4.8.1925

Noy-Lotan, S., Dgany, O., Lahmi, R., Marcoux, N., Krasnov, T., Yissachar, N., et al. (2009). Codanin-1, the protein encoded by the gene mutated in congenital dyserythropoietic anemia type I (CDAN1), is cell cycle-regulated. *Haematologica* 94, 629–637. doi: 10.3324/haematol.2008. 003327

Ogawa, L. M., and Baserga, S. J. (2017). Crosstalk between the nucleolus and the DNA damage response. *Mol. Biosyst.* 13, 443–455. doi: 10.1039/c6mb00740f

Palmblad, J., Sander, B., Bain, B., Klimkowska, M., and Björck, E. (2018). Congenital dyserythropoietic anemia type 1: a case with novel compound heterozygous mutations in the C15orf41 gene. *Am. J. Hematol.* doi: 10.1002/ ajh.25157 [Epub ahead of print].

Pop, R., Shearstone, J. R., Shen, Q., Liu, Y., Hallstrom, K., Koulnis, M., et al. (2010). A key commitment step in erythropoiesis is synchronized with the cell cycle clock through mutual inhibition between PU.1 and S-phase progression. *PLoS Biol.* 8:e1000484. doi: 10.1371/journal.pbio.1000484

Richards, S., Aziz, N., Bale, S., Bick, D., Das, S., Gastier-Foster, J., et al. (2015). Standards and guidelines for the interpretation of sequence variants: a joint consensus recommendation of the american college of medical genetics and genomics and the association for molecular pathology. *Genet. Med.* 17, 405–424. doi: 10.1038/gim.2015.30

Roy, N. B. A., and Babbs, C. (2019). The pathogenesis, diagnosis and management of CDA type I. *Br. J. Haematol.* 185, 436–449. doi: 10.1111/bjh.15817

Russo, R., Andolfo, I., Gambale, A., De Rosa, G., Manna, F., Arillo, A., et al. (2017). GATA1 erythroid-specific regulation of SEC23B expression and its implication in the pathogenesis of congenital dyserythropoietic anemia type II. *Haematologica* 102, e371–e374. doi: 10.3324/haematol.2016.162966

Russo, R., Andolfo, I., Manna, F., Gambale, A., Marra, R., Rosato, B. E., et al. (2018). Multi-gene panel testing improves diagnosis and management of patients with hereditary anemias. *Am. J. Hematol.* 93, 672–682. doi: 10.1002/ajh.2508

Russo, R., Langella, C., Esposito, M. R., Gambale, A., Vitiello, F., Vallefuoco, F., et al. (2013). Hypomorphic mutations of SEC23B gene account for mild phenotypes of congenital dyserythropoietic anemia type II. *Blood Cells Mol. Dis.* 51, 17–21. doi: 10.1016/j.bcmd.2013.02.003

Tamary, H., Shalev, H., Luria, D., Shaft, D., Zoldan, M., Shalmon, L., et al. (1996). Clinical features and studies of erythropoiesis in israeli bedouins with congenital dyserythropoietic anemia type I. *Blood* 87, 1763–1770.

6

CoDysAn: A Telemedicine Tool to Improve Awareness and Diagnosis for Patients with Congenital Dyserythropoietic Anemia

Cristian Tornador [1,2], Edgar Sánchez-Prados [3], Beatriz Cadenas [4,5,6], Roberta Russo [7,8], Veronica Venturi [9], Immacolata Andolfo [7,8], Ines Hernández-Rodriguez [10], Achille Iolascon [7,8] and Mayka Sánchez [1,9*]

[1] BloodGenetics S.L., Barcelona, Spain, [2] Teresa Moreto Foundation, Barcelona, Spain, [3] Bioinformatics for Health Sciences Master Programme, Universitat Pompeu Fabra, Barcelona, Spain, [4] Whole Genix SL., Barcelona, Spain, [5] Universitat de Vic-Universitat Central de Catalunya, Vic, Spain, [6] Iron Metabolism: Regulation and Diseases Group, Josep Carreras Leukaemia Research Institute, Campus Can Ruti, Barcelona, Spain, [7] Department of Molecular Medicine and Medical Biotechnologies, University of Naples Federico II, Naples, Italy, [8] CEINGE–Biotecnologie Avanzate, Naples, Italy, [9] Iron Metabolism: Regulation and Diseases Group, Department of Basic Sciences, Faculty of Medicine and Health Sciences, Universitat Internacional de Catalunya, Barcelona, Spain, [10] Haematology Service, Hospital Germans Trias i Pujol University Hospital, Oncology Catalan Institute, Barcelona, Spain

*Correspondence:
Mayka Sánchez
msanchezfe@uic.es

Congenital Dyserythropoietic Anemia (CDA) is a heterogeneous group of hematological disorders characterized by chronic hyporegenerative anemia and distinct morphological abnormalities of erythroid precursors in the bone marrow. In many cases, a final diagnosis is not achieved due to different levels of awareness for the diagnosis of CDAs and lack of use of advanced diagnostic procedures. Researchers have identified five major types of CDA: types I, II, III, IV, and X-linked dyserythropoietic anemia and thrombocytopenia (XLDAT). Proper management in CDA is still unsatisfactory, as the different subtypes of CDA have different genetic causes and different but overlapping patterns of signs and symptoms. For this reason, we developed a new telemedicine tool that will help doctors to achieve a faster diagnostic for this disease. Using open access code, we have created a responsive webpage named CoDysAn (**Co**ngenital **Dys**erythropoietic **An**emia) that includes practical information for CDA awareness and a step-by-step diagnostic tool based on a CDA algorithm. The site is currently available in four languages (Catalan, Spanish, Italian, and English). This telemedicine webpage is available at http://www.codysan.eu.

Keywords: telemedicine tool, congenital dyserythropoietic anemia, diagnosis, algorithm, hematological disease

INTRODUCTION

Congenital Dyserythropoietic Anemia (CDA) is a heterogeneous group of hematological disorders characterized by chronic hyporegenerative anemia and distinct morphological abnormalities of erythroid precursors in the bone marrow. Patients with CDA present congenital and chronic anemia of variable degree with a reticulocytosis not corresponding to the degree of anemia (ineffective erythropoiesis), jaundice and frequently splenomegaly and/or hepatomegaly (Iolascon et al., 2012, 2013).

Five classical types of CDAs (I–II–III–IV and XLTDA) have been defined based on bone marrow morphology. Among all types, CDA type II is the most common and well-known form. Genetically,

CDA type Ia (OMIN 224120) and CDA type Ib (OMIM 615631) are caused by mutations in codanin 1 (*CDAN1*) (chr 15q15.2) and *C15orf41* (chr15q14) genes, respectively (Dgany et al., 2002; Babbs et al., 2013). CDA type II (OMIM 224100) is due to pathogenic variants in Sec23 homolog B, coat complex II component (*SEC23B*) gene (chr20p11.23) (Bianchi et al., 2009; Schwarz et al., 2009). Few patients with CDA type III (OMIM 105600) have been described: they present the same mutation in the Kinesin Family Member 23 (*KIF23*) gene (chr15q23) (Liljeholm et al., 2013). CDA type IV (OMIM 613673) is due to mutations in the Kruppel Like Factor 1 (*KLF1*) gene (chr19p13.13) (Arnaud et al., 2010; Jaffray et al., 2013). Finally, X-linked dyserythropoietic anemia and thrombocytopenia (XLDAT) (OMIM 300367) is caused by mutations in transcription factor GATA Binding Protein 1 (*GATA1*) gene (chr Xp11.23) (Nichols et al., 2000; Del Vecchio et al., 2005). CDA types I and II are inherited in an autosomal recessive manner, CDA type III and IV present an autosomal dominant inheritance pattern and X-linked dyserythropoietic anemia with thrombocytopenia has an X-linked mode of inheritance.

Depending on the type of CDA, different treatments have been established. Allogenic bone marrow transplantation has been successfully employed in a few severe cases of CDAI and CDAII. CDA III patients may require a transfusion only during times of extreme anemia e.g., pregnancy or surgery. Treatment focuses on hemoglobin normalization with the administration of interferon (IFN) alpha is used with success in CDA I patients with *CDAN1* mutations; however, patients bearing a mutation in a different gene i.e., *C15ORF41* were unresponsive to this same treatment. Severe cases of fetal anemia associated with CDAI, CDAII, and XLTDA may require intrauterine transfusions. Blood iron levels should be closely monitored in CDA I, CDAII, and other CDA patients undergoing regular transfusions. In these cases, morbidity may be severe due to iron overload complications that can be fatal if left untreated (Gambale et al., 2016; Palmer et al., 2018); therefore, it is imperative to monitor iron overload and induce iron depletion, when needed, by iron chelation. This working classification of CDA is still in use in clinical practice; however, the identification of the mutated genes involved in the majority of CDA subgroups will improve the diagnostic possibilities and allow a better classification of CDA patients. At present, in many cases, a final diagnosis is not achieved due to different levels of awareness for the diagnosis of CDAs and lack of use of advanced diagnostic procedures. In addition, there are families that fulfill the general definition of CDAs, but do not conform to any of the classical CDA variants. Therefore, it is very plausible that new forms of CDA may exist. These new forms will be possibly identified if a proper diagnosed is achieved in each patient suspected with CDA. Toward this goal, we have developed a new telemedicine tool named CoDysAn (**Co**ngenital **Dys**erythropoietic **An**emia) for the management and diagnosis of patients with this disease.

The aim of CoDysAn webpage is to provide a freely accessible website where general public, patients and medical doctors can better understand and learn more about this disease. Moreover,

CoDysAn web page includes a diagnosis algorithm tool to ease the classification and diagnostic of CDA types.

METHODS

Patients and Validation

CoDysAn web algorithm has been developed with a set of 24 patients genetically diagnosed of different types of CDA (18 CDA type II, 1 CDA type Ib, 4 CDA type Ia, and 1 XLTDA) and with a set of 19 additional patients genetically diagnosed of non-CDA hereditable anemias including eight hereditary spherocytosis, four patients with pyruvate kinase defects, one patient with pyruvate kinase defect and a beta thalassemia trait, one patient with defects in hemolytic anemia due to adenylate kinase deficiency (AK1) gene, one patient with X-linked sideroblastic anemia, three patients with dehydrated hereditary stomatocytosis type 1 (DHS1) and one patient with dehydrated hereditary stomatocytosis type 2 (DHS2). A different set of 23 CDAII patients was utilized to independently validate the algorithm. Patients were previously reported (Iolascon et al., 2009; Schwarz et al., 2009; Russo et al., 2010, 2011, 2013, 2014, 2016, 2018; Unal et al., 2014; Andolfo et al., 2015, 2018; Di Pierro et al., 2015) and diagnosed at the Medical Genetics Unit of A.O.U. Federico II, CEINGE–Biotecnologie Avanzate (Napoli).

Design of Web Server

CoDysAn is implemented in PHP, HTML5, CSS, and Javascript. The web server is executed in a XAMPP. Network visualization and interactive exploration modules are based on several open-source projects: Bootstrap, jQuery and Filezilla. The source code of the diagnostic tool algorithm is implemented in php at http://www.codysan.eu/diagnostics-tool.html. It is integrated within this web page between lines 661 and 1,204 in four steps corresponding to the four steps of the form. The code can be checked by typing in a browser: "view-source: http://www.codysan.eu/diagnostics-tool.html."

Implementation

CoDysAn algorithm is based on the diagnostic workflow previously proposed (Iolascon et al., 2012; Gambale et al., 2016). This algorithm is based on hematological parameters depending on age and gender (**Table 1**). Age is split in three groups: from 0 to 6 months old; from 6 months to 12 years old; and older than 12 years. Hematological tested parameters include: hemoglobin levels, mean corpuscular volume (MCV), reticulocytes count and platelets count. Exclusion of other possible causes of anemia is also considered in the final step of the algorithm. References values for hematological data are adapted from general hematological reference books (Rabinovitch, 1990; Wakeman et al., 2007; Hoffman et al., 2018).

RESULTS

CoDySan Scope

Following previous experience of the group in developing telemedicine tools for management and diagnosis of patients (HIGHFERRITIN Web server http://highferritin.imppc.org/

TABLE 1 | Parameter thresholds used by the diagnostic CoDysAn algorithm.

Parameter		0–6 months	6 months to 12 years	>12 years	Units
Hemoglobin	M	9.5–18	11–15.5	13–17.5	g/dL
	F	9.5–18	11–15.5	12–16	
MCV*	M	77.5–111.5	74–89.5	80–100	fL
	F	77.5–111.5	74–89.5	80–100	
Reticulocytes	M	61–134	24–114	29–95	$\times 10^9$/L
	F	67–142	40–162	27–91	
Platelets	M	145–450	145–450	145–450	$\times 10^9$/L
	F	145–450	145–450	145–450	

MCV stands for Mean Corpuscular Volume. M stands for male and F stands for female.

tool) (Altes et al., 2014), we have developed CoDySan web tool. CoDySan is a user-friendly webpage for a better awareness on the rare hereditary hematological diseases, congenital dyserythropoietic anemias (CDAs). CoDySan webpage includes a step-by-step diagnostic algorithm based on **Figure 1**. The site is freely available at URL http://www.codysan.eu in four languages (Catalan, Spanish, Italian, and English).

Webpage Structure and Design

The CoDysAn website is currently containing seven sections (see **Supplementary Figure 1** to visualize several screenshots of different sections of CoDysAn webpage): A home or main webpage section including links to other sections of the site to make information more accessible; The CoDysAn section, where one can found information about congenital dyserythropoietic anemia (CDA) disease, the CoDysAn project as a whole research project, the privacy policy, cookies policy and medical disclaimer reminding that, as any other telemedicine project, CoDysAn diagnostic tool is a preliminary diagnostic test and expert medical doctors should be contacted for a conclusive diagnosis; The diagnostic section, including the CDA algorithm flowchart (**Figure 1**) and a step-by-step diagnostic tool with specific instructions on how to use it; The collaborators section, including links to the contributors for the CoDysAn project, patient associations and links to similar web tools, such as HIGHFERRITIN web server; A resource section, including news on the CoDysAn project, bibliographical references and reference values used for the diagnostic algorithm (see also **Table 1**); An opinion section containing a Google form that allows users to express their opinion and degree of satisfaction with the website; A contact section, where users can directly contact CoDysAn developers to address any doubt regarding the webpage.

Diagnostic Telemedicine Tool

The diagnostic algorithm used for setting up the CoDysAn diagnostic tool is depicted in **Figure 1**. A step-by-step and user-friendly form will progressively ask relevant patient information; in the first stage, age, gender and hemoglobin levels should be provided to discern if the patient has hyperhemoglobinemia (high hemoglobin values in regards to the reference value), anemia or if the values are inside the normal range, in which case the web tool will return a text indicating that there is no anemia.

Due to fluctuations in the hematological parameters, the algorithm correlates to the reference values for the hematological provided data (hemoglobin level, reticulocytes, platelets, etc.) according to age and gender, see **Table 1**. To simplify the algorithm, we have only considered three different age ranges, from 0 to 6 months, from 6 to 12 years, and older than 12 years old.

If anemia is detected, i.e., the hemoglobin levels are below the normal values for the indicated gender and age range, the algorithm will ask for three additional hematological parameters: mean corpuscular volume (MCV), reticulocytes count, and platelets count.

Users can change the input units of the provided hematological parameter. These values are converted to the international system of reference units and the value is used to check if the parameters are within range for their given thresholds (see **Table 1**).

Depending on the data provided, a new form will appear asking to exclude specific possible causes of macrocytic, normocytic or microcytic anemia. At least one alternative cause of anemia should be excluded to proceed with the diagnostic tool. In the following step, the user is asked to select additional patient's clinical or biochemical factors, such as binucleated erythroblasts, malformations or electron microscopy features.

Finally, depending on the provided information, CoDySan tool will return a result of clinical suspicion (any of the CDA types) if it applies, or a brief explanation if there is no clinical suspicion of CDA.

If a clinical suspicion of CDA is indicated, the user has the option to search for world-wide genetic laboratories that provide clinical diagnostic tests for a particular CDA gene via the button "Search Lab." The list of world-wide genetic laboratories is taken from the NCBI's Genetic Testing Registry (GTR) webpage (Rubinstein et al., 2013). There is also the possibility to refresh the webpage and perform a new diagnostic test via the button "New diagnostic."

Validation

The CodysAn algorithm has been designed with 43 patients with hereditable anemia, including 24 patients genetically diagnosed with different types of CDA (18 CDA type II, 1 CDA type Ib, 4 CDA type IIa, and 1 XLTDA) and 19 additional patients genetically diagnosed with non-CDA hereditable anemias. The algorithm achieved a specificity of 89.5% and a sensibility of 87.5%. An additional set of 23 patients (all CDA II) was utilized to validate the algorithm, which returned a specificity of 87%.

DISCUSSION

Telemedicine webpages and tools are significantly changing the way medical doctors and patients approach health care and diagnosis (Dinesen et al., 2016). CoDysAn telemedicine tool is a webpage intended to increase awareness about the rare disease CDA as, currently, patients suffering from this disease are under-diagnosed (Russo et al., 2014). The content of the webpage serves as an informative and training resource for the general public, patients and medical doctors. The use of this

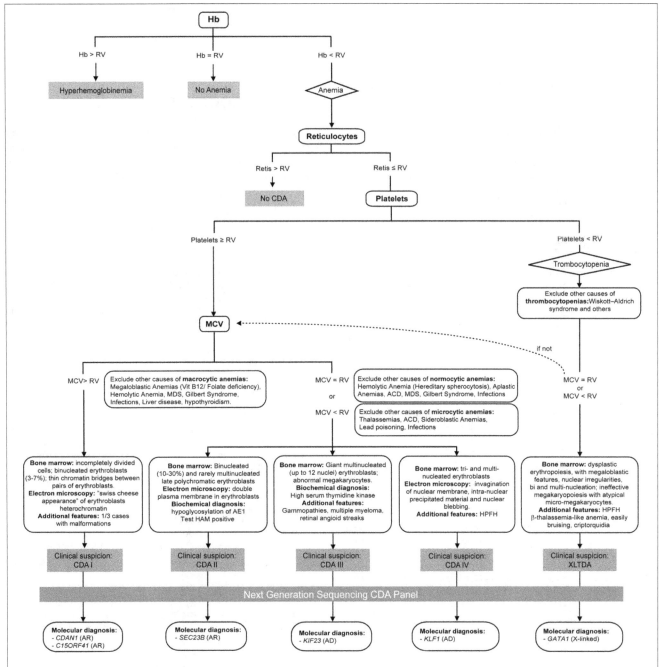

FIGURE 1 | Diagnostic algorithm used by the CoDysAn telemedicine tool. Hb, hemoglobin; RV, reference value; MCV, mean corpuscular volume; HPFH, hereditary persistence of fetal hemoglobin; AR, autosomal recessive; AD, autosomal dominant.

tool presents limits: patients should be considered as a whole entity and multiple biochemical determinations are needed due to daily parameters' variability within the same subject. Although hematological reference ranges are useful in results interpretation and in clinical decision-making, it should be borne in mind that variations within the population may affect some outcomes. CoDysAn incorporates a diagnostic algorithm that proved to be useful for a preliminary diagnostic. It will help medical doctors to know which molecular diagnostics they should request,

reducing time and effort necessary for the diagnostic of CDA and allowing a direct implementation of a proper treatment once reached a definitive molecular diagnosis. Few reference centers are now offering genetic diagnostic panels screening the six known genes causing CDA. CoDySan algorithm is connected to the NCBI Genetic Testing Registry (GTR) in a way to inform medical doctors about the existence of these accredited diagnostic centers to perform a complete genetic test, if required. This telemedicine tool aims to inform the general public and aid in the diagnosis of CDA. It is not intended as an attempt to practice medicine or provide specific medical advice and it should not be used to replace or overrule a qualified health care provider's judgment. Users should not rely upon this website for self-medication. We believe that CoDysAn webpage will positively contribute to improve medical and scientific communication on the anemia field.

AUTHOR CONTRIBUTIONS

MS designed the webpage, designed the study, and wrote the manuscript. ES-P, CT, and BC created the webpage and wrote the diagnostic algorithm. BC designed **Figure 1**. IA and RR translated the CoDysAn webpage to Italian. AI, IA, and RR

provided the patients data to test CoDysAn algorithm. VV wrote and revised the manuscript. IH-R helped with reference values and **Table 1**. All authors read and approved the final version of the manuscript.

ACKNOWLEDGMENTS

We would like to thank Nuria Centeno from UPF for Master Project advisor tasks and Francisco Fuster from Josep Carreras Leukaemia Research Institute for assistance with the opinion questionnaire. This work was performed in the context of the Experimental Sciences and Technology Ph.D. program of the University of Vic (UVic).

REFERENCES

Altes, A., Perez-Lucena, M. J., Bruguera, M., and Grp Iberico, F. (2014). Systematic approach to the diagnosis of hyperferritinemia. *Med. Clin. (Barc).* 142, 412–417. doi: 10.1016/j.medcli.2013.06.010

Andolfo, I., Russo, R., Manna, F., Shmukler, B. E., Gambale, A., Vitiello, G., et al. (2015). Novel Gardos channel mutations linked to dehydrated hereditary stomatocytosis (xerocytosis). *Am. J. Hematol.* 90, 921–926. doi: 10.1002/ajh.24117

Andolfo, I., Russo, R., Rosato, B. E., Manna, F., Gambale, A., Brugnara, C., et al. (2018). Genotype-phenotype correlation and risk stratification in a cohort of 123 hereditary stomatocytosis patients. *Am. J. Hematol.* 93, 1509–1517. doi: 10.1002/ajh.25276

Arnaud, L., Saison, C., Helias, V., Lucien, N., Steschenko, D., Giarratana, M. C., et al. (2010). A Dominant mutation in the gene encoding the erythroid transcription factor KLF1 causes a congenital dyserythropoietic anemia. *Am. J. Hum. Genet.* 87, 721–727. doi: 10.1016/j.ajhg.2010.10.010

Babbs, C., Roberts, N. A., Sanchez-Pulido, L., McGowan, S. J., Ahmed, M. R., Brown, J. M., et al. (2013). Homozygous mutations in a predicted endonuclease are a novel cause of congenital dyserythropoietic anemia type I. *Haematologica* 98, 1383–1387. doi: 10.3324/haematol.2013.089490

Bianchi, P., Fermo, E., Vercellati, C., Boschetti, C., Barcellini, W., Iurlo, A., et al. (2009). Congenital dyserythropoietic anemia type II (CDAII) is caused by mutations in the SEC23B gene. *Hum Mutat.* 30, 1292–1298. doi: 10.1002/humu.21077

Del Vecchio, G. C., Giordani, L., De Santis, A., and De Mattia, D. (2005). Dyserythropoietic anemia and thrombocytopenia due to a novel mutation in GATA-1. *Acta Haematol.* 114, 113–116. doi: 10.1159/000086586

Dgany, O., Avidan, N., Delaunay, J., Krasnov, T., Shalmon, L., Shalev, H., et al. (2002). Congenital dyserythropoietic anemia type I is caused by mutations in codanin-1. *Am. J. Hum. Genet.* 71, 1467–1474. doi: 10.1086/344781

Di Pierro, E., Russo, R., Karakas, Z., Brancaleoni, V., Gambale, A., Kurt, I., et al. (2015). Congenital erythropoietic porphyria linked to GATA1-R216W mutation: challenges for diagnosis. *Eur. J. Haematol.* 94, 491–497. doi: 10.1111/ejh.12452

Dinesen, B., Nonnecke, B., Lindeman, D., Toft, E., Kidholm, K., Jethwani, K., et al. (2016). Personalized telehealth in the future: a global research agenda. *J. Med. Internet Res.* 18:e53. doi: 10.2196/jmir.5257

Gambale, A., Iolascon, A., Andolfo, I., and Russo, R. (2016). Diagnosis and management of congenital dyserythropoietic anemias. *Expert Rev. Hematol.* 9, 283–296. doi: 10.1586/17474086.2016.1131608

Hoffman, R., Benz, E. J. Jr., Silberstein, L. E., Heslop, H., Weitz, J., and Anastasi, J. (2018). *Hematology: Basic Principles and Practice, 7th Edn.* Philadelphia, PA: Elsevier Saunders.

Iolascon, A., Esposito, M. R., and Russo, R. (2012). Clinical aspects and pathogenesis of congenital dyserythropoietic anemias: from morphology to molecular approach. *Haematologica* 97, 1786–1794. doi: 10.3324/haematol.2012.072207

Iolascon, A., Heimpel, H., Wahlin, A., and Tamary, H. (2013). Congenital dyserythropoietic anemias: molecular insights and diagnostic approach. *Blood* 122, 2162–2166. doi: 10.1182/blood-2013-05-468223

Iolascon, A., Russo, R., Esposito, M. R., Asci, R., Piscopo, C., Perrotta, S., et al. (2009). Molecular analysis of 42 patients with congenital dyserythropoietic anemia type II: new mutations in the SEC23B gene and a search for a genotype-phenotype relationship. *Haematologica* 95, 708–715. doi: 10.3324/haematol.2009.014985

Jaffray, J. A., Mitchell, W. B., Gnanapragasam, M. N., Seshan, S. V., Guo, X., Westhoff, C. M., et al. (2013). Erythroid transcription factor EKLF/KLF1 mutation causing congenital dyserythropoietic anemia type IV in a patient of Taiwanese origin: review of all reported cases and development of a clinical diagnostic paradigm. *Blood Cells Mol. Dis.* 51, 71–75. doi: 10.1016/j.bcmd.2013.02.006

Liljeholm, M., Irvine, A. F., Vikberg, A. L., Norberg, A., Month, S., Sandström, H., et al. (2013). Congenital dyserythropoietic anemia type III (CDA III) is caused by a mutation in kinesin family member, KIF23. *Blood* 121, 4791–4799. doi: 10.1182/blood-2012-10-461392

Nichols, K. E., Crispino, J. D., Poncz, M., White, J. G., Orkin, S. H., Maris, J. M., et al. (2000). Familial dyserythropoietic anaemia and thrombocytopenia due to an inherited mutation in GATA1. *Nat. Genet.* 24, 266–270. doi: 10.1038/73480

Palmer, W. C., Vishnu, P., Sanchez, W., Aqel, B., Riegert-Johnson, D., Seaman, L. A. K., et al. (2018). Diagnosis and management of genetic iron overload disorders. *J. Gen. Intern. Med.* 33, 2230–2236. doi: 10.1007/s11606-018-4669-2

Rabinovitch, A. (1990). Hematology reference ranges. *Arch. Pathol. Lab. Med.* 114:1189.

Rubinstein, W. S., Maglott, D. R., Lee, J. M., Kattman, B. L., Malheiro, A. J., Ovetsky, M., et al. (2013). The NIH genetic testing registry: a new, centralized database of genetic tests to enable access to comprehensive information and improve transparency. *Nucleic Acids Res.* 41, D925–D935. doi: 10.1093/nar/gks1173

Russo, R., Andolfo, I., Manna, F., De Rosa, G., De Falco, L., Gambale, A., et al. (2016). Increased levels of ERFE-encoding FAM132B in patients with congenital dyserythropoietic anemia type II. *Blood* 128, 1899–1902. doi: 10.1182/blood-2016-06-724328

Russo, R., Andolfo, I., Manna, F., Gambale, A., Marra, R., Rosato, B. E., et al. (2018). Multi-gene panel testing improves diagnosis and management of patients with hereditary anemias. *Am. J. Hematol.* 93, 672–682. doi: 10.1002/ajh.25058

Russo, R., Esposito, M. R., Asci, R., Gambale, A., Perrotta, S., Ramenghi, U., et al. (2010). Mutational spectrum in congenital dyserythropoietic anemia type II: identification of 19 novel variants in SEC23B gene. *Am. J. Hematol.* 85, 915–920. doi: 10.1002/ajh.21866

Russo, R., Gambale, A., Esposito, M. R., Serra, M. L., Troiano, A., De Maggio, I., et al. (2011). Two founder mutations in the SEC23B gene account for the relatively high frequency of CDA II in the Italian population. *Am. J. Hematol.* 86, 727–732. doi: 10.1002/ajh.22096

Russo, R., Gambale, A., Langella, C., Andolfo, I., Unal, S., and Iolascon, A. (2014). Retrospective cohort study of 205 cases with congenital dyserythropoietic anemia type II: definition of clinical and molecular spectrum and identification of new diagnostic scores. *Am. J. Hematol.* 89, E169–E175. doi: 10.1002/ajh.23800

Russo, R., Langella, C., Esposito, M. R., Gambale, A., Vitiello, F., Vallefuoco, F., et al. (2013). Hypomorphic mutations of SEC23B gene account for mild phenotypes of congenital dyserythropoietic anemia type II. *Blood Cells Mol. Dis.* 51, 17–21. doi: 10.1016/j.bcmd.2013.02.003

Schwarz, K., Iolascon, A., Verissimo, F., Trede, N. S., Horsley, W., Chen, W.,

et al. (2009). Mutations affecting the secretory COPII coat component SEC23B cause congenital dyserythropoietic anemia type II. *Nat. Genet.* 41, 936–940. doi: 10.1038/ng.405

Unal, S., Russo, R., Gumruk, F., Kuskonmaz, B., Cetin, M., Sayli, T., et al. (2014). Successful hematopoietic stem cell transplantation in a patient with congenital dyserythropoietic anemia type II. *Pediatr. Transplant.* 18, E130–E133. doi: 10.1111/petr.12254

Wakeman, L., Al-Ismail, S., Benton, A., Beddall, A., Gibbs, A., Hartnell, S., et al. (2007). Robust, routine haematology reference ranges for healthy adults. *Int. J. Lab. Hematol.* 29, 279–283. doi: 10.1111/j.1365-2257.2006.00883.x

7

The EPO-FGF23 Signaling Pathway in Erythroid Progenitor Cells: Opening a New Area of Research

Annelies J. van Vuren[1]*, Carlo A. J. M. Gaillard[2], Michele F. Eisenga[3], Richard van Wijk[4] and Eduard J. van Beers[1]

[1] Van Creveldkliniek, Department of Internal Medicine and Dermatology, University Medical Center Utrecht, Utrecht University, Utrecht, Netherlands, [2] Department of Internal Medicine and Dermatology, University Medical Center Utrecht, Utrecht University, Utrecht, Netherlands, [3] Department of Internal Medicine, Division of Nephrology, University Medical Center Groningen, University of Groningen, Groningen, Netherlands, [4] Department of Clinical Chemistry and Haematology, University Medical Center Utrecht, Utrecht University, Utrecht, Netherlands

*Correspondence:
Annelies J. van Vuren
A.J.vanVuren@umcutrecht.nl

We provide an overview of the evidence for an erythropoietin-fibroblast growth factor 23 (FGF23) signaling pathway directly influencing erythroid cells in the bone marrow. We outline its importance for red blood cell production, which might add, among others, to the understanding of bone marrow responses to endogenous erythropoietin in rare hereditary anemias. FGF23 is a hormone that is mainly known as the core regulator of phosphate and vitamin D metabolism and it has been recognized as an important regulator of bone mineralization. Osseous tissue has been regarded as the major source of FGF23. Interestingly, erythroid progenitor cells highly express FGF23 protein and carry the FGF receptor. This implies that erythroid progenitor cells could be a prime target in FGF23 biology. FGF23 is formed as an intact, biologically active protein (iFGF23) and proteolytic cleavage results in the formation of the presumed inactive C-terminal tail of FGF23 (cFGF23). FGF23-knockout or injection of an iFGF23 blocking peptide in mice results in increased erythropoiesis, reduced erythroid cell apoptosis and elevated renal and bone marrow erythropoietin mRNA expression with increased levels of circulating erythropoietin. By competitive inhibition, a relative increase in cFGF23 compared to iFGF23 results in reduced FGF23 receptor signaling and mimics the positive effects of FGF23-knockout or iFGF23 blocking peptide. Injection of recombinant erythropoietin increases FGF23 mRNA expression in the bone marrow with a concomitant increase in circulating FGF23 protein. However, erythropoietin also augments iFGF23 cleavage, thereby decreasing the iFGF23 to cFGF23 ratio. Therefore, the net result of erythropoietin is a reduction of iFGF23 to cFGF23 ratio, which inhibits the effects of iFGF23 on erythropoiesis and erythropoietin production. Elucidation of the EPO-FGF23 signaling pathway and its downstream signaling in hereditary anemias with chronic hemolysis or ineffective erythropoiesis adds to the understanding of the pathophysiology of these diseases and its complications; in addition, it provides promising new targets for treatment downstream of erythropoietin in the signaling cascade.

Keywords: FGF23, erythropoietin, anemia, osteoporosis, red blood cells

INTRODUCTION

At a concentration of 5 million red blood cells (RBC) per microliter blood, RBCs are the most abundant circulating cell type in humans (Eggold and Rankin, 2018). Normal erythropoiesis yields 200 billion RBCs every day, an equivalent of 40 mL of newly formed whole blood (Muckenthaler et al., 2017). Regulation of erythropoiesis in the bone marrow (BM) microenvironment depends on systemic and local factors controlling differentiation, proliferation and survival of the erythroid progenitor cells (EPC). Inherited RBC abnormalities might result in chronic hemolysis with an increased erythropoietic drive, or ineffective erythropoiesis, thereby challenging the erythropoietic system. Systemic erythropoietin (EPO) production plays a critical role in maintaining erythropoietic homeostasis under physiologic and pathologic conditions (Eggold and Rankin, 2018). Increasing evidence links EPO and erythropoiesis to skeletal homeostasis (Eggold and Rankin, 2018). First, there is a longstanding observation that patients with hemolysis have increased risk of skeletal pathology such as osteoporosis and osteonecrosis (Taher et al., 2010; Haidar et al., 2012; Eggold and Rankin, 2018; van Straaten et al., 2018). Second, removal of osteoblasts in mice resulted in increased loss of erythroid progenitors in the BM, followed by decreased amounts of hematopoietic stem cells with recovery after reappearance of osteoblasts, pointing to a critical role of osteoblasts in hemato- and erythropoiesis (Visnjic et al., 2004).

Erythropoietin, the core regulator of erythropoiesis, is an important regulator of fibroblast growth factor 23 (FGF23) production and cleavage (Clinkenbeard et al., 2017; Flamme et al., 2017; Daryadel et al., 2018; Hanudel et al., 2018; Rabadi et al., 2018; Toro et al., 2018). FGF23 is originally known as a bone-derived hormone and key player in phosphate and vitamin D metabolism. FGF23 seems to provide a link between bone mineralization and erythropoiesis (Clinkenbeard et al., 2017; Eggold and Rankin, 2018). FGF23 was first discovered as a regulator of phosphate metabolism, due to the association between hereditary phosphate wasting syndromes and *FGF23* mutations (ADHR Consortium, 2000). FGF23 induces phosphaturia, directly suppresses parathyroid hormone and the amount of $1,25(OH)_2D_3$ (active vitamin D) (Shimada et al., 2004; Quarles, 2012). FGF23 is secreted by osteocytes in response to vitamin D, parathyroid hormone and elevated levels of serum phosphate. Due to important alterations in phosphate balance in chronic kidney disease (CKD), most research on FGF23 up until now was focused on CKD (see section "EPO, Iron, CKD, and Inflammation Are Important Regulators of iFGF23

Cleavage") (Kanbay et al., 2017). However, a new, important role for FGF23 seems to exist as regulator of erythropoiesis.

Here, we review the interplay of EPO and FGF23 in the erythroid cells of the BM. We discuss that the action of FGF23 not only depends on the amount of intact FGF23 available, but also on the amount of FGF23 cleavage which is an important factor determining its efficacy. Elucidation of the role of the EPO-FGF23 signaling pathway in hereditary anemia and chronic hemolytic diseases will add to the understanding of the pathophysiology of the diseases, of bone mineralization disorders complicating chronic hemolytic diseases, and might provide new targets for treatment downstream of EPO. An overview of FGF23 production, cleavage and signaling is provided in **Figure 1**.

ANEMIA AND THE EPO SIGNALING CASCADE

Erythropoietin production by renal interstitial cells, and in a smaller amount by hepatocytes, plays a critical role in maintaining erythropoietic homeostasis. The primary physiological stimulus of increased *EPO* gene transcription is tissue hypoxia, which can augment circulating EPO up to a 1000-fold in states of severe hypoxia (Jelkmann, 1992; Ebert and Bunn, 1999). Under hypoxic conditions, *EPO* transcription is augmented by binding of hypoxia inducible factor (HIF)-2 to the *EPO* gene promoter. Under normoxic conditions prolyl hydroxylases (PHD) hydroxylate HIF1α and HIF2α, which associate with the von Hippel-Lindau tumor suppressor protein, targeting this complex for proteasomal degradation. Low iron or oxygen conditions inhibit hydroxylation by PHD2 (Ebert and Bunn, 1999; Schofield and Ratcliffe, 2004). EPO exerts its effect on early erythroid progenitors via the EPO receptor (EPOR), with a peak receptor number at the CFU-E (Colony Forming Unit-Erythroid) stage and a decline until absence of the receptor in late basophilic erythroblasts. EPOR signaling results in survival, proliferation, and terminal differentiation (Krantz, 1991; Muckenthaler et al., 2017; Eggold and Rankin, 2018).

Besides kidney and liver, EPO expression has also been reported in brain, lung, heart, spleen, and reproductive organs. Besides kidney and liver, only EPO produced by the brain was capable to functionally regulate erythropoiesis (Weidemann et al., 2009; Haase, 2010). More recently, it was discovered that local production of EPO by osteoprogenitors and osteoblasts in the BM microenvironment, under conditions of constitutive HIF stabilization, results in selective expansion of the erythroid lineage (Rankin et al., 2012; Eggold and Rankin, 2018). The role of osteoblastic EPO in the BM microenvironment under physiologic conditions is still under investigation (Shiozawa et al., 2010). The amount of circulating EPO is normal or elevated in most forms of hereditary anemia, although the amount is often relatively low for the degree of anemia (Caro et al., 1979; Rocha et al., 2005; Zeidler and Welte, 2007). EPO levels were generally elevated in β-thalassemia patients with large interpatient differences partly related to age (Sukpanichnant et al., 1997; O'Donnell et al., 2007; Singer et al., 2011; Butthep et al., 2015; Schotten et al., 2017). Sickle cell disease (SCD) patients had elevated serum EPO

Abbreviations: ADHR, autosomal dominant hypophosphatemic rickets; α-KL, α-klotho; BM, bone marrow; CKD, chronic kidney disease; EPC, erythroid progenitor cell; EPO, erythropoietin; EPOR, erythropoietin receptor; FGF, fibroblast growth factor; FGFR, fibroblast growth factor receptor; GalNT3, N-acetylgalactosaminyltransferase 3; HIF, hypoxia inducible factor; HIF-PHI, hypoxia inducible factor proline hydroxylase inhibitor; PHD, prolyl hydroxylase; RBC, red blood cell; rhEPO, recombinant erythropoietin; SCD, sickle cell disease; SPC, sutilisin-like proprotein convertase; TNAP, tissue non-specific alkaline phosphatase; WT, wild-type.

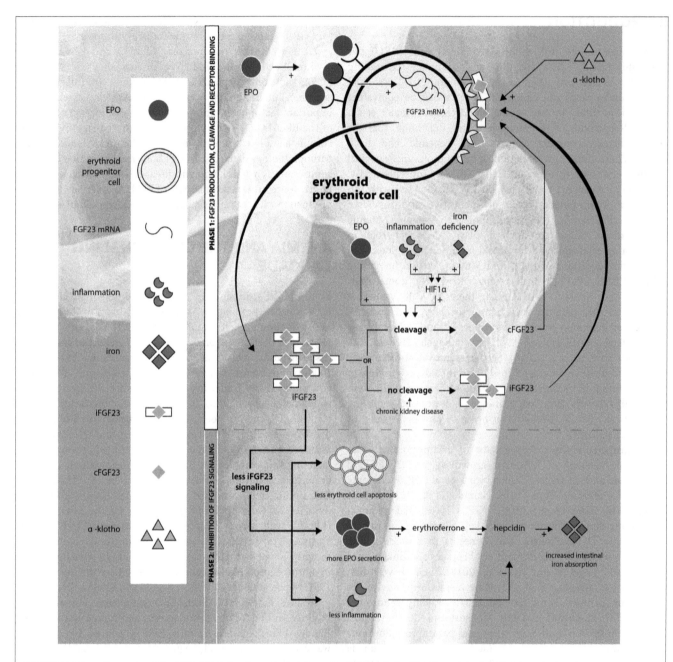

FIGURE 1 | Schematic overview of the EPO-FGF23 signaling pathway in the erythroid lineage in the BM. Phase 1 displays FGF23 production, the secretory process and FGFR binding; phase 2 summarizes the effects of inhibition of iFGF23 signaling.

concentrations ranging from the low end of expected for the degree of anemia to lower than expected (Pulte et al., 2014; Karafin et al., 2015). Off-label application of recombinant EPO (rhEPO) has been tried in selected patients to reduce transfusion requirements and improve quality of life. Responses varied and were unpredictable (Zachee et al., 1989; Singer et al., 2011; Fibach and Rachmilewitz, 2014; Han et al., 2017). Insight in components downstream of EPO in its signaling cascade might lead to insights in the EPO responsiveness in individual patients. FGF23 has shown to be one of those downstream components directly affecting erythropoiesis and providing feedback on EPO

production, as outlined in Section "Blockade of iFGF23 Signaling Results in More Erythropoiesis."

ERYTHROID PROGENITORS EXPRESS FGF23 IN RESPONSE TO EPO

Osseous tissue has been regarded as the major source of FGF23. Selective deletion of *FGF23* in early osteoblasts or osteocytes in a murine model demonstrated that both cell types significantly contribute to circulating FGF23. However, FGF23 was still detectable in serum after deletion of the *FGF23* gene in both osteoblasts and osteocytes: other, non-osseous, tissues contribute to circulating FGF23 (Clinkenbeard et al., 2016). It was shown that BM, specifically the early erythroid lineage, does significantly contribute to total circulating FGF23. In wild-type (WT) mice treated with marrow ablative carboplatin followed by a 3-day course of rhEPO, serum FGF23 was 40% lower compared to controls (Clinkenbeard et al., 2017). In WT mice, baseline FGF23 mRNA in BM was comparable with osseous tissue, but the amount of FGF23 protein in BM tissue was significantly higher. Hematopoietic stem cells and EPCs, including BFU-E (Burst Forming Unit-Erythroid), CFU-E and proerythroblasts, showed more than fourfold higher amounts of FGF23 mRNA compared with whole BM including lineage specific cells. FGF23 mRNA was shown to be transiently expressed during early erythropoiesis (Toro et al., 2018). EPCs do express FGF23 mRNA under physiologic conditions, however significant increases are observed in response to EPO (Clinkenbeard et al., 2017; Daryadel et al., 2018; Toro et al., 2018). RhEPO induced FGF23 mRNA expression in BM cells 24 h after injection (Daryadel et al., 2018). Indirect immunofluorescence staining with anti-mouse FGF23 antibodies and lineage specific markers showed intense staining of erythroid progenitors and mature erythroblasts (CD71$^+$ cells) of EPO-treated mice compared to controls (Daryadel et al., 2018).

Thus, erythroid cells of the BM significantly contribute to FGF23 production and FGF23 production is increased in response to EPO. As will be discussed in Sections "FGF23 Signaling Is Regulated by Cleavage of Intact FGF23" and "EPO, Iron, CKD, and Inflammation Are Important Regulators of iFGF23 Cleavage," the amount of cleavage of FGF23 is equally important and EPO has a strong effect on this as well.

FGF23 SIGNALING IS REGULATED BY CLEAVAGE OF INTACT FGF23

FGF23 is formed as a full-length, biologically active protein (iFGF23). Intact FGF23 is cleaved into two fragments: the inactive N-terminal fragment of FGF23 fails to co-immunoprecipitate with FGFR (FGF receptor) complexes, which suggests that the C-terminal fragment (cFGF23) mediates binding to the FGFR (Goetz et al., 2007, 2010; Courbebaisse et al., 2017). Only intact FGF23 (iFGF23) suppresses phosphate levels in mice through the FGF receptor 1 (FGFR1) (Shimada et al., 2002; Wolf and White, 2014). cFGF23 competes with iFGF23 for binding to the FGFR, and thereby antagonizes iFGF23 signaling in mice and rats (Goetz et al., 2010; Agoro et al., 2018). Treatment with cFGF23 increased the number of early and terminally differentiated BM erythroid cells and the colony forming capacity of early progenitors to the same amount as rhEPO. These data suggest that the outcome of rhEPO treatment resembles the effects of more cFGF23. Recently, it was shown that the cFGF23 fragment itself was able to induce heart hypertrophy in SCD patients (Courbebaisse et al., 2017), probably via FGFR4 and independent from a costimulatory signal (see section "Presence of α-Klotho Is Essential for Normal Erythropoiesis") (Faul et al., 2011).

Currently, two assays are available to measure iFGF23 and cFGF23: one assay that detects the C-terminal of FGF23 which measures both cFGF23 and (full-length) iFGF23 (Immunotopics/Quidel) and one assay that only detects iFGF23 (Kainos Laboratories) (Hanudel et al., 2018). Serum half-life time is approximately identical for both iFGF23 and cFGF23 ranging from 45 to 60 min (Khosravi et al., 2007).

So, although still subject of debate, proteolytic cleavage of iFGF23 seems to abrogate its activity by two mechanisms: reduction of the amount of iFGF23 and generation of an endogenous inhibitor, cFGF23 (Goetz et al., 2010). Therefore, measurement of both iFGF23 and cFGF23 is important: alterations in the iFGF23 to cFGF23 ratio lead to alterations of iFGF23 signaling efficacy.

Regulation of FGF23 secretion includes intracellular processing in the Golgi apparatus in which iFGF23 is partially cleaved within a highly conserved sutilisin-like proprotein convertase (SPC)-site by furin or prohormone convertase 1/3, 2, and 5/6 (**Figure 2**). Cleavage of iFGF23 generates two fragments: the C- and N-terminal peptide fragments (20 and 12 kDa) (Benet-Pages et al., 2004; Tagliabracci et al., 2014; Yamamoto et al., 2016). Competition between phosphorylation and O-glycosylation of the SPC-site in the secretory pathway of FGF23 is an important regulatory mechanism of cleavage (Tagliabracci et al., 2014). Secretion of iFGF23 requires O-glycosylation: the glycosyltransferase N-acetylgalactosaminyltransferase 3 (GalNT3) selectively exerts O-glycosylation of amino acid residues within or in the proximity of the SPC-site and blocks cleavage of iFGF23 (Kato et al., 2006). In contrast, phosphorylation of the SPC-site promotes FGF23 proteolysis indirectly by blocking O-glycosylation. The kinase Fam20C phosphorylates iFGF23 within the SPC-site, consequently reduces glycosylation and subsequently facilitates iFGF23 cleavage (Yamamoto et al., 2016).

Summarizing, a proportion of synthesized iFGF23 will be cleaved intracellularly before secretion, the amount of intracellular cleavage is determined by competition between glycosylation (GalNT3) and phosphorylation (Fam20C) (Martin et al., 2012; Tagliabracci et al., 2014; Yamamoto et al., 2016). Various factors regulate post-translational modification, these are described in Section "EPO, Iron, CKD, and Inflammation Are Important Regulators of iFGF23 Cleavage."

EPO, IRON, CKD, AND INFLAMMATION ARE IMPORTANT REGULATORS OF iFGF23 CLEAVAGE

Erythropoietin, iron, inflammation, and CKD have been identified as modifiers of iFGF23 cleavage. Notably, all these factors might co-exist in patients with hereditary anemia. The amount of cleavage is determined by alterations in GalNT3 and furin. Furin plays an important role in regulation of FGF23 cleavage in iron deficiency and inflammation (Silvestri et al., 2008; David et al., 2016), whereas under conditions of high EPO GalNT3 inhibition might augment cleavage (Hanudel et al., 2018).

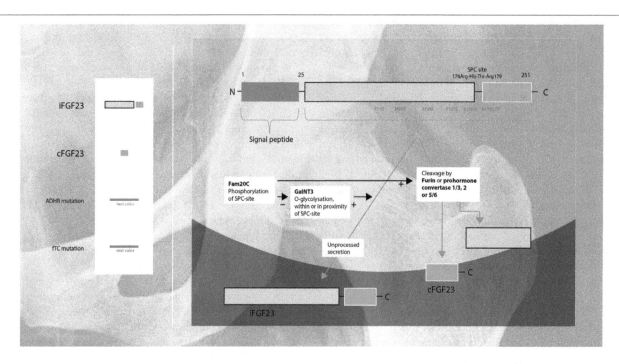

FIGURE 2 | Schematic overview of the regulation of FGF23 protein cleavage and secretion (Shimada et al., 2001; Saito and Fukumoto, 2009; Huang et al., 2013; Luo et al., 2019). FGF23 harbors a naturally-occurring proteolytic site at Arg176-XX-Arg179. O-Glycosylation within or in the proximity of this SPC-site of FGF23 by GalNT3 results in increased secretion of intact FGF23. Phosphorylation of the SPC-site by Fam20C indirectly promotes FGF23 cleavage by blocking O-glycosylation. ADHR is caused by mutations near the proteolytic site, that impairs proteolytic inactivation of FGF23 resulting in high levels of iFGF23 (Arg176Gln or Arg179Gln/Trp). FTC, is an autosomal recessive disorder, resulting from mutations in the FGF23 gene which lead to destabilization of the tertiary structure of FGF23 and rendering it susceptible to degradation (Ser71Gly, Met96Thr, Ser129Phe, and Phe157Leu). FTC, familial tumoral calcinosis; ADHR, autosomal dominant hypophosphatemic rickets.

Erythropoietin

Several studies report alterations of iFGF23 and cFGF23 after administration of rhEPO or under high endogenous EPO conditions, a summary is provided in the **Table 1** (Clinkenbeard et al., 2017; Flamme et al., 2017; Daryadel et al., 2018; Hanudel et al., 2018; Rabadi et al., 2018; Toro et al., 2018). Most experiments were carried out in animal models (rats and mice). Less information is available about the influence of EPO on the iFGF23/cFGF23 ratio in man.

In all animal studies one single injection or multiple-day regimen of rhEPO resulted in a significant increase in circulating cFGF23 (Clinkenbeard et al., 2017; Flamme et al., 2017; Daryadel et al., 2018; Hanudel et al., 2018; Toro et al., 2018). Increases in iFGF23 were less pronounced (Flamme et al., 2017; Hanudel et al., 2018; Toro et al., 2018), or absent (Daryadel et al., 2018), after a single injection of rhEPO. Multiple-day regimens resulted in small rises in iFGF23, less pronounced than the increase in cFGF23 (Clinkenbeard et al., 2017; Daryadel et al., 2018). EPO directly increased *FGF23* gene expression in murine hematopoietic cells (Flamme et al., 2017). Treatment of mice with an hematopoietic equipotent dose of a HIF-proline hydroxylase inhibitor (HIF-PH inhibitor) also led to a significant rise in plasma cFGF23, without an increase in circulating iFGF23. Increases in FGF23 expression after HIF-PH inhibitor treatment were mediated indirectly via EPO, as pre-administration of anti-EPO antibodies

opposed upregulation of circulating FGF23 (David et al., 2016; Flamme et al., 2017).

Effects of overexpression of endogenous EPO were investigated in a transgenic human EPO-overexpressing murine model. Results were in line with responses on rhEPO in mice: circulating cFGF23 and iFGF23 were significantly higher in EPO-overexpressing mice than in WT mice (Hanudel et al., 2018). Acute blood loss in mice, as a surrogate model for high endogenous EPO, also significantly increased circulating cFGF23, but not iFGF23 (Rabadi et al., 2018).

Only four studies (Clinkenbeard et al., 2017; Daryadel et al., 2018; Hanudel et al., 2018; Rabadi et al., 2018) explored effects of EPO on FGF23 in man. In all studies, rhEPO or a condition resulting in high endogenous EPO, increased circulating cFGF23, without (Daryadel et al., 2018; Hanudel et al., 2018) or with only minimal (Clinkenbeard et al., 2017) rise in circulating iFGF23. In a large cohort of 680 kidney transplant recipients higher EPO values were associated with increased cFGF23 values and not with iFGF23 values, independent of renal function (Hanudel et al., 2018)

Together, these data show that EPO (endogenous or exogenous) increases the total amount of circulating FGF23 (iFGF23 and cFGF23) and alters the iFGF23/cFGF23 ratio in favor of cFGF23.

It is uncertain which proteins mediate increased intracellular cleavage in the secretion pathway of iFGF23 in response to EPO.

TABLE 1 | Overview studies on the effects of erythropoietin (EPO) on FGF23.

Study	Model	rhEPO	iFGF23/cFGF23
Studies in animals			
Clinkenbeard et al., 2017, pp e427–e430	WT C57BL/6 mice	Three-day regimen with increasing doses rhEPO	Max. ±40x increase in serum cFGF23; ±2x increase in serum iFGF23. Increases in cFGF23 in dose-dependent way.
Rabadi et al., 2018, pp F132–F139	C57BL/6 mice with and without 10% loss of total blood volume	None	6 h: ± 4x increase in plasma cFGF23; no increase in iFGF23. cFGF23 values remained increased 48 h after blood loss.
Flamme et al., 2017, p. e0186979	Male Wistar rats	Single injection rhEPO	4–6 h: >10x increase in plasma cFGF23 (extrapolated); ±2x increase in plasma iFGF23 (extrapolated).
		Single injection high dose HIF-PH inhibitor	4–6 h: comparable with rhEPO. Pretreatment anti-EPO: cFGF23 response almost absent.
Toro et al., 2018	WT C57BL/6 mice	Single injection rhEPO	4 h: ±4x increase in plasma cFGF23; ± 2.5x increase in plasma iFGF23.
	Sprague-Dawley rats, hemorrhagic shock with 50–55% loss of total blood volume	None	24 h: ±5x increase in plasma cFGF23; ± 3.5x increase in plasma iFGF23.
Daryadel et al., 2018	WT C57BL/6 mice	Single injection rhEPO	24 h: ± 2x increase in plasma cFGF23; no increase in plasma iFGF23.
		4-day regimen rhEPO	4 days: increase in cFGF23 and iFGF23.
Hanudel et al., 2018	WT C57BL/6 mice with and without 0.2% adenine diet-induced CKD	Single injection rhEPO	6 h: *non-CKD* cFGF23 207→ 3289 pg/mL; *CKD* cFGF23 2056→ 9376 pg/mL. *Non-CKD* iFGF23 187→ 385 pg/mL; *CKDI* no significant rise in iFGF23.
	Transgenic Tg6 mice overexpressing human EPO	Transgenic EPO overexpression	cFGF23 *WT* 340 pg/mL; *Tg6* 3175 pg/mL. iFGF23 *WT* 317 pg/mL, *Tg6* 589 pg/mL.
Studies in man			
Clinkenbeard et al., 2017, pp e427–e430	4 patients with unexplained anemia	Single injection rhEPO	6–18 h: ±2x increase in serum cFGF23; ±1.5x increase in serum cFGF23.
Rabadi et al., 2018, pp F132–F139	131 patients admitted to ICU, categorized based on number of RBC transfusions in 48 h before admission	None	Number of blood transfusions was associated with plasma cFGF23.
Daryadel et al., 2018	28 healthy volunteers	Single injection rhEPO	24 h: significant increase in plasma cFGF23; plasma iFGF23 unchanged.
Hanudel et al., 2018	680 adult kidney transplant patients	None	Higher EPO values were significantly associated with increased cFGF23 and not with iFGF23; independent of renal function.

In mice, experiments investigating alterations in BM mRNA expression of GalNT3 after rhEPO injection were inconclusive (Daryadel et al., 2018). Meanwhile, in EPO-overexpressing mice, compared to WT mice, GalNT3 and prohormone convertase 5/6 mRNA expression were significantly decreased in bone and BM, no differences were observed in Fam20c and furin mRNA expression (Hanudel et al., 2018). Decreases in GalNT3 mRNA and absence of changes in furin and Fam20c mRNA expression were also observed in whole BM of mice after acute blood loss. However, the amount of GalNT3 mRNA expression in isolated erythroid precursors and mature erythroblasts (Ter119+ cells) of these mice was unchanged (Rabadi et al., 2018). So, decreased GalNT3 expression might increase cleavage in response to high EPO, although further study is needed to elucidate the contributory of GalNT3 and other, yet unknown, mechanisms in response to EPO.

Iron Deficiency

Iron deficiency in WT mice resulted in a significant increase of cFGF23, with a less pronounced or even absent increase in iFGF23 (Farrow et al., 2011b; Clinkenbeard et al., 2014; David et al., 2016; Hanudel et al., 2016). Treatment of iron deficiency in CKD mice resulted in a significant decrease in whole bone FGF23 (Clinkenbeard et al., 2017). Iron deficiency induced by iron chelation stabilized pre-existing HIF1α and increased FGF23 transcription (Farrow et al., 2011b; David et al., 2016). HIF1α inhibition partially blocked elevations in total FGF23, and inhibited cleavage of iFGF23 (David et al.,

2016). HIF1α stabilization under conditions of iron deficiency has been associated with upregulation of furin in liver cells (Silvestri et al., 2008).

Two large cohort studies support the relevance of the observations in mice in men. In a cohort of 2.000 pre-menopausal women serum iron was inversely correlated with cFGF23, but not with iFGF23 (Imel et al., 2016). And, associations between low iron parameters and high cFGF23 and iFGF23 values were found in a cohort of 3.780 elderly, with a more pronounced increase in cFGF23 (Bozentowicz-Wikarek et al., 2015).

Multiple studies examined the effects of distinct formulations of iron, oral and intravenous, in CKD patients on circulating cFGF23 and/or iFGF23 (Okada et al., 1983; Konjiki et al., 1994; Schouten et al., 2009a,b; Hryszko et al., 2012; Prats et al., 2013; Wolf et al., 2013; Block et al., 2015; Iguchi et al., 2015; Yamashita et al., 2017; Maruyama et al., 2018). Results have been inconclusive: interacting effects of rhEPO or endogenous high EPO might have influenced results. Moreover, the carbohydrate moieties of parenteral iron formulations themselves might lead to increased amounts of iFGF23 (Blazevic et al., 2014; Zoller et al., 2017).

In summary, iron deficiency leads to increased amounts of cFGF23 fragments. HIF1α stabilization plays an important role in upregulation of intracellular iFGF23 cleavage. Due to co-existence of anemia, erythropoiesis-related factors might influence the iron deficiency-FGF23 pathway. Observed differences in expression of proteins directly involved in the secretory process of FGF23, furin and GalNT3, suggest that EPO is not simply an intermediary between iron deficiency and FGF23: furin plays an important role in the upregulation of iFGF23 cleavage in iron deficiency, whereas EPO might act via GalNT3 inhibition as discussed in Section "Erythropoietin" (Hanudel et al., 2018).

Chronic Kidney Disease

Circulating total FGF23 rises progressively during early and intermediate stages of CKD and reaches levels of more than 1.000-times normal in advanced CKD. Elevated iFGF23 levels are considered as a compensatory mechanism for hyperphosphatemia, however regulation of FGF23 in CKD remains incompletely understood (Fliser et al., 2007; Gutierrez et al., 2009; Hanudel et al., 2018). Elevated total FGF23 is associated with progression of CKD (Fliser et al., 2007; Isakova et al., 2011; Portale et al., 2016), left ventricular hypertrophy (Faul et al., 2011), expression of IL-6 (Singh et al., 2016), impaired neutrophil recruitment (Rossaint et al., 2016), cardiovascular morbidity (Gutierrez et al., 2009; Faul et al., 2011; Mehta et al., 2016), and overall mortality (Isakova et al., 2011; Baia et al., 2013; Eisenga et al., 2017).

Besides the role of the kidney in clearance of iFGF23, CKD has also been identified as regulator of iFGF23 cleavage. Acute bilateral nephrectomy resulted in an immediate two-until threefold increase in iFGF23 levels with concomitant increase in iFGF23/cFGF23 ratio (Mace et al., 2015). In a murine CKD model, CKD was associated with less proteolytic cleavage of iFGF23 independent of iron status (Hanudel et al., 2016). Notably, iron deficiency, high endogenous EPO, or administration of rhEPO still resulted in increased total FGF23 production and cleavage in CKD (Hanudel et al., 2018).

So, CKD is associated with increased total FGF23 and alteration of the iFGF23/cFGF23 ratio in favor of iFGF23. As CKD progresses toward end-stage renal disease, the iFGF23/cFGF23 ratio will approximate 1:1 (Smith et al., 2012). Co-existence of iron deficiency or rhEPO administration still influence FGF23 secretion in CKD.

Inflammation

The association between FGF23 and inflammation has been reported in many diseases (Munoz Mendoza et al., 2012; Hanks et al., 2015; Holecki et al., 2015; Dounousi et al., 2016; Francis and David, 2016; Okan et al., 2016; Sato et al., 2016; Resende et al., 2017; Krick et al., 2018). Multiple inflammatory signaling pathways seem to interact closely to regulate FGF23 production and cleavage during acute or chronic inflammation. Additionally, other regulators of FGF23 expression and cleavage might develop under inflammatory conditions as inflammation-induced functional iron deficiency.

Regulation of FGF23 depends on chronicity of inflammation (David et al., 2016; Francis and David, 2016). In two murine models of acute inflammation, bone FGF23 mRNA expression and serum cFGF23 concentrations increased tenfold, without changes in iFGF23 (David et al., 2016). Increases in FGF23 mRNA were absent in the presence of NFκB (nuclear factor kappa-light-chain-enhancer of activated B cells, a canonical protein complex regulating many proinflammatory genes) inhibitor, which underlines the importance of the NFκB signaling pathway in regulation of FGF23 mRNA by pro-inflammatory stimuli (Ito et al., 2015). Co-treatment of bone cells with TNF or IL-1β and furin inhibitors resulted in increased levels of iFGF23, which suggests that increased cleavage of iFGF23 during acute inflammation is mediated by furin (McMahon et al., 2005; Ito et al., 2015; David et al., 2016). HIF1α was identified as an intermediate in FGF23 mRNA upregulation: iron deficiency and hypoxia only stabilized pre-existing HIF1α, where inflammation also led to increased cellular expression of HIF1α in bone cell lines (David et al., 2016).

Chronic inflammation resulted in increased amounts of total FGF23 with increased amounts of iFGF23. Chronic inflammation seems to exhaust or downregulate the FGF23 cleavage system (Francis and David, 2016).

In the presence of inflammation, development of functional iron deficiency (Stefanova et al., 2017), discussed in Section "Iron Deficiency," might contribute to increased cleavage of iFGF23 (David et al., 2016). The inflammatory cytokine IL-6 promotes hepcidin transcription in hepatocytes via the IL-6 receptor and subsequent activation of JAK tyrosine kinases and signal transducer and transcription activator 3 complexes that bind to the hepcidin promotor. Additionally, activin B stimulates formation of hepcidin transcriptional complexes via the BMP (bone morphogenetic protein)/SMAD signaling pathway (Verga Falzacappa et al., 2007; Besson-Fournier et al., 2012; Canali et al., 2016; Muckenthaler et al., 2017). Hepcidin controls the inflow of iron from enterocytes, the reticuloendothelial system and hepatocytes into the circulation via regulation of the expression of iron exporter ferroportin (Ganz, 2011). Upregulation of hepcidin redistributes iron to the reticuloendothelial system at the expense of FGF23 producing cells including RBC precursor cells, osteocytes, and osteoblasts. Moreover, inflammation induces proteins that scavenge and relocate iron, including lactoferrin, lipocalin 2, haptoglobin, and hemopexin. These proteins contribute to inflammation-induced functional iron deficiency (Soares and Weiss, 2015).

Summarizing, inflammation does augment both FGF23 expression and its cleavage, by increased HIF1α expression and stabilization and increased furin activity, but also via hepcidin-induced functional iron deficiency and subsequent non-hypoxic HIF1α stabilization.

BLOCKADE OF iFGF23 SIGNALING RESULTS IN MORE ERYTHROPOIESIS

The effects of iFGF23 signaling have been studied by direct infusion of rh-iFGF23 (Daryadel et al., 2018), and by blockage of iFGF23 signaling by knockout (Coe et al., 2014), or rh-cFGF23 injection (Agoro et al., 2018). FGF23-knockout mice displayed severe bone abnormalities, reduced lymphatic organ size, including spleen and thymus and elevated erythrocyte counts with increased RBC distribution width and reduced mean cell volume, and mean corpuscular hemoglobin (Coe et al., 2014). Knockout of the *FGF23* gene in mice resulted in a relative increase in hematopoietic stem cells, with decreased apoptosis, increased proliferative capacity of hematopoietic stem cells *in vitro* to form erythroid colonies, and an increased number of immature (pro-E, Ter119^{+med}, CD71$^{=hi}$) and mature erythroid cells (Ter119^{+hi}) in BM and peripheral blood. Hematopoietic changes were also observed in fetal livers, underlining the importance of FGF23 in hematopoietic stem cell generation and differentiation during embryonic development independent of the BM microenvironment. EPO, HIF1α, and HIF2α mRNA expression were significantly increased in BM, liver and kidney of FGF23-knockout mice, and the EPO receptor was upregulated on isolated BM mature erythroid cells. On the other hand, EPO, HIF1α, and HIF2α mRNA expression in osseous tissue was decreased; which might be explained by the remarkably lower osteoblast numbers in FGF23-knockout mice. Administration of rh-iFGF23 in WT mice resulted in a rapid decrease in erythropoiesis and a significant decrease in circulating EPO. *In vitro* administration of iFGF23 to FGF23-knockout BM-derived erythropoietic cells normalized erythropoiesis, normalized HIF, and EPO mRNA abundance and normalized EPOR expression (Coe et al., 2014). Alterations of EPO expression in response to iFGF23 were also observed by others: injection of rh-iFGF23 in mice reduced kidney EPO mRNA levels with 50% within 30 min, persisting over 24 h (Daryadel et al., 2018).

Inhibition of iFGF23 signaling with rh-cFGF23 in CKD mice resulted in decreased erythroid cell apoptosis, upregulation of renal and BM HIF1α and subsequent EPO mRNA expression, elevated serum EPO levels and amelioration of iron deficiency. Inflammatory markers and liver hepcidin mRNA expression

declined after iFGF23 blockage (Agoro et al., 2018). Lower hepcidin expression might have followed directly from decreases in inflammation, however, might also have resulted from increased EPO expression (Wang et al., 2017).

Interestingly, the increase in erythropoiesis after iFGF23 inhibition resembles the effects of α-klotho inhibition as outlined in Section "Presence of α-Klotho Is Essential for Normal Erythropoiesis" (Xu et al., 2017). In summary, current studies underline the importance of FGFR signaling by FGF23 for early erythropoiesis.

PRESENCE OF α-KLOTHO IS ESSENTIAL FOR NORMAL ERYTHROPOIESIS

Murine BM erythroid cells (Ter119^{+}) express the FGF23 receptors FGFR1, 2, and 4, and a small amount of FGFR3 (Coe et al., 2014). The FGFR1, that among others regulates phosphaturia, needs three components to be activated: the FGFR itself, iFGF23, and α-klotho (α-KL). α-KL, first described as an aging suppressor (Kuro-o et al., 1997), forms a complex with FGFR1 subgroup c, FGFR3 subgroup c or FGFR4 thereby selectively increasing the affinity of these FGFRs to FGF23 (Kurosu et al., 2006; Urakawa et al., 2006). α-KL simultaneously tethers FGFR and FGF23 to create proximity and stability (Chen et al., 2018). Membrane-bound α-KL is predominantly expressed in kidney, parathyroid gland and brain choroid plexus, however, shed α-KL ectodomain seems to function as an on-demand cofactor (Chen et al., 2018). There is expression of α-KL mRNA in BM, including BM erythroid cells (Ter119^{+}), spleen and fetal liver cells (Coe et al., 2014; Vadakke Madathil et al., 2014). The importance of α-KL for hematopoietic stem cell development and erythropoiesis was demonstrated in α-KL-knockout mice. Knockout of the α-KL gene resulted in a significant increase in erythropoiesis with significant increases in immature pro-erythroblasts and a relatively mature fraction of erythroblasts. *In vitro* α-KL-knockout BM cells generated more erythroid colonies than BM cells of WT mice. EPO mRNA expression was significantly upregulated in α-KL-knockout mice kidney, BM and liver cells, along with upregulation of HIF1α and HIF2α (Vadakke Madathil et al., 2014). Effects of α-KL-knockout are remarkably similar to effects of iFGF23 blockade or knockout. This suggests that α-KL is indeed an essential cofactor for FGF23 signaling in the regulation of erythropoiesis. However, if the link between less α-KL and more EPO involves less iFGF23 signaling remains to be proven. Besides EPO, iron load seems to influence α-KL. Iron overload decreased renal expression of α-KL at mRNA and protein level; iron chelation suppressed the downregulation of α-KL via angiotensin II (Saito et al., 2003).

Recent studies showed that FGF23 has various effects on many tissues in an α-KL-dependent way, but might also act in an α-KL-independent way especially under pathological conditions. The mechanism by which FGF23 activates the FGFR2 independent of α-KL on leukocytes and the FGFR4 independent of α-KL on cardiomyocytes is still unclear (Grabner et al., 2015; Grabner and Faul, 2016; Rossaint et al., 2016).

In conclusion, α-KL seems to be essential for FGF23 signaling in erythropoiesis, as α-KL-knockout resembles the effects of iFGF23 blockade or knockout on erythroid cell development.

FGF23 EXPRESSION IN HEREDITARY ANEMIA

Currently, information about the abundance of the EPO-FGF23 pathway in hereditary anemia is limited to two studies: one study in β-thalassemia mice and one study in SCD patients. β-thalassemia intermedia mice are characterized by anemia, iron overload and high endogenous EPO. FGF23 mRNA expression in bone and BM of thalassemia intermedia mice were elevated, reaching expression levels of endogenous EPO-overexpressing, polycythemic mice. The amount of circulating iFGF23 was significantly elevated compared to WT mice (436 versus 317 pg/mL), although the increase in iFGF23 was small compared to the increase in total circulating FGF23 (3129 versus 340 pg/mL in WT mice) (Hanudel et al., 2018). Circulating FGF23 levels were measured in 77 SCD patients, no EPO measurements were available (Courbebaisse et al., 2017). Serum ferritin concentrations and estimated glomerular filtration rate were significantly higher in SCD patients than in the control group. Mean plasma cFGF23 concentrations were significantly higher in SCD patients than in healthy controls (563 versus 55 RU/mL). The magnitude of multiplication of cFGF23 in SCD patients compared to healthy controls was comparable with the multiplication of cFGF23 observed after rhEPO (**Table 1**). In 75% of the SCD patients cFGF23 values were above the upper limit of normal, whereas in only 10% of the SCD patients iFGF23 values were above the upper limit of normal. Unfortunately, the association between the iFGF23/cFGF23 ratio, EPO and the extent of erythropoiesis was not evaluated.

The first study underlines that the EPO-FGF23 pathway is upregulated in β-thalassemia intermedia and can be upregulated under iron-overloaded conditions. The second study suggests that FGF23 production and cleavage are increased in SCD, if EPO or inflammation, or another factor, is the most important driving force remains to be investigated.

The activity of the EPO-FGF23 pathway in other hereditary anemias, including BM failure syndromes, with distinct amounts of hemolysis and ineffective hematopoiesis, accompanied by distinct elevations in circulating EPO, remains to be investigated. Besides activity of the pathway, the contribution of other factors influencing FGF23 signaling in hereditary anemias, including inflammation and iron load, remains to be investigated. Moreover, the role of the individual FGFRs and α-KL in FGF23 signaling in hereditary anemia is currently unknown.

IFGF23 DIRECTLY IMPAIRS BONE MINERALIZATION

The mineral ultrastructure of bone is crucial for its mechanical and biological properties. Non-collagenous proteins, as osteocalcin and osteopontin, are secreted during osteoid mineralization (Gericke et al., 2005). Loss of function of either or both osteocalcin and highly phosphorylated osteopontin significantly reduces crystal thickness and results in altered crystal shape (Poundarik et al., 2018). Tissue non-specific alkaline phosphatase (TNAP) is anchored to the membranes of osteoblasts and chondrocytes and to matrix vesicles released by both cells, and degrades pyrophosphate (PPi) to Pi. Pyrophosphate is an inhibitor of bone mineralization, and the regulation of pyrophosphate by TNAP controls continuous extracellular mineralization of apatite crystals. TNAP deficiency leads to accumulation of pyrophosphate, thereby decreasing mineralization (Rader, 2017).

FGF23 and EPO, are known regulators of bone mineralization, and are discussed in Section "Fibroblast Growth Factor 23." Finally, we discuss the contribution of these factors to defective bone mineralization in chronic diseases of erythropoiesis.

Fibroblast Growth Factor 23

Both gain and loss of function mutations in the *FGF23* gene result in bone mineralization disorders (**Table 2**). Gain of function mutations in *FGF23* cause autosomal dominant hypophosphatemic rickets (AHDR), a disease marked by severe decreased bone mineral density (Benet-Pages et al., 2005; Farrow et al., 2011a; Goldsweig and Carpenter, 2015). The metabolic mirror of ADHR is familial tumoral calcinosis, which is associated with pathologic increase of bone mineral density and is caused by loss of function mutations in the *FGF23* or *GalNT3* gene (Farrow et al., 2011a; Goldsweig and Carpenter, 2015). So, disturbances in FGF23, either primary (congenital) or secondary (e.g., in response to high EPO), ultimately result in bone mineralization deficits.

FGF23 seems to act auto- and/or paracrine in the bone environment (Murali et al., 2016b). A model has been proposed for a local role of FGF23 signaling in bone mineralization, independent of α-KL, via FGFR3. Local FGF23 signaling in osteocytes results in suppression of TNAP transcription, which leads to decreased degradation, and subsequent accumulation, of pyrophosphate and suppression of inorganic phosphate production. Both directly reduce bone mineralization. Osteopontin secretion is indirectly downregulated by FGF23 signaling: lower availability of extracellular phosphate suppresses osteopontin expression (Murali et al., 2016b). Although, acting locally, also high systemically circulating FGF23 could modulate pyrophosphate metabolism (Murali et al., 2016a,b; Andrukhova et al., 2018). Moreover, alterations in vitamin D metabolism contribute to impaired bone mineralization in response to iFGF23. $1,25(OH)_2D_3$ inhibits bone mineralization locally in osteoblasts and osteocytes via stimulation of transcription and subsequent expression of presumably inadequately phosphorylated osteopontin (Lieben et al., 2012; Murali et al., 2016b).

So, iFGF23 signaling results directly in impaired bone mineralization via TNAP suppression. Notably, current knowledge is based on FGF23-knockout models, thereby not reflecting the interplay of iFGF23 and cFGF23 (Murali et al., 2016a,b; Andrukhova et al., 2018).

TABLE 2 | FGF23-related disorders.

Disease	Locus	Inheritance pattern	Genetic defect	FGF23 function	iFGF23	cFGF23	TmP/GFR	Serum calcium	Serum phosphate	Urinary phosphate	1,25(OH)$_2$D	PTH	Bone features	Erythropoiesis
ADHR (OMIM 193100)	12p13.3	AD	R176Q, R179Q/W	GoF	= or ↑	↑ or =	↓	=	↓	↑	= or ↓	= or ↑	Bone deformities including varus deformity lower extremities, rachitic rosary, craniosynostosis, short stature; bone pain, bone fractures.	IDA, or low serum iron, associated with elevated FGF23 in ADHR.
fTC (OMIM 211900)	12p13.3	AR	S71G, M96T, S129F, F157L	LoF	= or ↓	↑	↑	=	↑	↓	= or ↑	= or ↓	Tumoral calcinosis, or ectopic calcifications, hyperostosis, vascular calcifications.	Not reported.

Summary of laboratory parameters and clinical characteristics of disorders associated with gain of function (ADHR) (ADHR Consortium, 2000; Imel et al., 2007, 2011; Huang et al., 2013; Acar et al., 2017; Clinkenbeard and White, 2017; Michalus and Rusinska, 2018; Luo et al., 2019) and loss of function (fTC) mutations (Ramnitz et al., 1993; Araya et al., 2005; Larsson et al., 2005a,b; Bergwitz et al., 2009; Huang et al., 2013; Clinkenbeard and White, 2017; Luo et al., 2019) in the FGF23 gene. AD, autosomal dominant; ADHRs, autosomal dominant hypophosphatemic rickets; AR, autosomal recessive; FGF23, fibroblast growth factor 23; fTC, familial tumoral calcinosis; GoF, gain of function; IDA, iron deficiency anemia; LoF, loss of function; PTH, parathyroid hormone; TmP/GFR, tubular maximum reabsorption rate of phosphate per glomerular filtration rate.

Erythropoietin

In addition to its role in erythropoiesis, EPO regulates bone homeostasis. Mice overexpressing endogenous EPO developed severe osteopenia (Hiram-Bab et al., 2015). Treatment of WT mice with rhEPO for ten days resulted in a significant reduction in trabecular bone volume and increased bone remodeling. Similar changes in bone volume were observed after increased endogenous EPO expression due to induction of acute hemolysis (Singbrant et al., 2011; Suda, 2011). Despite these observations, the action of EPO on bone homeostasis remains controversial. Effects might be dose-dependent: supraphysiologic EPO concentrations induced mineralization (Shiozawa et al., 2010; Holstein et al., 2011; Rolfing et al., 2012; Sun et al., 2012; Betsch et al., 2014; Guo et al., 2014; Wan et al., 2014; Eggold and Rankin, 2018), whereas low endogenous overexpression or moderate exogenous doses of EPO impaired bone formation via EPOR signaling (Shiozawa et al., 2010; Singbrant et al., 2011; Hiram-Bab et al., 2015; Rauner et al., 2016). Whether excess cFGF23, in response to EPO, is capable to neutralize α-KL independent osseous signaling of iFGF23, is currently unknown. We hypothesize that supraphysiologic EPO concentrations suppress the iFGF23/cFGF23 ratio to a level where the amount of cFGF23 is sufficient to fully prevent signaling of iFGF23 by competitive inhibition at the FGFR3. This resembles the hypermineralization observed in patients with elevated cFGF23 in familial tumoral calcinosis based on a *GalNT3* mutation (Ramnitz et al., 2016).

Bone Mineralization in Disorders of Erythropoiesis

Impaired bone mineralization, osteoporosis, is an important complication of chronic disorders affecting erythropoiesis (Valderrabano and Wu, 2018). The etiology of low bone mass is multifactorial including marrow expansion, various endocrine causes, direct iron toxicity, side effects of iron chelation therapy, lack of physical activity and genetic factors (Tzoulis et al., 2014; De Sanctis et al., 2018). In SCD and thalassemia bone abnormalities have been attributed mainly to marrow expansion (Valderrabano and Wu, 2018), although a linear correlation between circulating EPO levels and degree of bone demineralization in patients with identical diseases lacked (Steer et al., 2017). Eighty percent of adult SCD patients had an abnormal low bone mineral density (Sarrai et al., 2007), and up to 90% of β-thalassemia patients had an elevated fracture risk (Christoforidis et al., 2007; Wong et al., 2016). More recently, among children and young adults receiving regular transfusions and adequate iron chelation therapy Z-scores were within the normal range (Christoforidis et al., 2007; Wong et al., 2016). The role of transfusions in correction of bone mineral density underlines the importance of EPO signaling in the etiology of bone disease.

Currently, it is unknown what the extent is of the contribution of high EPO and subsequent lowering the iFGF23/cFGF23 ratio, to impaired bone mineralization in patients with chronic disorders of erythropoiesis. We suggest that iFGF23 excreted by BM erythroid cells might act on the surrounding osteocytes and osteoblasts in an auto- and/or paracrine way which will impair bone mineralization via TNAP suppression, subsequent pyrophosphate accumulation, and indirect downregulation of ostopontin (Murali et al., 2016a,b; Andrukhova et al., 2018). Hypothetically, rhEPO therapy in selected patients might increase EPO levels toward adequately elevated EPO levels, with further decline in the iFGF23/cFGF23 ratio, ultimately turning the balance toward increased bone mineralization.

SUMMARY AND FUTURE DIRECTIONS

We have outlined the importance of the EPO-FGF23 signaling pathways in erythroid cell development and bone mineralization. Both the amount of iFGF23 and its cleavage product cFGF23 determine signaling capacity. Insight in the activity of the EPO-FGF23 signaling pathway in rare hereditary anemias with varies degrees of hemolysis and ineffective erythropoiesis and varying circulating EPO concentrations, will add to the understanding of the pathophysiology and bone complications of these diseases.

Currently, two therapeutic agents are under development, or already registered, interfering with the EPO-FGF23 axis: FGF23 antagonists (KRN23; a therapeutic antibody against the C-terminus of FGF23) and FGFR1 inhibitor (BGJ-398; a small molecule pan-FGF kinase inhibitor) (Luo et al., 2019). Both agents have been tested for disorders characterized by high iFGF23 concentrations: tumor-induced osteomalacia (iFGF23 secreting tumors), or x-linked hyperphosphatemia (PHEX mutation results in high iFGF23).

Administration of rhEPO decreases the iFGF23/cFGF23 ratio, inhibiting apoptosis in erythroid cells. However, both EPO and an increase in the absolute amount of iFGF23 impair bone mineralization. Hypothetically, application of selective iFGF23 antagonists, or cFGF23 agonists, might bypass non-FGF23 related side-effects of rhEPO by regulating a more downstream component of the EPO-FGF23 pathway.

Uncertainties exist regarding (long-term) application of FGF23 antagonists or FGFR1 inhibitors in human. Thereby, the influence of FGF23, and pharmacological manipulation of FGF23, on energy metabolism is unclear. FGF23 is along with FGF21 and FGF19, both clearly associated with energy metabolism, grouped as endocrine FGFs (Luo et al., 2019).

Moreover, iFGF23 serves as a proinflammatory paracrine factor, secreted mainly by M1 proinflammatory macrophages (Hanks et al., 2015; Holecki et al., 2015; Han et al., 2016; Agoro et al., 2018; Wallquist et al., 2018). Oxygen supply in inflamed tissues is often very limited (Imtiyaz and Simon, 2010; Eltzschig and Carmeliet, 2011). This inflammation-induced hypoxia leads to increased expression of EPOR in macrophages, suppresses inflammatory macrophage signaling and promotes resolution of inflammation (Liu et al., 2015; Luo et al., 2016). In response on EPO, a substantial increase in cFGF23 compared to iFGF23 might antagonize the pro-inflammatory effects of iFGF23 or even promote development of a M2-like phenotype, characterized by immunoregulatory capacities (Rees, 2010; Liu et al., 2015; Eggold and Rankin, 2018). Several forms of hemolytic hereditary anemias present with chronic (low-grade) inflammation, which might play an important role in the vascular complications of these diseases (Frenette, 2002; Belcher et al., 2003, 2005; Aggeli et al., 2005; Rees et al., 2010; Rocha et al., 2011; Atichartakarn et al., 2014). Theoretically, cFGF23 agonists might diminish inflammation in these patients and improve clinical outcomes.

In conclusion, although first discovered as phosphate regulator, FGF23 is an important regulator of erythropoiesis being part of the EPO-FGF23 signaling pathway. A new area of research is open to extent our knowledge about FGF23 biology beyond the kidney. Experimental research is required to identify the molecular and cellular players of the EPO-FGF23 signaling pathway and the role of the various FGFRs in erythropoiesis. Thereby, to determine the clinical relevance of the pathway in patients with alterations in erythropoiesis, we propose measuring iFGF23, cFGF23, and EPO levels in patients with various forms of dyserythropoietic or hemolytic anemia, and relating these values to inflammation, bone health and vasculopathic complications.

AUTHOR CONTRIBUTIONS

All authors listed have made a substantial, direct and intellectual contribution to the work, and approved it for publication.

REFERENCES

Acar, S., Demir, K., and Shi, Y. (2017). Genetic causes of rickets. J. Clin. Res. Pediatr. Endocrinol. 9, 88–105. doi: 10.4274/jcrpe.2017.S008

ADHR Consortium (2000). Autosomal dominant hypophosphataemic rickets is associated with mutations in FGF23. Nat. Genet. 26, 345–348. doi: 10.1038/81664

Aggeli, C., Antoniades, C., Cosma, C., Chrysohoou, C., Tousoulis, D., Ladis, V., et al. (2005). Endothelial dysfunction and inflammatory process in transfusion-dependent patients with beta-thalassemia major. Int. J. Cardiol. 105, 80–84. doi: 10.1016/j.ijcard.2004.12.025

Agoro, R., Montagna, A., Goetz, R., Aligbe, O., Singh, G., Coe, L. M., et al. (2018). Inhibition of fibroblast growth factor 23 (FGF23) signaling rescues renal anemia. FASEB J. 32, 3752–3764. doi: 10.1096/fj.201700667R

Andrukhova, O., Schuler, C., Bergow, C., Petric, A., and Erben, R. G. (2018). Augmented fibroblast growth factor-23 secretion in bone locally contributes to impaired bone mineralization in chronic kidney disease in mice. Front. Endocrinol. 9:311. doi: 10.3389/fendo.2018.00311

Araya, K., Fukumoto, S., Backenroth, R., Takeuchi, Y., Nakayama, K., Ito, N., et al. (2005). A novel mutation in fibroblast growth factor 23 gene as a cause of tumoral calcinosis. J. Clin. Endocrinol. Metab. 90, 5523–5527. doi: 10.1210/jc.2005-0301

Atichartakarn, V., Chuncharunee, S., Archararit, N., Udomsubpayakul, U., and Aryurachai, K. (2014). Intravascular hemolysis, vascular endothelial cell activation and thrombophilia in splenectomized patients with hemoglobin E/beta-thalassemia disease. Acta Haematol. 132, 100–107. doi: 10.1159/000355719

Baia, L. C., Humalda, J. K., Vervloet, M. G., Navis, G., Bakker, S. J., de Borst, M. H., et al. (2013). Fibroblast growth factor 23 and cardiovascular mortality after kidney transplantation. Clin. J. Am. Soc. Nephrol. 8, 1968–1978. doi: 10.2215/CJN.01880213

Belcher, J. D., Bryant, C. J., Nguyen, J., Bowlin, P. R., Kielbik, M. C., Bischof, J. C., et al. (2003). Transgenic sickle mice have vascular inflammation. *Blood* 101, 3953–3959. doi: 10.1182/blood-2002-10-3313

Belcher, J. D., Mahaseth, H., Welch, T. E., Vilback, A. E., Sonbol, K. M., Kalambur, V. S., et al. (2005). Critical role of endothelial cell activation in hypoxia-induced vasoocclusion in transgenic sickle mice. *Am. J. Physiol. Heart Circ. Physiol.* 288, H2715–H2725. doi: 10.1152/ajpheart.00986.2004

Benet-Pages, A., Lorenz-Depiereux, B., Zischka, H., White, K. E., Econs, M. J., and Strom, T. M. (2004). FGF23 is processed by proprotein convertases but not by PHEX. *Bone* 35, 455–462. doi: 10.1016/j.bone.2004.04.002

Benet-Pages, A., Orlik, P., Strom, T. M., and Lorenz-Depiereux, B. (2005). An FGF23 missense mutation causes familial tumoral calcinosis with hyperphosphatemia. *Hum. Mol. Genet.* 14, 385–390. doi: 10.1093/hmg/ddi034

Bergwitz, C., Banerjee, S., Abu-Zahra, H., Kaji, H., Miyauchi, A., Sugimoto, T., et al. (2009). Defective O-glycosylation due to a novel homozygous S129P mutation is associated with lack of fibroblast growth factor 23 secretion and tumoral calcinosis. *J. Clin. Endocrinol. Metab.* 94, 4267–4274. doi: 10.1210/jc.2009-0961

Besson-Fournier, C., Latour, C., Kautz, L., Bertrand, J., Ganz, T., Roth, M. P., et al. (2012). Induction of activin B by inflammatory stimuli up-regulates expression of the iron-regulatory peptide hepcidin through Smad1/5/8 signaling. *Blood* 120, 431–439. doi: 10.1182/blood-2012-02-411470

Betsch, M., Thelen, S., Santak, L., Herten, M., Jungbluth, P., Miersch, D., et al. (2014). The role of erythropoietin and bone marrow concentrate in the treatment of osteochondral defects in mini-pigs. *PLoS One* 9:e92766. doi: 10.1371/journal.pone.0092766

Blazevic, A., Hunze, J., and Boots, J. M. (2014). Severe hypophosphataemia after intravenous iron administration. *Neth. J. Med.* 72, 49–53.

Block, G. A., Fishbane, S., Rodriguez, M., Smits, G., Shemesh, S., Pergola, P. E., et al. (2015). A 12-week, double-blind, placebo-controlled trial of ferric citrate for the treatment of iron deficiency anemia and reduction of serum phosphate in patients with CKD Stages 3-5. *Am. J. Kidney Dis.* 65, 728–736. doi: 10.1053/j.ajkd.2014.10.014

Bozentowicz-Wikarek, M., Kocelak, P., Owczarek, A., Olszanecka-Glinianowicz, M., Mossakowska, M., Skalska, A., et al. (2015). Plasma fibroblast growth factor 23 concentration and iron status. Does the relationship exist in the elderly population? *Clin. Biochem.* 48, 431–436. doi: 10.1016/j.clinbiochem.2014.12.027

Butthep, P., Wisedpanichkij, R., Jindadamrongwech, S., and Fucharoen, S. (2015). Elevated erythropoietin and cytokines levels are related to impaired reticulocyte maturation in thalassemic patients. *Blood Cells Mol. Dis.* 54, 170–176. doi: 10.1016/j.bcmd.2014.11.007

Canali, S., Core, A. B., Zumbrennen-Bullough, K. B., Merkulova, M., Wang, C. Y., Schneyer, A. L., et al. (2016). Activin B Induces Noncanonical SMAD1/5/8 Signaling via BMP Type I Receptors in Hepatocytes: evidence for a Role in Hepcidin Induction by Inflammation in Male Mice. *Endocrinology* 157, 1146–1162. doi: 10.1210/en.2015-1747

Caro, J., Brown, S., Miller, O., Murray, T., and Erslev, A. J. (1979). Erythropoietin levels in uremic nephric and anephric patients. *J. Lab. Clin. Med.* 93, 449–458.

Chen, G., Liu, Y., Goetz, R., Fu, L., Jayaraman, S., Hu, M. C., et al. (2018). alpha-Klotho is a non-enzymatic molecular scaffold for FGF23 hormone signalling. *Nature* 553, 461–466. doi: 10.1038/nature25451

Christoforidis, A., Kazantzidou, E., Tsatra, I., Tsantali, H., Koliakos, G., Hatzipantelis, E., et al. (2007). Normal lumbar bone mineral density in optimally treated children and young adolescents with beta-thalassaemia major. *Hormones* 6, 334–340. doi: 10.14310/horm.2002.1111030

Clinkenbeard, E. L., Cass, T. A., Ni, P., Hum, J. M., Bellido, T., Allen, M. R., et al. (2016). Conditional Deletion of Murine Fgf23: interruption of the normal skeletal responses to phosphate challenge and rescue of genetic hypophosphatemia. *J. Bone Miner. Res.* 31, 1247–1257. doi: 10.1002/jbmr.2792

Clinkenbeard, E. L., Farrow, E. G., Summers, L. J., Cass, T. A., Roberts, J. L., Bayt, C. A., et al. (2014). Neonatal iron deficiency causes abnormal phosphate metabolism by elevating FGF23 in normal and ADHR mice. *J. Bone Miner. Res.* 29, 361–369. doi: 10.1002/jbmr.2049

Clinkenbeard, E. L., Hanudel, M. R., Stayrook, K. R., Appaiah, H. N., Farrow, E. G., Cass, T. A., et al. (2017). Erythropoietin stimulates murine and human fibroblast growth factor-23, revealing novel roles for bone and

bone marrow. *Haematologica* 102, e427–e430. doi: 10.3324/haematol.2017.167882

Clinkenbeard, E. L., and White, K. E. (2017). Heritable and acquired disorders of phosphate metabolism: etiologies involving FGF23 and current therapeutics. *Bone* 102, 31–39. doi: 10.1016/j.bone.2017.01.034

Coe, L. M., Madathil, S. V., Casu, C., Lanske, B., Rivella, S., and Sitara, D. (2014). FGF-23 is a negative regulator of prenatal and postnatal erythropoiesis. *J. Biol. Chem.* 289, 9795–9810. doi: 10.1074/jbc.M113.527150

Courbebaisse, M., Mehel, H., Petit-Hoang, C., Ribeil, J. A., Sabbah, L., Tuloup-Minguez, V., et al. (2017). Carboxy-terminal fragment of fibroblast growth factor 23 induces heart hypertrophy in sickle cell disease. *Haematologica* 102, e33–e35. doi: 10.3324/haematol.2016.150987

Daryadel, A., Bettoni, C., Haider, T., Imenez Silva, P. H., Schnitzbauer, U., Pastor-Arroyo, E. M., et al. (2018). Erythropoietin stimulates fibroblast growth factor 23 (FGF23) in mice and men. *Pflugers Arch.* 470, 1569–1582. doi: 10.1007/s00424-018-2171-7

David, V., Martin, A., Isakova, T., Spaulding, C., Qi, L., Ramirez, V., et al. (2016). Inflammation and functional iron deficiency regulate fibroblast growth factor 23 production. *Kidney Int.* 89, 135–146. doi: 10.1038/ki.2015.290

De Sanctis, V., Soliman, A. T., Elsefdy, H., Soliman, N., Bedair, E., Fiscina, B., et al. (2018). Bone disease in beta thalassemia patients: past, present and future perspectives. *Metabolism* 80, 66–79. doi: 10.1016/j.metabol.2017.09.012

Dounousi, E., Torino, C., Pizzini, P., Cutrupi, S., Panuccio, V., D'Arrigo, G., et al. (2016). Intact FGF23 and alpha-Klotho during acute inflammation/sepsis in CKD patients. *Eur. J. Clin. Invest.* 46, 234–241. doi: 10.1111/eci.12588

Ebert, B. L., and Bunn, H. F. (1999). Regulation of the erythropoietin gene. *Blood* 94, 1864–1877.

Eggold, J. T., and Rankin, E. B. (2018). Erythropoiesis, EPO, macrophages, and bone. *Bone* 119, 36–41. doi: 10.1016/j.bone.2018.03.014

Eisenga, M. F., van Londen, M., Leaf, D. E., Nolte, I. M., Navis, G., Bakker, S. J. L., et al. (2017). C-terminal fibroblast growth factor 23, iron deficiency, and mortality in renal transplant recipients. *J. Am. Soc. Nephrol.* 28, 3639–3646. doi: 10.1681/ASN.2016121350

Eltzschig, H. K., and Carmeliet, P. (2011). Hypoxia and inflammation. *N. Engl. J. Med.* 364, 656–665. doi: 10.1056/NEJMra0910283

Farrow, E. G., Imel, E. A., and White, K. E. (2011a). Miscellaneous non-inflammatory musculoskeletal conditions. Hyperphosphatemic familial tumoral calcinosis (FGF23, GALNT3 and alphaKlotho). *Best Pract. Res. Clin. Rheumatol.* 25, 735–747. doi: 10.1016/j.berh.2011.10.020

Farrow, E. G., Yu, X., Summers, L. J., Davis, S. I., Fleet, J. C., Allen, M. R., et al. (2011b). Iron deficiency drives an autosomal dominant hypophosphatemic rickets (ADHR) phenotype in fibroblast growth factor-23 (Fgf23) knock-in mice. *Proc. Natl. Acad. Sci. U.S.A.* 108, E1146–E1155. doi: 10.1073/pnas.1110905108

Faul, C., Amaral, A. P., Oskouei, B., Hu, M. C., Sloan, A., Isakova, T., et al. (2011). FGF23 induces left ventricular hypertrophy. *J. Clin. Invest* 121, 4393–4408. doi: 10.1172/JCI46122

Fibach, E., and Rachmilewitz, E. A. (2014). Does erythropoietin have a role in the treatment of beta-hemoglobinopathies? *Hematol. Oncol. Clin. North Am.* 28, 249–263. doi: 10.1016/j.hoc.2013.11.002

Flamme, I., Ellinghaus, P., Urrego, D., and Kruger, T. (2017). FGF23 expression in rodents is directly induced via erythropoietin after inhibition of hypoxia inducible factor proline hydroxylase. *PLoS One* 12:e0186979. doi: 10.1371/journal.pone.0186979

Fliser, D., Kollerits, B., Neyer, U., Ankerst, D. P., Lhotta, K., Lingenhel, A., et al. (2007). Fibroblast growth factor 23 (FGF23) predicts progression of chronic kidney disease: the Mild to Moderate Kidney Disease (MMKD) Study. *J. Am. Soc. Nephrol.* 18, 2600–2608. doi: 10.1681/ASN.2006080936

Francis, C., and David, V. (2016). Inflammation regulates fibroblast growth factor 23 production. *Curr. Opin. Nephrol. Hypertens.* 25, 325–332. doi: 10.1097/MNH.0000000000000232

Frenette, P. S. (2002). Sickle cell vaso-occlusion: multistep and multicellular paradigm. *Curr. Opin. Hematol.* 9, 101–106. doi: 10.1097/00062752-200203000-00003

Ganz, T. (2011). Hepcidin and iron regulation, 10 years later. *Blood* 117, 4425–4433. doi: 10.1182/blood-2011-01-258467

Gericke, A., Qin, C., Spevak, L., Fujimoto, Y., Butler, W. T., Sorensen, E. S., et al. (2005). Importance of phosphorylation for osteopontin regulation of biomineralization. *Calcif. Tissue Int.* 77, 45–54. doi: 10.1007/s00223-004-1288-1

Goetz, R., Beenken, A., Ibrahimi, O. A., Kalinina, J., Olsen, S. K., Eliseenkova, A. V., et al. (2007). Molecular insights into the klotho-dependent, endocrine mode of action of fibroblast growth factor 19 subfamily members. *Mol. Cell Biol.* 27, 3417–3428. doi: 10.1128/MCB.02249-06

Goetz, R., Nakada, Y., Hu, M. C., Kurosu, H., Wang, L., Nakatani, T., et al. (2010). Isolated C-terminal tail of FGF23 alleviates hypophosphatemia by inhibiting FGF23-FGFR-Klotho complex formation. *Proc. Natl. Acad. Sci. U.S.A.* 107, 407–412. doi: 10.1073/pnas.0902006107

Goldsweig, B. K., and Carpenter, T. O. (2015). Hypophosphatemic rickets: lessons from disrupted FGF23 control of phosphorus homeostasis. *Curr. Osteoporos. Rep.* 13, 88–97. doi: 10.1007/s11914-015-0259-y

Grabner, A., Amaral, A. P., Schramm, K., Singh, S., Sloan, A., Yanucil, C., et al. (2015). Activation of cardiac fibroblast growth factor receptor 4 causes left ventricular hypertrophy. *Cell Metab.* 22, 1020–1032. doi: 10.1016/j.cmet.2015.09.002

Grabner, A., and Faul, C. (2016). The role of fibroblast growth factor 23 and Klotho in uremic cardiomyopathy. *Curr. Opin. Nephrol. Hypertens.* 25, 314–324. doi: 10.1097/MNH.0000000000000231

Guo, L., Luo, T., Fang, Y., Yang, L., Wang, L., Liu, J., et al. (2014). Effects of erythropoietin on osteoblast proliferation and function. *Clin. Exp. Med.* 14, 69–76. doi: 10.1007/s10238-012-0220-7

Gutierrez, O. M., Januzzi, J. L., Isakova, T., Laliberte, K., Smith, K., Collerone, G., et al. (2009). Fibroblast growth factor 23 and left ventricular hypertrophy in chronic kidney disease. *Circulation* 119, 2545–2552. doi: 10.1161/CIRCULATIONAHA.108.844506

Haase, V. H. (2010). Hypoxic regulation of erythropoiesis and iron metabolism. *Am. J. Physiol. Renal Physiol.* 299, F1–F13. doi: 10.1152/ajprenal.00174.2010

Haidar, R., Mhaidli, H., Musallam, K. M., and Taher, A. T. (2012). The spine in beta-thalassemia syndromes. *Spine* 37, 334–339. doi: 10.1097/BRS.0b013e31821bd095

Han, J., Zhou, J., Kondragunta, V., Zhang, X., Molokie, R. E., Gowhari, M., et al. (2017). Erythropoiesis-stimulating agents in sickle cell anaemia. *Br. J. Haematol.* 182, 602–605. doi: 10.1111/bjh.14846

Han, X., Li, L., Yang, J., King, G., Xiao, Z., and Quarles, L. D. (2016). Counter-regulatory paracrine actions of FGF-23 and 1,25(OH)2 D in macrophages. *FEBS Lett.* 590, 53–67. doi: 10.1002/1873-3468.12040

Hanks, L. J., Casazza, K., Judd, S. E., Jenny, N. S., and Gutierrez, O. M. (2015). Associations of fibroblast growth factor-23 with markers of inflammation, insulin resistance and obesity in adults. *PLoS One* 10:e0122885. doi: 10.1371/journal.pone.0122885

Hanudel, M. R., Chua, K., Rappaport, M., Gabayan, V., Valore, E., Goltzman, D., et al. (2016). Effects of dietary iron intake and chronic kidney disease on fibroblast growth factor 23 metabolism in wild-type and hepcidin knockout mice. *Am. J. Physiol. Renal Physiol.* 311, F1369–F1377. doi: 10.1152/ajprenal.00281.2016

Hanudel, M. R., Eisenga, M. F., Rappaport, M., Chua, K., Qiao, B., Jung, G., et al. (2018). Effects of erythropoietin on fibroblast growth factor 23 in mice and humans. *Nephrol. Dial. Transplant.* doi: 10.1093/ndt/gfy189 [Epub ahead of print].

Hiram-Bab, S., Liron, T., Deshet-Unger, N., Mittelman, M., Gassmann, M., Rauner, M., et al. (2015). Erythropoietin directly stimulates osteoclast precursors and induces bone loss. *FASEB J.* 29, 1890–1900. doi: 10.1096/fj.14-259085

Holecki, M., Chudek, J., Owczarek, A., Olszanecka-Glinianowicz, M., Bozentowicz-Wikarek, M., Dulawa, J., et al. (2015). Inflammation but not obesity or insulin resistance is associated with increased plasma fibroblast growth factor 23 concentration in the elderly. *Clin. Endocrinol.* 82, 900–909. doi: 10.1111/cen.12759

Holstein, J. H., Orth, M., Scheuer, C., Tami, A., Becker, S. C., Garcia, P., et al. (2011). Erythropoietin stimulates bone formation, cell proliferation, and angiogenesis in a femoral segmental defect model in mice. *Bone* 49, 1037–1045. doi: 10.1016/j.bone.2011.08.004

Hryszko, T., Rydzewska-Rosolowska, A., Brzosko, S., Koc-Zorawska, E., and Mysliwiec, M. (2012). Low molecular weight iron dextran increases fibroblast

growth factor-23 concentration, together with parathyroid hormone decrease in hemodialyzed patients. *Ther. Apher. Dial.* 16, 146–151. doi: 10.1111/j.1744-9987.2011.01037.x

Huang, X., Jiang, Y., and Xia, W. (2013). FGF23 and phosphate wasting disorders. *Bone Res.* 1, 120–132. doi: 10.4248/BR201302002

Iguchi, A., Kazama, J. J., Yamamoto, S., Yoshita, K., Watanabe, Y., Iino, N., et al. (2015). Administration of ferric citrate hydrate decreases circulating FGF23 Levels independently of serum phosphate levels in hemodialysis patients with iron deficiency. *Nephron* 131, 161–166. doi: 10.1159/000440968

Imel, E. A., Hui, S. L., and Econs, M. J. (2007). FGF23 concentrations vary with disease status in autosomal dominant hypophosphatemic rickets. *J. Bone Miner. Res.* 22, 520–526. doi: 10.1359/jbmr.070107

Imel, E. A., Liu, Z., McQueen, A. K., Acton, D., Acton, A., Padgett, L. R., et al. (2016). Serum fibroblast growth factor 23, serum iron and bone mineral density in premenopausal women. *Bone* 86, 98–105. doi: 10.1016/j.bone.2016.03.005

Imel, E. A., Peacock, M., Gray, A. K., Padgett, L. R., Hui, S. L., and Econs, M. J. (2011). Iron modifies plasma FGF23 differently in autosomal dominant hypophosphatemic rickets and healthy humans. *J. Clin. Endocrinol. Metab.* 96, 3541–3549. doi: 10.1210/jc.2011-1239

Imtiyaz, H. Z., and Simon, M. C. (2010). Hypoxia-inducible factors as essential regulators of inflammation. *Curr. Top. Microbiol. Immunol.* 345, 105–120. doi: 10.1007/82_2010_74

Isakova, T., Xie, H., Yang, W., Xie, D., Anderson, A. H., Scialla, J., et al. (2011). Fibroblast growth factor 23 and risks of mortality and end-stage renal disease in patients with chronic kidney disease. *JAMA* 305, 2432–2439. doi: 10.1001/jama.2011.826

Ito, N., Wijenayaka, A. R., Prideaux, M., Kogawa, M., Ormsby, R. T., Evdokiou, A., et al. (2015). Regulation of FGF23 expression in IDG-SW3 osteocytes and human bone by pro-inflammatory stimuli. *Mol. Cell Endocrinol.* 399, 208–218. doi: 10.1016/j.mce.2014.10.007

Jelkmann, W. (1992). Erythropoietin: structure, control of production, and function. *Physiol. Rev.* 72, 449–489. doi: 10.1152/physrev.1992.72.2.449

Kanbay, M., Vervloet, M., Cozzolino, M., Siriopol, D., Covic, A., Goldsmith, D., et al. (2017). Novel Faces of Fibroblast Growth Factor 23 (FGF23): iron deficiency, inflammation, insulin resistance, left ventricular hypertrophy, proteinuria and acute kidney injury. *Calcif. Tissue Int.* 100, 217–228. doi: 10.1007/s00223-016-0206-7

Karafin, M. S., Koch, K. L., Rankin, A. B., Nischik, D., Rahhal, G., Simpson, P., et al. (2015). Erythropoietic drive is the strongest predictor of hepcidin level in adults with sickle cell disease. *Blood Cells Mol. Dis.* 55, 304–307. doi: 10.1016/j.bcmd.2015.07.010

Kato, K., Jeanneau, C., Tarp, M. A., Benet-Pages, A., Lorenz-Depiereux, B., Bennett, E. P., et al. (2006). Polypeptide GalNAc-transferase T3 and familial tumoral calcinosis. Secretion of fibroblast growth factor 23 requires O-glycosylation. *J. Biol. Chem.* 281, 18370–18377. doi: 10.1074/jbc.M602469200

Khosravi, A., Cutler, C. M., Kelly, M. H., Chang, R., Royal, R. E., Sherry, R. M., et al. (2007). Determination of the elimination half-life of fibroblast growth factor-23. *J. Clin. Endocrinol. Metab.* 92, 2374–2377. doi: 10.1210/jc.2006-2865

Konjiki, O., Fukaya, S., Kanou, H., Imamura, T., Iwamoto, T., and Takasaki, M. (1994). A case of hypophosphatemia induced by intravenous administration of saccharated iron oxide. *Nihon Ronen Igakkai Zasshi* 31, 805–810. doi: 10.3143/geriatrics.31.805

Krantz, S. B. (1991). Erythropoietin. *Blood* 77, 419–434.

Krick, S., Grabner, A., Baumlin, N., Yanucil, C., Helton, S., Grosche, A., et al. (2018). Fibroblast growth factor 23 and Klotho contribute to airway inflammation. *Eur. Respir. J.* 52:1800236. doi: 10.1183/13993003.00236-2018

Kuro-o, M., Matsumura, Y., Aizawa, H., Kawaguchi, H., Suga, T., Utsugi, T., et al. (1997). Mutation of the mouse klotho gene leads to a syndrome resembling ageing. *Nature* 390, 45–51. doi: 10.1038/36285

Kurosu, H., Ogawa, Y., Miyoshi, M., Yamamoto, M., Nandi, A., Rosenblatt, K. P., et al. (2006). Regulation of fibroblast growth factor-23 signaling by klotho. *J. Biol. Chem.* 281, 6120–6123. doi: 10.1074/jbc.C500457200

Larsson, T., Davis, S. I., Garringer, H. J., Mooney, S. D., Draman, M. S., Cullen, M. J., et al. (2005a). Fibroblast growth factor-23 mutants causing familial tumoral calcinosis are differentially processed. *Endocrinology* 146, 3883–3891.

Larsson, T., Yu, X., Davis, S. I., Draman, M. S., Mooney, S. D., Cullen, M. J., et al. (2005b). A novel recessive mutation in fibroblast growth factor-23 causes familial tumoral calcinosis. *J. Clin. Endocrinol. Metab.* 90, 2424–2427. doi: 10.1210/jc.2004-2238

Lieben, L., Masuyama, R., Torrekens, S., Van Looveren, R., Schrooten, J., Baatsen, P., et al. (2012). Normocalcemia is maintained in mice under conditions of calcium malabsorption by vitamin D-induced inhibition of bone mineralization. *J. Clin. Invest.* 122, 1803–1815. doi: 10.1172/JCI45890

Liu, Y., Luo, B., Shi, R., Wang, J., Liu, Z., Liu, W., et al. (2015). Nonerythropoietic erythropoietin-derived peptide suppresses adipogenesis, inflammation, obesity and insulin resistance. *Sci. Rep.* 5:15134. doi: 10.1038/srep15134

Luo, B., Gan, W., Liu, Z., Shen, Z., Wang, J., Shi, R., et al. (2016). Erythropoietin signaling in macrophages promotes dying cell clearance and immune tolerance. *Immunity* 44, 287–302. doi: 10.1016/j.immuni.2016.01.002

Luo, Y., Ye, S., Li, X., and Lu, W. (2019). Emerging structure-function paradigm of endocrine FGFs in metabolic diseases. *Trends Pharmacol. Sci.* 40, 142–153. doi: 10.1016/j.tips.2018.12.002

Mace, M. L., Gravesen, E., Hofman-Bang, J., Olgaard, K., and Lewin, E. (2015). Key role of the kidney in the regulation of fibroblast growth factor 23. *Kidney Int.* 88, 1304–1313. doi: 10.1038/ki.2015.231

Martin, A., David, V., and Quarles, L. D. (2012). Regulation and function of the FGF23/klotho endocrine pathways. *Physiol. Rev.* 92, 131–155. doi: 10.1152/physrev.00002.2011

Maruyama, N., Otsuki, T., Yoshida, Y., Nagura, C., Kitai, M., Shibahara, N., et al. (2018). Ferric citrate decreases fibroblast growth factor 23 and improves erythropoietin responsiveness in hemodialysis patients. *Am. J. Nephrol.* 47, 406–414. doi: 10.1159/000489964

McMahon, S., Grondin, F., McDonald, P. P., Richard, D. E., and Dubois, C. M. (2005). Hypoxia-enhanced expression of the proprotein convertase furin is mediated by hypoxia-inducible factor-1: impact on the bioactivation of proproteins. *J. Biol. Chem.* 280, 6561–6569. doi: 10.1074/jbc.M413248200

Mehta, R., Cai, X., Lee, J., Scialla, J. J., Bansal, N., Sondheimer, J. H., et al. (2016). Association of fibroblast growth factor 23 with atrial fibrillation in chronic kidney disease, from the chronic renal insufficiency cohort study. *JAMA Cardiol.* 1, 548–556. doi: 10.1001/jamacardio.2016.1445

Michalus, I., and Rusinska, A. (2018). Rare, genetically conditioned forms of rickets: Differential diagnosis and advances in diagnostics and treatment. *Clin. Genet.* 94, 103–114. doi: 10.1111/cge.13229

Muckenthaler, M. U., Rivella, S., Hentze, M. W., and Galy, B. (2017). A Red Carpet for Iron Metabolism. *Cell* 168, 344–361. doi: 10.1016/j.cell.2016.12.034

Munoz Mendoza, J., Isakova, T., Ricardo, A. C., Xie, H., Navaneethan, S. D., Anderson, A. H., et al. (2012). Fibroblast growth factor 23 and Inflammation in CKD. *Clin. J. Am. Soc. Nephrol.* 7, 1155–1162. doi: 10.2215/CJN.13281211

Murali, S. K., Andrukhova, O., Clinkenbeard, E. L., White, K. E., and Erben, R. G. (2016a). Excessive Osteocytic Fgf23 secretion contributes to pyrophosphate accumulation and mineralization defect in hyp mice. *PLoS Biol.* 14:e1002427. doi: 10.1371/journal.pbio.1002427

Murali, S. K., Roschger, P., Zeitz, U., Klaushofer, K., Andrukhova, O., and Erben, R. G. (2016b). FGF23 regulates bone mineralization in a 1,25(OH)2 D3 and Klotho-Independent Manner. *J. Bone Miner. Res.* 31, 129–142. doi: 10.1002/jbmr.2606

O'Donnell, A., Premawardhena, A., Arambepola, M., Allen, S. J., Peto, T. E., Fisher, C. A., et al. (2007). Age-related changes in adaptation to severe anemia in childhood in developing countries. *Proc. Natl. Acad. Sci. U.S.A.* 104, 9440–9444. doi: 10.1073/pnas.0703424104

Okada, M., Imamura, K., Iida, M., Fuchigami, T., and Omae, T. (1983). Hypophosphatemia induced by intravenous administration of Saccharated iron oxide. *Klin. Wochenschr.* 61, 99–102. doi: 10.1007/BF01496662

Okan, G., Baki, A. M., Yorulmaz, E., Dogru-Abbasoglu, S., and Vural, P. (2016). Fibroblast growth factor 23 and placental growth factor in patients with psoriasis and their relation to disease severity. *Ann. Clin. Lab. Sci.* 46, 174–179.

Portale, A. A., Wolf, M. S., Messinger, S., Perwad, F., Juppner, H., Warady, B. A., et al. (2016). Fibroblast Growth Factor 23 and Risk of CKD Progression in Children. *Clin. J. Am. Soc. Nephrol.* 11, 1989–1998. doi: 10.2215/CJN.02110216

Poundarik, A. A., Boskey, A., Gundberg, C., and Vashishth, D. (2018). Biomolecular regulation, composition and nanoarchitecture of bone mineral. *Sci. Rep.* 8:1191. doi: 10.1038/s41598-018-19253-w

Prats, M., Font, R., Garcia, C., Cabre, C., Jariod, M., and Vea, A. M. (2013). Effect of ferric carboxymaltose on serum phosphate and C-terminal FGF23 levels in non-dialysis chronic kidney disease patients: post-hoc analysis of a prospective study. *BMC Nephrol.* 14:167. doi: 10.1186/1471-2369-14-167

Pulte, E. D., McKenzie, S. E., Caro, J., and Ballas, S. K. (2014). Erythropoietin levels in patients with sickle cell disease do not correlate with known inducers of erythropoietin. *Hemoglobin* 38, 385–389. doi: 10.3109/03630269.2014.967868

Quarles, L. D. (2012). Role of FGF23 in vitamin D and phosphate metabolism: implications in chronic kidney disease. *Exp. Cell Res.* 318, 1040–1048. doi: 10.1016/j.yexcr.2012.02.027

Rabadi, S., Udo, I., Leaf, D. E., Waikar, S. S., and Christov, M. (2018). Acute blood loss stimulates fibroblast growth factor 23 production. *Am. J. Physiol. Renal Physiol.* 314, F132–F139. doi: 10.1152/ajprenal.00081.2017

Rader, B. A. (2017). Alkaline phosphatase, an unconventional immune protein. *Front. Immunol.* 8:897. doi: 10.3389/fimmu.2017.00897

Ramnitz, M. S., Gafni, R. I., and Collins, M. T. (1993). "Hyperphosphatemic Familial Tumoral Calcinosis," in *GeneReviews((R))*, eds M. P. Adam, H. H. Ardinger, R. A. Pagon, S. E. Wallace, L. J. H. Bean, K. Stephens, et al. (Seattle, WA: University of Washington, Seattle).

Ramnitz, M. S., Gourh, P., Goldbach-Mansky, R., Wodajo, F., Ichikawa, S., Econs, M. J., et al. (2016). Phenotypic and genotypic characterization and treatment of a cohort with familial tumoral calcinosis/hyperostosis-hyperphosphatemia syndrome. *J. Bone Miner. Res.* 31, 1845–1854. doi: 10.1002/jbmr.2870

Rankin, E. B., Wu, C., Khatri, R., Wilson, T. L., Andersen, R., Araldi, E., et al. (2012). The HIF signaling pathway in osteoblasts directly modulates erythropoiesis through the production of EPO. *Cell* 149, 63–74. doi: 10.1016/j.cell.2012.01.051

Rauner, M., Franke, K., Murray, M., Singh, R. P., Hiram-Bab, S., Platzbecker, U., et al. (2016). Increased EPO levels are associated with bone loss in mice Lacking PHD2 in EPO-Producing Cells. *J. Bone Miner. Res.* 31, 1877–1887. doi: 10.1002/jbmr.2857

Rees, A. J. (2010). Monocyte and macrophage biology: an overview. *Semin. Nephrol.* 30, 216–233. doi: 10.1016/j.semnephrol.2010.03.002

Rees, D. C., Williams, T. N., and Gladwin, M. T. (2010). Sickle-cell disease. *Lancet* 376, 2018–2031. doi: 10.1016/S0140-6736(10)61029-X

Resende, A. L., Elias, R. M., Wolf, M., Dos Reis, L. M., Graciolli, F. G., Santos, G. D., et al. (2017). Serum levels of fibroblast growth factor 23 are elevated in patients with active Lupus nephritis. *Cytokine* 91, 124–127. doi: 10.1016/j.cyto.2016.12.022

Rocha, S., Costa, E., Catarino, C., Belo, L., Castro, E. M., Barbot, J., et al. (2005). Erythropoietin levels in the different clinical forms of hereditary spherocytosis. *Br. J. Haematol.* 131, 534–542. doi: 10.1111/j.1365-2141.2005.05802.x

Rocha, S., Costa, E., Rocha-Pereira, P., Ferreira, F., Cleto, E., Barbot, J., et al. (2011). Erythropoiesis versus inflammation in Hereditary Spherocytosis clinical outcome. *Clin. Biochem.* 44, 1137–1143. doi: 10.1016/j.clinbiochem.2011.06.006

Rolfing, J. H., Bendtsen, M., Jensen, J., Stiehler, M., Foldager, C. B., Hellfritzsch, M. B., et al. (2012). Erythropoietin augments bone formation in a rabbit posterolateral spinal fusion model. *J. Orthop. Res.* 30, 1083–1088. doi: 10.1002/jor.22027

Rossaint, J., Oehmichen, J., Van Aken, H., Reuter, S., Pavenstadt, H. J., Meersch, M., et al. (2016). FGF23 signaling impairs neutrophil recruitment and host defense during CKD. *J. Clin. Invest.* 126, 962–974. doi: 10.1172/JCI83470

Saito, K., Ishizaka, N., Mitani, H., Ohno, M., and Nagai, R. (2003). Iron chelation and a free radical scavenger suppress angiotensin II-induced downregulation of klotho, an anti-aging gene, in rat. *FEBS Lett.* 551, 58–62. doi: 10.1016/S0014-5793(03)00894-9

Saito, T., and Fukumoto, S. (2009). Fibroblast Growth Factor 23 (FGF23) and disorders of phosphate metabolism. *Int. J. Pediatr. Endocrinol.* 2009:496514. doi: 10.1155/2009/496514

Sarrai, M., Duroseau, H., D'Augustine, J., Moktan, S., and Bellevue, R. (2007). Bone mass density in adults with sickle cell disease. *Br. J. Haematol.* 136, 666–672. doi: 10.1111/j.1365-2141.2006.06487.x

Sato, H., Kazama, J. J., Murasawa, A., Otani, H., Abe, A., Ito, S., et al. (2016). Serum Fibroblast Growth Factor 23 (FGF23) in patients with rheumatoid arthritis. *Intern. Med.* 55, 121–126. doi: 10.2169/internalmedicine.55.5507

Schofield, C. J., and Ratcliffe, P. J. (2004). Oxygen sensing by HIF hydroxylases. *Nat. Rev. Mol. Cell Biol.* 5, 343–354. doi: 10.1038/nrm1366

Schotten, N., Laarakkers, C. M., Roelofs, R. W., Origa, R., van Kraaij, M. G., and Swinkels, D. W. (2017). EPO and hepcidin plasma concentrations in blood donors and beta-thalassemia intermedia are not related to commercially tested plasma ERFE concentrations. *Am. J. Hematol.* 92, E29–E31. doi: 10.1002/ajh.24636

Schouten, B. J., Doogue, M. P., Soule, S. G., and Hunt, P. J. (2009a). Iron polymaltose-induced FGF23 elevation complicated by hypophosphataemic osteomalacia. *Ann. Clin. Biochem.* 46, 167–169. doi: 10.1258/acb.2008.008151

Schouten, B. J., Hunt, P. J., Livesey, J. H., Frampton, C. M., and Soule, S. G. (2009b). FGF23 elevation and hypophosphatemia after intravenous iron polymaltose: a prospective study. *J. Clin. Endocrinol. Metab.* 94, 2332–2337. doi: 10.1210/jc.2008-2396

Shimada, T., Kakitani, M., Yamazaki, Y., Hasegawa, H., Takeuchi, Y., Fujita, T., et al. (2004). Targeted ablation of Fgf23 demonstrates an essential physiological role of FGF23 in phosphate and vitamin D metabolism. *J. Clin. Invest.* 113, 561–568. doi: 10.1172/JCI19081

Shimada, T., Mizutani, S., Muto, T., Yoneya, T., Hino, R., Takeda, S., et al. (2001). Cloning and characterization of FGF23 as a causative factor of tumor-induced osteomalacia. *Proc. Natl. Acad. Sci. U.S.A.* 98, 6500–6505. doi: 10.1073/pnas.101545198

Shimada, T., Muto, T., Urakawa, I., Yoneya, T., Yamazaki, Y., Okawa, K., et al. (2002). Mutant FGF-23 responsible for autosomal dominant hypophosphatemic rickets is resistant to proteolytic cleavage and causes hypophosphatemia in vivo. *Endocrinology* 143, 3179–3182. doi: 10.1210/endo.143.8.8795

Shiozawa, Y., Jung, Y., Ziegler, A. M., Pedersen, E. A., Wang, J., Wang, Z., et al. (2010). Erythropoietin couples hematopoiesis with bone formation. *PLoS One* 5:e10853. doi: 10.1371/journal.pone.0010853

Silvestri, L., Pagani, A., and Camaschella, C. (2008). Furin-mediated release of soluble hemojuvelin: a new link between hypoxia and iron homeostasis. *Blood* 111, 924–931. doi: 10.1182/blood-2007-07-100677

Singbrant, S., Russell, M. R., Jovic, T., Liddicoat, B., Izon, D. J., Purton, L. E., et al. (2011). Erythropoietin couples erythropoiesis, B-lymphopoiesis, and bone homeostasis within the bone marrow microenvironment. *Blood* 117, 5631–5642. doi: 10.1182/blood-2010-11-320564

Singer, S. T., Vichinsky, E. P., Sweeters, N., and Rachmilewitz, E. (2011). Darbepoetin alfa for the treatment of anaemia in alpha- or beta- thalassaemia intermedia syndromes. *Br. J. Haematol.* 154, 281–284. doi: 10.1111/j.1365-2141.2011.08617.x

Singh, S., Grabner, A., Yanucil, C., Schramm, K., Czaya, B., Krick, S., et al. (2016). Fibroblast growth factor 23 directly targets hepatocytes to promote inflammation in chronic kidney disease. *Kidney Int.* 90, 985–996. doi: 10.1016/j.kint.2016.05.019

Smith, E. R., Cai, M. M., McMahon, L. P., and Holt, S. G. (2012). Biological variability of plasma intact and C-terminal FGF23 measurements. *J. Clin. Endocrinol. Metab.* 97, 3357–3365. doi: 10.1210/jc.2012-1811

Soares, M. P., and Weiss, G. (2015). The Iron age of host-microbe interactions. *EMBO Rep.* 16, 1482–1500. doi: 10.15252/embr.201540558

Steer, K., Stavnichuk, M., Morris, M., and Komarova, S. V. (2017). Bone health in patients with hematopoietic disorders of bone marrow origin: systematic review and meta- analysis. *J. Bone Miner. Res.* 32, 731–742. doi: 10.1002/jbmr.3026

Stefanova, D., Raychev, A., Arezes, J., Ruchala, P., Gabayan, V., Skurnik, M., et al. (2017). Endogenous hepcidin and its agonist mediate resistance to selected infections by clearing non-transferrin-bound iron. *Blood* 130, 245–257. doi: 10.1182/blood-2017-03-772715

Suda, T. (2011). Hematopoiesis and bone remodeling. *Blood* 117, 5556–5557. doi: 10.1182/blood-2011-03-344127

Sukpanichnant, S., Opartkiattikul, N., Fucharoen, S., Tanphaichitr, V. S., Hasuike, T., and Tatsumi, N. (1997). Difference in pattern of erythropoietin response between beta-thalassemia/hemoglobin E children and adults. *Southeast Asian J. Trop. Med. Public Health* 28(Suppl. 3), 134–137.

Sun, H., Jung, Y., Shiozawa, Y., Taichman, R. S., and Krebsbach, P. H. (2012). Erythropoietin modulates the structure of bone morphogenetic protein 2-engineered cranial bone. *Tissue Eng. Part A* 18, 2095–2105. doi: 10.1089/ten.TEA.2011.0742

Tagliabracci, V. S., Engel, J. L., Wiley, S. E., Xiao, J., Gonzalez, D. J., Nidumanda Appaiah, H., et al. (2014). Dynamic regulation of FGF23 by Fam20C phosphorylation, GalNAc-T3 glycosylation, and furin proteolysis. *Proc Natl Acad Sci U S A* 111, 5520–5525. doi: 10.1073/pnas.1402218111

Taher, A. T., Musallam, K. M., Karimi, M., El-Beshlawy, A., Belhoul, K., Daar, S., et al. (2010). Overview on practices in thalassemia intermedia management aiming for lowering complication rates across a region of endemicity: the OPTIMAL CARE study. *Blood* 115, 1886–1892. doi: 10.1182/blood-2009-09-243154

Toro, L., Barrientos, V., Leon, P., Rojas, M., Gonzalez, M., Gonzalez-Ibanez, A., et al. (2018). Erythropoietin induces bone marrow and plasma fibroblast growth factor 23 during acute kidney injury. *Kidney Int.* 93, 1131–1141. doi: 10.1016/j.kint.2017.11.018

Tzoulis, P., Ang, A. L., Shah, F. T., Berovic, M., Prescott, E., Jones, R., et al. (2014). Prevalence of low bone mass and vitamin D deficiency in beta-thalassemia major. *Hemoglobin* 38, 173–178. doi: 10.3109/03630269.2014.905792

Urakawa, I., Yamazaki, Y., Shimada, T., Iijima, K., Hasegawa, H., Okawa, K., et al. (2006). Klotho converts canonical FGF receptor into a specific receptor for FGF23. *Nature* 444, 770–774. doi: 10.1038/nature05315

Vadakke Madathil, S., Coe, L. M., Casu, C., and Sitara, D. (2014). Klotho deficiency disrupts hematopoietic stem cell development and erythropoiesis. *Am. J. Pathol.* 184, 827–841. doi: 10.1016/j.ajpath.2013.11.016

Valderrabano, R. J., and Wu, J. Y. (2018). Bone and blood interactions in human health and disease. *Bone* 119, 65–70. doi: 10.1016/j.bone.2018.02.019

van Straaten, S., Verhoeven, J., Hagens, S., Schutgens, R., van Solinge, W., van Wijk, R., et al. (2018). Organ involvement occurs in all forms of hereditary haemolytic anaemia. *Br. J. Haematol.* doi: 10.1111/bjh.15575 [Epub ahead of print].

Verga Falzacappa, M. V., Vujic Spasic, M., Kessler, R., Stolte, J., Hentze, M. W., and Muckenthaler, M. U. (2007). STAT3 mediates hepatic hepcidin expression and its inflammatory stimulation. *Blood* 109, 353–358. doi: 10.1182/blood-2006-07-033969

Visnjic, D., Kalajzic, Z., Rowe, D. W., Katavic, V., Lorenzo, J., and Aguila, H. L. (2004). Hematopoiesis is severely altered in mice with an induced osteoblast deficiency. *Blood* 103, 3258–3264. doi: 10.1182/blood-2003-11-4011

Wallquist, C., Mansouri, L., Norrback, M., Hylander, B., Jacobson, S. H., Larsson, T. E., et al. (2018). Associations of fibroblast growth factor 23 with markers of inflammation and leukocyte transmigration in chronic kidney disease. *Nephron* 138, 287–295. doi: 10.1159/000485472

Wan, L., Zhang, F., He, Q., Tsang, W. P., Lu, L., Li, Q., et al. (2014). EPO promotes bone repair through enhanced cartilaginous callus formation and angiogenesis. *PLoS One* 9:e102010. doi: 10.1371/journal.pone.0102010

Wang, C. Y., Core, A. B., Canali, S., Zumbrennen-Bullough, K. B., Ozer, S., Umans, L., et al. (2017). Smad1/5 is required for erythropoietin-mediated suppression of hepcidin in mice. *Blood* 130, 73–83. doi: 10.1182/blood-2016-12-759423

Weidemann, A., Kerdiles, Y. M., Knaup, K. X., Rafie, C. A., Boutin, A. T., Stockmann, C., et al. (2009). The glial cell response is an essential component of hypoxia-induced erythropoiesis in mice. *J. Clin. Invest.* 119, 3373–3383. doi: 10.1172/JCI39378

Wolf, M., Koch, T. A., and Bregman, D. B. (2013). Effects of iron deficiency anemia and its treatment on fibroblast growth factor 23 and phosphate homeostasis in women. *J. Bone Miner. Res.* 28, 1793–1803. doi: 10.1002/jbmr.1923

Wolf, M., and White, K. E. (2014). Coupling fibroblast growth factor 23 production and cleavage: iron deficiency, rickets, and kidney disease. *Curr. Opin. Nephrol. Hypertens.* 23, 411–419. doi: 10.1097/01.mnh.0000447020.74593.6f

Wong, P., Fuller, P. J., Gillespie, M. T., and Milat, F. (2016). Bone disease in Thalassemia: a molecular and clinical overview. *Endocr. Rev.* 37, 320–346. doi: 10.1210/er.2015-1105

Xu, Y., Peng, H., and Ke, B. (2017). alpha-klotho and anemia in patients with chronic kidney disease patients: a new perspective. *Exp. Ther. Med.* 14, 5691–5695. doi: 10.3892/etm.2017.5287

Yamamoto, H., Ramos-Molina, B., Lick, A. N., Prideaux, M., Albornoz, V., Bonewald, L., et al. (2016). Posttranslational processing of FGF23 in osteocytes during the osteoblast to osteocyte transition. *Bone* 84, 120–130. doi: 10.1016/j.bone.2015.07.055

Yamashita, K., Mizuiri, S., Nishizawa, Y., Kenichiro, S., Doi, S., and Masaki, T. (2017). Oral iron supplementation with sodium ferrous citrate reduces the serum intact and c-terminal fibroblast growth factor 23 levels of maintenance haemodialysis patients. *Nephrology* 22, 947–953. doi: 10.1111/nep.12909

Zachee, P., Staal, G. E., Rijksen, G., De Bock, R., Couttenye, M. M., and De Broe, M. E. (1989). Pyruvate kinase deficiency and delayed clinical response to recombinant human erythropoietin treatment. *Lancet* 1, 1327–1328. doi: 10.1016/S0140-6736(89)92718-9

Zoller, H., Schaefer, B., and Glodny, B. (2017). Iron-induced hypophosphatemia: an emerging complication. *Curr. Opin. Nephrol. Hypertens.* 26, 266–275. doi: 10.1097/MNH.0000000000000329

Zeidler, C., and Welte, K. (2007). Hematopoietic growth factors for the treatment of inherited cytopenias. *Semin. Hematol.* 44, 133–137. doi: 10.1053/j.seminhematol.2007.04.003

8

Clinical and Molecular Spectrum of Glucose-6-Phosphate Isomerase Deficiency: Report of 12 New Cases

Elisa Fermo[1]*, Cristina Vercellati[1], Anna Paola Marcello[1], Anna Zaninoni[1], Selin Aytac[2], Mualla Cetin[2], Ilaria Capolsini[3], Maddalena Casale[4], Sabrina Paci[5], Alberto Zanella[1], Wilma Barcellini[1] and Paola Bianchi[1]

[1] UOC Ematologia, UOS Fisiopatologia delle Anemie, Fondazione IRCCS Ca' Granda Ospedale Maggiore Policlinico di Milano, Milan, Italy, [2] Department of Pediatric Hematology, Faculty of Medicine, Hacettepe University, Ankara, Turkey, [3] Pediatric Oncohematology Section with BMT, Santa Maria della Misericordia Hospital, Perugia, Italy, [4] Department of Woman, Child and General and Special Surgery, University of Campania "Luigi Vanvitelli", Naples, Italy, [5] Dipartimento di Pediatria, ASST Santi Paolo e Carlo, Presidio Ospedale San Paolo Universita' di Milano, Milan, Italy

*Correspondence:
Elisa Fermo
elisa.fermo@policlinico.mi.it

Glucose-6-phosphate isomerase (GPI, EC 5.3.1.9) is a dimeric enzyme that catalyzes the reversible isomerization of glucose-6-phosphate to fructose-6-phosphate, the second reaction step of glycolysis. GPI deficiency, transmitted as an autosomal recessive trait, is considered the second most common erythro-enzymopathy of anaerobic glycolysis, after pyruvate kinase deficiency. Despite this, this defect may sometimes be misdiagnosed and only about 60 cases of GPI deficiency have been reported. GPI deficient patients are affected by chronic non-spherocytic hemolytic anemia of variable severity; in rare cases, intellectual disability or neuromuscular symptoms have also been reported. The gene locus encoding GPI is located on chromosome 19q13.1 and contains 18 exons. So far, about 40 causative mutations have been identified. We report the clinical, hematological and molecular characteristics of 12 GPI deficient cases (eight males, four females) from 11 families, with a median age at admission of 13 years (ranging from 1 to 51); eight of them were of Italian origin. Patients displayed moderate to severe anemia, that improves with aging. Splenectomy does not always result in the amelioration of anemia but may be considered in transfusion-dependent patients to reduce transfusion intervals. None of the patients described here displayed neurological impairment attributable to the enzyme defect. We identified 13 different mutations in the *GPI* gene, six of them have never been described before; the new mutations affect highly conserved residues and were not detected in 1000 Genomes and HGMD databases and were considered pathogenic by several mutation algorithms. This is the largest series of GPI deficient patients so far reported in a single study. The study confirms the great heterogeneity of the molecular defect and provides new insights on clinical and molecular aspects of this disease.

Keywords: red cell disorders, chronic hemolytic anemias, red cell metabolism, glucose-6-phosphate isomerase deficiency, glycolysis

INTRODUCTION

Glucose-6-phosphate isomerase (GPI, EC 5.3.1.9) is a dimeric enzyme that catalyzes the reversible isomerization of glucose-6-phosphate (G6P) to fructose-6-phosphate (F6P), the second reaction step of glycolysis (Kugler and Lakomek, 2000). In addition to the catalytic function of the dimeric enzyme, the monomeric form of GPI has been shown to act as a cytokine, its activities including neuroleukin (Gurney et al., 1986), myofibril-bound serine-protease inhibitor (Cao et al., 2000), autocrine motility factor (Watanabe et al., 1996), and the maturation and differentiation factor (Xu et al., 1996). More recently an unexpected relationship between GPI and phosphatidate phosphatase 1 (PAP1) activity involved in glycerolipid biosynthesis has also been reported (Haller et al., 2010).

Glucose-6-phosphate isomerase deficiency (OMIM 172400), transmitted as an autosomal recessive trait, is considered the second most common erythro-enzymopathy of anaerobic glycolysis, after pyruvate kinase deficiency. GPI deficient patients are affected by mild to severe chronic non-spherocytic hemolytic anemia (CNSHA); in rare cases intellectual disabilty or neuromuscular symptoms have also been reported (Van Biervliet et al., 1975; Kahn et al., 1978; Zanella et al., 1980; Schröter et al., 1985; Shalev et al., 1993; Jamwal et al., 2017).

The gene locus encoding GPI is located on chromosome 19q13.1 and contains 18 exons (Walker et al., 1995). So far, about 60 cases of GPI deficiency have been described, and more than 40 mutations have been reported at the nucleotide level (Kugler and Lakomek, 2000; Clarke et al., 2003; Repiso et al., 2006; Zhu et al., 2015; Manco et al., 2016; Jamwal et al., 2017; Zaidi et al., 2017; Kedar et al., 2018; Mojzikova et al., 2018). Missense mutations are the most common, but non-sense and splicing mutations have also been observed.

In this paper we report the clinical and molecular characterization of 12 patients affected by GPI deficiency: six new mutations of the GPI gene have been found and related to the clinical pattern. Long term follow-up allowed us to describe the clinical spectrum of the GPI deficiency from infancy to adulthood.

PATIENTS AND METHODS

Patients

Twelve patients (eight males and four females) from 11 families, with a median age at admission of 13 years (ranging from 1 to 51) were studied; eight were of Italian origin, two were Turkish, one from Pakistan and one from Romania.

Hematological and Enzyme Assays

Blood samples were collected after obtaining written informed consent from the patients and approval from the Institutional Ethical Committee. For patients under the age of 18, written informed consent was obtained from the parents. All the diagnostic procedures and investigations were performed in accordance with the Helsinki Declaration of 1975. Routine hematological investigations were carried out according to Dacie

and Lewis (2001): complete blood count, reticulocyte count, bilirubin, serum ferritin levels, screening for abnormal/unstable hemoglobins, direct antiglobulin test. To exclude red cell membrane disorders, RBC morphology and red cell osmotic fragility tests were evaluated in all cases. When possible EMA binding tests (Bianchi et al., 2012), red cell protein content by SDS–PAGE analyses (Mariani et al., 2008), and RBC deformability analyses by LoRRca MaxSis (Laser-Assisted Optical Rotational Cell Analyzer, Mechatronics, NL) (Zaninoni et al., 2018) were performed. RBC enzymes activities were determined according to Beutler et al. (1977). The diagnosis of GPI deficiency was made through the exclusion of the most common causes of hemolytic anemia, by the demonstration of a reduced GPI activity in the probands or in the parents, and by the identification of homozygous or compound heterozygous mutations in the GPI gene.

Molecular Analysis

Genomic DNA was extracted from leukocytes collected from peripheral blood, using standard manual methods (Sambrook et al., 1989). The entire codifying region and intronic flanking regions of the GPI gene were analyzed by direct sequencing (ABI PRISM 310 Genetic Analyzer, Applied Biosystems, Warrington, United Kingdom) using the Big Dye Terminator Cycle Sequencing Kit (Applied Biosystems, Warrington, United Kingdom).

When available, total RNA was isolated from leucocytes using TRIzol (Life Technologies, Paisley, United Kingdom) and reverse transcribed to cDNA using random hexamer primers and AMV reverse transcriptase. The entire GPI cDNA was amplified by PCR and automatically sequenced. (RefSeq: ENST00000356487, UniProt P06744). **Table 1** reports the primers used for molecular analysis.

To clarify the pathogenetic effect of the genotype identified in patient seven and to exclude other concomitant causes of hemolysis, the DNA sample of the patient was

---

TABLE 1 | Primers used for DNA analysis of GPI gene.

1F	CGCCCACGCGCCTCGCT	1R	GCCCCCGCCTCCAGACC
2F	TCTTCTGGGAACAGCTCCTG	2R	GAGGAGGTGACTGAGGTCTA
3F	CGTCTGTCTGTCTCATTGGG	3R	GGTGAAGACACAGGGTGATG
4F	TGTCTAGTGGATAGAGGGCC	4R	CCCCTCCCTTAAGCTGCA
5F	CCAGGACACGGCAGTAATGA	5R	ACAGCCAGGTCCCATCCCTG
6F	GTCTGGGCACTGTTGGTCC	6R	CCAAAAGGGACCAATGGCCA
7F	GTCACTGTCACTGACCTGCA	7R	CCGCCTTCACTTCCAACTTC
8F	CTCAGAACCAAGGACTGGGA	8R	ATCCACCAGACCTACGAACC
9F	TCACGGAGCACAGCTCCCT	9R	GCTAGGTATGCAGCAGGTAC
10F	GTGCAAGACCAGGGACAGG	10R	GCATGATGTTCAGGGACACAA
11F	GCCTTCCTTCGTTGCAGAAG	11R	GCAGGATGAGTGGGAGCTG
12F	CTCTGCCAAGTGCTGGCCA	12R	AATGGGGCAAAGAGCTCCTG
13F	TTACAGGCTTGAGCCACTGC	13R	ACTGTGGTCACCCACATGAC
14F	GGAGGGAAAGGATCTTCCAG	14R	GCCAACCAATGCACCAGGTT
15F	GAAGTACCAGGCGGTCTTGT	15R	CCCATTCTGTAGGACAAGCC
16F	ACCTGCACGTCTCAGCCTC	17R	GTGGTATGAGGAAGGGTGTAA
18F	TAGGGGAGGGCCGGGAATA	18R	CCACAACCAGAGGGTGCTL

further analyzed on an NGS-targeted panel designed by SureDesign software (Agilent Technologies, Santa Clara, CA, United States), containing 40 genes associated with congenital hemolytic anemias. Libraries were obtained by the HaloPlexHS Target Enrichment System Kit and sequenced on a MiSeq platform (Illumina, San Diego, CA, United States).

RESULTS

Table 2 reports the main clinical and hematological data in the 12 GPI deficient patients at the time of diagnosis. In 10/12 patients, extensive clinical data, family history, and laboratory data were available, with a median follow-up of 18 years (ranging from 2 to 40 years).

Consanguinity was confirmed in one Turkish patient and suspected in another two families originating from small Italian villages. Despite the onset of anemia reported at birth or early infancy, the median age of diagnosis varied greatly, half of the cases in fact were diagnosed in adulthood (18 to 51 years) (**Figure 1**). Six patients were misdiagnosed before receiving the correct diagnosis of GPI in this study: the most common diagnostic errors were hereditary spherocytosis (four cases), thalassemia (one case), or G6PD deficiency (one case). None of the patients showed neurological symptoms attributable to GPI deficiency. Growth and intellectual disability were reported only in case 5, affected by phenylketonuria' (PKU), untreated during infancy. Case 12 had a concomitant G6PD deficiency (0.6 IU/gHb; ref. ranges: 7.2–9.6).

All the patients displayed chronic macrocytic anemia before splenectomy, with median Hb levels during follow-up of 9.4 g/dL (range 8–11.3); median VGM 119 fL (84.8–127.8), MCHC 32.1 g/dL (28.6–33), increased absolute reticulocyte number (210×10^9/L, range 113–660) and increased unconjugated bilirubin. Recurrent drastic drops down of Hb levels (median 5.4 g/dL, 2.7–6.2) were reported during infection/aplastic crisis in five patients.

In 8/12 cases, information on iron status was available, serum ferritin levels were increased in most patients (median 353 ng/mL, 90–2356), two of them requiring chelation therapy due to iron overload.

All the patients displayed a normal osmotic fragility and EMA-binding test. RBC morphology, available in 9/12 patients, was unremarkable although not comparable to normal subjects; a few spherocytes, stomatocytes (ranging from 3 to 10%), echinocytes (3 to 4%), rare ovalocytes or target cells were reported. A more compromised RBC morphology was observed in the splenectomized patients (**Figure 2**). In six patients, RBC deformability was investigated by LoRRca Osmoscan analysis. Interestingly, all the them showed an altered enlarged Osmoscan curve associated with significantly increased Omin (median 156, range 126–176, $p < 0.001$) and, even more, Ohyper (median 527, range 439–579, $p < 0.001$). EImax and AUC values were decreased compared to the controls (**Figure 3**).

All the patients but one displayed a reduced GPI activity (from 10 to 40% of low normal reference range). In case 8, who showed

TABLE 2 | Clinical and hematological data in the 12 GPI deficient patients at the time of the diagnosis.

Pt	Age	Sex	Neon. Jaun.	Extx	Tx	Tot. n.	Splenect. (age)	Colecyst. (age)	Hb g/dL	Retics 10⁹/L	Hb g/dL	Retics 10⁹/L	MCV (fL)	Unc. Bil (mg/dL)	SF (ng/mL)
									Pre-splenectomy		Post-splenectomy				
1	2	M	Yes	No	Occasional	4	No	No	6.1'–10.2	231	–	–	103	1.1	n.a.
2	6	F	No	No	Occasional	2	No	No	6.2'–11.6	166	–	–	94.9	n.a.	n.a.
3	40	M	Yes	Yes	Occasional	n.a.	Yes (9)	No	n.a.	n.a.	11.5	445	126.5	3.56	2356
4	8	F	No	No	Occasional	n.a.	Yes (7)	Yes (7)	9.4	113	10	364	105.1	3–11.9	488
5	1	M	Yes	Yes	Occasional	10	No	No	10	n.a.	–	–	102	5	202
6	51	F	No	no	Occasional	9	Yes (17)	Yes (18)	n.a.	n.a.	10.5	170	119	3,18	353
7	3	M	No	No	Occasional	n.a.	No	No	11.7	347	–	–	127.8	0.93	210
8	1	M	Yes	Yes (2)	Regular (4w)	n.a.	No	No	8.5	410	–	–	84.8	2	n.a.
9	18	F	No	No	Regular* (4w)	>50	Yes (6)	Yes	5.4'–8.9	210	9.4	1420	127	13.4 (post)	1123
10	23	M	No	No	Regular* (4w)	>30	Yes (3)	Yes	2.7'–8.4	660	9.2	1740	123	8.2 (post)	185
11	18	M	No	No	No	0	No	No	10.8	200	–	–	103.3	4.3	n.a.
12	46	M	Yes	No	No	0	Yes (45)	No	8.0	126	13.9	342	101.6	2.7	n.a.
Ref. values									12–16	16–84	12–16	16–84	78–99	<0.75	30–400

Tx, transfusions; SF, serum ferritin; n.a., not available; *, case 9: every 4 weeks until splenectomy then occasional; case 10 every 4 week until splenectomy; ' = during hemolytic crises.

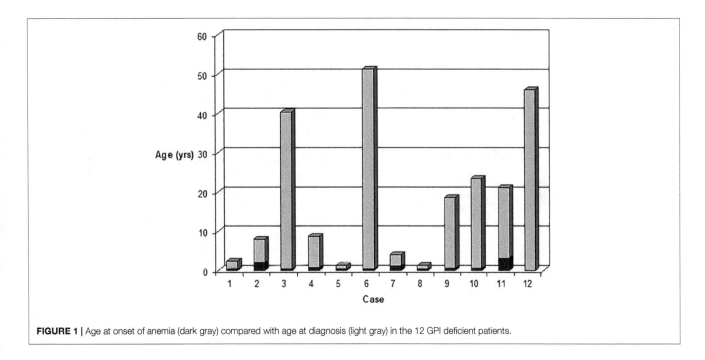

FIGURE 1 | Age at onset of anemia (dark gray) compared with age at diagnosis (light gray) in the 12 GPI deficient patients.

normal GPI activity, the diagnosis was reached by studying the GPI activity in the parents.

Glucose-6-Phosphate Isomerase Deficiency in Infancy

No intrauterine growth retardation and/or fetal distress were observed in this series of patients prior to birth. Information on the neonatal period was available in 11 patients. Five of them displayed anemia at birth, the remaining six in early infancy (all before 3 years of age). Neonatal jaundice was present in five patients, three of whom required exchange transfusion. During childhood all patients but two needed blood transfusions: three of them regularly with a transfusion interval of 4 to 8 weeks. The other patients were occasionally transfused in concomitance of hemolytic crises due to infections.

Glucose-6-Phosphate Isomerase Deficiency and Splenectomy

Six patients were splenectomized, all of them before the diagnosis of GPI deficiency. Only one patient recovered from anemia; in the remaining cases, although resulting only in a slight increase of Hb levels (0.5–1 g/dL), splenectomy greatly reduced or even eliminated transfusion requirement.

Interestingly, in some patients a considerable increase of the reticulocyte counts and unconjugated bilirubin was observed after splenectomy. No thrombotic events have been reported in the six splenectomized patients, since their surgeries.

Molecular Heterogeneity of Glucose-6-Phosphate Isomerase Deficiency

Table 3 reports the biochemical and molecular data of the GPI deficient patients.

Thirteen different missense mutations were found in the GPI gene, six of them never described before (c.145G>C, p.Gly49Arg; c.269T>C, p.Ile90Thr; c.307C>G, p.Leu103Val; c.311 G>A, p.Arg104Gln; c.839T>G, p.Ile280Ser; c.921C>A, p.Phe307Leu) (**Figure 4**).

All the new mutations affect highly conserved residues, and were predicted to have pathogenic effects by Polyphen-2, Mutation Taster, and M-CAP (**Table 4**).

Seven patients were homozygote and four compounds heterozygotes for two different mutations. In patient 7, despite the sequencing of the entire *GPI* codifying region, intronic flanking regions and promoter, we were able to find only one mutation at the heterozygous level (p.Arg472His), transmitted by the mother. In addition, we detected the polymorphism c.489A>G [synonymous variant p.Gly163=, rs1801015, GMAF 0.20070 (G), ExAC 0.11116], transmitted by the father. No other pathogenetic mutations were detected by the NGS targeted sequencing of 40 genes associated with congenital hemolytic anemias, confirming that *GPI* deficiency was the only cause of anemia in this patient. cDNA analysis in the proband and his parents revealed a loss of heterozygosity, with only the maternal allele present at the cDNA level, suggesting that the paternal allele was not expressed or rapidly degraded. Despite this, we did not find a difference in clinical severity in these patients with respect to the other GPI patients carrying two missense mutations.

DISCUSSION

The present cohort of GPI deficient patients represents the largest series so far described in a single study, collecting retrospective information and follow-up data over a median period of 18 years. All the cases were never reported before, consistently increasing the number of GPI patients reported

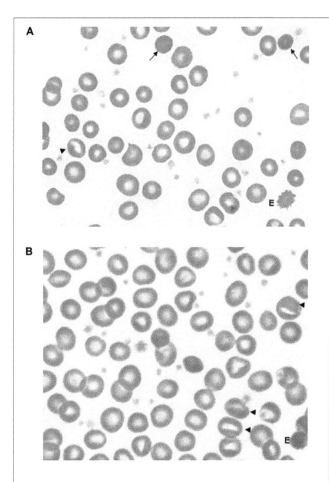

FIGURE 2 | Peripheral red cell morphology from a non-splenectomized **(A)** and from a splenectomized **(B)** GPI patient (May-Grünwald's Giemsa staining). Anisopoikilocytosis with presence of rare spherocytes (arrows), stomatocytes (triangles), more evident after splenectomy, rare echinocytes (E). The increased platelet number in panel **(B)** is due to splenectomy, some large and vacuolated platelets are likely due to EDTA anticoagulant.

in literature (Kugler and Lakomek, 2000; Clarke et al., 2003; Repiso et al., 2006; Warang et al., 2012; Adama van Scheltema et al., 2015; Zhu et al., 2015; Manco et al., 2016; Jamwal et al., 2017; Zaidi et al., 2017; Burger et al., 2018; Kedar et al., 2018; Mojzikova et al., 2018).

Despite the fact that GPI deficiency is considered the second most frequent RBC enzymopathy of anaerobic glycolysis after pyruvate kinase, the exact frequency of this disorder is not known and a diagnosis is often difficult to reach; this may be due to the lack of availability of the enzymatic assay, performed only in a few specialized centers, or because of the lack of knowledge about some rare disorders for which specific tests are not considered during laboratory investigations (Bianchi et al., 2018; Kedar et al., 2018; Sonaye et al., 2018). Moreover, due to the similarity in clinical presentation with other congenital hemolytic anemias, an exact diagnosis is often delayed.

An increasing number of new diagnoses might be expected in the coming years due to the advent of new NGS technologies that allow the simultaneous analysis of multiple genes associated to

rare/very rare hemolytic anemias. At least three additional GPI-deficient patients have been reported in the literature in the last 2 years using these technologies (Jamwal et al., 2017; Kedar et al., 2018; Russo et al., 2018).

The possibility to evaluate a consistent group of patients from infancy to adulthood allowed us to describe the clinical picture of GPI deficiency, which is characterized by the onset of chronic macrocytic anemia at birth or early infancy, reticulocytosis, jaundice and splenomegaly associated with mild hepatomegaly; in all the patients in which the information was available, pregnancy was uneventful with normal growth development.

This clinical pattern is in line with cases previously described by our group (Baronciani et al., 1996); however, in some patients a more severe clinical presentation, i.e., hydrops fetalis, has been reported (Ravindranath et al., 1987; Adama van Scheltema et al., 2015).

Neuromuscular impairment or mental retardation are rare complication sometimes reported in GPI deficiency (Van Biervliet et al., 1975; Kahn et al., 1978; Zanella et al., 1980; Shalev et al., 1993; Kugler et al., 1998; Jamwal et al., 2017), as well as in other glycolytic enzyme defects caused by ubiquitously expressed genes (i.e., phosphoglycerate kinase deficiency, phosphofructokinase deficiency or triosephosphate isomerase deficiency). The link between GPI deficiency and neuromuscular dysfunction has not been fully established, and has been attributed to the fact that the monomeric form of GPI is identical to neuroleukin (NLK), a neurotrophic factor that supports the survival of embryonic spinal neurons, skeletal neurons and sensory neurons; however, the proposed hypothesis on the molecular mechanism leading to a neuromuscular dysfunction are in some cases contradictory (Kugler et al., 1998; Repiso et al., 2005). Actually, only three GPI deficient cases with neurological impairment were characterized at molecular level: two of them were homozygous for mutations p.Arg347Cys and p.Arg347His, respectively, and one was compound heterozygous for mutations p.His20Pro and p.Leu339Pro (Beutler et al., 1997; Kugler et al., 1998; Jamwal et al., 2017). A large number of cases with mutations affecting amino acid Arg347 (including two in our series) have been reported with only hematological involvement, suggesting that other possible confounding factors, independent from enzyme deficiency itself, such as kernicterus (Jamwal et al., 2017) or other genetic defects in consanguineous families, may contribute to the clinical phenotype.

A long follow-up time allowed us to shine light on other possible features of GPI deficiency not yet clearly reported in literature: (a) increased sensitivity to infections that result in a dramatic drop-down of hemoglobin levels persisting also in adults, (b) a low response to splenectomy resulting only in a slight increase of Hb levels, however eliminating or reducing the transfusion requirement in all patients, (c) a tendency to increase the reticulocyte number after splenectomy, probably due to selective sequestration of younger GPI defective erythrocytes by the spleen as previously hypothesized in PK deficiency (Mentzer et al., 1971; Matsumoto et al., 1972).

Increased sensitivity to infections was reported in other GPI cases (Helleman and Van Biervliet, 1976; Repiso et al., 2006; Manco et al., 2016; Kedar et al., 2018), making this aspect relevant

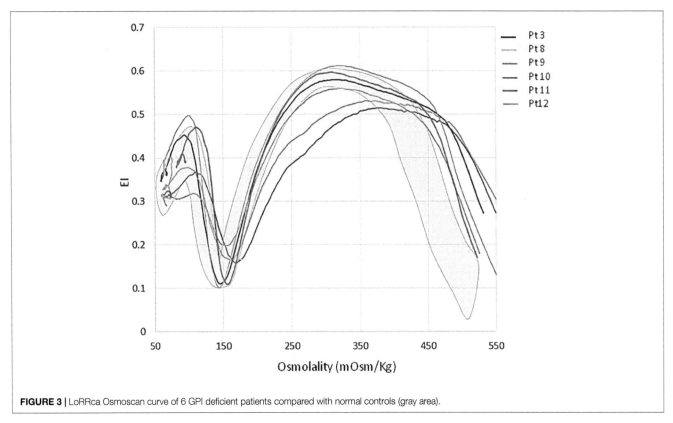

FIGURE 3 | LoRRca Osmoscan curve of 6 GPI deficient patients compared with normal controls (gray area).

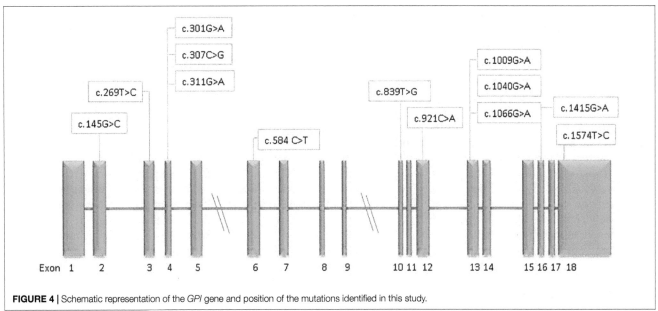

FIGURE 4 | Schematic representation of the *GPI* gene and position of the mutations identified in this study.

in the follow-up, suggesting that adequate vaccination coverage should be considered.

As previously reported, GPI-deficient red cells produce an altered Osmoscan profile (LoRRca analyzer), characterized by a right enlarged opened curve (Zaninoni et al., 2018). These findings, which result in a statistically significative increase of Ohyper values, offer an initial laboratory screen for patients with this rare enzyme defect. A possible explanation may reside in

an increased red cell volume, or a cellular overhydrated state resulting in cell swelling of an origin not yet investigated.

Increased thrombotic risk after splenectomy, clearly demonstrated in hereditary xerocytosis, and in overhydrated stomatocytosis (Fermo et al., 2017; Iolascon et al., 2017) has recently been reported in some enzyme defects i.e., pyruvate kinase deficiency) (Grace et al., 2018). No thrombotic events have been reported in the analyzed series, or in the GPI deficient

TABLE 3 | Biochemical and molecular data of the GPI deficient patients.

Pt	GPI activity (IU/gHb)	Residual activity %	Mutation	Effect
1	6	10%	**c.145G>C/c.921C>A**	**p.Gly49Arg/p.Phe307Leu**
2	10.5	19%	**c.311 G>A**/c.584C>T	**p.Arg104Gln**/p.Thr195Ile
3	18	32%	**c.307C>G/c.307C>G**	**p.Leu103Val/p.Leu103Val**
4	15.7	28%	c.301G>A/c.1009G>A	p.Val101Met/p.Ala337Thr
5	13.3	24%	c.1009G>A/c.1009G>A	p.Ala337Thr/p.Ala337Thr
6	14.3	26%	c.584C>T/c.584C>T	p.Thr195Ile/p.Thr195Ile
7	16	29%	c.489A>G (rs1801015)/c.1415G>A	LOH/p.Arg472His
8	54.6	98%	**c.269T>C/**c.1066G>A	**p.Ile90Thr/**p.Asp356Asn
9	22	40%	c.1040G>A/c.1040G>A	p.Arg347His/p.Arg347His
10	17	30%	c.1040G>A/c.1040G>A	p.Arg347His/p.Arg347His
11	20.2	36.5%	**c.839T>G/c.839T>G**	**p.Ile280Ser/p.Ile280Ser**
12	4.8	9%	c.1574 T>C/c.1574 T>C	p. Ile525Thr/p.Ile525Thr
Ref. range	55,3–72,3			

Percentage of residual GPI activity was calculated on the lower reference value. New mutations are reported in bold.

TABLE 4 | List of new variants identified.

HGVS coding	HGVS protein	GPI structure	Exon	Status	Polyphen-2	M-CAP	MAF1000G	MAF ExAC	RefSeqID
c.145G>C	Gly49Arg	Lβ1-β2	2	Het	1.000 (0.00; 1.00) D	0.358 P	–	–	–
c.269T>C	p.Ile90Thr	Lα6-Turn	3	Het	1.000 (0.00; 1.00) D	0.343 P	–	–	–
c.307C>G	p.Leu103Val	α8	4	Hom	0.649 (0.87; 0.91) PD	0.479 P	–	–	–
c.311 G>A	p.Arg104Gln	Lα8-b4	4	Het	0.544 (0.88; 0.91) PD	0.577 P	–	–	–
c.839T>G	p.Ile280Ser	α21	10	Hom	1.000 (0.00; 1.00) D	0.611 P	–	–	–
c.921C>A	p.Phe307Leu	α23	12	Het	1.000 (0.00; 1.00) D	0.383 P	–	A = 0.000008	rs754782152

Polyphen-2 analysis (HumDiv) PD, possibly damaging; D, probably damaging; in bracket sensitivity, specificity; M-CAP P, possibly pathogenetic (ref. Jagadeesh et al., 2016). Recommended pathogenicity threshold: Polyphen-2 > 0.8 (with misclassified pathogenetic variants 31%); M-CAP > 0.025 (with misclassified pathogenetic variants 5%).

cases reported in literature; however, we cannot exclude that this information might be lost at follow up.

Information on iron status and erythropoietic activity in GPI deficiency is scant, although it is known that iron overload may frequently occur in other more common glycolytic enzymopathies as a consequence of various factors, including hyperhaemolysis or ineffective erythropoiesis. Only iron stores (ferritin levels) were available in the present series and found to be elevated in four of seven patients, underlying the need of monitoring iron status in this disease.

Glucose-6-phosphate isomerase deficiency shows a wide molecular heterogeneity with more than 40 mutations in the GPI gene currently listed in the Human Gene Mutation Database[1]. Most of them are missense, covering about 93% of the total mutations identified, with only a few splicing, nonsense or frameshift mutations (Kugler and Lakomek, 2000; Manco et al., 2016). This is in line with the findings in our series, where all the different mutations identified were missense. Despite this, loss of heterozygosity at the cDNA level in patient 7, who did not show the second causative mutation, neither by Sanger sequencing nor by NGS targeted sequencing, may suggest that in GPI deficiency some drastic molecular abnormalities escape the conventional screening techniques. Interestingly, patient 7 carried the paternal allele on the silent polymorphic variant c.489A>G (p.Gly163=),

that is located in the third nucleotide of exon 6. Although we did not perform functional *in vitro* analysis of this silent mutation, we cannot exclude that the variant, although polymorphic, may interfere with the normal splicing, resulting in an unstable mRNA, rapidly degraded.

Despite the molecular heterogeneity, some recurrent mutations have been identified in GPI deficiency. This is the case of missense mutations affecting the amino acid Arg347, here detected in two brothers of Turkish origin (c.1040G>A, p.Arg347His) and already reported in literature in other unrelated patients of different ethnical origins (Walker et al., 1993; Repiso et al., 2006; Lin et al., 2009); another mutation at the same codon (c.1039 C>T, p. Arg347Cys) has also been described (Xu and Beutler, 1994; Lin et al., 2009), suggesting the presence of a mutational hotspot (Repiso et al., 2005). Arg347 is a highly conserved residue (GERP 5.65), falling in the region responsible for GPI dimerization. It has been hypothesized that a mutation in these residues causes a loss of GPI capability to dimerize, making the enzyme more susceptible to thermolability; actually, kinetic studies performed in a mutant enzyme from an homozygous p.Arg347His patient, showed that the Km for G6P and for F6P were not altered, but the thermostability was drastically reduced (Repiso et al., 2005).

---

[1] www.hgmd.cf.ac.uk

Different than expected and previously reported in literature (Walker et al., 1993; Repiso et al., 2005) the cases in this series carrying mutation p.Arg347His did not show a drastic reduction of GPI activity (30–40% of residual activity vs. 18% reported by others); this could be explained by technical variability in the enzymatic assay, or by the very high number of reticulocytes found in our patients at the time of the assay, which may display an higher enzyme activity than mature red cells (Beutler et al., 1977). Other recurrent mutations found in this series were p.Thr195Ile and p.Val101Met, already reported in Italian patients by Baronciani et al. (1996).

CONCLUSION

In conclusion, the study confirms the great heterogeneity of the molecular defect and provides new insights on clinical and molecular aspects of this disease.

AUTHOR CONTRIBUTIONS

EF and PB performed the molecular analysis, analyzed the results, prepared and revised the manuscript. CV, AM, and AnZ performed the hematologic and biochemical investigations. SA, MuC, IC, MaC, SP, AlZ, and WB performed the patient follow-up and revision of the manuscript.

REFERENCES

Adama van Scheltema, P. N., Zhang, A., Ball, L. M., Steggerda, S. J., van Wijk, R., Fransen van de Putte, D. E., et al. (2015). Successful treatment of fetal hemolytic disease due to glucose phosphate isomerase deficiency (GPI) using repeated intrauterine transfusions: a case report. *Clin. Case Rep.* 3, 862–865. doi: 10.1002/ccr3.358

Baronciani, L., Zanella, A., Bianchi, P., Zappa, M., Alfinito, F., Iolascon, A., et al. (1996). Study of the molecular defects in glucose phosphate isomerase-deficient patients affected by chronic hemolytic anemia. *Blood* 88, 2306–2310.

Beutler, E., Blume, K. G., Kaplan, J. C., Lohr, G. W., Ramot, B., and Valentine, W. N. (1977). International Committee for Standardization in Haematology: recommended methods for red-cell enzyme analysis. *Br. J. Haematol.* 35, 331–340. doi: 10.1111/j.1365-2141.1977.tb00589.x

Beutler, E., West, C., Britton, H. A., Harris, J., and Forman, L. (1997). Glucosephosphate isomerase (GPI) deficiency mutations associated with hereditary nonspherocytic hemolytic anemia (HNSHA). *Blood Cells Mol. Dis.* 23, 402–409. doi: 10.1006/bcmd.1997.0157

Bianchi, P., Fermo, E., Glader, B., Kanno, H., Agarwal, A., Barcellini, W., et al. (2018). Addressing the diagnostic gaps in pyruvate kinase deficiency: consensus recommendations on the diagnosis of pyruvate kinase deficiency. *Am. J. Hematol.* [Epub ahead of print].

Bianchi, P., Fermo, E., Vercellati, C., Marcello, A. P., Porretti, L., Cortelezzi, A., et al. (2012). Diagnostic power of laboratory tests for hereditary spherocytosis: a comparison study in 150 patients grouped according to molecular and clinical characteristics. *Haematologica* 97, 516–523. doi: 10.3324/haematol. 2011.052845

Burger, N. C. M., van Wijk, R., Bresters, D., and Schell, E. A. (2018). A novel mutation of glucose phosphate isomerase (GPI) causing severe neonatal anemia due to GPI deficiency. *J. Pediatr. Hematol. Oncol.* 41, e186–e189. doi: 10.1097/ MPH.0000000000001393

Cao, M. J., Osatomi, K., Matsude, R., Ohkubo, M., Hara, K., and Ishihara, K. (2000). Purification of a novel serine proteinase inhibitor from skeletal muscle of white croaker (*Argyrosomus argentatus*). *Biochem. Biophys. Res. Commun.* 272, 485–489. doi: 10.1006/bbrc.2000.2803

Clarke, J. L., Vulliamy, T. J., Roper, D., Mesbah-Namin, S. A., Wild, B. J., Walker, J. I., et al. (2003). Combined glucose-6-phosphate dehydrogenase and glucosephosphate isomerase deficiency can alter clinical outcome. *Blood Cells Mol. Dis.* 30, 258–263. doi: 10.1016/s1079-9796(03)00027-5

Dacie, J. V., and Lewis, S. M. (2001). *Practical Haematology*, 9th Edn. London: Churchill Livingston.

Fermo, E., Vercellati, C., Marcello, A. P., Zaninoni, A., van Wijk, R., and Mirra, N. (2017). Hereditary xerocytosis due to mutations in PIEZO1 gene associated with heterozygous pyruvate kinase deficiency and beta-thalassemia trait in two unrelated families. *Case Rep. Hematol.* 2017:2769570. doi: 10.1155/2017/ 2769570

Grace, R. F., Bianchi, P., van Beers, E. J., Eber, S. W., Glader, B., Yaish, H. M., et al. (2018). Clinical spectrum of pyruvate kinase deficiency: data from the pyruvate kinase deficiency natural history study. *Blood* 131, 2183–2192. doi: 10.1182/blood-2017-10-810796

Gurney, M. E., Heinrich, S. P., Lee, M. R., and Yin, H. S. (1986). Molecular cloning and expression of neuroleukin, a neurotrophic factor for spinal and sensory neurons. *Science* 234, 566–573.

Haller, J. F., Smith, C., Liu, D., Zheng, H., Tornheim, K., Ham, G.-S., et al. (2010). Isolation of novel animal cell linesisomerase reveals mutations in glucose-6-phosphate defective in glycerolipid biosynthesis. *J. Biol. Chem.* 285, 866–877. doi: 10.1074/jbc.M109.068213

Helleman, P. W., and Van Biervliet, J. P. (1976). Haematological studies in a new variant of glucosephosphate isomerase deficiency (GPI Utrecht). *Helv. Paediatr. Acta* 30, 525–536.

Iolascon, A., Andolfo, I., Barcellini, W., Corcione, F., Garçon, L., De Franceschi, L., et al. (2017). Recommendations regarding splenectomy in hereditary hemolytic anemias. *Haematologica* 102, 1304–1313. doi: 10.3324/haematol.2016.161166

Jagadeesh, K. A., Wenger, A. M., Berger, M. J., Guturu, H., Stenson, P. D., Cooper, D. N., et al. (2016). M-CAP eliminates a majority of variants of uncertain significance in clinical exomes at high sensitivity. *Nat. Genet.* 48, 1581–1586. doi: 10.1038/ng.3703

Jamwal, M., Aggarwal, A., Das, A., Maitra, A., Sharma, P., Krishnan, S., et al. (2017). Next-generation sequencing unravels homozygous mutation in glucose-6-phosphate isomerase, GPIc.1040G> A (p.Arg347His) causing hemolysis in an Indian infant. *Clin. Chim. Acta* 468, 81–84. doi: 10.1016/j.cca.2017.02.012

Kahn, A., Buc, H. A., Girot, R., Cottreau, D., and Griscelli, C. (1978). Molecular and functional anomalies in two new mutant glucose-phosphate-insomerase variants with enzyme deficiency and chronic hemolysis. *Hum. Genet.* 40, 293–304. doi: 10.1007/bf00272190

Kedar, P. S., Gupta, V., Dongerdiye, R., Chiddarwar, A., Warang, P., and Madkaikar, M. R. (2018). Molecular diagnosis of unexplained haemolytic anaemia using targeted next-generation sequencing panel revealed (p.Ala337Thr) novel mutation in GPI gene in two Indian patients. *J. Clin. Pathol.* 2019, 81–85. doi: 10.1136/jclinpath-2018-205420

Kugler, W., Breme, K., Laspe, P., Muirhead, H., Davies, C., Winkler, H., et al. (1998). Molecular basis of neurological dysfunction coupled with haemolytic anaemia in human glucose-6-phosphate isomerase (GPI) deficiency. *Hum. Genet.* 103, 450–454. doi: 10.1007/s004390050849

Kugler, W., and Lakomek, M. (2000). Glucose-6-phosphate isomerase deficiency. *Bailliere's Best. Pract. Res. Clin. Haematol.* 13, 89–101. doi: 10.1053/beha.1999. 0059

Lin, H. Y., Kao, Y. H., Chen, S. T., and Meng, M. (2009). Effects of inherited mutations on catalytic activity and structural stability of human glucose-6-phosphate isomerase expressed in *Escherichia coli. Biochim. Biophys. Acta* 1794, 315–323. doi: 10.1016/j.bbapap.2008.11.004

Manco, L., Bento, C., Victor, B. L., Pereira, J., Relvas, L., Brito, R. M., et al. (2016). Hereditary nonspherocytic hemolytic anemia caused by red cell glucose-6-phosphate isomerase (GPI) deficiency in two Portuguese patients: clinical features and molecular study. *Blood Cells Mol. Dis.* 60, 18–23. doi: 10.1016/j. bcmd.2016.06.002

Mariani, M., Barcellini, W., Vercellati, C., Marcello, A. P., Fermo, E., Pedotti, P., et al. (2008). Clinical and hematologic features of 300 patients affected by hereditary spherocytosis grouped according to the type of the membrane protein defect. *Haematologica* 93, 1310–1317. doi: 10.3324/haematol.12546

Matsumoto, N., Ishihara, T., Nakashima, K., Miwa, S., Uchino, F., and Kondo, M. (1972). Sequestration and destruction of reticulocytes in the spleen in pyruvate kinase deficiency hereditary non-spherocytic hemolytic anemia. *Nippon Ketsueki Gakkai zasshi* 35, 525–537.

Mentzer, W. C. Jr., Baehner, R. L., Schmidt-Schonbeth, H., Robinson, S. H., and Nathan, D. G. (1971). Selective reticulocyte destruction in erythrocyte pyruvate kinase deficiency. *J. Clin. Invest.* 5, 0688–699.

Mojzikova, R., Koralkova, P., Holub, D., Saxova, Z., Pospisilova, D., Prochazkova, D., et al. (2018). Two novel mutations (p.(Ser160Pro) and p.(Arg472Cys) causing glucose-6-phosphate isomerase deficiency are associated with erythroid dysplasia and inappropriately suppressed hepcidin. *Blood Cells Mol. Dis.* 69, 23–29. doi: 10.1016/j.bcmd.2017.04.003

Ravindranath, Y., Paglia, D. E., Warrier, I., Valentine, W., Nakatani, M., and Brockway, R. A. (1987). Glucose phosphate isomerase deficiency as a cause of hydrops fetalis. *N. Engl. J. Med.* 316, 258–261. doi: 10.1056/nejm198701293160506

Repiso, A., Oliva, B., Vives Corrons, J. L., Carreras, J., and Climent, F. (2005). Glucose phosphate isomerase deficienvy: enzymatic and familial characterization of Arg346His mutation. *Biochim. Biophys. Acta* 1740, 467–471. doi: 10.1016/j.bbadis.2004.10.008

Repiso, A., Oliva, B., Vives-Corrons, J. L., Beutler, E., Carreras, J., and Climent, F. (2006). mRed cell glucose phosphate isomerase (GPI): a molecular study of three novel mutations associated with hereditary nonspherocytic hemolytic anemia. *Hum. Mutat.* 27:1159. doi: 10.1002/humu.9466

Russo, R., Andolfo, I., Manna, F., Gambale, A., Marra, R., Rosato, B. E., et al. (2018). Multi-gene panel testing improves diagnosis and management of patients with hereditary anemias. *Am. J. Hematol.* 93, 672–682. doi: 10.1002/ajh.25058

Sambrook, J., Fritsch, E. F., and Maniatis, T. (1989). *Molecular Cloning. A Laboratory Manual.* New York, NY: Cold Spring Harbor Laboratory Press.

Schröter, W., Eber, S. W., Bardosi, A., Gahr, M., Gabriel, M., and Sitzmann, F. C. (1985). Generalised glucosephosphate isomerase (GPI) deficiency causing haemolytic anaemia, neuromuscular symptoms and impairment of granulocyte function: a new syndrome due to a new stable GPI variant with diminished specifc activity (GPI Homburg). *Eur. J. Paediatr.* 144, 301–305. doi: 10.1007/bf00441768

Shalev, O., Shalev, R. S., Forman, L., and Beutler, E. (1993). GPI mount scopus ± a variant of glucose-phosphate isomerase defciency. *Ann. Hematol.* 67, 197–200. doi: 10.1007/bf01695868

Sonaye, R., Sombans, S., and Ramphul, K. (2018). A case report of congenital non-spherocytic hemolytic anemia in a patient from India. *Cureus* 2018:e2478. doi: 10.7759/cureus.2478

Van Biervliet, J. P., Van Milligen-Boersma, L., and Staal, G. E. (1975). A new variant of glucosephosphate isomerase deficiency (GPI-Utrecht). *Clin. Chim. Acta* 65, 157–165. doi: 10.1016/0009-8981(75)90103-5

Walker, J. I. H., Layton, D. M., Bellingham, A. J., Morgan, M. J., and Faik, P. (1993). DNA sequence abnormalities in human glucose 6-phosphate isomerase deficiency. *Hum. Mol. Gen.* 2, 327–329. doi: 10.1093/hmg/2.3.327

Walker, J. I. H., Morgan, M. J., and Faik, P. (1995). Structure and organization of the human glucose phosphate isomerase gene (GPI). *Genomics* 29, 261–265. doi: 10.1006/geno.1995.1241

Warang, P., Kedar, P., Ghosh, K., and Colah, R. B. (2012). Hereditary non-spherocytic hemolytic anemia and severe glucose phosphate isomerase deficiency in an Indian patient homozygous for the L487F mutation in the human GPI gene. *Int. J. Hematol.* 96, 263–267. doi: 10.1007/s12185-012-1122-x

Watanabe, H., Takehana, K., Date, M., Shinozaki, T., and Raz, A. (1996). Tumor cell autocrine motility factor is the neuroleukin/phosphohexose isomerase polypeptide. *Cancer Res.* 56, 2960–2963.

Xu, W., and Beutler, E. (1994). The characterization of gene mutations for human glucose phosphate isomerase deficiency associated with chronic haemolytic anemia. *J. Clin. Invest.* 94, 2326–2329. doi: 10.1172/jci117597

Xu, W., Seiter, K., Feldman, E., Ahmed, T., and Chiao, J. W. (1996). The differentiation and maturation meditator for human myeloid leukemia cells shares homology with neuroleukin or phosphoglucose isomerise. *Blood* 87, 4502–4506.

Zaidi, A. U., Kedar, P., Koduri, P. R., Goyette, G. W. Jr., Buck, S., Paglia, D. E., et al. (2017). Glucose phosphate isomerase (GPI) Tadikonda: characterization of a novel Pro340Ser mutation. *Pediatr. Hematol. Oncol.* 34, 449–454. doi: 10.1080/08880018.2017.1383541

Zanella, A., Izzo, C., Rebulla, P., Perroni, L., Mariani, M., Canestri, G., et al. (1980). The first stable variant of erythrocyte glucose-phosphate isomerase associated with severe hemolytic anemia. *Am. J. Hematol.* 9, 1–11. doi: 10.1002/ajh.2830090102

Zaninoni, A., Fermo, E., Vercellati, C., Consonni, D., Marcello, A. P., Zanella, A., et al. (2018). Use of laser assisted optical rotational cell analyzer (LoRRca MaxSis) in the diagnosis of RBC membrane disorders, enzyme defects, and congenital dyserythropoietic anemias: a monocentric study on 202 patients. *Front. Physiol.* 9:451. doi: 10.3389/fphys.2018.00451

Zhu, X., Petrovski, S., Xie, P., Ruzzo, E. K., Lu, Y. F., McSweeney, K. M., et al. (2015). Whole-exome sequencing in undiagnosed genetic diseases: interpreting 119 trios. *Genet. Med.* 17, 774–781. doi: 10.1038/gim.2014.191

9

Receptor for Advanced Glycation End Products Antagonism Blunts Kidney Damage in Transgenic Townes Sickle Mice

Emmanuelle Charrin[1,2], Camille Faes[1,2], Amandine Sotiaux[1,2], Sarah Skinner[1,2], Vincent Pialoux[1,2,3], Philippe Joly[1,2,4], Philippe Connes[1,2,3] and Cyril Martin[1,2*]

[1]Interuniversity Laboratory of Human Movement Biology, University Claude Bernard Lyon 1, University of Lyon, Lyon, France, [2]Laboratory of Excellence "GR-Ex", Paris, France, [3]Institut Universitaire de France, Paris, France, [4]Groupement Hospitalier Est, UF "Biochimie des Pathologies érythrocytaires" Centre de Biologie Est, CHU de Lyon, Lyon, France

*Correspondence:
Cyril Martin
cyril.martin@univ-lyon1.fr

A large proportion of adult patients with sickle cell disease (SCD) develops kidney disease and is at a high risk of mortality. The contribution of advanced glycation end products and their receptor (AGE/RAGE) axis has been established in the pathogenesis of multiple kidney diseases. The aim of the present study was to determine the implication of RAGE in the development of SCD-related kidney complications in a mouse model of SCD, as this has never been investigated. 8-week-old AA (normal) and SS (homozygous SCD) Townes mice were treated with a specific RAGE antagonist (RAP) or vehicle (NaCl). After 3 weeks of treatment, red blood cell count, hematocrit, and hemoglobin levels were significantly higher in RAP-treated SS mice. Reticulocyte count and sickle cell count were reduced in RAP-SS compared to their NaCl-treated littermates. The lower NADPH oxidase activity in the kidney of RAP-treated mice compared to NaCl-treated mice suggests limited ROS production. RAP-treated SS mice had decreased NF-κB protein expression and activation as well as reduced TNF-α mRNA expression in the kidney. Glomerular area, interstitial fibrosis, tubular iron deposits, and KIM-1 protein expression were significantly reduced after RAP treatment. In conclusion, this study provides evidence supporting the pathogenic role of RAGE in kidney injuries in sickle cell mice.

Keywords: sickle cell disease, RAGEs, kidney, Townes mice, oxidative stress, inflammation

INTRODUCTION

Sickle cell disease (SCD) is one of the most common severe monogenic disorders worldwide. Mutated intra-erythrocytic hemoglobin S results from the substitution of valine for glutamic acid on the sixth codon of the β-globin gene (HBB) and leads to the formation of sickle-shaped red blood cells (RBCs) (Ballas and Mohandas, 1996). The homozygous disease is characterized by increased RBC fragility, decreased RBC deformability, and increased endothelial adhesion, which promote chronic hemolytic anemia and painful vaso-occlusive crises (VOC) (Rees et al., 2010; Connes et al., 2018). An imbalanced redox state and chronic inflammation also participate in the development of vasculopathy and multiple organ damage (Wood et al., 2008; Sparkenbaugh and Pawlinski, 2013; Conran and Belcher, 2018; van Beers and van Wijk, 2018). Due to its high rate of oxygen consumption and functional features, the kidney is particularly vulnerable in SCD patients. It has been estimated that 16–18% of overall mortality in patients with SCD is attributed to chronic renal failure (Platt et al., 1994). Renal manifestations of the disease include altered renal hemodynamics, renal and glomerular enlargement, and tubular deposits of iron that ultimately contribute to the development of chronic kidney disease (Nath and Hebbel, 2015).

Under oxidative conditions, advanced glycation end products (AGEs) are generated by non-enzymatic glycation and oxidation of proteins and lipids in the Maillard reaction (Singh et al., 2001). Beyond their valuable role as well-established markers of oxidative stress (Genuth et al., 2005; Koyama et al., 2007; Meerwaldt et al., 2008), it has been demonstrated that AGEs contribute to the pathophysiology of organ complications in diabetes mellitus and other chronic inflammatory diseases (Miyata et al., 1998; Huebschmann et al., 2006; Guo et al., 2012), partially through oxidative stress mechanisms/pathways (Genuth et al., 2005; Koyama et al., 2007; Meerwaldt et al., 2008). The accumulation of AGEs has been shown to participate in renal filtration alteration and glomerulopathy (Ahmed, 2005; Tan et al., 2007). The underlying molecular mechanisms involve enhanced production of pro-inflammatory cytokines, adhesion molecules, and oxidants following the activation of AGEs receptors (RAGEs) (Rojas et al., 2000; Ahmed, 2005; Goldin et al., 2006).

Although numerous SCD-related kidney complications are consistent with tissue damage induced by RAGE activation, such as albuminuria (Wendt et al., 2003), focal segmental glomerulosclerosis (Tanji et al., 2000; Wendt et al., 2003), and fibrosis (Cooper, 2004), the possible role of this receptor in the pathogenesis of SCD has been poorly investigated. To date, only two studies have reported increased plasma AGEs concentrations in children and adults with homozygous SCD at steady state with no further increase during VOC (Somjee et al., 2005; Nur et al., 2010). More recently, a third study reported increased level of AGEs in the skin of SCD patients compared to controls but the authors found no association with the clinical status of the patients (Kashyap et al., 2018). To test the hypothesis that RAGE may contribute to the development of kidney damage in SCD, we investigated the effects of RAGE inhibition on the kidney of a transgenic mouse model of SCD (Townes) expressing exclusively human sickle hemoglobin. Histological sections of the kidney, pro-inflammatory molecule expression, oxidative stress markers, and hematological parameters were analyzed in SCD mice treated with a specific antagonist peptide of RAGE.

MATERIALS AND METHODS

Animals

We have established a colony of Townes sickle mice in our laboratory, originally purchased from the Jackson Laboratory (Bar Harbor, ME, USA). Mouse genotypes were confirmed by PCR. Townes mice have both human α- and β-globin genes knocked into the mouse locus, allowing the generation of littermates AA (healthy controls) and SS (homozygous SCD) mice (Wu et al., 2006). A total of 44 mice (21 females and 23 males) aged 8–9 weeks were used and maintained on a 12-h light–dark cycle with food and water *ad libitum*. The guidelines from the French Ministry of Agriculture for experimental procedures and the Institute for Laboratory Animal Research (National Academy of Sciences, USA) were followed and the protocol was approved by the regional animal care committee (#DR2013-46, Rhône-Alpes, France).

Experimental Design

To determine the role of RAGE in SCD pathophysiology, RAGE antagonist peptide (RAP; 5 mg kg^{-1}, #553031, Merck Millipore, Molsheim, France) was administered in 8- to 9-week-old AA and SS mice *via* intraperitoneal (IP) injection, 5 days per week for 3 weeks, as previously proposed (Arumugam et al., 2012). Saline solution (NaCl 0.9%) IP injection was used as a control.

Tissue Sampling

The day after the last injection, mice were anesthetized with an IP injection of pentobarbital (50 mg/kg, Dolethal®, Vétoquinol, Lure, France) and blood was collected by a retro-orbital venipuncture into EDTA tubes for hematological analysis. Mice were euthanatized by exsanguination with a 0.9% NaCl transcardial perfusion for 70 s. One kidney was collected and immediately frozen in liquid nitrogen for oxidative stress and qRT-PCR analyses. The second kidney was conditioned for histology (*vide infra*).

Hematology

An ABX Micros 60 automat (Horiba, Montpellier, France) was used for the following hematological measurements: hematocrit (Hct); red blood cell (RBC) count; hemoglobin concentration; mean corpuscular volume (MCV); RBC distribution width (RDW); mean corpuscular hemoglobin concentration (MCHC); mean corpuscular hemoglobin (MCH); white blood cell (WBC) count; lymphocyte, monocyte, and granulocyte counts. The percentage of reticulocytes and sickle cells was blindly assessed on smears stained with brilliant cresyl blue (860867, Sigma-Aldrich, St-Louis, MO, USA) by two investigators under a light microscope (BX43 Microscope, Olympus, Tokyo, Japan).

qRT-PCR for Cytokines mRNA Expression

Total mRNA from kidney was isolated using Tri Reagent LS (Euromedex, Souffelweyersheim, France) according to the manufacturer's instructions, purified with DNase I (EN0525, ThermoFisher scientific, Waltham, MA, USA), and concentrated at 80 ng.µl^{-1}. One thousand nanograms per sample of total mRNA were reverse transcribed to cDNA with the reverse transcriptase RNase Hminus (Promega, Madison, WI, USA) using oligo (T)15 (Eurogentec, Seraing, Belgium). RT calibration was done in the presence of 80 pg. of a synthetic external and non-homologous poly(A) Standard RNA (SmRNA) used to normalize the reverse transcription of mRNAs of biological samples (Morales and Bezin, patent WO2004.092414). Real-time qPCR analysis was performed on a Rotor-Gene Q system (Qiagen, Venlo, Netherlands) by using the Rotor-Gene SYBR® green PCR kit (Qiagen, Venlo, Netherlands). The thermal profiles consisted of 15 min at 95°C for denaturing followed by 45 cycles of amplifications (15 s at 94°C for denaturation, 30 s at 58°C for annealing and, 6 s at 72°C for extension). Results obtained for the targeted mRNAs were normalized against the SmRNA. The primer pair used was: *Tumor necrosis factor-α* (TNF-α; M13049.1) forward 5′ CTG TAG CCC ACG TCG TAG C 3′, reverse 5′ TTG AGA TCC ATG CCG TTG 3′ (97 bp), *Interleukine-1β* (IL-1β; NM 008361.3) forward 5′ TTG ACG GAC CCC AAA AGA T 3′, reverse 5′ AGC TGG ATG CTC TCA TCA GG 3′ (73 bp); Interleukine-6 (IL-6; M24221) forward 5′ GCT ACC AAA CTG GAT ATA ATC AGG A 3′, reverse 5′ CCA GGT AGC TAT GGT ACT CCA GAA 3′ (78 bp); *Vascular cell adhesion molecule-1* (VCAM-1; NM 011693.2) forward 5′ TGG TGA AAT GGA ATC TGA ACC 3′, reverse 5′ CCC AGA TGG TGG TTT CCT T 3′ (86 bp).

Oxidative Stress and Antioxidant Assessment

Kidney was homogenized (10%, w/v) in PBS 1X + EDTA 0.5 mM in ice. After centrifugation at 12,000 g for 10 min at 4°C, the supernatant was collected for measurement of oxidative stress markers. Homogenate aliquots were stored at −80°C. Protein concentrations were determined using the BCA protein assays Kit (Novagen, Darmstadt, Germany) in accordance with the manufacturer's instructions. All of the chemicals used for oxidative stress measurements were purchased from Sigma-Aldrich (St-Louis, MO, USA) and spectrophotometric measurements were performed on TECAN Infinite 2000 plate reader (Männedorf, Switzerland). Results were standardized per mg of total protein. Glutathione peroxidase (GPx) activity was determined by the modified method of Paglia and Valentine (Paglia and Valentine, 1967). GPx activity was determined by measuring the rate of NADPH extinction after addition of glutathione reductase, reduced glutathione and NADPH using hydrogen peroxide (H_2O_2) as substrate as previously described (Charrin et al., 2015). NADPH oxidase activity was quantified as the formation rate of formazan blue from nitroblue tetrazolium and the superoxide radicals produced by NADPH oxidase in the presence of NADPH.

Histology

The kidneys were harvested and fixed in a 4% paraformaldehyde (Sigma-Aldrich, St Louis, MO, USA) in a 0.1 M phosphate buffer solution for 2 h. They were then incubated in 25% sucrose (Sigma-Aldrich, St Louis, MO, USA) for 24 h for cryopreservation and gently frozen in −40°C isopentane (VWR, West Chester, PA, USA) before storage at −80°C. Seven-micrometer sections were cut and stained with hematoxylin-eosin, Masson's trichrome, and Perl's Blue. All observations in light microscopy were performed using a light microscope Olympus BX43 (Olympus Corporation, Tokyo, Japan), images were captured with a video camera SC30 (Olympus Corporation, Tokyo, Japan) coupled to an image analysis system (AnalySIS® getIT! 5.1; Olympus Soft Imaging Solutions GmbH, Münster, Germany). The area of 50 glomeruli per mouse was measured using Image J.

Immunostaining

Briefly, antigen retrieval was performed by immersing frozen sections in 0.01 M citrate buffer (pH 6.0), at 95°C for 25 min. Slides were then incubated in blocking solution (TBS + 3% donkey serum) at room temperature for 1 h 30 min. Endogenous biotin and peroxidase activity were blocked before staining, by using commercial avidin/biotin and peroxidase kits, respectively (Vector Lab, Burlingame, CA, USA). Slides were incubated overnight at 4°C with the following primary antibodies: rabbit polyclonal anti-NF-κB p65 (sc-372, dilution 1:200, Santa Cruz Biotechnology, CA), mouse monoclonal anti-phosphorylated NF-κB p65 Ser536 (sc-136,548, dilution 1:200, Santa Cruz Biotechnology), or rat monoclonal anti-KIM1 (sc-53,769, dilution 1:50, Santa Cruz Biotechnology). After washing, sections were then incubated with a biotinylated donkey anti-rabbit (711-065-152, dilution 1:2,000; Jackson Immuno-Research, Suffolk, UK), donkey anti-mouse (715-065-150, dilution 1:5,000; Jackson Immuno-Research), or donkey anti-rat antibody (712-065-153, dilution 1:2,000; Jackson Immuno-Research). Exposure was performed with the avidin-biotin enzyme complex (Vectastain Elite ABC standard peroxidase Kit; Vector Lab, Burlingame, CA, USA) and the substrate 3,3′-diaminobenzidine (DAB Peroxidase Substrate Kit; Vector Lab, Burlingame, CA, USA). ImageJ® software with the "Immunoratio" plugin was used to semi-quantify NF-κB p65, phosphorylated NF-κB p65 Ser536, and KIM-1 expression in 30–50 randomly selected cortical areas. This score was measured by determining the total tissue area on the original picture while the DAB-positive area was defined using ImageJ's automatic threshold on the DAB component, obtained as previously described (Tuominen et al., 2010).

Statistics

Statistical analyses were performed using Statistica Software (Tulsa, OK, USA). All variables were tested for normality and variance homogeneity. Data were analyzed using two-way ANOVA followed by planned comparisons or Student's *t*-test when appropriate. A "*p*-value" inferior to 0.05 was considered statistically significant. The data were expressed as means ± SD.

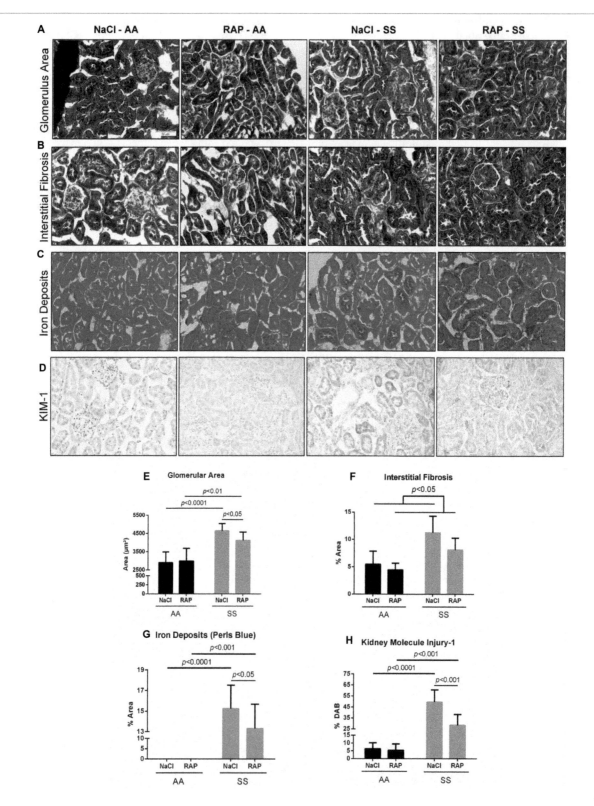

FIGURE 1 | Histopathological analysis of changes in morphology of 11- to 12-week-old AA and SS mice kidneys after 3 weeks of treatment with RAGE antagonist peptide. Representative images with Masson's trichrome staining **(A,B)** for determining glomerular area and interstitial fibrosis and Perl's Blue staining **(C)** for determining iron deposits **(D)** representative images of KIM-1 stained kidney sections. Magnification: ×400. Quantification of glomerular area **(E)**, interstitial fibrosis **(F)**, tubular iron deposits **(G)**, and KIM-1 expression **(H)**. Values are means ± SD. NaCl-AA (n = 6; three females and three males), RAP-AA (n = 6; four females and two males), NaCl-SS (n = 7; three females and four males), RAP-SS (n = 7; three females and four males). Scale bar = 50 μm.

RESULTS

Receptor for Advanced Glycation End Product Blockade Blunts Kidney Damage in SS mice

Renal histology as assessed by Masson's trichrome staining revealed glomerular hypertrophy demonstrated by higher glomerular area ($p < 0.05$; **Figures 1A,E**) and higher interstitial fibrosis ($p < 0.05$; **Figures 1B,F**) in SS compared to AA mice. Remarkably, RAGE inhibition lowered the glomerular area in SS mice ($p < 0.05$; **Figures 1A,E**). In addition, an overall treatment effect on interstitial fibrosis was detectable in the RAP-treated group compared with the NaCl-treated group ($p < 0.05$; **Figures 1B,F**). Marked accumulation of iron deposits was observed on kidney sections of SS mice stained by Perl's Blue compared to their AA littermates ($p < 0.01$; **Figures 1C,G**) but the number of iron-positive tubules was significantly decreased in RAP-SS compared to NaCl-SS mice (**Figures 1C,G**). Finally, while tubular and glomerular accumulation of KIM-1 was exacerbated in SS compared to AA mice, RAGE blockade blunted KIM-1 immunostaining in SS when compared to NaCl-SS mice (**Figures 1D,H**). Results were similar between male and female mice (data not shown).

Receptor for Advanced Glycation End Product Inhibition Modulates NAPDH Oxidase and Glutathione Peroxidase Activity in SS mice

We next examined whether NADPH oxidase – which can be activated by RAGE (Wautier et al., 2001) – was modulated by RAGE antagonist peptide (RAP) treatment in the kidney of sickle cell mice. Both NADPH oxidase and GPx activities were reduced in the kidney of RAP-SS compared to NaCl-SS mice ($p < 0.05$; **Figure 2**).

Blockade With Receptor for Advanced Glycation End Product Antagonist Peptide Decreases Kidney Inflammation

To further understand the role of RAGE on kidney pathophysiology in sickle cell mice, we assessed NF-κB protein expression and TNF-α genic expression, key pro-inflammatory molecule acting downstream of the RAGE pathway. After 3 weeks of treatment, phosphorylated NF-κBp65 Ser536 staining was lower ($p < 0.05$) in RAP-SS compared to NaCl-SS mice (**Figures 3A,B**). RAP treatment did not significantly change ($p = 0.06$) total NF-κBp65 expression on SS mice kidney sections in comparison with their NaCl-treated littermates (**Figures 3C,D**). Finally, TNF-α mRNA expression was five times greater in the kidney of NaCl-SS (**Table 1**) than in NaCl-AA mice. In contrast, TNF-α mRNA was significantly reduced in RAP-SS kidney ($p < 0.05$; **Table 1**) compared with that of NaCl-SS. The seemingly present increase in TNF-α mRNA after RAP is not significant in the AA group. No significant difference was detected for IL-1, IL-6,

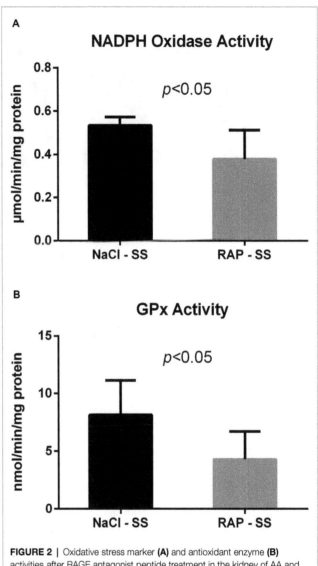

FIGURE 2 | Oxidative stress marker **(A)** and antioxidant enzyme **(B)** activities after RAGE antagonist peptide treatment in the kidney of AA and SS mice. Values are means ± SD. GPx, Glutathione Peroxidase. NaCl-SS ($n = 7$; three females and four males), RAP-SS ($n = 7$; three females and four males).

and VCAM-1 mRNA expression in SS group after RAP treatment (**Table 1**).

Receptor for Advanced Glycation End Product Inhibition Limits Anemia

Hematological changes are detailed in **Figure 4**. MCV, RDW, MCH, WBCs, and reticulocyte count were significantly higher in the SS group while MCHC, hematocrit, RBCs, and hemoglobin level were lower in SS mice than in their AA littermates (**Table 2, Figure 4**). In RAP-treated SS mice, there was no treatment effect on WBCs (**Table 2**). However, RBC count and hemoglobin level were increased ($p < 0.05$; **Figures 4A–C**). Sickle cell percentage as well as reticulocyte count decreased in RAP-treated SS compared to NaCl-SS mice ($p < 0.05$; **Figures 4D,E**).

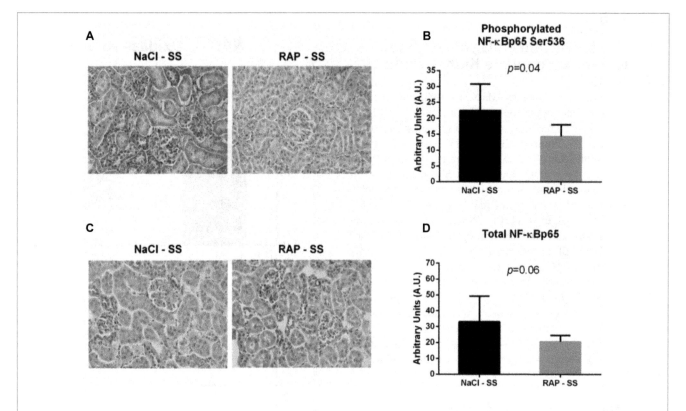

FIGURE 3 | Effect of RAP treatment on protein and mRNA expression of molecules acting downstream of the RAGE signaling pathway. Kidney sections from NaCl-SS and RAP-SS mice were subjected to immunohistochemistry using anti-NF-κBp65 IgG (A) and anti-phosphorylated NF-κBp65 Ser 536 IgG (B), Magnification: ×400. Staining score (C,D) was determined using ImageJ plugin "Immunoratio". Values are means ± SD. NaCl-SS (n = 7; three females and four males), RAP-SS (n = 7; three females and four males).

TABLE 1 | Renal mRNA expression of inflammatory and adhesion cell markers in NaCl- or RAP-treated AA and SS mice.

	NaCl-AA	RAP-AA	NaCl-SS	RAP-SS
TNF-α (No. of copies)	50.1 ± 49.5	110.4 ± 88.7	247.3 ± 187.2*	132.9 ± 105.4$
IL-1β (No. of copies)	261.0 ± 173.7	232.8 ± 89.6	578.9 ± 254.9	602.2 ± 299.9†
IL-6 (No. of copies)	93.3 ± 97.8	36.0 ± 25.6	113.6 ± 59.8	185.1 ± 191.0
VCAM-1 (No. of copies)	4905.5 ± 4601.6	7716.9 ± 2556.3	13790.8 ± 6839.5	25046.9 ± 19009.7†

IL-1β, Interleukin-1β; IL-6, Interleukin-6; VCAM-1, Vascular Cell Adhesion Molecule-1.
*$p < 0.01$ vs. NaCl-AA; †$p < 0.05$ vs. RAP-AA; $$p < 0.05$ vs. NaCl-SS.
NaCl-AA (n = 6; three females and three males), RAP-AA (n = 6; four females and two males), NaCl-SS (n = 7; three females and four males), RAP-SS (n = 7; three females and four males).

DISCUSSION

The current study aimed to investigate the effect of RAGE inhibition on markers of kidney damage as well as on markers of oxidative stress and inflammation in the kidney of homozygous sickle mice. In support of our hypothesis, the results of the present study demonstrated for the first time that a RAGE blockade (1) dampened kidney damage, as evidenced by reduced glomerular hypertrophy, interstitial fibrosis, iron deposition, and KIM-1 protein expression in SS mice; (2) reduced the activation of both NADPH oxidase and NF-κBp65 acting downstream of the AGE/RAGE signaling pathway; (3) increased hematocrit, RBC count, and hemoglobin level, and decreased reticulocyte count and sickle cell count in SS mice.

While SS mice displayed common renal manifestations of SCD, i.e., glomerular hypertrophy (Elfenbein et al., 1974; Bhathena and Sondheimer, 1991), interstitial fibrosis (Walker et al., 1971; Alhwiesh, 2014), iron overload (Walker et al., 1971; Buckalew and Someren, 1974), and KIM-1 overexpression (Sundaram et al., 2011; Hamideh et al., 2014) – a specific marker of tubular injuries – RAP treatment minimized kidney injuries in these mice. Our findings are in agreement with those of a previous study performed in diabetic mice where administration of soluble RAGE reduced glomerular area (Wendt et al., 2003). In nephropathies, it was reported that glomerular hypertrophy results from podocyte hypertrophy and extracellular matrix (ECM) accumulation (Li et al., 2007), and RAGE activation was shown to contribute to both of these pathological

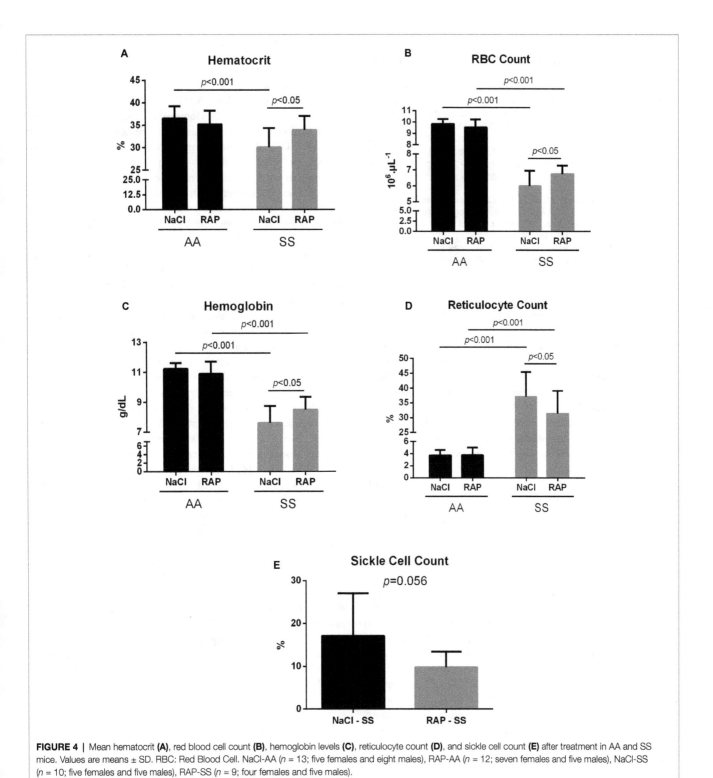

FIGURE 4 | Mean hematocrit **(A)**, red blood cell count **(B)**, hemoglobin levels **(C)**, reticulocyte count **(D)**, and sickle cell count **(E)** after treatment in AA and SS mice. Values are means ± SD. RBC: Red Blood Cell. NaCl-AA (n = 13; five females and eight males), RAP-AA (n = 12; seven females and five males), NaCl-SS (n = 10; five females and five males), RAP-SS (n = 9; four females and five males).

changes (Liebisch et al., 2014; Zhao et al., 2014). Through the inhibition of the expression of the protein NIPP1, AGE/RAGE interaction induced cell cycle arrest and concomitant podocyte hypertrophy. Interestingly, the activation of this pathway was NF-κB/TNF-α dependent (Liebisch et al., 2014). Similarly, ECM accumulation has been shown to be mediated by the AGE/RAGE axis and the NF-κB signaling pathway, which are involved in ECM synthesis and myofibroblast differentiation (Zhao et al., 2014). Thus, both glomerular hypertrophy and interstitial fibrosis – which also results from ECM accumulation in the interstitium and myofibroblast differentiation (Farris and Colvin, 2012) – may be sustained

TABLE 2 | Hematological indices in NaCl- or RAP-treated AA and SS mice.

	NaCl-AA	RAP-AA	NaCl-SS	RAP-SS
MCV (fl)	37.2 ± 2.5	37.2 ± 2.0	50.6 ± 4.1*	50.2 ± 2.2[†]
RDW (%)	15.3 ± 0.6	15.3 ± 1.1	23.0 ± 2.1*	22.4 ± 1.5[†]
MCHC (g dl⁻¹)	31.3 ± 0.8	30.9 ± 1.7	25.3 ± 0.9*	25.2 ± 0.8[†]
MCH (pg)	12.0 ± 0.9	11.5 ± 0.5	12.8 ± 0.9*	12.7 ± 0.7[†]
WBC (10³ μl⁻¹)	4.8 ± 1.2	4.2 ± 1.9	43.2 ± 6.7*	47.7 ± 11.0[†]
Lymphocytes (10³ μl⁻¹)	3.6 ± 0.8	3.3 ± 1.5	38.1 ± 6.1*	42.9 ± 9.3[†]
Monocytes (10³ μl⁻¹)	0.4 ± 0.2	0.3 ± 0.2	2.2 ± 0.8*	1.9 ± 0.8[†]
Granulocytes (10³ μl⁻¹)	0.9 ± 0.4	0.6 ± 0.3	2.9 ± 1.4*	2.9 ± 1.9[†]

Values are presented as means ± SD. MCV, Mean corpuscular volume; RDW, Red blood cell distribution width; MCHC, Mean corpuscular hemoglobin concentration; MCH, Mean corpuscular hemoglobin; WBC, White blood cell.

*p < 0.001 vs. NaCl-AA; †p < 0.001 vs. RAP-AA.

NaCl-AA (n = 13; five females and eight males), RAP-AA (n = 12; seven females and five males), NaCl-SS (n = 10; five females and five males), RAP-SS (n = 9; four females and five males).

by AGE/RAGE/NF-κB signaling in sickle cell mice. Nevertheless, additional quantitative measurements on the expression of fibrosis markers (i.e., Col1α1, α-SMA, Vimentin, Fibronectin) are required to confirm this assumption. Tubular iron deposition is a common feature of SCD, as free plasma HbS pass through the glomerular filtration barrier and are incorporated into renal tubules (Nath and Hebbel, 2015). As iron deposits in the cortex of SCD patients were associated with intravascular hemolysis, one could hypothesize that the decrease in tubular iron deposits measured in our SS mice might be related to the reduced anemia we observed after RAP treatment. Interestingly, we observed an increase in hematocrit, RBC count, and hemoglobin level and a decrease in reticulocyte count in RAP-treated sickle mice that could suggest that RAGE may play a significant role in anemia. This finding could most likely be explained by decreased hemolysis rather than increased erythropoietic process, as a previous study reported a role of AGEs in the pathophysiology of chronic hemolysis-associated organ complications in SCD (Nur et al., 2010). Nevertheless, further studies are required to elucidate the role of the AGE/RAGE pathway on hemolytic processes. Finally, KIM-1 is commonly used to assess acute tubular injury as it is expressed specifically on damaged tubules but is undetectable in healthy ones (van Timmeren et al., 2007). In a recent study, urinary KIM-1 levels were reduced in diabetic RAGE-KO mice compared to diabetic wildtype mice (Thallas-Bonke et al., 2013), which is consistent with the results in the present study. Furthermore, KIM-1 has been shown to be associated with renal fibrosis and inflammation (Humphreys et al., 2013), which further supports the implication of the RAGE signaling pathway in SCD-related kidney disease.

Considerable evidence demonstrates increased oxidative stress in sickle cell disease (Chirico and Pialoux, 2012; Charrin et al., 2016). The primary mechanism by which RAGE generates oxidative stress is *via* the activation of NADPH oxidase (Gao et al., 2008). The downward RAP treatment effect on renal NADPH oxidase activity could suggest blunted basal oxidative stress in mice treated with RAGE antagonist that may explain the lower GPx activity in RAP-SS compared to vehicle-SS mice.

This hypothesis is supported by previous work showing reduced NADPH oxidase activity and nitrotyrosine levels in a glomerulosclerosis mouse model either knocked-out for RAGE or treated with soluble RAGEs (sRAGEs) (Guo et al., 2008). In these mice, RAGE blockade also improved albuminuria and limited glomerular sclerosis. Additionally, other studies reported decreased intracellular reactive oxygen species (ROS) after inhibition of RAGE with either RAGE-shRNA in renal fibroblasts (Chen et al., 2010) or RAGE antibody in renal mesangial cells (Ide et al., 2010). Collectively, our data strongly suggest that RAGE blockade is likely to ameliorate oxidative stress status in the kidney of sickle mice and may further support the hypothesis of a reduced anemia after RAP treatment.

As inflammation plays a key role in the pathophysiology of SCD (Hoppe, 2014) and is potentiated by RAGE activation (Goldin et al., 2006), we assessed protein expression of a key inflammatory molecule, i.e., NF-κBp65, and one of its target genes (i.e., TNF-α) at the mRNA level (**Figure 3, Table 1**). In the kidney of our vehicle-SS Townes mice, the high gene expression of pro-inflammatory cytokine TNF-α strengthens the assumption of a renal pro-inflammatory state in SCD (Akohoue et al., 2007; Hebbel et al., 2009; Krishnan et al., 2010). Interestingly, RAP treatment dampened phosphorylated NF-κBp65 expression in our SS mice. Consistent with this, it was reported that blockade of RAGE with either soluble RAGE or FPS-ZM1 suppressed NF-κB pathway in a murine model of systolic overload-induced heart failure (Liu et al., 2016). In addition, Flyvbjerg et al. reported a decrease in renal NF-κB expression along with an overall improvement of kidney function after treatment with RAGE antibody in obese Type 2 diabetic mice (Flyvbjerg et al., 2004). Thus, in the present study, inhibition of NF-κB in RAP-SS mice could explain the reduction of TNF-α mRNA levels to close to the levels observed in healthy mice. In line with this observation, recent studies showed decreased cardiac TNF-α mRNA expression in a mouse model of inflammatory heart disease knocked-out for RAGE (Bangert et al., 2016) and lower hepatic TNF-α mRNA in RAGE−/− mice after ischemia/reperfusion injury (Zeng et al., 2009). A similar drop in aortic TNF-α mRNA occurred in sinoaortic denervated rats treated with sRAGEs, acting as a decoy for RAGE (Wu et al., 2013). In this context, our data suggest that RAGE inhibition could weaken pro-inflammatory processes in the kidney of sickle cell mice.

In conclusion, our data suggest that specific inhibition of RAGE could blunt anemia-related markers. Both RAP-mediated reduced oxidative stress markers and decreased pro-inflammatory molecule expression might take part in reducing the hemolytic process as well as the glomerular hypertrophy, interstitial fibrosis, and iron deposits in the kidney of sickle cell mice. Although further studies are warranted to elucidate the role of RAGE on kidney function in sickle cell disease, our data demonstrate that this receptor seems to be an important pathogenic factor in the development of renal changes in SCD mice. Only one clinical grade antagonist of RAGE (Azeliragon: TTP488) has been tested in Alzheimer's disease patients only, in Phase I, II

(Burstein et al., 2014, BMC Neurobiol.), and III clinical trials (NCT02080364, Clinicaltrial.gov). Results of Phase III are not available at this time.

Limitations

Our study has some limitations. The study was primarily designed to investigate acute effects of RAGE inhibition on sickle cell mice. Therefore, no functional nor mechanistic experiments were performed and thus no definitive conclusions about kidney function can be drawn.

REFERENCES

Ahmed, N. (2005). Advanced glycation endproducts—role in pathology of diabetic complications. *Diabetes Res. Clin. Pract.* 67, 3–21. doi: 10.1016/j.diabres.2004.09.004

Akohoue, S. A., Shankar, S., Milne, G. L., Morrow, J., Chen, K. Y., Ajayi, W. U., et al. (2007). Energy expenditure, inflammation, and oxidative stress in steady-state adolescents with sickle cell anemia. *Pediatr. Res.* 61, 233–238. doi: 10.1203/pdr.0b013e31802d7754

Alhwiesh, A. (2014). An update on sickle cell nephropathy. *Saudi J. Kidney Dis. Transpl.* 25, 249–265. doi: 10.4103/1319-2442.128495

Arumugam, T., Ramachandran, V., Gomez, S. B., Schmidt, A. M., and Logsdon, C. D. (2012). S100P-derived RAGE antagonistic peptide reduces tumor growth and metastasis. *Clin. Cancer Res.* 18, 4356–4364. doi: 10.1158/1078-0432.CCR-12-0221

Ballas, S. K., and Mohandas, N. (1996). Pathophysiology of vaso-occlusion. *Hematol. Oncol. Clin. North Am.* 10, 1221–1239. doi: 10.1016/S0889-8588(05)70396-8

Bangert, A., Andrassy, M., Müller, A.-M., Bockstahler, M., Fischer, A., Volz, C. H., et al. (2016). Critical role of RAGE and HMGB1 in inflammatory heart disease. *Proc. Natl. Acad. Sci. USA* 113, E155–E164. doi: 10.1073/pnas.1522288113

Bhathena, D. B., and Sondheimer, J. H. (1991). The glomerulopathy of homozygous sickle hemoglobin (SS) disease: morphology and pathogenesis. *J. Am. Soc. Nephrol.* 1, 1241–1252.

Buckalew, V. M., and Someren, A. (1974). Renal manifestations of sickle cell disease. *Arch. Intern. Med.* 133, 660–669. doi: 10.1001/archinte.1974.00320160154014

Burstein, A. H., Grimes, I., Galasko, D. R., Aisen, P. S., Sabbagh, M., and Mjalli, A. M. (2014). Effect of TTP488 in patients with mild to moderate Alzheimer's disease. *BMC Neurol.* 14:12. doi: 10.1186/1471-2377-14-12

Charrin, E., Aufradet, E., Douillard, A., Romdhani, A., Souza, G. D., Bessaad, A., et al. (2015). Oxidative stress is decreased in physically active sickle cell SAD mice. *Br. J. Haematol.* 168, 747–756. doi: 10.1111/bjh.13207

Charrin, E., Ofori-Acquah, S. F., Nader, E., Skinner, S., Connes, P., Pialoux, V., et al. (2016). Inflammatory and oxidative stress phenotypes in transgenic sickle cell mice. *Blood Cells Mol. Dis.* 62, 13–21. doi: 10.1016/j.bcmd.2016.10.020

Chen, S.-C., Guh, J.-Y., Hwang, C.-C., Chiou, S.-J., Lin, T.-D., Ko, Y.-M., et al. (2010). Advanced glycation end-products activate extracellular signal-regulated kinase via the oxidative stress-EGF receptor pathway in renal fibroblasts. *J. Cell. Biochem.* 109, 38–48. doi: 10.1002/jcb.22376

Chirico, E. N., and Pialoux, V. (2012). Role of oxidative stress in the pathogenesis of sickle cell disease. *IUBMB Life* 64, 72–80. doi: 10.1002/iub.584

Connes, P., Renoux, C., Romana, M., Abkarian, M., Joly, P., Martin, C., et al. (2018). Blood rheological abnormalities in sickle cell anemia. *Clin. Hemorheol. Microcirc.* 68, 165–172. doi: 10.3233/CH-189005

Conran, N., and Belcher, J. D. (2018). Inflammation in sickle cell disease. *Clin. Hemorheol. Microcirc.* 68, 263–299. doi: 10.3233/CH-189012

Cooper, M. E. (2004). Importance of advanced glycation end products in diabetes-associated cardiovascular and renal disease. *Am. J. Hypertens.* 17, 31S–38S. doi: 10.1016/j.amjhyper.2004.08.021

Elfenbein, I. B., Patchefsky, A., Schwartz, W., and Weinstein, A. G. (1974). Pathology of the glomerulus in sickle cell anemia with and without nephrotic syndrome. *Am. J. Pathol.* 77, 357–374.

Farris, A. B., and Colvin, R. B. (2012). Renal interstitial fibrosis: mechanisms and evaluation in: current opinion in nephrology and hypertension. *Curr. Opin. Nephrol. Hypertens.* 21, 289–300. doi: 10.1097/MNH.0b013e3283521cfa

AUTHOR CONTRIBUTIONS

EC and CM participated in the design of the study. EC, CF, and AS performed the experiments. EC, CF, SS, VP, PJ, PC, and CM wrote the manuscript.

ACKNOWLEDGMENTS

We thank Patrice Del Carmine for technical support.

Flyvbjerg, A., Denner, L., Schrijvers, B. F., Tilton, R. G., Mogensen, T. H., Paludan, S. R., et al. (2004). Long-term renal effects of a neutralizing RAGE antibody in obese type 2 diabetic mice. *Diabetes* 53, 166–172. doi: 10.2337/diabetes.53.1.166

Gao, X., Zhang, H., Schmidt, A. M., and Zhang, C. (2008). AGE/RAGE produces endothelial dysfunction in coronary arterioles in type 2 diabetic mice. *Am. J. Physiol. Heart Circ. Physiol.* 295, H491–H498. doi: 10.1152/ajpheart.00464.2008

Genuth, S., Sun, W., Cleary, P., Sell, D. R., Dahms, W., Malone, J., et al. (2005). Glycation and carboxymethyllysine levels in skin collagen predict the risk of future 10-year progression of diabetic retinopathy and nephropathy in the diabetes control and complications trial and epidemiology of diabetes interventions and complications participants with type 1 diabetes. *Diabetes* 54, 3103–3111. doi: 10.2337/diabetes.54.11.3103

Goldin, A., Beckman, J. A., Schmidt, A. M., and Creager, M. A. (2006). Advanced glycation end products sparking the development of diabetic vascular injury. *Circulation* 114, 597–605. doi: 10.1161/CIRCULATIONAHA.106.621854

Guo, J., Ananthakrishnan, R., Qu, W., Lu, Y., Reiniger, N., Zeng, S., et al. (2008). RAGE mediates podocyte injury in adriamycin-induced glomerulosclerosis. *J. Am. Soc. Nephrol.* 19, 961–972. doi: 10.1681/ASN.2007101109

Guo, W. A., Knight, P. R., and Raghavendran, K. (2012). The receptor for advanced glycation end products and acute lung injury/acute respiratory distress syndrome. *Intensive Care Med.* 38, 1588–1598. doi: 10.1007/s00134-012-2624-y

Hamideh, D., Raj, V., Harrington, T., Li, H., Margolles, E., Amole, F., et al. (2014). Albuminuria correlates with hemolysis and NAG and KIM-1 in patients with sickle cell anemia. *Pediatr. Nephrol.* 29, 1997–2003. doi: 10.1007/s00467-014-2821-8

Hebbel, R. P., Vercellotti, G. M., and Nath, K. A. (2009). A systems biology consideration of the vasculopathy of sickle cell anemia: the need for multi-modality chemo-prophylaxis. *Cardiovasc. Hematol. Disord. Drug Targets* 9, 271–292. doi: 10.2174/1871529X10909040271

Hoppe, C. C. (2014). Inflammatory mediators of endothelial injury in sickle cell disease. *Hematol. Oncol. Clin. North Am.* 28, 265–286. doi: 10.1016/j.hoc.2013.11.006

Huebschmann, A. G., Regensteiner, J. G., Vlassara, H., and Reusch, J. E. B. (2006). Diabetes and advanced glycoxidation end products. *Diabetes Care* 29, 1420–1432. doi: 10.2337/dc05-2096

Humphreys, B. D., Xu, F., Sabbisetti, V., Grgic, I., Naini, S. M., Wang, N., et al. (2013). Chronic epithelial kidney injury molecule-1 expression causes murine kidney fibrosis. *J. Clin. Invest.* 123, 4023–4035. doi: 10.1172/JCI45361

Ide, Y., Matsui, T., Ishibashi, Y., Takeuchi, M., and Yamagishi, S. (2010). Pigment epithelium-derived factor inhibits advanced glycation end product-elicited mesangial cell damage by blocking NF-κB activation. *Microvasc. Res.* 80, 227–232. doi: 10.1016/j.mvr.2010.03.015

Kashyap, L., Alsaheel, A., Ranck, M., Gardner, R., Maynard, J., and Chalew, S. A. (2018). Sickle cell disease is associated with elevated levels of skin advanced glycation endproducts. *J. Pediatr. Hematol. Oncol.* 40, 285–289. doi: 10.1097/MPH.0000000000001128

Koyama, Y., Takeishi, Y., Arimoto, T., Niizeki, T., Shishido, T., Takahashi, H., et al. (2007). High serum level of pentosidine, an advanced glycation end product (AGE), is a risk factor of patients with heart failure. *J. Card. Fail.* 13, 199–206. doi: 10.1016/j.cardfail.2006.11.009

Krishnan, S., Setty, Y., Betal, S. G., Vijender, V., Rao, K., Dampier, C., et al. (2010). Increased levels of the inflammatory biomarker C reactive protein at baseline are associated with childhood sickle cell vasocclusive crises. *Br. J. Haematol.* 148, 797–804. doi: 10.1111/j.1365-2141.2009.08013.x

Li, J. J., Kwak, S. J., Jung, D. S., Kim, J.-J., Yoo, T.-H., Ryu, D.-R., et al. (2007). Podocyte biology in diabetic nephropathy. *Kidney Int. Suppl.* 106, S36–S42. doi: 10.1038/sj.ki.5002384

Liebisch, M., Bondeva, T., Franke, S., Daniel, C., Amann, K., and Wolf, G. (2014). Activation of the receptor for advanced glycation end products induces nuclear inhibitor of protein phosphatase-1 suppression. *Kidney Int.* 86, 103–117. doi: 10.1038/ki.2014.3

Liu, Y., Yu, M., Zhang, Z., Yu, Y., Chen, Q., Zhang, W., et al. (2016). Blockade of receptor for advanced glycation end products protects against systolic overload-induced heart failure after transverse aortic constriction in mice. *Eur. J. Pharmacol.* 791, 535–543. doi: 10.1016/j.ejphar.2016.07.008

Meerwaldt, R., Links, T., Zeebregts, C., Tio, R., Hillebrands, J.-L., and Smit, A. (2008). The clinical relevance of assessing advanced glycation endproducts accumulation in diabetes. *Cardiovasc. Diabetol.* 7:29. doi: 10.1186/1475-2840-7-29

Miyata, T., Ishiguro, N., Yasuda, Y., Ito, T., Nangaku, M., Iwata, H., et al. (1998). Increased pentosidine, an advanced glycation end product, in plasma and synovial fluid from patients with rheumatoid arthritis and its relation with inflammatory markers. *Biochem. Biophys. Res. Commun.* 244, 45–49. doi: 10.1006/bbrc.1998.8203

Nath, K. A., and Hebbel, R. P. (2015). Sickle cell disease: renal manifestations and mechanisms. *Nat. Rev. Nephrol.* 11, 161–171. doi: 10.1038/nrneph.2015.8

Nur, E., Brandjes, D. P., Schnog, J.-J. B., Otten, H.-M., Fijnvandraat, K., Schalkwijk, C. G., et al. (2010). Plasma levels of advanced glycation end products are associated with haemolysis-related organ complications in sickle cell patients. *Br. J. Haematol.* 151, 62–69. doi: 10.1111/j.1365-2141.2010.08320.x

Paglia, D. E., and Valentine, W. N. (1967). Studies on the quantitative and qualitative characterization of erythrocyte glutathione peroxidase. *J. Lab. Clin. Med.* 70, 158–169.

Platt, O. S., Brambilla, D. J., Rosse, W. F., Milner, P. F., Castro, O., Steinberg, M. H., et al. (1994). Mortality in sickle cell disease–life expectancy and risk factors for early death. *N. Engl. J. Med.* 330, 1639–1644. doi: 10.1056/NEJM199406093302303

Rees, D. C., Williams, T. N., and Gladwin, M. T. (2010). Sickle-cell disease. *Lancet* 376, 2018–2031. doi: 10.1016/S0140-6736(10)61029-X

Rojas, A., Romay, S., González, D., Herrera, B., Delgado, R., and Otero, K. (2000). Regulation of endothelial nitric oxide synthase expression by albumin-derived advanced glycosylation end products. *Circ. Res.* 86, e50–e54. doi: 10.1161/01.RES.86.3.e50

Singh, R., Barden, A., Mori, T., and Beilin, L. (2001). Advanced glycation end-products: a review. *Diabetologia* 44, 129–146. doi: 10.1007/s001250051591

Somjee, S. S., Warrier, R. P., Thomson, J. L., Ory-Ascani, J., and Hempe, J. M. (2005). Advanced glycation end-products in sickle cell anaemia. *Br. J. Haematol.* 128, 112–118. doi: 10.1111/j.1365-2141.2004.05274.x

Sparkenbaugh, E., and Pawlinski, R. (2013). Interplay between coagulation and vascular inflammation in sickle cell disease. *Br. J. Haematol.* 162, 3–14. doi: 10.1111/bjh.12336

Sundaram, N., Bennett, M., Wilhelm, J., Kim, M.-O., Atweh, G., Devarajan, P., et al. (2011). Biomarkers for early detection of sickle nephropathy. *Am. J. Hematol.* 86, 559–566. doi: 10.1002/ajh.22045

Tan, A. L. Y., Forbes, J. M., and Cooper, M. E. (2007). AGE, RAGE, and ROS in diabetic nephropathy. *Semin. Nephrol.* 27, 130–143. doi: 10.1016/j.semnephrol.2007.01.006

Tanji, N., Markowitz, G. S., Fu, C., Kislinger, T., Taguchi, A., Pischetsrieder, M., et al. (2000). Expression of advanced glycation end products and their cellular receptor RAGE in diabetic nephropathy and nondiabetic renal disease. *J. Am. Soc. Nephrol.* 11, 1656–1666.

Thallas-Bonke, V., Coughlan, M. T., Tan, A. L., Harcourt, B. E., Morgan, P. E., Davies, M. J., et al. (2013). Targeting the AGE-RAGE axis improves renal function in the context of a healthy diet low in advanced glycation end-product content. *Nephrology* 18, 47–56. doi: 10.1111/j.1440-1797.2012.01665.x

Tuominen, V. J., Ruotoistenmäki, S., Viitanen, A., Jumppanen, M., and Isola, J. (2010). ImmunoRatio: a publicly available web application for quantitative image analysis of estrogen receptor (ER), progesterone receptor (PR), and Ki-67. *Breast Cancer Res.* 12:R56. doi: 10.1186/bcr2615

van Beers, E. J., and van Wijk, R. (2018). Oxidative stress in sickle cell disease; more than a DAMP squib. *Clin. Hemorheol. Microcirc.* 68, 239–250. doi: 10.3233/CH-189010

van Timmeren, M. M., van den Heuvel, M. C., Bailly, V., Bakker, S. J. L., van Goor, H., and Stegeman, C. A. (2007). Tubular kidney injury molecule-1 (KIM-1) in human renal disease. *J. Pathol.* 212, 209–217. doi: 10.1002/path.2175

Walker, B. R., Alexander, F., Birdsall, T. R., and Warren, R. L. (1971). Glomerular lesions in sickle cell nephropathy. *JAMA* 215, 437–440. doi: 10.1001/jama.1971.03180160037009

Wautier, M.-P., Chappey, O., Corda, S., Stern, D. M., Schmidt, A. M., and Wautier, J.-L. (2001). Activation of NADPH oxidase by AGE links oxidant stress to altered gene expression via RAGE. *Am. J. Physiol. Endocrinol. Metab.* 280, E685–E694. doi: 10.1152/ajpendo.2001.280.5.E685

Wendt, T. M., Tanji, N., Guo, J., Kislinger, T. R., Qu, W., Lu, Y., et al. (2003). RAGE drives the development of glomerulosclerosis and implicates podocyte activation in the pathogenesis of diabetic nephropathy. *Am. J. Pathol.* 162, 1123–1137. doi: 10.1016/S0002-9440(10)63909-0

Wood, K. C., Hsu, L. L., and Gladwin, M. T. (2008). Sickle cell disease vasculopathy: a state of nitric oxide resistance. *Free Radic. Biol. Med.* 44, 1506–1528. doi: 10.1016/j.freeradbiomed.2008.01.008

Wu, F., Feng, J.-Z., Qiu, Y.-H., Yu, F.-B., Zhang, J.-Z., Zhou, W., et al. (2013). Activation of receptor for advanced glycation end products contributes to aortic remodeling and endothelial dysfunction in sinoaortic denervated rats. *Atherosclerosis* 229, 287–294. doi: 10.1016/j.atherosclerosis.2013.04.033

Wu, L.-C., Sun, C.-W., Ryan, T. M., Pawlik, K. M., Ren, J., and Townes, T. M. (2006). Correction of sickle cell disease by homologous recombination in embryonic stem cells. *Blood* 108, 1183–1188. doi: 10.1182/blood-2006-02-004812

Zeng, S., Dun, H., Ippagunta, N., Rosario, R., Zhang, Q. Y., Lefkowitch, J., et al. (2009). Receptor for advanced glycation end product (RAGE)-dependent modulation of early growth response-1 in hepatic ischemia/reperfusion injury. *J. Hepatol.* 50, 929–936. doi: 10.1016/j.jhep.2008.11.022

Zhao, J., Randive, R., and Stewart, J. A. (2014). Molecular mechanisms of AGE/RAGE-mediated fibrosis in the diabetic heart. *World J. Diabetes* 5, 860–867. doi: 10.4239/wjd.v5.i6.860

10

Glutaraldehyde – A Subtle Tool in the Investigation of Healthy and Pathologic Red Blood Cells

Asena Abay[1,2†], Greta Simionato[1,3†], Revaz Chachanidze[1,4], Anna Bogdanova[5], Laura Hertz[1,3], Paola Bianchi[6], Emile van den Akker[2], Marieke von Lindern[2], Marc Leonetti[4], Giampaolo Minetti[7], Christian Wagner[1,8] and Lars Kaestner[1,3*

[1] Dynamics of Fluids, Department of Experimental Physics, Saarland University, Saarbrücken, Germany, [2] Landsteiner Laboratory, Sanquin, Amsterdam, Netherlands, [3] Theoretical Medicine and Biosciences, Saarland University, Homburg, Germany, [4] Université Grenoble Alpes, CNRS, Grenoble INP, LRP, Grenoble, France, [5] Red Blood Cell Research Group, Institute of Veterinary Physiology, Vetsuisse Faculty and the Zurich Center for Integrative Human Physiology (ZIHP), University of Zurich, Zurich, Switzerland, [6] UOC Ematologia, UOS Fisiopatologia delle Anemie, Fondazione IRCCS Ca' Granda Ospedale Maggiore Policlinico, Milan, Italy, [7] Laboratory of Biochemistry, Department of Biology and Biotechnology, University of Pavia, Pavia, Italy, [8] Physics and Materials Science Research Unit, University of Luxembourg, Luxembourg City, Luxembourg

*Correspondence:
Lars Kaestner
lars_kaestner@me.com

[†] *These authors have contributed equally to this work*

Glutaraldehyde is a well-known substance used in biomedical research to fix cells. Since hemolytic anemias are often associated with red blood cell shape changes deviating from the biconcave disk shape, conservation of these shapes for imaging in general and 3D-imaging in particular, like confocal microscopy, scanning electron microscopy or scanning probe microscopy is a common desire. Along with the fixation comes an increase in the stiffness of the cells. In the context of red blood cells this increased rigidity is often used to mimic malaria infected red blood cells because they are also stiffer than healthy red blood cells. However, the use of glutaraldehyde is associated with numerous pitfalls: (i) while the increase in rigidity by an application of increasing concentrations of glutaraldehyde is an analog process, the fixation is a rather digital event (all or none); (ii) addition of glutaraldehyde massively changes osmolality in a concentration dependent manner and hence cell shapes can be distorted; (iii) glutaraldehyde batches differ in their properties especially in the ratio of monomers and polymers; (iv) handling pitfalls, like inducing shear artifacts of red blood cell shapes or cell density changes that needs to be considered, e.g., when working with cells in flow; (v) staining glutaraldehyde treated red blood cells need different approaches compared to living cells, for instance, because glutaraldehyde itself induces a strong fluorescence. Within this paper we provide documentation about the subtle use of glutaraldehyde on healthy and pathologic red blood cells and how to deal with or circumvent pitfalls.

Keywords: glutaraldehyde, erythrocytes, hemolytic anemia, fixation, cell shapes, stiffness, osmolality, batch variation

INTRODUCTION

Besides its application as disinfectant and medication, glutaraldehyde is used in biomedical research to fix cells. The principle behind the fixation is the binding of glutaraldehyde to nucleophiles of which the amino groups are the most abundant but binding to, e.g., sulfhydryl groups also occurs (Griffiths, 1993). The result is a crosslinking of the proteins of the cell (Kawahara et al., 1997),

Figure 1. Approximately 45–50 years ago, glutaraldehyde and its properties were a hot research topic (Richards and Knowles, 1968; Hardy et al., 1969; Robertson and Schultz, 1970; Morel et al., 1971; Gillett and Gull, 1972; Rasmussen and Albrechtsen, 1974; Squier et al., 1976). Such studies mention the abundance of this molecule in monomeric and polymeric form, discussing the formation of polymers at high temperatures and arguing the influence of monomers and polymers in fixation efficiency. Nowadays glutaraldehyde is "only" used as a tool to fix cells. Especially for rare red blood cell (RBC)-related diseases, cell shape is an important diagnostic parameter and fixation is an approach to circumvent the subtle sample transportation challenge (Makhro et al., 2016; Hertz et al., 2017). However, a large variety of protocols exist due to laboratory specific customs and habits. Even for the storage of the glutaraldehyde a non-representative poll among collaborators revealed storage from room temperature, refrigerated to frozen conditions.

Along with the fixation comes an increase in the stiffness of the cells. In the context of RBCs this increased rigidity is often used to mimic malaria infected RBCs because they are also stiffer than healthy RBCs (Aingaran et al., 2012). Furthermore, hydrodynamic studies on blood flow and RBC interactions use glutaraldehyde as a parameter to change cellular rigidity, supposing a gradual concentration dependent process increases the stiffness of the cells.

Here we summarize properties and provide original data of glutaraldehyde's action on RBCs and stress the parameters that are important in particular in respect to RBC related pathologies

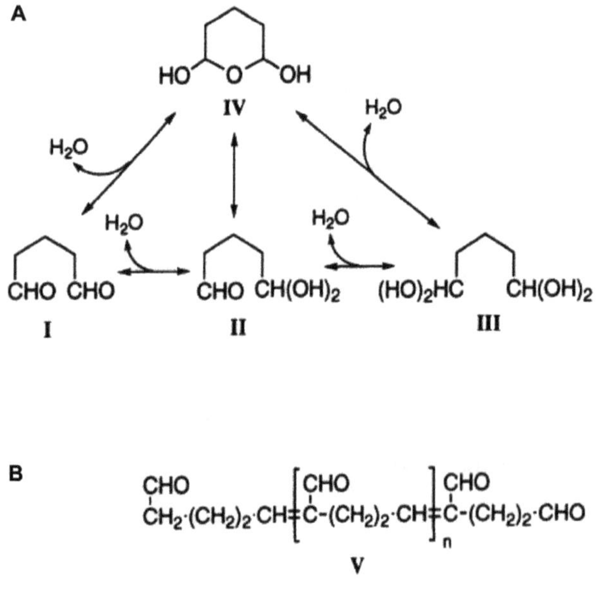

to avoid pitfalls and to allow data reproducibility as well as interlaboratory-comparability.

MATERIALS AND METHODS

Blood Collection

Donors and patients were enrolled in the study after signing an informed consent. The procedure is approved by the local ethics committee (approval no. 51/18) and was performed in accordance with the Helsinki international ethical standards on human experimentation. Venous blood was collected into EDTA coated tubes (1.6 mg/ml). RBCs were isolated from the whole blood by washing (centrifugation, $380 \times g$, 5 min) 3 times with PBS (Sigma, Germany).

Glutaraldehyde Supply

Partly because this paper reflects a collaborative project including partners at different locations and partly by purpose, different sources of glutaraldehyde have been used throughout this study. The source (supplier), the mode of storage and in which experiments/measurements they were used in are summarized in **Table 1**.

RBC Stability Test

PBS solutions (39.4 ml) with various concentrations of glutaraldehyde (various suppliers) were prepared in 50 ml tubes. Packed RBCs (600 μl) were pipetted slowly into the solution. The large tube and the high solution/cell volume ratio (65:1) was chosen to make sure the sample had sufficient volume to fix as individual cells and would not form aggregates. The tubes were placed on a tube roller for 1 h to allow for glutaraldehyde to fix. After the fixation procedure, glutaraldehyde was removed by washing the cells 3 times with PBS and resuspended in the same solution. To test the "stability" of the cells the supernatant was spectroscopically tested for hemoglobin to identify the portion of lysed cells. For the spectrophotometry each tube was resuspended completely until the whole sample appeared homogenous. Three milliliter from each sample were placed into a new tube and centrifuged at $500 \times g$ for 5 min to get a clear distinction between the pellet and the supernatant. One milliliter from the supernatant was placed in a spectrometer cuvette and was diluted 1:3 with PBS to ensure the hemoglobin absorption value is within the limits of the spectrophotometer (Red Tide, Ocean Optics, Netherlands). The hemoglobin absorption peak of the Soret band at about 420 nm was observed and compared between the samples. As a 100% hemolysis reference, healthy RBCs were lysed with distilled water to measure the total hemoglobin content.

Spectroscopy

To determine the ratio of glutaraldehyde monomers and polymers, UV-absorption spectroscopy was performed at room temperature. The extinction peaks are at 280 nm for monomers and at around 235 nm for polymers (Morel et al., 1971). To determine the monomer-polymer ratio, putative 1% glutaraldehyde samples were prepared in water. Spectra were recorded on these samples for wavelengths from 200 nm to

FIGURE 1 | The structure of glutaraldehyde. **(A)** The molecular structure of glutaraldehyde in non-concentrated aqueous solution and the possible conversion paths. **(B)** The principal structure of glutaraldehyde in aqueous solution in the current theory in biochemistry. This figure is a reprint from Kawahara et al. (1997).

TABLE 1 | Sources of glutaraldehyde and in which measurements they were used.

Supplier and grade	Mode of storage	Measurements used
Sigma, grade I, 25% in H_2O	$-20°C$; more than one year of storage, thawed for every use	**Figures 2A,C**; batch 1 in **Figures 3B, 4B,C**
Merck 25% in H_2O	Refrigerated	**Figure 2B**
Sigma, grade I, 25% in H_2O	$-20°C$; fresh batch	**Figures 3A,C, 5, 6B,D, 7B, 8**; batch 2 in **Figures 3B, 4B,C**; dashed line in **Figure 4A**; bold lines in **Figure 6A**
Merck 25% in H_2O	room temperature for more than one year	batch 3 in **Figures 3B, 4B,C**; solid line in **Figure 4A**
Sigma, grade I, 50% in H_2O	$-20°C$, aliquoted upon delivery	batch 4 in **Figures 4B,C**; thin lines in **Figure 6A**
Fluka 25% in H_2O	room temperature for more than one year	**Figures 7A, 9**

350 nm on Thermo Scientific Evolution 220 (Thermo Fisher, United States). To measure trypan blue's absorption spectra, 0.01% trypan blue (Sigma-Aldrich, United States) solution was prepared in PBS and recorded for wavelengths from 200 to 750 nm. The hemoglobin absorption spectrum was measured as detailed before (Kaestner et al., 2006).

The emission and excitation spectra of the glutaraldehyde induced fluorescence was measured with a Jasco FP-6500 spectrofluorometer (Jasco, Germany). RBCs were fixed with 1% glutaraldehyde from different batches for one hour, washed three times in PBS and resuspended in PBS to the concentration of 0.01125% to avoid excessive scattering. For the emission spectra measurements, excitation was set to 450 nm and the fluorescence was recorded in the range from 480 nm to 750 nm. For the excitation spectra, emission was set to 540 nm and the excitation scanned from 350 nm to 500 nm.

Elongation Index

To compare the mechanical properties of RBCs treated with various concentrations of glutaraldehyde, their elongation index was measured by LoRRca Maxsis (Mechatronics, Netherlands). Samples were treated as outlined above (2.2 RBC stability test). For each case 25 µl of 45% cell suspension in PBS were mixed with 5 ml of polyvinylpyrrolidone buffer (PVP, Mechatronics, Netherlands). The range of set shear was 1 to 30 Pa.

Atomic Force Spectroscopy

In order to investigate the variation between cells at certain concentrations of glutaraldehyde, atomic force microscopy (AFM) was employed. All measurements were performed in PBS with the JPK Nanowizard 3 (Bruker, Germany) setup coupled with a microscope. Effective Young's modulus of cells was measured through force-distance curves. The variety of cantilevers of MLCT model (Bruker AFM Probes, United States) with different nominal spring constants as well as different indentation forces were tested in order to adapt measurement conditions for each glutaraldehyde concentration. Prior to the measurements cells were immobilized on the substrate with Cell-Tak (Corning, United States). Force mapping was performed for 3–5 cells of each population on a grid of 32 × 32 points, corresponding to a 10 µm × 10 µm map. Force-distance curves were acquired at the indentation rate of 5 µm/s. Curves were

analyzed according to the Hertz model, implemented in the JPK software. The Poisson ratio was set to 0.5.

Measurement of Osmolality

Glutaraldehyde was added to PBS for osmolality measurements. The osmometer (Type 6, Loser Messtechnik, Germany) was checked for zero display with distilled water prior to each measurement. Glutaraldehyde solutions in PBS with various concentrations were diluted 1:10 to have a 110 µl sample.

Density Measurements

The densities of glutaraldehyde treated cells were determined by adjusting the density of solutions they were suspended in. In an Eppendorf tube with treated cells, the percentage of OptiPrep (Stemcell Technologies, Canada) was adjusted slowly to match the density of treated cells. To determine the cell density values, tubes with known concentration of OptiPrep were centrifuged at 500 × g. In the case where the density of the solution matched the density of the cells, no sedimentation was observed after centrifugation.

Sample Preparation for Microscopy

Ten microliters of blood were diluted 1 to 10 in PBS and directly added to 1 ml of 1% or 0.1% glutaraldehyde in PBS. Additional samples were prepared in order to study the stability of RBCs shapes within the spherocyte-discocyte-echinocyte scale in fixative solutions. The samples were prepared by suspending 30 µl of whole blood in 1 ml NaCl solutions with different osmolality. A hypotonic solution (131 mosmol/kg H_2O) was used to form spherocytes, a hypertonic solution (800 mosmol/kg H_2O) for echinocytes and an isotonic solution (290 mosmol/kg H_2O) was used for discocytes. After inducing the shape transformations, 20 µl of each cell suspension were fixed in 1 ml of the respective NaCl solutions supplemented with 1% or 0.1% glutaraldehyde. Since the addition of 1% glutaraldehyde increases the osmolality of the solutions, extra samples were fixed in respective NaCl solutions that were diluted in order to keep the same final osmolality after addition of 1% glutaraldehyde. Samples were kept in rotation (Grantbio, United Kingdom) for 1 h at room temperature. Consequently, cells were washed three times by addition of 1 ml of each respective original solution and centrifuged at 735 × g for 3 min. Finally, cells were resuspended in 1 ml of their original solution. Brightfield images of both live and fixed cells were acquired with a 50× objective (LU Plan 50×, NA = 0.55) on an inverted microscope (Eclipse TE2000-S, Nikon, Japan).

Staining Procedures

Eosin-5'-maleimide (EMA) membrane staining was performed on both fresh and glutaraldehyde fixed RBCs. Two microliters of blood were added to 50 µl EMA (5 mg/ml) supplemented with 10 mM CaCl₂ and incubated at room temperature for 2 hours in rotation (Suemori et al., 2015). Samples were washed 3 times with 1 ml of Tyrode solution, containing in mM: 135 NaCl, 5.4 KCl, 5 glucose, 1 MgCl₂, 1.5 CaCl₂ and 10 HEPES, pH 7.4, each time spun at 300 × g for 2 min. Cells were resuspended in 1 ml of Tyrode solution and imaged in confocal microscopy with a 100x oil objective (Plan Apo TIRF, NA = 1.49, Nikon, Japan) and an excitation wavelength of 488 nm. Glutaraldehyde induced fluorescence was examined at an excitation wavelength of 647 nm.

Some of the samples were fluorescently labeled for 3D image acquisition with confocal microscopy. Staining of the cell membrane was performed either with CellMask™ Deep Red (Life Technologies, United States) or with PKH67 (Sigma-Aldrich, United States). Living cells were stained for comparison with fixed samples. CellMask staining was performed by adding 1 µl of CellMask stock solution (0.5 µg/ml) into the RBCs suspension followed by incubation for 5 min and 3 washes prior to resuspension in 1 ml PBS. For PKH67, 10 µl of packed cells were stained with 0.5 µl PKH67 as recommended by the manufacturer and incubated at room temperature for 5 min. 3 washes followed before resuspension in 1 ml PBS. Living cells were resuspended in PBS supplemented with 0.1% bovine serum albumin.

Flow Cytometry

Fixed cells were used for immunofluorescence tests performed by flow cytometry on cord blood to measure fetal hemoglobin (HbF) content. Ten microliters of whole cord blood were fixed for 10 min in either 0.05% or 1% glutaraldehyde in PBS. An appropriate staining buffer suggested by the company (BD Biosciences, United States) was used for next steps. After one wash, cells were permeabilized with 0.1% Triton X-100 (Sigma-Aldrich, United States) solution for 10 min. Cells were then washed and incubated with FITC mouse anti-human fetal hemoglobin antibody (BD Biosciences, United States) for 20 min at room temperature. After washes, cells were finally resuspended in 500 µl of staining buffer and 100,000 events were recorded by flow cytometry (Gallios Flow Cytometer, Beckman Coulter, United States). Each stained sample was measured together with its respective unstained fixed sample used as a negative control. Living cells were also analyzed for comparison. Plots were obtained with the software FlowJo V10 (BD Biosciences, United States).

3D Imaging

Cells were placed between two glass cover slips (24 mm × 60 mm) with a suspension of beads with a 20 µm diameter used as spacers between the cover slips. A 60× oil objective (CFI Plan Apochromat Lambda 60× Oil, NA = 1.4) of an inverted microscope (Eclipse Ti, Nikon, Japan) was used to image. Cells were scanned using a diode laser emitting at 647 nm (LU-NV Laser Unit, Nikon, Japan) in a z-range of 20 µm with steps of 300 nm. A spinning disk-based confocal head (CSU-W1, Yokogawa Electric Corporation, Japan) was used to generate the images. 3D reconstruction was later performed with a Matlab R2017b (MathWorks, United States) routine.

Examination of Autofluorescence Quenching

To test the quenching of glutaraldehyde autofluorescence, fixed cells were permeabilized with 1 ml 0.1% Triton X-100 for 10 min, washed and resuspended in 1 ml PBS. Two hundred microliter of cell suspension were added to 800 µl of 0.4% trypan blue (Sigma-Aldrich, United States) in PBS. After 15 min of incubation at room temperature, cells were washed twice and imaged as described before.

Scanning Electron Microscopy (SEM)

Fixed samples in 1% glutaraldehyde solution (Fluka, Germany) were centrifuged on circular glass coverslips (10 mm, Schott, Germany) for 6 min at 40 × g in a cytocentrifuge (Cytospin 2 SHANDON, United States). Sample slides were immediately resuspended in PBS to avoid sample drying and washed 3 times to remove any glutaraldehyde residues. Post fixation was done for 30 min in a solution containing 1% osmium tetroxide in PBS, followed by 3 washes in PBS, 5 min each. Samples were dehydrated in increasing ethanol concentrations: 30 min in 70% ethanol, 30 min in 80% ethanol and overnight in 100% ethanol. Cells were dried in a critical point drying (Bal-tec CPD030, United States), mounted on aluminum stubs and sputter coated with 4 nm platinum (Safematic CCU-010, Switzerland). SEM (Zeiss Supra 50 VP, Germany) imaging was performed at 10 kV with a secondary electron detector for a 5000× magnification.

RESULTS

Fixation vs. Modulation of Stiffness

The protocols so far published are confusing concerning the application of the glutaraldehyde concentration because they range from 0.0005% to 8% (Morel et al., 1971; Tong and Caldwell, 1995; Guo et al., 2014) and all use the term "to fix cells" upon the application of glutaraldehyde.

Basing on the assumption that fixed cells may be conserved for a long time (ideally months or even years) with no morphological changes or lysis of the cells, we investigated the shelf life by treating samples with various glutaraldehyde concentrations kept at 4°C for 6 days. Every 2 days the supernatant sample was prepared to measure the free hemoglobin content in the suspensions. It correlates directly to the amount of lysed cells in the samples. **Figure 2A** reveals glutaraldehyde's seemingly digital (all or none) fixation property. Percentages above 0.01% showed almost no hemoglobin in the supernatant. At lower concentrations, increase in glutaraldehyde percentage increase

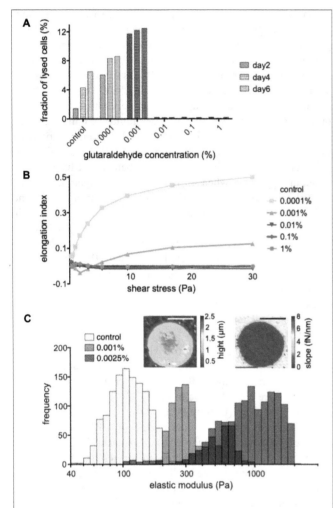

FIGURE 2 | Dependence of fixation and rigidity on the glutaraldehyde concentration. **(A)** Hemolysis of RBC in suspension without and with the specified concentrations of glutaraldehyde 2, 4 and 6 days after withdrawal/initial treatment. Living RBCs (leftmost columns) show an increased hemolysis over time which is further increased with increasing glutaraldehyde concentrations (0.0001 and 0.001%) until the cells reach a fixed state (0.01% to 1% glutaraldehyde). **(B)** Measurements of the elongation index for living RBCs vs. populations treated with 0.0001, 0.001, 0.01, 0.1, and 1% glutaraldehyde. **(C)** Histograms for the determination of the elastic modules of living RBCs vs. their treatment with 0.001 and 0.0025% glutaraldehyde. Please note that the histograms partly overlap, e.g., the brown appearing columns represent the overlap of the orange and gray columns. The inset are illustrate the AFM measurements. The images show a RBC fixed with 0.0025% glutaraldehyde. The color code of the left image depicts the height/thickness of the cell, while the right image represents slopes of force-displacement curves. Scale bars indicate 5 μm. Please note that the indicated glutaraldehyde concentrations in all panels are batch-specific and not of general validity.

the hemolysis rate compared to unfixed control cells until glutaraldehyde reaches a concentration were RBCs are fixed.

To probe the stiffness of glutaraldehyde-treated RBCs we used an ektacytometer, LoRRca, a routine tool to investigate hemolytic anemias (Zaninoni et al., 2018). **Figure 2B** reveals that very low concentrations of glutaraldehyde (here: 0.0001%) resemble the mechanical behavior of living cells, while concentrations

above 0.01% glutaraldehyde are (in agreement with **Figure 2A**) indistinguishable in their elongation index plot. Interestingly, 0.001% glutaraldehyde shows indeed a curve/behavior in between the two extreme conditions. Using atomic force spectroscopy, we had a closer look in the latter range and compared living RBCs with 0.001 and 0.0025% glutaraldehyde treated RBCs (**Figure 2C**). On the one hand this plot shows that indeed the cell populations are shifted in their elastic module in dependence of the glutaraldehyde concentration. On the other hand, one can also notice a wide and overlapping spread of the elastic modulus (please note the logarithmic scale).

Correction for Osmolality

Changes in the osmotic pressure result in highly deformed shapes, which lead to the formation of flattened discocytes with a clear shrunk appearance. We came across artificially deformed cells when we fixed RBCs of a patient with pyruvate kinase deficiency (**Figure 3A**). The shrinkage of the RBCs is proportional to the concentration of the glutaraldehyde (**Figures 3B,C**) and although the osmolality increase of glutaraldehyde solution scales linearly with its concentration, there are severe differences between glutaraldehyde batches as outlined in **Figure 3B**. While the change in osmolality might not be relevant in certain cell types in terms of morphology (Machado, 1967; Bone and Denton, 1971; Rasmussen, 1974), for RBCs we observed that the osmolality is essential for shape preservation (**Figure 3C**).

We are aware of the fact that glutaraldehyde may not be osmotically active. It is an uncharged, rather hydrophobic molecule that crosses the membrane, as it clearly reacts with intracellular proteins with a fast kinetics. Whether an osmotic effect could be present and relevant depends on the differential permeability of the membrane to glutaraldehyde itself and to water. Glutaraldehyde appears to act rapidly and to fix RBCs within 1 s (Sutera and Mehrjardi, 1975). Water fluxes across the RBC membrane are also fast owing to the presence of aquaporin. So the two permeabilities may be seen as to be approximately equivalent. Yet it is unknown if, and to what extent these parameters change in the time frame of glutaraldehyde reacting with the membrane, for instance affecting its own permeability coefficient and/or that of aquaporin, not to mention all the other protein-mediated transport systems of the RBC membrane. In the literature it is also argued that the buffer osmolality plays a more important role than the osmolality increase caused by glutaraldehyde addition (Barnard, 1976; González-Aguilar, 1982). Despite of all this, we have nonetheless observed that osmolality compensation by dilution of the buffer is essential for the preservation of shapes within the spherocyte-discocyte-echinocyte range, especially when glutaraldehyde is used in the high concentration range.

For discocytes, as they are the most stable shape for the cells, the range of tolerable osmolality is wide. Discocytes can preserve their shape for osmolality values between 210 and 380 mosmol/kg H_2O. Ideally 290 mosmol/kg H_2O is the aimed osmolality for most media, and it was also the osmolality value that fixation solutions were corrected for within this study. However, rare cell shapes are a lot more sensitive to

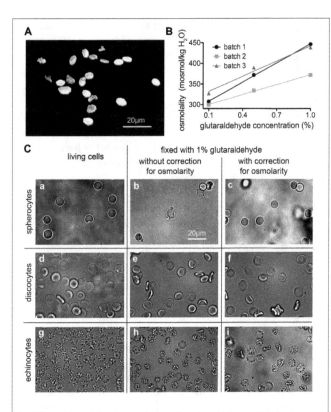

FIGURE 3 | Osmolality changes induced by glutaraldehyde. **(A)** Patient sample (pyruvate kinase deficiency) fixed in 1% glutaraldehyde without correction for osmolarity (495 mosmol/kg H_2O). The resulting dehydrated cells have a flat aspect and borders and are spiky like in echinocytes. **(B)** Relation between nominal glutaraldehyde concentration and osmolality in PBS for three different batches of glutaraldehyde. **(C)** RBCs shapes are drastically influenced by osmolality. Spherocytes can only preserve their shape for about 127 to 145 mosmol/kg H_2O **(a–c)**. Although for the uncorrected 1% glutaraldehyde fixation **(b)**, one would expect a shrinkage of the cell, we observed a high percentage of lysis with only a few cells left. Discocytes **(d–f)** can preserve their shape for osmolality values between 210 and 380 mosmol/kg H_2O. 290 mosmol/kg H_2O is the aimed osmolality for most mediums and it was the osmolality value that fixation solutions were corrected to be for this study. For the echinocytes **(g–i)** a more pronounced shrinkage can be seen in uncorrected 1% glutaraldehyde solution **(h)**. The detailed osmolalities are (in mosmol/kg H_2O) for **(a)**: 131; **(b)**: 214; **(c)**: 122; **(d)**: 291; **(e)**: 389; **(f)**: 292; **(g)**: 802; **(h)**: 877; **(i)**: 774. Please note that the indicated glutaraldehyde concentrations in all panels are batch-specific and not of general validity.

osmolality changes. For example; spherocytes can only preserve their shape for about 127 to 145 mosmol/kg H_2O, which is a much narrower range.

Monomers and Polymers

In a glutaraldehyde solution monomers and polymers coexist (compare **Figure 1**). Both monomers and polymers have different "fixation properties." In particular, the higher efficiency in crosslinking due to monomers or polymers is discussed controversially (Richards and Knowles, 1968; Hardy et al., 1969; Robertson and Schultz, 1970; Gillett and Gull, 1972). While preparation/purification to yield pure monomeric and polymeric solutions requires a certain

preparation effort, the analysis of differences or variations of cell ultrastructure in electron microscopy (Bessis, 1974) goes far beyond the frame of this report. However, it is of interest to evaluate the particular composition of glutaraldehyde, which can be measured by UV-absorption spectroscopy as indicated in **Figure 4A** depicting the large variety of glutaraldehyde solutions used in our laboratories. The ratio of absorbance between 280 nm (monomer, **Figure 4B**) and 235 nm (polymer) can be taken as the monomer-polymer ratio (**Figure 4C**). Our results show indeed that glutaraldehyde polymerization can vary between batches. Change over time, in particular when stored at room temperature is the most likely cause for the differing ratios. In addition and independent of the polymerization, we found variations in the concentration of different glutaraldehyde batches for nominal equal concentrations as indicated by the optical density of the monomer peak depicted in **Figure 4B**. Therefore, it is important to document both, the monomer to polymer ratio of glutaraldehyde as well as the peak of the monomer concentration as a reference.

Handling Pitfalls

When RBCs are pipetted into a glutaraldehyde solution they are believed to be fixed within 1 s (Sutera and Mehrjardi, 1975). This means that if the pipetting creates a considerable flow (compare also Wiegmann et al., 2017), the cellular shape adaptation to flow (Lanotte et al., 2016; Quint et al., 2017) is also conserved, which is a deviation from RBC shape in stasis (**Figure 5**) and must be regarded as an artifact. The cells marked by red circles in **Figure 5** include knizocytes (trilobes), a clear indication for flow induced cell shape changes (Lanotte et al., 2016). Gentle pipetting is compulsory when fixing with 1% or higher glutaraldehyde concentrations. In addition a pre-dilution in saline solution of the blood sample to a hematocrit of 5% or lower proved to be helpful, due to a decrease in the viscosity of the suspension (Eckmann et al., 2000) and thus a decrease in shear stress on the cells.

In microfluidics, glutaraldehyde treated cells are often used to test deformability-based cell sorting devices, as well as to study flow of non-deformable particles (Holmes et al., 2014; Tomaiuolo et al., 2015). One common problem that often occurs while working with fixed cells is the increased sedimentation rate due to higher density of cells. This disadvantage can be improved upon by using a lower glutaraldehyde concentration for fixation. The density of cells that have been fixed with 1% was measured to be 1.21 g/ml whereas the density for 0.1% fixed cells is 1.18 g/ml, while the average cell density of living cells is 1.10 g/ml. We considered two possible reasons that could explain the increase in density of cells post-fixation: either the cross-linking caused a decrease in the cell volume (cellular dehydration), or the binding of the glutaraldehyde molecules on the cell increased the mass of the cell. Since glutaraldehyde has molar density of 0.933 g/ml (Zang et al., 2016), which is lower than both surrounding medium and the healthy cell density (1.1 g/ml), the addition of glutaraldehyde molecules to the cell membrane is unlikely to increase the density of the cell. From the density measurements

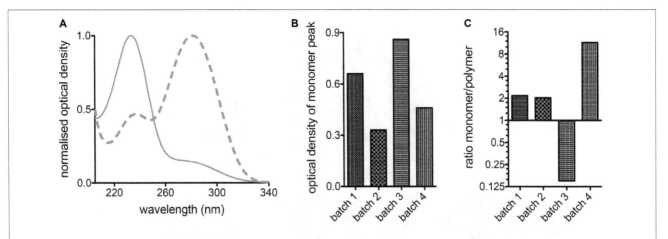

FIGURE 4 | Batch variations of glutaraldehyde. **(A)** Normalized absorption spectra of two different batches of glutaraldehyde in distilled water. The solid line shows predominantly the monomere peak, whereas the highest band of the dashed line represents the polymers. **(B)** Comparison of the monomer absorption peak for 4 batches of glutaraldehyde with nominally the same concentration of 1% in distilled water. **(C)** Ratio between monomers and polymers derived from 1% glutaraldehyde solutions in distilled water for 4 different batches of glutaraldehyde.

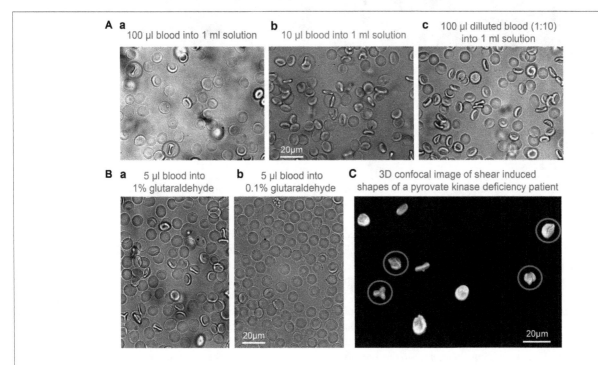

FIGURE 5 | Shear induced artifacts during glutaraldehyde fixation. **(A)** Representative fixation examples in 1% glutaraldehyde solution in dependence of the sample preparation. **(a)** 100 μl of whole blood pipetted into a 1% glutaraldehyde solution; **(b)** 10 μl of whole blood pipetted into a 1% glutaraldehyde solution; **(c)** 100 μl of a 1:10 diluted blood suspension pipetted into a 1% glutaraldehyde solution. Circles indicate knizocytes and arrows otherwise deformed RBCs. **(B)** Representative fixation examples of 5 μl whole blood in **(a)** 1% glutaraldehyde and **(b)** 0.1% glutaraldehyde. **(C)** Patient sample (pyruvate kinase deficiency) fixed in 1% glutaraldehyde with cells showing shear induced artifacts as the knizocytes marked with circles. Please note that the indicated glutaraldehyde concentrations in all panels are batch-specific and not of general validity.

we can calculate that 1% glutaraldehyde fixation results in approximately 9% volume decrease, whereas 0.1% fixation results in approximately 7%. A possibility to counterbalance the increase in density is the adaptation of the density of the suspension, e.g., by using OptiPrep (Stemcell Technologies, Vancouver, BC, Canada).

Glutaraldehyde Induced Fluorescence and Staining of Fixed Cells

Staining of fixed RBCs requires to consider both the possible interference of hemoglobin with fluorescent dyes (Kaestner et al., 2006) and the fluorescence induced by glutaraldehyde. Although the autofluorescence of the glutaraldehyde itself is negligible it

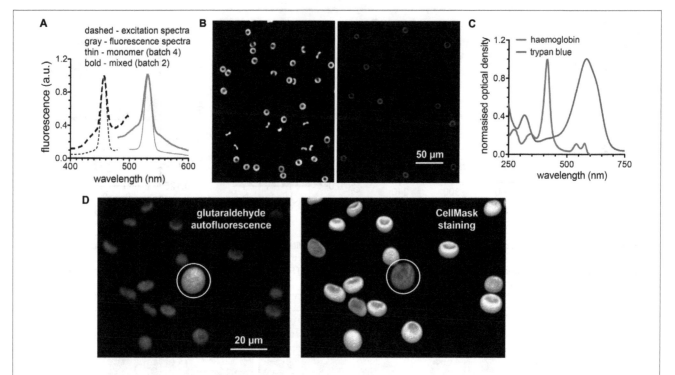

FIGURE 6 | Fluorescence induced by glutaraldehyde fixation. **(A)** Normalized excitation and fluorescence spectra of a RBC suspension fixed with 1%
glutaraldehyde. **(B)** Confocal images of RBC fixed with 1% glutaraldehyde before (left image) and after (right image) suspending the cells in trypan blue solution.
(C) Normalized absorption spectra of hemoglobin and trypan blue to spectrally judge fluorescence quenching. **(D)** 3D images of RBCs fixed with 1% glutaraldehyde.
Left image shows the autofluorescence based on the excitation wavelength of 561 nm (no excitation of CellMask). Right image shows the CellMask fluorescence of
the same cells excited with a wavelength of 647 nm (only residual glutaraldehyde induced fluorescence). The yellow circle marks a white blood cell. Please note that
the indicated glutaraldehyde concentrations in all panels are batch-specific and not of general validity.

forms fluorescent entities upon binding to peptides and proteins (Lee et al., 2013).

To judge the fluorescence induced by glutaraldehyde, the excitation and emission spectra of the glutaraldehyde fixed RBCs is presented in **Figure 6A**. We present spectra of cell suspensions fixed with 2 different batches of glutaraldehyde. For the almost exclusive monomeric glutaraldehyde (batch 4 in **Figure 4C**), the induced fluorescence contains distinct narrow bands (thin lines in **Figure 6A**), whereas the mixture of monomers and polymers (batch 2 in **Figure 4C**) gives in addition to the monomer band a wide band fluorescence background (bold lines in **Figure 6A**), exceeding the range of the spectra measured. This demonstrates that the induced fluorescence can be a problem in immunofluorescence staining (see also below), also considering the wide spectral range of the induced fluorescence, in particular in the presence of glutaraldehyde polymers. Especially when quantitative fluorescence intensity measurements are required, it is crucial to take the glutaraldehyde induced fluorescence into account. Therefore, we present a previously described method to quench the fluorescence by addition of trypan blue (Loike and Silverstein, 1983). Confocal sections of glutaraldehyde fixed RBCs (excitation at 488 nm) in the absence and presence of trypan blue are exemplified in **Figure 6B**. Although the fluorescence signal is reduced, it could not be completely excluded. To evaluate the putative effect of trypan blue, the absorption spectrum is depicted in **Figure 6C**.

Additionally, the absorption spectrum of hemoglobin is plotted in **Figure 6C**.

To evaluate the putative use of the glutaraldehyde induced fluorescence for RBC imaging we present in **Figure 6D** 3D-images of glutaraldehyde fixed and CellMask stained cells. While the left image in **Figure 6D** predominantly presents glutaraldehyde induced fluorescence, the right image depicts mainly CellMask fluorescence. To highlight the special properties of RBCs we choose an image that contains by chance a white blood cell (marked with a yellow circle in **Figure 6D**).

To further illustrate the scenario of interaction between glutaraldehyde and the staining of proteins of interest we present two prominent examples of (i) a cytosolic protein and (ii) a membrane protein. (i): We performed flow cytometric measurements of living RBCs and fixed cells with different concentrations of glutaraldehyde with and without additional staining of the (cytosolic) hemoglobin F (**Figure 7A**). Induced fluorescence is high at 1% glutaraldehyde but lower at decreased concentrations. Furthermore, flow cytometry data reveal higher fluorescence for samples kept in glutaraldehyde for longer time (several hours, data not shown). Moreover, cells showed different fluorescence intensities within the same sample, underlining different glutaraldehyde binding amounts between individual cells. This might reflect cell protein content, which varies between cells, e.g., in dependence of RBC age (Kaestner and Minetti, 2017). Additionally, we observe the effect that long staining with

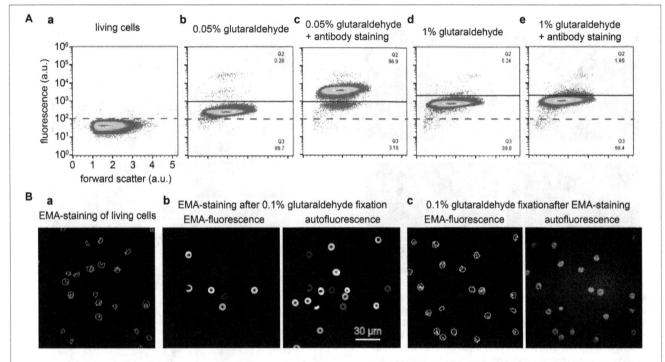

FIGURE 7 | Staining of glutaraldehyde fixed samples. **(A)** Flow cytometric analysis of cord RBCs for the detection of cytosolic fetal hemoglobin F. Panels **(a–e)** are plotted at the same scale as annotated in panel **(a)**. **(a)**: unstained control RBCs; **(b)**: cord blood fixed with 0.05% glutaraldehyde; **(c)**: cord blood fixed with 0.05% glutaraldehyde and consecutively stained with an antibody against hemoglobin F; **(d)**: cord blood fixed with 1% glutaraldehyde; **(e)**: cord blood fixed with 1% glutaraldehyde and consecutively stained with an antibody against hemoglobin F. **(B)** Eosin-5′-maleimide (EMA) staining of RBCs. **(a)**: EMA staining of living cells induces cell shape changes. **(b)**: EMA staining of 0.1% glutaraldehyde fixed RBCs, the left image is excited at 488 nm, the excitation peak of EMA with only residual glutaraldehyde induced fluorescence. The right image is excited at 647 nm where no EMA fluorescence is induced but the residual glutaraldehyde induced fluorescence is sufficient to image RBCs. Both images reveal a very heterogeneous fluorescence, whereas the fluorescence intensity is inverted, i.e., cells with a high EMA fluorescence show a low glutaraldehyde induced fluorescence and vice versa. **(c)**: 0.1% glutaraldehyde fixation of EMA stained cells, the images are recorded under the same conditions as in **(b)**. The left image depicts a similar pattern as the living cells presented in **(a)**, while the right image shows the glutaraldehyde induced fluorescence. Please note that the indicated glutaraldehyde concentrations in all panels are batch-specific and not of general validity.

high (1%) concentrations of glutaraldehyde prevents binding of the antibodies (**Figures 7Aa–e**). However, hemoglobin F antibodies (FITC) can distinctively be identified in 0.05% glutaraldehyde fixation. (ii): We imaged RBCs stained with EMA, which binds to the amino group of Lys-430 on RBCs membrane Band 3 protein and it is commonly used to estimate Band 3 protein abundance. **Figure 7B** compares images of living cells (**Figure 7Ba**), EMA staining after 0.1% glutaraldehyde fixation (**Figure 7Bb**) and fixation with 0.1% glutaraldehyde after EMA staining (**Figure 7Bc**).

Also the choice of the particular dye might be influenced by the glutaraldehyde. This statement goes beyond the obvious spectral selection presented above. For illustration we tested two types of cell membrane fluorescent staining dyes both on living and fixed cells: PKH dyes proved to be reliable for RBC *in vivo* staining for several weeks (Wang et al., 2013); CellMask is a popular dye to stain RBC *in vitro* (Flormann et al., 2017). While for living cells we observed a homogeneous membrane staining, the dyes did not always show to be ideal on fixed cells. PKH26 as well as PKH67 in particular resulted in the formation of visible "filaments" forming at the cell membrane (**Figure 8**). For CellMask we occasionally noticed the formation of small accumulations of dye in certain fixed samples, when staining at

low concentrations. Such an inconsistent effect could be due to the monomer/polymer ratio of the glutaraldehyde affecting the crosslinking of cells.

Special Emphasis on Sickle Cell Disease

Since glutaraldehyde consumes oxygen during its reaction with compounds (Johnson, 1987), we investigated if a glutaraldehyde induced deoxygenation could cause hemoglobin crystallization in sickle cell disease patients, transforming discocytes containing oxygenated hemoglobin into sickle cells. To this end we fixed oxygenated and deoxygenated RBCs of a sickle cell disease patient with 1% of glutaraldehyde and performed scanning electron microscopy (SEM). The resulting SEM images are presented in **Figure 9**, clearly showing discocytes in oxygenated cells (**Figure 9A**) and sickled cells in deoxygenated RBCs (**Figure 9B**) of the same patient.

DISCUSSION

Fixation vs. Modulation of Stiffness

Previous literature gives different meanings to the concept of "fixation": conservation of cells (Nowakowski and Luckham,

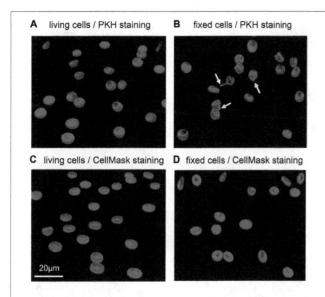

FIGURE 8 | Representative confocal 3D-images of membrane stained RBCs. **(A)** and **(B)** show RBCs stained with PKH67, while **(C)** and **(D)** are stained with CellMask deep red. **(A)** and **(C)** depict living RBCs, while **(B)** and **(D)** contain cells fixed in 1% glutaraldehyde. The red arrows point to the filaments formed in fixed RBCs stained with PKH67. Please note that the indicated glutaraldehyde concentration in panels **(B)** and **(D)** are batch-specific and not of general validity.

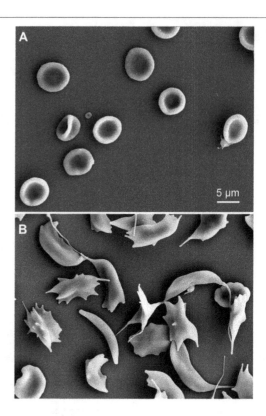

FIGURE 9 | Scanning electron microscopy images of RBCs of a sickle cell disease patient. **(A)** oxygenated cells fixed with 1% glutaraldehyde. **(B)** deoxygenated RBCs (8 h in a hypoxic glove box with 0.2% PO₂) of the same sickle cell disease patient as in **(A)** also fixed with 1% glutaraldehyde. Please note that the indicated glutaraldehyde concentrations in all panels are batch-specific and not of general validity.

2002; Faivre et al., 2006; Karon et al., 2012) and regulation of cellular rigidity (Guo et al., 2014; Tong and Caldwell, 1995). This study emphasizes the subtle difference between the two concepts as presented in **Figures 2A,B**. Fixation of cells with glutaraldehyde and increase in cellular stiffness are two different pairs of shoes. Fixation can be thought of as a binary state (all or none), whereas rigidity can be roughly regulated at low glutaraldehyde concentrations, as shown by ektacytometry (**Figure 2B**) and atomic force spectroscopy (**Figure 2C**). However, for the latter application one should avoid the term "fixation," because instead of being fixed, cells are rather more fragile (**Figure 2A**). Please note that the concentrations of glutaraldehyde given in **Figure 2** and in the results sections can't be regarded as general numbers, because the batch to batch differences (**Figure 4** and discussion below), probably highly influenced by the ratio of monomers and polymers, have a tremendous influence on the fixation properties. Furthermore, glutaraldehyde appears to have a toxic effect on the cells for 0.0001 and 0.001% concentrations (**Figure 2A**), since they exhibited more lysis than the control case (living cells). The toxicity effect also can explain the increase of lysis from a 0.0001 to 0.001%.

Correction for Osmolality

Unlike some other types of cells, RBC morphology is highly sensitive to several parameters, e.g., mechanical stress, pH changes, addition of chemical agents and osmolality differences. Because of such changes, RBC shapes are thoroughly studied in blood diseases, where genetic mutations and/or impaired cell functions affect cell shapes (Ponder, 1948; Delaunay, 2004;

Diez-Silva et al., 2010; Fermo et al., 2017). This implies that morphological analysis must be performed on reliable samples. Cell fixation is an ideal step when working with rare anemias, where patients' samples often need to be investigated in specialized laboratories and may be stored before the analysis can be performed (**Figure 3B**). It is well known that RBC shapes are sensitive to osmolality (Reinhart et al., 2015). Adding 1% glutaraldehyde to a given solution increases the osmolality by approximately 100 mosmol/kg H₂O, which results for physiological solutions in a relevant osmolality change of approximately 30%. Even if fixation occurs within seconds, the osmotic pressure difference allows water to flow in or out of the cell, affecting the shape that will be fixed. Such a water flow is also observed at higher glutaraldehyde concentrations, where the increase in osmolality is proportionally higher while fixation occurs faster (data not shown). Our results show that each shape has a different tolerance to osmolality, spherocytes being the most fragile and unstable shape (**Figure 3A**). Therefore the evaluation of spherocytes underlines the importance of osmolality correction in the fixative. If the osmolality is particularly high, discocytes appear flattened and borders slightly spiky, resembling echinocytes. Cells do not fully deform into echinocytes probably because of the simultaneous crosslinking of glutaraldehyde while dehydration occurs. In the case of discocytes, a judgment on fixed shape quality becomes generally more difficult because the shape change is less evident and often subjective to the observer. Therefore we see a need for automated (unbiased) cell shape analysis algorithms. A visual inspection is not enough for comparison with living cells, even in 3D imaging. We can, however, mention that cells fixed in 1% corrected glutaraldehyde resemble cells fixed in 0.1% glutaraldehyde, where the osmotic imbalance after addition of glutaraldehyde to the buffer is minimal (10 mosmol/kg H_2O). Therefore we suggest to verify the osmolality of the fixative solution before fixation of any samples, particularly when dealing with patients that display shape deformations, e.g., hereditary spherocytosis, sickle cell disease or pyruvate kinase deficiency. Such diseased RBCs might be more severely affected by environmental changes, like osmolarity, than healthy discocytes.

Monomers and Polymers

Glutaraldehyde solutions are mixtures of monomers and polymers as outlined in **Figure 4**. We did not investigate the advantages and disadvantages of monomers and polymers for the fixation of RBCs but this topic was previously discussed controversially (Richards and Knowles, 1968; Hardy et al., 1969; Robertson and Schultz, 1970). However, it is evident that the ratio of monomers and polymers can vary between different glutaraldehyde batches (**Figure 4C**), but the ratio can easily be determined by UV-absorption spectroscopy. Previous studies (Gillett and Gull, 1972; Rasmussen and Albrechtsen, 1974; Prentø, 1995) demonstrated that the storage temperature of glutaraldehyde is among the most important parameters for a stable preservation of the stock solution. Rasmussen (1974) has tested different storage temperatures, concluding that glutaraldehyde is most stable at −20°C. The higher the temperature, the faster the increase in polymer formation. However, we point out that the uncontrolled formation of polymers in the stock solution will affect the impact of glutaraldehyde on osmolality, therefore making it necessary to check the osmolality increase for every prepared solution before applying osmolality correction.

Handling Pitfalls

As stated before, RBC morphology is affected by mechanical stress, e.g., flow, to which RBCs adapt by changing their shapes into hydrodynamic ones. Pipetting results in shear of RBCs, which leads to the formation and fixation of flow shapes like knizocytes (also referred to as trilobes) (Lanotte et al., 2016), known to form at high shear rates (**Figure 5**). This highlights that the speed of fixation is extremely fast, knowing that RBCs in flow relax to the static shape in between 100 ms (Amirouche et al., 2017) and 1 s (Braunmüller et al., 2011). We observed knizocytes when fixing with 1% glutaraldehyde, but not when fixing with lower concentrations, hinting to a slower fixation for lower concentrations. Such distortions of the regular cell shape can cause confusion when diseased RBCs are under investigation (**Figure 5C**). To avoid the presence of flow induced shapes, we found it is sufficient to dilute the blood sample to hematocrits of 5% in a solution of lower viscosity, e.g., PBS.

Staining of Fixed Cells

The fluorescence induced by glutaraldehyde is significant and covers a wide range of wavelengths (**Figures 6A, 7A**), which can be essential for the fluorescence measurement as exemplified by the measurement of hemoglobin F in cord blood RBCs using flow cytometry (**Figure 7A**) or by staining for Band 3 protein with EMA (**Figure 7B**). Although glutaraldehyde induced fluorescence can in principle be used to image RBCs (**Figures 6B,D**), the 3D-reconstruction reveals that fluorescence intensity is limited and does not reach dedicated staining such as CellMask staining (**Figure 6D**).

However, for fluorescent staining of membrane proteins that do not require permeabilization of the RBCs we recommend to first perform the membrane staining followed by the fixation. Already the staining of Band 3 protein with EMA showed severe inconsistencies that are likely to result from the fact that glutaraldehyde also binds to amino groups, i.e., EMA needs to compete with glutaraldehyde for putative binding sites (compare **Figure 7Bb**). If this is already evident for the highly abundant Band 3 protein, we expect even more severe effects for less abundant proteins and their detection using antibodies.

According to the application needed, we recommend to fix cells shortly if the autofluorescence signal is not desirable, meaning few minutes, using low concentrations to avoid higher autofluorescence than the signal coming from a specific staining. Using monomeric glutaraldehyde, the autofluorescence induced is in a narrower spectral range compared to polymeric glutaraldehyde (**Figure 6B**). This results in a several fold reduced autofluorescence at the popular laser line 488 nm, which is also advantageous in respect to the absorption properties of both hemoglobin and trypan blue (**Figure 6C**). Quenching tests revealed trypan blue to be efficient, however, not completely eliminating the signal (**Figures 6C,D**).

Membrane staining showed to be different between living and fixed cells (**Figure 8**). While CellMask is toxic at high concentrations on living cells, PKH dyes might not provide an appropriate staining on fixed cells, even at low glutaraldehyde concentrations. PKH consists of a fluorescent dye incorporated in a long aliphatic chain that inserts into membrane lipids. Due to the presence of glutaraldehyde crosslinking the membrane proteins, it might be that PKH cannot be appropriately inserted into the membrane, giving the formation of protrusions that affect the quality of the staining (**Figure 8B**). CellMask is an amphipathic molecule linked to a charged dye that can be used both for the staining of living and fixed cells and resulted in fact in a more efficient labeling of fixed cells with any tested concentration of glutaraldehyde.

Sickle Cells

Generally, the effect of O_2 consumption during glutaraldehyde fixation is clearly visible in RBCs suspension, which upon fixation become darker, as a consequence of methemoglobin formation (Guillochon et al., 1986). However, up to 1% of glutaraldehyde based fixation of sickle cells we could not detect any sickling as outlined in **Figure 9A** and therefore we like to exclude hemoglobin crystallization due to deoxygenation.

CONCLUSION

In this section we will provide general recommendations to use glutaraldehyde to fix or rigidify RBCs. Due to glutaraldehyde variations between commercial providers, batch to batch variations and conversions of glutaraldehyde during storage time, these recommendations can hardly provide particular numbers neither for the minimal glutaraldehyde concentration to fix or rigidify the cells nor for the exact osmolality compensation. Instead we recommend procedures to consider, with the aim to ease glutaraldehyde use.

(i) We recommend to store glutaraldehyde at −20°C in aliquots to avoid unnecessary thawing of the whole bottle for each use. Use these aliquots to prepare fresh solutions before treating the cells. This allows a maximal consistency within a series of measurements in a particular laboratory over time.

(ii) The glutaraldehyde concentration to be used depends on the purpose und needs to be determined for the particular application and the particular glutaraldehyde batch. If fixation is required, a quick control can be done by washing the cells in distilled water prior to experiments. Fully fixed, fully non-deformable cells, will not lyse or have any morphological changes (test the supernatant for hemoglobin). In general, concentrations between 0.05 and 0.1%, fix cells but do not require osmolality compensation, limit the induced fluorescence as well as the increase in the density of cells. However, attention should be given, because fixation is not immediate but take longer time. In contrast, concentrations of glutaraldehyde around 1% require an osmotic compensation (see below) and if induced fluorescence is not a hindering aspect, 1% glutaraldehyde provides a sound fixation and is ideal for electron microscopy applications, where often even higher percentages of glutaraldehyde are used as these methods are physically more abrasive to the cells compared to optical imaging. Additionally, we like to mention the opportunity to set a fixation at a rather

low glutaraldehyde concentration, e.g., 0.05 – 0.1% and increase the concentration in a second step to 1% to avoid insufficient glutaraldehyde content.

(iii) We suggest to measure the osmolality of the glutaraldehyde containing solution and correct it by diluting the suspension buffer when fixing with 0.5% or higher concentrations of glutaraldehyde.

(iv) It is recommended to check the monomer/polymer ratio of the glutaraldehyde using a spectrometer and provide this ratio in the publications as a way to help interlaboratory comparability.

(v) It is necessary to consider the appropriate staining dye and its concentration in relation to the induced autofluorescence. If cell shapes are considered, the autofluorescence is rather advantageous. Staining based on the recognition of protein structures (antibodies) or relying on the access to intracellular structures have to be handled with care and should pre-tested on glutaraldehyde treated positive controls to show the feasibility. Trypan blue can be used to quench the autofluorescence. Staining of membrane proteins (e.g., using dyes or cluster of differentiation antibodies) should be performed prior to fixation.

AUTHOR CONTRIBUTIONS

All authors listed have made a substantial, direct and intellectual contribution to the work, and approved it for publication.

ACKNOWLEDGMENTS

We would like to thank Dr. Rob van Zwieten and Martijn Veldthuis for assistance with the LoRRca, Matthias Jourdain and Prof. Gregor Jung for assistance with the fluorescence spectroscopy and Dr. Thomas Fischer for helpful comments and a critical discussion of the manuscript.

REFERENCES

Aingaran, M., Zhang, R., Law, S. K., Peng, Z., Undisz, A., Meyer, E., et al. (2012). Host cell deformability is linked to transmission in the human malaria parasite *Plasmodium falciparum*. *Cell. Microbiol.* 14, 983–993. doi: 10.1111/j.1462-5822.2012.01786.x

Amirouche, A., Ferrigno, R., and Faivre, M. (2017). Impact of channel geometry on the discrimination of mechanically impaired red blood cells in passive microfluidics. *Proceedings* 1:512. doi: 10.3390/proceedings1040512

Barnard, T. (1976). An empirical relationship for the formulation of glutaraldehyde-based fixatives. *J. Ultrastruct. Res.* 54, 478–786.

Bessis, M. (1974). *Corpuscles*. Berlin: Springer-Verlag.

Bone, Q., and Denton, E. J. (1971). The osmotic effects of electron microscope fixatives. *J. Cell Biol.* 49, 571–581. doi: 10.1083/jcb.49.3.571

Braunmüller, S., Schmid, L., and Franke, T. (2011). Dynamics of red blood cells and vesicles in microchannels of oscillating width. *J. Phys. Condens. Matter* 23:184116. doi: 10.1088/0953-8984/23/18/184116

Delaunay, J. (2004). The hereditary stomatocytoses: genetic disorders of the red cell membrane permeability to monovalent cations. *Semin. Hematol.* 41, 165–172. doi: 10.1053/j.seminhematol.2004.02.005

Diez-Silva, M., Dao, M., Han, J., Lim, C. T., and Suresh, S. (2010). Shape and biomechanical characteristics of human red blood cells in health and disease. *MRS Bull.* 35, 382–388. doi: 10.1557/mrs2010.571

Eckmann, D. M., Bowers, S., Stecker, M., and Cheung, A. T. (2000). Hematocrit, volume expander, temperature, and shear rate effects on blood viscosity. *Anesth. Analg.* 91, 539–545. doi: 10.1097/00000539-200009000-00007

Faivre, M., Abkarian, M., Bickraj, K., and Stone, H. A. (2006). Geometrical focusing of cells in a microfluidic device: an approach to separate blood plasma. *Biorheology* 43, 147–159.

Fermo, E., Bogdanova, A., Petkova-Kirova, P., Zaninoni, A., Marcello, A. P., Makhro, A., et al. (2017). "GardosChannelopathy": a variant of hereditary *Stomatocytosis* with complex molecular regulation. *Sci. Rep.* 7:1744. doi: 10.1038/s41598-017-01591-w

Flormann, D., Aouane, O., Kaestner, L., Ruloff, C., Misbah, C., Podgorski, T., et al. (2017). The buckling instability of aggregating red blood cells. *Sci. Rep.* 7:7928. doi: 10.1038/s41598-017-07634-6

Gillett, R., and Gull, K. (1972). Glutaraldehyde-its purity and stability. *Histochemie* 30, 162–167. doi: 10.1007/bf01444063

González-Aguilar, F. (1982). Cell volume preservation and the reflection coefficient in chemical fixation. *J. Ultrastruct. Res.* 80, 354–362. doi: 10.1016/s0022-5320(82)80048-8

Griffiths, G. (ed.) (1993). "Fine-structure preservation," in *Fine Structure Immunocytochemistry*, (Berlin: Springer), 9–25. doi: 10.1007/978-3-642-77095-1_2

Guillochon, D., Esclade, L., and Thomas, D. (1986). Effect of glutaraldehyde on haemoglobin: oxidation-reduction potentials and stability. *Biochem. Pharmacol.* 35, 317–323. doi: 10.1016/0006-2952(86)90532-0

Guo, Q., Duffy, S. P., Matthews, K., Santoso, A. T., Scott, M. D., and Ma, H. (2014). Microfluidic analysis of red blood cell deformability. *J. Biomech.* 47, 1767–1776. doi: 10.1016/j.jbiomech.2014.03.038

Hardy, P. M., Nicholls, A. C., and Rydon, H. N. (1969). The nature of glutaraldehyde in aqueous solution. *J. Chem. Soc. D* 1969, 565–566. doi: 10.1039/c29690000565

Hertz, L., Huisjes, R., Llaudet-Planas, E., Petkova-Kirova, P., Makhro, A., Danielczok, J. G., et al. (2017). Is increased intracellular calcium in red blood cells a common component in the molecular mechanism causing anemia? *Front. Physiol.* 8:673. doi: 10.3389/fphys.2017.00673

Holmes, D., Whyte, G., Bailey, J., Vergara-Irigaray, N., Ekpenyong, A., Guck, J., et al. (2014). Separation of blood cells with differing deformability using deterministic lateral displacement(†). *Interface Focus* 4:20140011. doi: 10.1098/rsfs.2014.0011

Johnson, T. J. (1987). Glutaraldehyde fixation chemistry: oxygen-consuming reactions. *Eur. J. Cell Biol.* 45, 160–169.

Kaestner, L., and Minetti, G. (2017). The potential of erythrocytes as cellular aging models. *Cell Death Differ.* 24, 1475–1477. doi: 10.1038/cdd.2017.100

Kaestner, L., Tabellion, W., Weiss, E., Bernhardt, I., and Lipp, P. (2006). Calcium imaging of individual erythrocytes: problems and approaches. *Cell Calcium* 39, 13–19. doi: 10.1016/j.ceca.2005.09.004

Karon, B. S., van Buskirk, C. M., Jaben, E. A., Hoyer, J. D., and Thomas, D. D. (2012). Temporal sequence of major biochemical events during blood bank storage of packed red blood cells. *Blood Transfus.* 10, 453–461. doi: 10.2450/2012.0099-11

Kawahara, J.-I., Ishikawa, K., Uchimaru, T., and Takaya, H. (1997). "Chemical cross-linking by glutaraldehyde between amino groups: its mechanism and effects," in *Polymer Modification*, eds G. Swift, C. E. Carraher, and C. N. Bowman (Boston, MA: Springer), 119–131. doi: 10.1007/978-1-4899-1477-4_11

Lanotte, L., Mauer, J., Mendez, S., Fedosov, D. A., Fromental, J.-M., Claveria, V., et al. (2016). Red cells' dynamic morphologies govern blood shear thinning under microcirculatory flow conditions. *Proc. Natl. Acad. Sci. U.S.A.* 113, 13289–13294. doi: 10.1073/pnas.1608074113

Lee, K., Choi, S., Yang, C., Wu, H.-C., and Yu, J. (2013). Autofluorescence generation and elimination: a lesson from glutaraldehyde. *Chem. Commun.* 49, 3028–3030. doi: 10.1039/c3cc40799c

Loike, J. D., and Silverstein, S. C. (1983). A fluorescence quenching technique using trypan blue to differentiate between attached and ingested glutaraldehyde-fixed red blood cells in phagocytosing murine macrophages. *J. Immunol. Methods* 57, 373–379. doi: 10.1016/0022-1759(83)90097-2

Machado, A. B. (1967). Straight OsO4 versus glutaraldehyde-OsO4 in sequence as fixatives for the granular vesicles in sympathetic axons of the rat pineal body. *Stain Technol.* 42, 293–300. doi: 10.3109/10520296709115028

Makhro, A., Huisjes, R., Verhagen, L. P., Mañú Pereira, M. D. M., Llaudet-Planas, E., Petkova-Kirova, P., et al. (2016). Red cell properties after different modes of blood transportation. *Front. Physiol.* 7:288. doi: 10.3389/fphys.2016.00288

Morel, F. M., Baker, R. F., and Wayland, H. (1971). Quantitation of human red blood cell fixation by glutaraldehyde. *J. Cell Biol.* 48, 91–100. doi: 10.1083/jcb.48.1.91

Nowakowski, R., and Luckham, P. (2002). Imaging the surface details of red blood cells with atomic force microscopy. *Surface Interface Anal.* 33, 118–121. doi: 10.1002/sia.1174

Ponder, E. (1948). *Hemolysis and Related Phenomena*. New York, NY: Grune & Stratton.

Prentø, P. (1995). Glutaraldehyde for electron microscopy: a practical investigation of commercial glutaraldehydes and glutaraldehyde-storage conditions. *Histochem. J.* 27, 906–913. doi: 10.1007/bf00173845

Quint, S., Christ, A. F., Guckenberger, A., Himbert, S., Kaestner, L., Gekle, S., et al. (2017). 3D tomography of cells in micro-channels. *Appl. Phys. Lett.* 111:103701. doi: 10.1063/1.4986392

Rasmussen, K. E. (1974). Fixation in aldehydes. A study on the influence of the fixative, buffer, and osmolarity upon the fixation of the rat retina. *J. Ultrastruct. Res.* 46, 87–102. doi: 10.1016/s0022-5320(74)80024-9

Rasmussen, K.-E., and Albrechtsen, J. (1974). Glutaraldehyde. The influence of pH, temperature, and buffering on the polymerization rate. *Histochemistry* 38, 19–26. doi: 10.1007/bf00490216

Reinhart, S. A., Schulzki, T., and Reinhart, W. H. (2015). Albumin reverses the echinocytic shape transformation of stored erythrocytes. *Clin. Hemorheol. Microcirc.* 60, 437–449. doi: 10.3233/CH-141899

Richards, F. M., and Knowles, J. R. (1968). Glutaraldehyde as a protein cross-linking reagent. *J. Mol. Biol.* 37, 231–233. doi: 10.1016/0022-2836(68)90086-7

Robertson, E. A., and Schultz, R. L. (1970). The impurities in commercial glutaraldehyde and their effect on the fixation of brain. *J. Ultrastruct. Res.* 30, 275–287. doi: 10.1016/s0022-5320(70)80063-6

Squier, C. A., Hart, J. S., and Churchland, A. (1976). Changes in red blood cell volume on fixation in glutaraldehyde solutions. *Histochemistry* 48, 7–16. doi: 10.1007/bf00489711

Suemori, S., Wada, H., Nakanishi, H., Tsujioka, T., Sugihara, T., and Tohyama, K. (2015). Analysis of hereditary elliptocytosis with decreased binding of eosin-5-maleimide to red blood cells. *BioMed Res. Int.* 2015:451861. doi: 10.1155/2015/451861

Sutera, S. P., and Mehrjardi, M. H. (1975). Deformation and fragmentation of human red blood cells in turbulent shear flow. *Biophys. J.* 15, 1–10. doi: 10.1016/S0006-3495(75)85787-0

Tomaiuolo, G., Carciati, A., Caserta, S., and Guido, S. (2015). Blood linear viscoelasticity by small amplitude oscillatory flow. *Rheol. Acta* 55, 485–495. doi: 10.1007/s00397-015-0894-3

Tong, X., and Caldwell, K. D. (1995). Separation and characterization of red blood cells with different membrane deformability using steric field-flow fractionation. *J. Chromatogr. B Biomed. Appl.* 674, 39–47. doi: 10.1016/0378-4347(95)00297-0

Wang, J., Wagner-Britz, L., Bogdanova, A., Ruppenthal, S., Wiesen, K., Kaiser, E., et al. (2013). Morphologically homogeneous red blood cells present a heterogeneous response to hormonal stimulation. *PLoS One* 8:e67697. doi: 10.1371/journal.pone.0067697

Wiegmann, L., de Zélicourt, D. A., Speer, O., Muller, A., Goede, J. S., Seifert, B., et al. (2017). Influence of standard laboratory procedures on measures of erythrocyte damage. *Front. Physiol.* 8:731. doi: 10.3389/fphys.2017.00731

Zang, Q., Mansouri, K., Williams, A. J., Judson, R. S., Allen, D. G., Casey, W. M., et al. (2016). In silico prediction of physicochemical properties of environmental chemicals using molecular fingerprints and machine learning. *J. Chem. Inf. Model.* 57, 36–49. doi: 10.1021/acs.jcim.6b00625

Zaninoni, A., Fermo, E., Vercellati, C., Consonni, D., Marcello, A. P., Zanella, A., et al. (2018). Use of laser assisted optical rotational cell analyzer (LoRRcaMaxSis) in the diagnosis of RBC membrane disorders, enzyme defects, and congenital dyserythropoietic anemias: a monocentric study on 202 patients. *Front. Physiol.* 9:451. doi: 10.3389/fphys.2018.00451

11

PIEZO1 Hypomorphic Variants in Congenital Lymphatic Dysplasia Cause Shape and Hydration Alterations of Red Blood Cells

Immacolata Andolfo[1,2]*, Gianluca De Rosa[1,2], Edoardo Errichiello[3], Francesco Manna[1,2], Barbara Eleni Rosato[1,2], Antonella Gambale[1,2], Annalisa Vetro[4], Valeria Calcaterra[5], Gloria Pelizzo[6], Lucia De Franceschi[7], Orsetta Zuffardi[3], Roberta Russo[1,2] and Achille Iolascon[1,2]

[1] Department of Molecular Medicine and Medical Biotechnologies, University of Naples Federico II, Naples, Italy, [2] CEINGE, Biotecnologie Avanzate, Naples, Italy, [3] Department of Molecular Medicine, University of Pavia, Pavia, Italy, [4] Pediatric Neurology, Neurogenetics and Neurobiology Unit and Laboratories, Department of Neuroscience, A. Meyer Children's Hospital, University of Florence, Florence, Italy, [5] Pediatric Unit, Department of Maternal and Children's Health, Fondazione IRCCS Policlinico San Matteo, University of Pavia, Pavia, Italy, [6] Department of Pediatric Surgery, Children's Hospital "G. Di Cristina", ARNAS Civico-Di Cristina-Benfretelli, Palermo, Italy, [7] Department of Medicine, University of Verona, Verona, Italy

*Correspondence:
Immacolata Andolfo
andolfo@ceinge.unina.it

PIEZO1 is a cation channel activated by mechanical force. It plays an important physiological role in several biological processes such as cardiovascular, renal, endothelial and hematopoietic systems. Two different diseases are associated with alteration in the DNA sequence of *PIEZO1*: (i) dehydrated hereditary stomatocytosis (DHS1, #194380), an autosomal dominant hemolytic anemia caused by gain-of-function mutations; (ii) lymphatic dysplasia with non-immune fetal hydrops (LMPH3, #616843), an autosomal recessive condition caused by biallelic loss-of-function mutations. We analyzed a 14-year-old boy affected by severe lymphatic dysplasia already present prenatally, with peripheral edema, hydrocele, and chylothoraces. By whole exome sequencing, we identified compound heterozygosity for *PIEZO1*, with one splicing and one deletion mutation, the latter causing the formation of a premature stop codon that leads to mRNA decay. The functional analysis of the erythrocytes of the patient highlighted altered hydration with the intracellular loss of the potassium content and structural abnormalities with anisopoikilocytosis and presence of both spherocytes and stomatocytes. This novel erythrocyte trait, sharing features with both hereditary spherocytosis and overhydrated hereditary stomatocytosis, complements the clinical features associated with loss-of-function mutations of *PIEZO1* in the context of the generalized lymphatic dysplasia of LMPH3 type.

Keywords: *PIEZO1*, lymphedema, red blood cell alterations, overhydration, stomatocytosis, spherocytosis

BACKGROUND

PIEZO1 gene encodes for the mechanoreceptor PIEZO1, a selective cation channel activated by mechanical force (Coste et al., 2010), with several different functions, such as regulation of urinary osmolarity (Martins et al., 2016), control of blood pressure (Wang et al., 2016), or sensor of epithelial cell crowding and stretching (Gudipaty et al., 2017). PIEZO1 is expressed in developing blood and lymphatic vessels and plays a key role in blood vessel formation (Andolfo et al., 2013; Li et al., 2014; Ranade et al., 2014). Two different diseases are associated with PIEZO1 mutations: (i) dehydrated hereditary stomatocytosis 1 (DHS1), hemolytic anemia caused by gain-of-function mutations (Zarychanski et al., 2012; Andolfo et al., 2013); (ii) autosomal recessive generalized lymphatic dysplasia with non-immune fetal hydrops (LMPH3) caused by biallelic, loss-of-function mutations (Fotiou et al., 2015; Lukacs et al., 2015). The two diseases are completely different: DHS1 affects red blood cells (RBCs) while LMPH3 is characterized by widespread lymphedema. The only shared phenotype is the presence of perinatal edema (Andolfo et al., 2016; Martin-Almedina et al., 2018).

Several animal models for PIEZO1 were generated. Piezo1-deficient mice die in utero at mid-gestation due to defective vasculogenesis (Cahalan et al., 2015). Thus, another model was developed by a specific deletion in the hematopoietic system (Vav1-P1cKO mice). Interestingly, hematological analysis of Vav1-P1cKO mice revealed elevated MCV and MCH and reduced MCHC (Cahalan et al., 2015). RBCs exhibited increased osmotic fragility, suggesting that Piezo1-deficient erythrocytes were overhydrated. Recently, zebrafish models have also been created. Morpholino-knockdown of Piezo1 expression in *Danio rerio* was reported to result in severe anemia (Faucherre et al., 2014; Shmukler et al., 2015). However, the phenotype observed in the morpholino-knockdown model was not present in an independent zebrafish model carrying a predicted truncated form of Piezo1 (Shmukler et al., 2015). The debate on the phenotype observed in the two different models is still open (Shmukler et al., 2016).

Patients with homozygous loss-of-function mutations in human PIEZO1 show lymphatic dysplasia and an asymptomatic, fully compensated, very mild hemolytic state (Fotiou et al., 2015; Lukacs et al., 2015). Of note, a comprehensible hematological characterization of the anemia carried by patients with *PIEZO1* loss-of-function mutations has not yet been performed. We herein characterized the hematological phenotype of a patient with *PIEZO1* biallelic mutations and lymphatic dysplasia, identifying a new nosological erythrocyte alteration.

CASE PRESENTATION

Patient II.1 (**Figure 1A**) is a 17-years-old male child affected by non-immune hydrops fetalis and congenital lymphatic dysplasia. During pregnancy, a fetal pleural effusion (32 weeks) was observed. The proband was born at 38 weeks by cesarean section. Birth parameters showed a low Apgar score (5/8) with breathing difficulties treated by continuous positive airway pressure, axial hypotonia, peripheral edema, hydrocele, hypoglycemia, and normal auxologic parameters (weight 3.650 Kg; length 53 cm; and head circumference 36 cm). The hemogram resulted normal for age, and total hyperbilirubinemia was observed (13.2 mg/dL) treated by phototherapy. During childhood, a hydrocelectomy (2-years-old) and a scrotum reduction surgery (14-years-old) were performed. At 14 years, a lower limb lymphoscintigraphy was executed, showing distinctive changes of a severe bilateral

lymphovascular disease. Particularly, the patient highlighted poor asymmetrical uptake of tracer in the groin at 45 min (almost in the right limb) with evidence of rerouting in the scrotum at 2 h. At 15 years, a thoracentesis was performed to reduce the excess of fluid because of respiratory failure due to restrictive lung disease. The cytological analyses highlighted the presence of chylous fluid. After 1 week the chylous edema was re-observed at X-ray. Due to the worsening of respiratory disease at 16 years, magnetic resonance imaging was performed. The analysis showed an impairment of the chylothoraces and reoccurrence of the hydrocele (**Figure 1B**). Currently, the proband presents a progressive worsening of the respiratory function.

The other family members are healthy expect for the mother of the proband (I.2) that showed an iron deficiency anemia due to imbalanced diet supplies negative for hemoglobinopathies.

PIEZO1 Mutational Analysis

We performed WES on the proband and the parents, highlighting the presence of two variants within *PIEZO1* gene: the nucleotide substitution c.6165-7G>A in the intron 42–43, annotated in 1000 Genomes database (rs141011459) with a minor allele frequency (MAF) = 0.0004; the novel nucleotide deletion c.5725delA that results in the frameshift variant p.Arg1909Glufs*12 (**Figure 1A**). According to the recessive pattern of inheritance, the proband showed a compound heterozygous genotype. Indeed, the father, I.1, carried the variant c.6165-7G>A, while the mother, I.2, carried the variant c.5725delA. We also extended the analysis to additional unaffected subjects: the patient's brother, II.2, carried the variant c.6165-7G>A, while the sister, II.3, carried the variant c.5725delA.

To evaluate the possible effect of the frameshift variant on mRNA processing, we sequenced the *PIEZO1* cDNA of the proband. Amplification of the specific exon region, encompassing the mutation, of *PIEZO1* cDNA highlighted the selective expression of the wild-type allele, while the c.5725delA allele was not expressed, demonstrating its decay (**Figure 2A**). Human Splicing Finder web-tool predicted for the splicing variant c.6165-7G>A the creation of a new "branch point motif," and two exon splicing enhancer (ESE) motifs for SRp40 protein. High sensitivity analysis of the exon regions encompassing the intronic variant (exons 42–44), using the Agilent 4200 TapeStation system (**Supplementary Data Sheet S1**), demonstrated that the proband and the father expressed about the 4 and 36%, respectively, of PIEZO1 cDNA compared to the control (**Figure 2B**).

Characterization of PIEZO1 Expression

To further evaluate the role of PIEZO1 variants, we assessed gene expression in all the family members, as well as in a subset of healthy controls (HCs). A significant decrease of *PIEZO1* expression in the proband compared to those revealed in the HCs was observed, and a minor decrease (about 50%) of mRNA levels in both parents was detected compared to HCs (**Figure 2C**). Nevertheless, immunoblot analysis on RBCs membranes highlighted a marked decrease of PIEZO1 protein in the proband compared to the HCs expression with about 30% of expression (**Figure 2D**). The parents showed also a decrease of PIEZO1 level with 47 and 65% of PIEZO1 expression

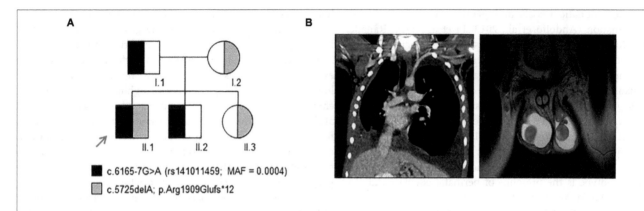

FIGURE 1 | Genetic study and clinical findings. **(A)** The inheritance pattern of c.6165-7G>A and c.5725delA variants in *PIEZO1* in the family here analyzed. The proband (II.1) is a compound heterozygous for these variants. The red arrow indicates the proband. **(B)** Magnetic resonance image of the proband (II.1) showing chylothoraces and hydrocele.

for mother and father, respectively. Additionally, we evaluated the expression of other RBC membrane proteins, including Band 3 and Stomatin, altered in hereditary spherocytosis (HS) and overhydrated hereditary stomatocytosis (OHS). Proband showed a similar amount of both proteins compared to the HCs (**Figure 2E**).

Osmotic Fragility Analysis

The ektacytometry analysis was performed for the proband and his parents. As shown in **Figure 3A**, the proband (II.1) exhibited an ektacytometry curve with right shift compared to the curve obtained from the HCs, indicating overhydration of the erythrocytes. The mother (I.2) showed a right shift of the osmolarity curve similar to those observed in the proband. Conversely, the osmolarity curve of the father I.1 was in the range of the controls with a slight right shift of the curve compared to both the proband II.1 and the subject I.2.

Potassium Content Evaluation

We measured extracellular and intracellular potassium levels in fresh blood samples from all family members, and HCs. The proband (II:1) and his mother (I.2) showed a decrease of potassium content compared to the HC, while the father (I.1) showed intracellular [K+] comparable to HC (**Figure 3B**). The analysis of K+ plasmatic levels showed increased levels in the proband and his parents compared to the HC.

Peripheral Blood Smear Examination

The hemogram showed a slight reduction of the Hb content with normal MCV and decreased MCH and MCHC values (**Supplementary Table S1**). The RDW resulted increased while the reticulocytes count was normal (**Supplementary Table S1**). Accurate analysis of the peripheral blood (PB) smear of the proband revealed marked anisopoikolocytosis, hypocromia, several spherocytes, some stomatocytes, some mushroom−shaped RBCs, several RBCs fragmentation and debris (**Figure 3C**).

DISCUSSION

PIEZO1 gene encodes for the mechanoreceptor PIEZO1, a selective cation channel activated by mechanical force (Coste et al., 2010; Kim et al., 2012; Ge et al., 2015; Gnanasambandam et al., 2015; Andolfo et al., 2016; Dubin et al., 2017; Hyman et al., 2017; Zhao et al., 2017). In human, the first disease associated with mutations in *PIEZO1* was the DHS1 (Zarychanski et al., 2012; Andolfo et al., 2013). In erythrocytes, PIEZO1 regulates cell volume homeostasis, and gain-of-function mutations in DHS1 are causative of alterations of the RBC membrane permeability to monovalent cations Na+ and K+, with consequent alterations of the intracellular cationic content and cell volume (Albuisson et al., 2013; Bae et al., 2013; Archer et al., 2014; Sandberg et al., 2014; Shmukler et al., 2014; Imashuku et al., 2016). Generally, DHS1 patients show hemolytic anemia, with high reticulocyte count, the tendency to macrocytosis, and mild jaundice (Zarychanski et al., 2012; Andolfo et al., 2018b). The second condition associated with *PIEZO1* mutations is the lymphatic dysplasia. Two recent reports have described homozygous or compound heterozygous mutations in *PIEZO1* in families with LMPH3 (Fotiou et al., 2015; Lukacs et al., 2015). These cases exhibited full body edema and severe facial swelling. Most patients also presented intestinal lymphangiectasia, growth retardation, seizures, microcephaly, and intellectual disability. Loss-of-function mutations in *PIEZO1* also account for hydrops fetalis, chylothorax, and chronic pleural effusions with persistent lymphedema of legs, torso, and face. The cosegregating homozygous and compound heterozygous *PIEZO1* mutations in these families included non-sense, missense, and splice donor site mutations (Fotiou et al., 2015; Lukacs et al., 2015). Regarding the hematological framework, some of these patients were not anemic and exhibited normal hematological indices, including MCV (Lukacs et al., 2015).

The patient herein described shared some similar characteristics with the other LMPH3 patients until described such as hydrops fetalis, chylothorax, and chronic pleural effusions with persistent lymphedema. On the other hand, our patient showed peculiar characteristics: the hydrocele never

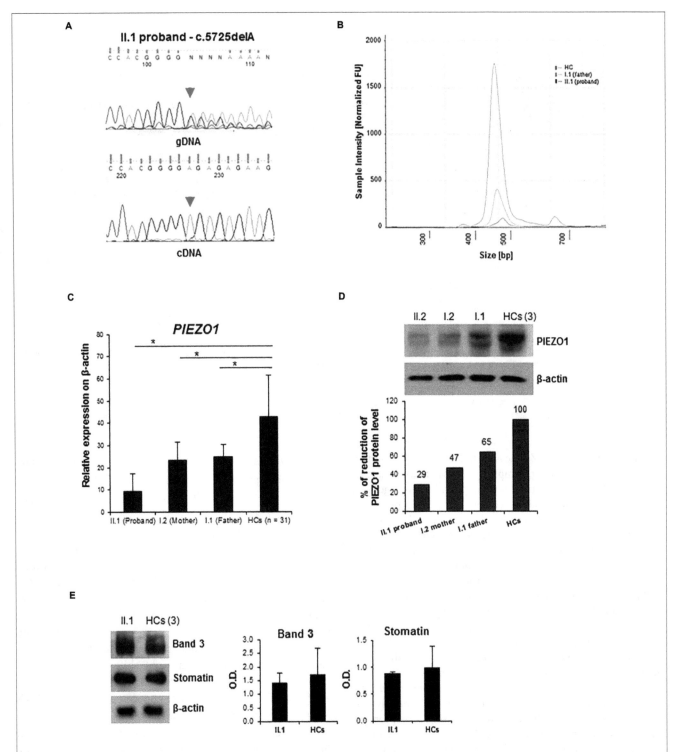

FIGURE 2 | Characterization of *PIEZO1* mutations: cDNA study and membrane proteins expression analysis. **(A)** Electropherograms showing sequencing analysis of the PIEZO1 variant c.5725delA in the proband. Genomic DNA (gDNA) and cDNA sequences are shown. **(B)** DNA electrophoresis profile of the PIEZO1 cDNA fragment encompassing exons 42–44 of the proband (green line), the father (orange line), and the control (blu line) by 4200 TapeStation system. The electropherogram shows the size distribution and the intensity of the detected bands of RT-PCR. **(C)** *PIEZO1* mRNA level normalized to *GAPDH* in the proband II.1 compared to his parents, I.1 and I.2 and the HCs (n = 30). Data are presented as a mean ± SD. *p-value < 0.05. **(D)** Immunoblot showing PIEZO1 protein expression normalized to β-actin in the proband II.1 compared to his parents, I.1 and I.2 and the HCs (pool of n = 3). Densitometric analysis of one representative western blotting is shown. **(E)** Immunoblot analysis of RBCs membrane proteins, Band 3 (Anion Exchanger 1) and Stomatin (Erythrocyte Membrane Protein 7.2), in the proband II.1 compared to the HCs (pool of n = 3). Protein levels are normalized to β-actin. Densitometric analysis of two separate western blotting is shown. Data are presented as a mean ± SD.

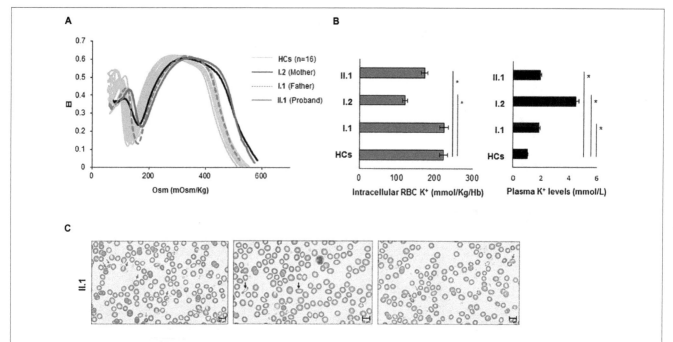

FIGURE 3 | Characterization of the hematological phenotype. **(A)** The red cell deformability index was measured as a function of increasing osmolarity of RBCs from proband II.1 (red line), from mother I.2 (black line), from father I.1 (orange dotted line), and internal HCs (light blue lines). Values are means +/– SE of two independent experiments. Elongation index (EI) **(B)** intracellular K+ content (expressed as mmol/Kg/Hb) of blood from II.1, I.1, I.2 subjects, and from HC (the graph with gray bars). Plasma K+ content (expressed as mmol/L of whole blood) of blood from II.1, I.1, I.2 subjects, and from HC (the graph with black bars) *p-value < 0.05. **(C)** Peripheral blood smear (May-Grünwald Giemsa stain 40×) examination of the proband II.1 showing marked anisopoikilocytosis. Blue arrows indicate fragmented cells; red arrows indicate stomatocytes; green arrows indicate spherocytes; black arrows indicate ovalocytes; orange arrows indicate mushroom cells.

observed in the other *PIEZO1* loss-of-function patients, and the absence of facial swelling, lymphangiectasia, and intellectual disability. Of note, the proband is a compound heterozygous for a splicing variant and a coding deletion that causes a premature stop codon. We demonstrated the decay of the allele carrying the deletion variant, and the massive reduction of expression of the allele carrying the splicing variant. The combination of the two variants causes a substantial reduction of both mRNA and protein expression of PIEZO1 in the proband.

PIEZO1 is a highly polymorphic gene that has a very large tolerance for both missense and loss-of-function variants and has a lot of variations. The variable expressivity of both DHS1 and lymphatic dysplasia could be explained with the combination of multiple disease-causing alleles or their combination with polymorphic variants (Lupski, 2012; Lacroix et al., 2018). Indeed, we previously demonstrated that multiple modifier *PIEZO1* variants could account for highly variable clinical expressivity in DHS1, with subsequent difficulties in establishing the appropriate genotype/phenotype correlation (Andolfo et al., 2018a,b). Of note, the patient showed a peculiar phenotype characterized by peripheral edema, hydrocele, and chylothoraces. Furthermore, even if the blood count seems only slightly altered with a mild reduction of the Hb, and decreased MCH and MCHC values, the RDW resulted increased despite the reticulocytes count was normal. According to the increased RDW, the PB smear of the proband revealed anisopoikilocytosis, hypocromia, with the presence of some spherocytes, mushroom—shaped RBCs, stomatocytes, erythrocytes' fragmentation, and debris. Moreover,

the ektacytometry analysis revealed a right shift of the right arm of the osmolarity curve indicating mild overhydration of RBCs, without the decreased DImax typical of HS. Finally, the ionic flux assay indicated increased plasma [K+] and decreased intracellular [K+] as in OHS. Thus, our patient seems to present pathological traits of the erythrocyte with some characteristics shared with hereditary spherocytosis as spherocytes at PB smear and normal MCV and several features of overhydrated hereditary stomatocytosis as stomatocytes at PB, decreased MCHC, normal Dimax, right shift of the osmolarity curve, and decreased intracellular potassium. The mother showed a similar, but less pronounced, right shift of the osmolarity curve. This finding could be caused by the iron deficiency anemia that is known to alter the deformability of RBCs (Vayá et al., 2005; Brandão et al., 2009).

Of note, Vav1-P1cKO mice with specific deletion of *Piezo1* in the hematopoietic system showed a slight increase of RDW and reduced MCHC confirming overhydration of RBCs as seen in our patient (Cahalan et al., 2015). Moreover, morpholino-knockdown of Piezo1 in zebrafish showed the erythroid phenotype of fragile, spherocytic, dysmorphic cells also like our patient (Shmukler et al., 2015).

In conclusion, the proband presents an alteration of the structure and the ionic content of erythrocytes caused by the two hypomorphic variants in *PIEZO1*. We speculate that the substantial decreased expression of PIEZO1 could be compensated by overactivation of other cation channels/pumps that act by compensating the hematological phenotype. Patients affected by lymphedema caused by mutations in *PIEZO1* could benefit in future of therapy by Yoda1, a novel small synthetic molecule specific activator of PIEZO1 (Cahalan et al., 2015; Lacroix et al., 2018), or by gene therapy by selective insertion of the gene in the lymphatic system, or by *in vivo* target gene activation via CRISPR/CAS9 mediated *trans-*epigenetic modulation.

AUTHOR CONTRIBUTIONS

IA, RR, and AI designed and conducted the study, and prepared the manuscript. GDR performed the western blotting analysis and contributed to the preparation of the manuscript. EE and AV performed the preparation of the WES libraries and the NGS analysis. FM and BER performed the molecular analysis and collection of the samples. AG, VC, and GP contributed to take care of the patients. LDF performed the ionic flux data analysis. RR performed the mutational analysis. OZ designed and supervised the NGS analysis and also provided a critical evaluation of the study.

REFERENCES

Albuisson, J., Murthy, S. E., Bandell, M., Coste, B., Louis-Dit-Picard, H., Mathur, J., et al. (2013). Dehydrated hereditary stomatocytosis linked to gain-of-function mutations in mechanically activated piezo1 ion channels. *Nat. Commun.* 4:1884. doi: 10.1038/ncomms2899

Andolfo, I., Alper, S. L., De Franceschi, L., Auriemma, C., Russo, R., De Falco, L., et al. (2013). Multiple clinical forms of dehydrated hereditary stomatocytosis arise from mutations in PIEZO1. *Blood* 121, 3925–3935. doi: 10.1182/blood-2013-02-482489

Andolfo, I., Manna, F., De Rosa, G., Rosato, B. E., Gambale, A., Tomaiuolo, G., et al. (2018a). PIEZO1-R1864H rare variant accounts for a genetic phenotype-modifier role in dehydrated hereditary stomatocytosis. *Haematologica* 103, e94–e97. doi: 10.3324/haematol.2017.180687

Andolfo, I., Russo, R., Rosato, B. E., Manna, F., Gambale, A., Brugnara, C., et al. (2018b). Genotype-phenotype correlation and risk stratification in a cohort of 123 hereditary stomatocytosis patients. *Am. J. Hematol.* 93, 1509–1517. doi: 10.1002/ajh.25276

Andolfo, I., Russo, R., Gambale, A., and Iolascon, A. (2016). New insights on hereditary erythrocyte membrane defects. *Haematologica* 101, 1284–1294. doi: 10.3324/haematol.2016.142463

Archer, N. M., Shmukler, B. E., Andolfo, I., Vandorpe, D. H., Gnanasambandam, R., Higgins, J. M., et al. (2014). Hereditary xerocytosis revisited. *Am. J. Hematol.* 89, 1142–1146. doi: 10.1002/ajh.23799

Bae, C., Gnanasambandam, R., Nicolai, C., Sachs, F., and Gottlieb, P. A. (2013). Xerocytosis is caused by mutations that alter the kinetics of the mechanosensitive channel PIEZO1. *Proc. Natl. Acad. Sci. U.S.A.* 110, E1162–E1168. doi: 10.1073/pnas.1219777110

Brandão, M. M., Castro Mde, L., Fontes, A., Cesar, C. L., Costa, F. F., and Saad, S. T. (2009). Impaired red cell deformability in iron deficient subjects. *Clin. Hemorheol. Microcirc.* 43, 217–221. doi: 10.3233/CH-2009-1211

Cahalan, S. M., Lukacs, V., Ranade, S. S., Chien, S., Bandell, M., and Patapoutian, A. (2015). Piezo1 links mechanical forces to red blood cell volume. *eLife* 22:4. doi: 10.7554/eLife.07370

Coste, B., Mathur, J., Schmidt, M., Earley, T. J., Ranade, S., Petrus, M. J., et al. (2010). Piezo1 and Piezo2 are essential components of distinct mechanically activated cation channels. *Science* 330, 55–60. doi: 10.1126/science.1193270

Dubin, A. E., Murthy, S., Lewis, A. H., Brosse, L., Cahalan, S. M., Grandl, J., et al. (2017). Endogenous piezo1 can confound mechanically activated channel identification and characterization. *Neuron* 94, 266–270. doi: 10.1016/j.neuron.2017.03.039

Faucherre, A., Kissa, K., Nargeot, J., Mangoni, M. E., and Jopling, C. (2014). Piezo1 plays a role in erythrocyte volume homeostasis. *Haematologica* 99, 70–75. doi: 10.3324/haematol.2013.086090

Fotiou, E., Martin-Almedina, S., Simpson, M. A., Lin, S., Gordon, K., Brice, G., et al. (2015). Novel mutations in PIEZO1 cause an autosomal recessive generalized lymphatic dysplasia with non-immune hydrops fetalis. *Nat. Commun.* 6:8085. doi: 10.1038/ncomms9085

Ge, J., Li, W., Zhao, Q., Li, N., Chen, M., Zhi, P., et al. (2015). Architecture of the mammalian mechanosensitive Piezo1 channel. *Nature* 527, 64–69. doi: 10.1038/nature15247

Gnanasambandam, R., Bae, C., Gottlieb, P. A., and Sachs, F. (2015). Ionic Selectivity and Permeation Properties of Human PIEZO1 Channels. *PLoS One* 8:e0125503. doi: 10.1371/journal.pone.0125503

Gudipaty, S. A., Lindblom, J., Loftus, P. D., Redd, M. J., Edes, K., Davey, C. F., et al. (2017). Mechanical stretch triggers rapid epithelial cell division through Piezo1. *Nature* 543, 118–121. doi: 10.1038/nature21407

Hyman, A. J., Tumova, S., and Beech, D. J. (2017). Piezo1 channels in vascular development and the sensing of shear stress. *Curr. Top Membr.* 2017, 37–57. doi: 10.1016/bs.ctm.2016.11.001

Imashuku, S., Muramatsu, H., Sugihara, T., Okuno, Y., Wang, X., Yoshida, K., et al. (2016). PIEZO1 gene mutation in a Japanese family with hereditary high phosphatidylcholine hemolytic anemia and hemochromatosis-induced diabetes mellitus. *Int. J. Hematol.* 104, 125–129. doi: 10.1007/s12185-016-1970-x

Kim, S. E., Coste, B., Chadha, A., Cook, B., and Patapoutian, A. (2012). The role of *Drosophila* piezo in mechanical nociception. *Nature* 483, 209–212. doi: 10.1038/nature10801

Lacroix, J. J., Botello-Smith, W. M., and Luo, Y. (2018). Probing the gating mechanism of the mechanosensitive channel Piezo1 with the small molecule yoda1. *Nat. Commun.* 9:2029. doi: 10.1038/s41467-018-04405-3

Li, J., Hou, B., Tumova, S., Muraki, K., Bruns, A., Ludlow, M. J., et al. (2014). Piezo1 integration of vascular architecture with physiological force. *Nature* 515, 279–283. doi: 10.1038/nature13701

Lukacs, V., Mathur, J., Mao, R., Bayrak-Toydemir, P., Procter, M., Cahalan, S. M., et al. (2015). Impaired PIEZO1 function in patients with a novel autosomal recessive congenital lymphatic dysplasia. *Nat. Commun.* 6:8329. doi: 10.1038/ncomms9329

Lupski, J. R. (2012). Digenic inheritance and mendelian disease. *Nat. Genet.* 44, 1291–1292. doi: 10.1038/ng.2479

Martin-Almedina, S., Mansour, S., and Ostergaard, P. (2018). Human phenotypes caused by piezo1 mutations one gene, two overlapping phenotypes? *J. Physiol.* 596, 985–992. doi: 10.1113/JP275718

Martins, J. R., Penton, D., Peyronnet, R., Arhatte, M., Moro, C., Picard, N., et al. (2016). Piezo1-dependent regulation of urinary osmolarity. *Pflugers Arch.* 468, 1197–1206. doi: 10.1007/s00424-016-1811-z

Ranade, S. S., Qiu, Z., Woo, S.-H., Hur, S. S., Murthy, S. E., Cahalan, S. M., et al. (2014). Piezo1, a mechanically activated ion channel, is required for vascular development in mice. *Proc. Natl. Acad. Sci. U.S.A.* 111, 10347–10352. doi: 10.1073/pnas.1409233111

Sandberg, M. B., Nybo, M., Birgens, H., and Frederiksen, H. (2014). Hereditary xerocytosis and familial haemolysis due to mutation in the piezo1 gene: a simple diagnostic approach. *Int. Jnl. Lab Hematol.* 36, e62–e65. doi: 10.1111/ijlh.12172

Shmukler, B. E., Huston, N. C., Thon, J. N., Ni, C. W., Kourkoulis, G., Lawson, N. D., et al. (2015). Homozygous knockout of the piezo1 gene in the zebrafish is not associated with anemia. *Haematologica* 100, e483–e485. doi: 10.3324/haematol.2015.132449

Shmukler, B. E., Lawson, N. D., Paw, B. H., and Alper, S. L. (2016). Authors response to "comment on: homozygous knockout of the piezo1 gene in the zebrafish is not associated with anemia". *Haematologica* 101:e39. doi: 10.3324/haematol.2015.137810

Shmukler, B. E., Vandorpe, D. H., Rivera, A., Auerbach, M., Brugnara, C., and Alper, S. L. (2014). Dehydrated stomatocytic anemia due to the heterozygous mutation R2456H in the mechanosensitive cation channel PIEZO1: a case report. *Blood Cells Mol. Dis.* 52, 53–54. doi: 10.1016/j.bcmd.2013.07.015

Vayá, A., Simó, M., Santaolaria, M., Todolí, J., and Aznar, J. (2005). Red blood cell deformability in iron deficiency anaemia. *Clin. Hemorheol. Microcirc.* 33, 75–80.

Wang, S., Chennupati, R., Kaur, H., Iring, A., Wettschureck, N., and Offermanns, S. (2016). Endothelial cation channel PIEZO1 controls blood pressure by mediating flow-induced ATP release. *J. Clin. Invest.* 126, 4527–4536. doi: 10.1172/JCI87343

Zarychanski, R., Schulz, V. P., Houston, B. L., Maksimova, Y., Houston, D. S., Smith, B., et al. (2012). Mutations in the mechanotransduction protein piezo1 are associated with hereditary xerocytosis. *Blood* 120, 1908–1915. doi: 10.1182/blood-2012-04-422253

12

Red Blood Cell Membrane Conductance in Hereditary Haemolytic Anaemias

Polina Petkova-Kirova[1], Laura Hertz[2,3], Jens Danielczok[2], Rick Huisjes[4], Asya Makhro[5], Anna Bogdanova[5], Maria del Mar Mañú-Pereira[6], Joan-Lluis Vives Corrons[7], Richard van Wijk[4] and Lars Kaestner[2,3]*

[1] Institute of Molecular Cell Biology, Saarland University, Homburg, Germany, [2] Theoretical Medicine and Biosciences, Saarland University, Homburg, Germany, [3] Experimental Physics, Saarland University, Saarbrücken, Germany, [4] Department of Clinical Chemistry & Haematology, University Medical Center Utrecht, Utrecht, Netherlands, [5] Red Blood Cell Research Group, Institute of Veterinary Physiology, Vetsuisse Faculty, Zurich Center for Integrative Human Physiology (ZIHP), University of Zürich, Zurich, Switzerland, [6] Vall d'Hebron Research Institute, Vall d'Hebron University Hospital, Barcelona, Spain, [7] Red Blood Cell Defects and Hematopoietic Disorders Unit, Josep Carreras Leukaemia Research Institute, Barcelona, Spain

*Correspondence:
Lars Kaestner
lars_kaestner@me.com

Congenital haemolytic anaemias are inherited disorders caused by red blood cell membrane and cytoskeletal protein defects, deviant hemoglobin synthesis and metabolic enzyme deficiencies. In many cases, although the causing mutation might be known, the pathophysiology and the connection between the particular mutation and the symptoms of the disease are not completely understood. Thus effective treatment is lagging behind. As in many cases abnormal red blood cell cation content and cation leaks go along with the disease, by direct electrophysiological measurements of the general conductance of red blood cells, we aimed to assess if changes in the membrane conductance could be a possible cause. We recorded whole-cell currents from 29 patients with different types of congenital haemolytic anaemias: 14 with hereditary spherocytosis due to mutations in α-spectrin, β-spectrin, ankyrin and band 3 protein; 6 patients with hereditary xerocytosis due to mutations in Piezo1; 6 patients with enzymatic disorders (3 patients with glucose-6-phosphate dehydrogenase deficiency, 1 patient with pyruvate kinase deficiency, 1 patient with glutamate-cysteine ligase deficiency and 1 patient with glutathione reductase deficiency), 1 patient with β-thalassemia and 2 patients, carriers of several mutations and a complex genotype. While the patients with β-thalassemia and metabolic enzyme deficiencies showed no changes in their membrane conductance, the patients with hereditary spherocytosis and hereditary xerocytosis showed largely variable results depending on the underlying mutation.

Keywords: haemolytic anemia, patch-clamp, electrophysiology, hereditary spherocytosis, hereditary xerocytosis

INTRODUCTION

Haemolytic anaemias, characterized by the abnormal breakdown of red blood cells (RBCs), could be either acquired or inherited. The latter are a diverse group of diseases that could be classified based on the affected RBC component into membranopathies, haemoglobinopathies, and enzymopathies (Dhaliwal et al., 2004). Membranopathies are presented by hereditary spherocytosis (HS), hereditary elliptocytosis (HE) and its aggravated form pyropoikilocytosis (HPP) with defective structural membrane and cytoskeletal proteins (Iolascon et al., 2003) and by the largely heterogeneous group of stomatocytosis divided in a most general way, but not exhaustively, into overhydrated stomatocytosis (OHSt), cryohydrocytosis (CHC) and some types of familial pseudohyperkalaemia (FP) (overhydrated RBCs) and dehydrated stomatocytosis (DHSt) (hereditary xerocytosis (HX)) (dehydrated RBCs) with defective ion channels or transporters (Iolascon et al., 2003; Bruce et al., 2009). Haemoglobinopathies are presented by β-thalassemia (Cao and Galanello, 2010) and sickle cell disease (Ware et al., 2017) with defective hemoglobin and enzymopathies are presented most commonly by glucose-6-phosphate dehydrogenase deficiency (G6PD) (Luzzatto et al., 2016) and pyruvate kinase deficiency (PKD) (Zanella et al., 2005) but also by glutamate-cysteine ligase (γ-glutamylcysteine synthetase) (GCL) deficiency (Ristoff and Larsson, 1998) and glutathione reductase deficiency (van Zwieten et al., 2014). Although much is known so far, especially regarding the defective genes related to hereditary haemolytic anaemias, there are still questions, whose answers would lead to a much better understanding of the disease and possibly to a more effective treatment. A recurrent issue is if a changed membrane conductance, resulting from primary mutated channels or secondary adapted ones, does contribute to the various phenotypes. Most of the research has been done on membranopathies, understandable, primarily on the ones linked to mutations in ion channels or transporters such as band 3 protein, Rh-associated glycoprotein (RhAG), the glucose transporter GLUT1, Piezo1 and the Gardos channel (KCNN4) and accompanied by abnormal RBC cation content and disrupted volume homeostasis (Badens and Guizouarn, 2016). However, although on most occasions, the RBC cation content linked to the particular mutation has been extensively described (e.g., Stewart et al., 2011 for R730C in band 3 protein or Fermo et al., 2017 for R352H in the Gardos channel) and the defective channels, when known, expressed and studied in heterologous systems (e.g., Glogowska et al., 2017 for a number of Piezo1 mutations) with a few exceptions (Stewart et al., 2011; Andolfo et al., 2013; Shmukler et al., 2014; Fermo et al., 2017; Rotordam et al., 2018), direct electrophysiological measurements of membrane conductance in mutated RBCs have been scarce.

Thus, within the CoMMiTMenT project, by direct RBCs electrophysiological measurements in physiological solutions, we aimed to investigate whether RBC membrane conductance changes are accompanying HS due to mutations in the SPTA1 gene (coding for α-spectrin), SPTB (β-spectrin), ANK1 (ankyrin), and SLC4A1 (band 3 protein); HX due to mutations in PIEZO1; enzymatic disorders due to glucose-6-phosphate dehydrogenase

deficiency (G6PD), pyruvate kinase deficiency (PKD), glutamate-cysteine ligase (γ-glutamylcysteine synthetase) (GCL) deficiency, glutathione reductase deficiency and β-thalassemia.

MATERIALS AND METHODS

Patients

Patients diagnosed with different types of haemolytic anemia were enrolled in the study after signing an informed consent. Patients' data were handled anonymously as outlined in the ethics agreements. These agreements were approved by the Medical Ethical Research Board (MERB) of the University Medical Center Utrecht, the Netherlands (UMCU) under reference code 15/426M "Disturbed ion homeostasis in hereditary hemolytic anemia" and by the Ethical Committee of Clinical Investigations of Hospital Clinic, Spain (IDIBAPS) under reference code 2013/8436. Exclusion criteria were erythrocyte transfusion in the past 90 days, age below 3 years and/or bodyweight lower than 18 kg. Blood from healthy control donors was anonymously obtained using the approved medical ethical protocol of 07/125 Mini Donor Dienst, also approved by the MERB of UMCU. The blood of the patient/patients and the healthy donor anti-coagulated in heparin was shipped overnight from the University Medical Center Utrecht (Utrecht, Netherlands) or from Institut d'Investigacions Biomèdiques August Pi i Sunyer/Hospital Clínic de Barcelona (Barcelona, Spain) to Saarland University (Homburg, Germany) without additional cooling as previously tested/simulated (Makhro et al., 2016). All patients included in the study were genetically screened for mutations by next-generation sequencing and diagnosed with the following types of anemia: 14 patients were diagnosed with HS (due to mutations in α-spectrin, β-spectrin, ankyrin and band 3 protein), using golden standard techniques (EMA-binding, osmotic gradient ektacytometry and osmotic fragility test), 6 patients were diagnosed with hereditary xerocytosis (due to mutations in Piezo 1), 6 patients had enzymatic disorders (3 patients with glucose-6-phosphate dehydrogenase deficiency, 1 patient with pyruvate kinase deficiency, 1 patient with glutamate-cysteine ligase deficiency and 1 patient with glutathione reductase deficiency), 1 patient had β-thalassemia and 2 were carriers of several mutations and a complex genotype. The genotype of the patients with HS, HX and of the two patients with several mutations is given in **Table 1**. The numbering of the patients and the corresponding healthy controls is kept consistent with previous research (Hertz et al., 2017) studying the same patient group.

Patch Clamp Analysis

Patch-clamp whole-cell measurements were performed with a NPC-16 Patchliner (Nanion Technologies, Munich, Germany) as previously described (Petkova-Kirova et al., 2018). Briefly, the resistance of the chips was between 5 and 8 MΩ with internal and external solutions as follows (in mM): KCl 70, KF 70, NaCl 10, HEPES 10, EGTA 3, CaCl$_2$ 1.2 to give free $[Ca^{2+}]_i$ = 120 nM, pH = 7.2 adjusted with KOH (internal) and NaCl 140, KCl 4, MgCl$_2$ 5, CaCl$_2$ 2, D-glucose 5, HEPES 10, pH = 7.3 adjusted

TABLE 1 | Patients overview.

Patient	Clinical presentation	Genotype	Current compared to transportation control	Current compared to general control
P18.1	**HS (α-spectrin)**	**c.2755G > T (p.Glu919); α^{LELY}**	**Current ↑**	**Current ↑**
P19.1	**HS (α-spectrin)**	**c.678G > A (p.Glu227fs); α^{LELY}**	**Current ↑ (not statistically significant)**	**Current ↑**
P15.1	HS (α-spectrin)	c.4339-99C > T p.(?)	No change	No change
P20.1	HS (α-spectrin)	c.[4339-99C > T; c.4347G > T] p.[(?; Lys1449Asn)]	No change	No change
P17.1 (splenectomized)	HS (ankyrin)	c.341C > T (p.Pro114Leu)	Current ↓ *	No change
P17.2	HS (ankyrin)	c.341C > T (p.Pro114Leu)	Current ↓ *	No change
P11.1	HS (ankyrin)	c.1943delC;c.2042delC (p.Ala648fs;p.Ala681fs)	No change	No change
P13.1	HS (ankyrin)	c.344T > C (p.Leu115Pro)	No change	No change
P13.2	HS (ankyrin)	c.344T > C (p.Leu115Pro)	No change	No change
P14.1	HS (ankyrin)	c.2559-2A > G (splicing)	No change	No change
P10.1	HS (β-spectrin)	c.2470C > T (p.Gln824)	Outward current ↓↓ *	No change
P21.1	HS (β-spectrin)	c.3449G > A (p.Trp1150)	No change	No change
P12.1	HS (band 3 protein)	c.2348T > A (p.Ile783Asn)	Current ↓	Inward current ↓
P16.1	HS (band 3 protein)	c.2057 + 1G > A (splicing)	No change	No change
P11.1	**SPTB**	**c.154delC; p.Arg52fs + RHAG c.808G > A; p.Val270Ile**	**Current ↑**	**Current ↑**
P22.1	**SPTA1**	**c.460_462dupTTG; p.Leu154dup + PKLR c.1687G > A; p.Gly563Ser + del3.7Kb HBA**	**Current ↑**	**Current ↑**
Family 1				
P51.3	HX	c. 7367G > A p.Arg2456His	No change	No change
P51.4	HX	c. 7367G > A p.Arg2456His	No change	No change
Family 2				
P53.3	HX	c. 6262C > G, p. Arg2088Gly	No change	No change
P53.2	HX	c. 6262C > G, p. Arg2088Gly	No change	No change
Family 3				
P50.2	HX	c.1276T > C p. Cys426Arg	No change	Outward current ↑ *
Family 4				
P52.1	**HX**	**c.7483_7488dupCTGGAG p.2495_2496dupLeuGlu**	**Current ↓**	**Current ↓**
P40.1	G6PD		No change	No change
P41.1	G6PD		No change	No change
P42.1	G6PD		No change	No change
P43.1	GCLD		No change	No change
P44.1	GRD		No change	No change
P45.1	PKD		No change	No change
P60.1	β-thalassemia		No change	No change

An upward arrow indicates an increase in current and a downward arrow indicates a decrease in current compared to the respective control. Two arrows label an extreme change in the designated direction. Patients that show a change in current compared to both the transportation and a general control are given in bold. Asterisks mark a deviation commented on in the main text. HS, hereditary spherocytosis; SPTB, β-spectrin; SPTA1, α-spectrin; HX, hereditary xerocytosis; GCLD, glutamate-cysteine ligase deficiency; GRD, glutathione reductase deficiency; PKD, pyruvate kinase deficiency.

with NaOH (external). Gigaseals were considered successful if exceeding 5 GΩ. Gigaseal formation was facilitated by the use of a seal enhancing solution as recommended by the Patchliner manufacturer and containing (in mM): NaCl 80, KCl 3, MgCl$_2$ 10, CaCl$_2$ 35, HEPES 10, pH = 7.3 adjusted with NaOH. Whole-cell configuration was achieved by negative pressure suction pulses between −45 mbar and −150 mbar and its formation judged by the appearance of sharp capacitive transients. Whole-cell patch-clamp recordings were conducted at room temperature using voltage steps from −100 to 100 mV for 500 ms in 20 mV increments at 5 s intervals, the holding potential being set at −30 mV. Data are presented as current density (current divided by capacitance, the latter estimated at the time of attaining the whole-cell configuration and by using a short test pulse of 10 mV, 5 ms) and given as means ± SEMs (n denotes number of cells and N – number of patients). Significant differences are determined based on an unpaired t-test and Welch's correction for unequal variances, when needed, with * denoting $p < 0.05$.

RESULTS

Whole-cell patch clamp measurements were performed to assess possible differences in the membrane conductance of hereditary anemia patients compared to healthy controls. Regarding controls, we have compared the currents measured from the RBCs of our patients once with their transportation control, i.e., currents measured from the RBCs of a healthy subject, whose blood was delivered together with the blood of the patient, and once with a general, pooled, control, i.e., currents measured from the cells of all healthy subjects delivered throughout the study (**Table 1**). The rational for this 'double comparison' is provided in the discussion. Throughout the whole study, accordingly in the manuscript, the abbreviation "P" stands for patient and "C" stands for a control, healthy subject.

Hereditary Spherocytosis

Studied were patients with pathogenic mutations in *SPTA1* (α-spectrin) (4 patients: P15.1, P18.1, P19.1, P20.1), *SPTB* (β-spectrin) (2 patients: P10.1 and P21.1), *ANK1* (ankyrin) (6 patients: P11.1, P13.1, P13.2, P14.1, P17.1, and P17.2), and *SLC4A1* (band 3 protein) (2 patients: P12.1 and P16.1), whose blood was delivered and, respectively, recorded from together with the blood of a healthy subject (transportation control). While no changes in the membrane conductance, nor in membrane capacitance (0.69 pA/pF general control vs. 0.63 pA/pF patients, $p > 0.05$; 0.65 pA/pF transportation control vs. 0.63 pA/pF patients; $p > 0.05$) were revealed with patients taken altogether (**Figure 1**), differences were observed in certain patients' groups as well as linked to particular mutations **Figures 3–5**). Thus patients with mutations in SPTA1 (4 patients), showed no significant differences compared to healthy controls delivered at the same days (4 healthy subjects) (**Figure 2A**) or compared to a control pooled over all healthy subjects included in the study (27 healthy subjects) (**Figure 2B**). Capacitances were not different either (0.67 pA/pF patients vs. 0.68 pA/pF transportation control, $p > 0.05$; 0.67 pA/pF patients

vs. 0.69 pA/pF general control; $p > 0.05$). However, the two patients, heterozygous for the *SPTA1* mutation and carrying at the same time an α^{LELY} allele showed an increase in their inward current (**Figure 3**). **Figures 3Aa,Ba** consider the particular *SPTA1* α^{LELY} patients [patient P18.1 (10 cells) and patient P19.1 (6 cells), respectively] vs. their transportation controls [C18 (6 cells) and C19 (7 cells), respectively]. **Figures 3Ab,Bb** compare the particular *SPTA1* α^{LELY} patients [P18.1 (10 cells) and P19.1 (6 cells) vs. a control pooled over all the cells of all healthy subjects included in the study (175 cells)]. **Figures 3Ac,Ad,Bc,Bd** present raw current traces recorded from the RBCs of a healthy subject (**Figures Ac,Bc**), P18.1 (**Figure 3Ad**), and P19.1 (**Figure 3Bd**). None of the two patients showed any difference in capacitance compared with the general or with its transportation control (0.59 pA/pF P18.1 vs. 0.74 pA/pF C18, $p > 0.05$; 0.59 pA/pF P18.1 vs. 0.69 pA/pF general control, $p > 0.05$; 0.66 pA/pF P19.1 vs. 0.58 pA/pF C19, $p > 0.05$; 0.66 pA/pF P19.1 vs. 0.69 pA/pF general control, $p > 0.05$). Furthermore, while HS patients with underlying defects in *ANK1* (6 patients) showed no significant differences neither in their currents, nor in their capacitances (0.67 pA/pF patients vs. 0.63 pA/pF transportation control, $p > 0.05$; 0.67 pA/pF patients vs. 0.69 pA/pF general control; $p > 0.05$) compared to the control group [**Figure 4Aa** considered are the control healthy subjects delivered together with the patients (4 healthy subjects) and **Figure 4Ab** considered are all healthy subjects included in the study (27 healthy subjects)], there was a family of patients P17.1 (splenectomized) and P17.2 (with spleen) in whom an *ANK1* mutation [c.341C > T (p.Pro114Leu)] was associated with a decreased membrane conductance when compared to their own controls (**Figures 4Ba,Ca**, respectively) but not when compared to the pooled control of all healthy cells (**Figures 4Bb,Cb**, respectively). Comparison of the capacitances of P17.1 and P17.2 with their controls as well as the capacitance of C17 with the general control is as follows: 0.67 pA/pF P17.1 vs. 0.525 pA/pF C17, $p > 0.05$; 0.67 pA/pF P17.1 vs. 0.69 pA/pF general control, $p > 0.05$; 0.62 pA/pF P17.2 vs. 0.525 pA/pF C17, $p > 0.05$; 0.62 pA/pF P17.2 vs. 0.69 pA/pF general control,

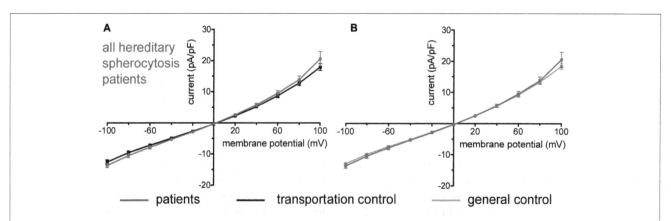

FIGURE 1 | Whole-cell recordings of ion currents from RBCs of healthy donors and HS patients. Compared are the I/V-curves of all HS patients (N = 14) with the I/V curves of their transportation controls (N = 12) **(A)** and with the I/V curves of all healthy subjects delivered throughout the study (N = 27) **(B)**, where N denotes number of healthy subjects or HS patients. No changes were observed in capacitance either with the transportation (0.63 pA/pF patients vs. 0.65 pA/pF transportation control; $p > 0.05$) or with the general control (0.63 pA/pF patients vs. 0.69 pA/pF general control; $p > 0.05$). Currents were elicited by voltage steps from −100 to 100 mV for 500 ms in 20 mV increments at V_h = −30 mV. Data are expressed as mean current density ± SEMs.

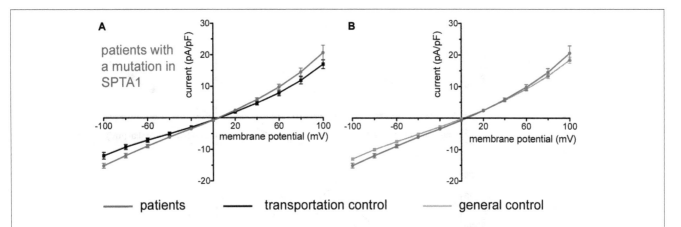

FIGURE 2 | Whole-cell recordings of ion currents from RBCs of healthy donors and HS patients with α-spectrin mutations. Compared are the I/V-curves of all HS patients with α-spectrin mutations ($N = 4$) with the I/V curves of their own transportation controls ($N = 4$) **(A)** and with the I/V curves of all healthy subjects delivered throughout the study ($N = 27$) **(B)**, where N denotes the number of healthy subjects or HS patients. No changes were observed in capacitance either with the transportation (0.67 pA/pF patients vs. 0.68 pA/pF control; $p > 0.05$) or with the general control (0.67 pA/pF patients vs. 0.69 pA/pF control; $p > 0.05$). Currents were elicited by voltage steps from –100 to 100 mV for 500 ms in 20 mV increments at $V_h = -30$ mV. Data are expressed as mean current density ± SEMs.

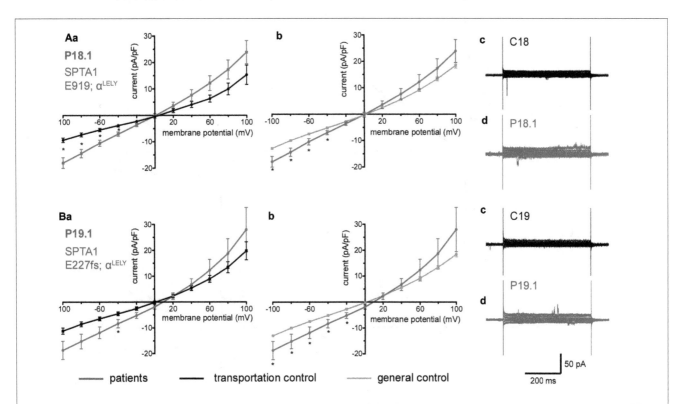

FIGURE 3 | Whole-cell recordings of ion currents from RBCs of healthy donors and HS patients with α-spectrin mutations and carrying at the same time an α^{LELY} allele. Compared are the I/V curves of P18.1 ($n = 10$) with its own transportation control C18 ($n = 6$) **(Aa)** as well as with a general control ($n = 175$) **(Ab)**, where n denotes the number of cells from the patient or the controls. As examples raw current traces recorded from the RBCs of a healthy donor (C18), whose blood was delivered together with the blood of P18.1 **(Ac)** and of patient P18.1 **(Ad)** are presented. Capacitances were not any different either with the transportation control (0.59 pA/pF P18.1 vs. 0.74 pA/pF C18; $p > 0.05$) or with the general control (0.59 pA/pF patient vs. 0.69 pA/pF control; $p > 0.05$). Compared are the I/V curves of P19.1 ($n = 6$) with its own transportation control C19 ($n = 7$) **(Ba)** as well as with a general control ($n = 175$) **(Bb)**, where n denotes the number of cells from the patient or the controls. As examples raw current traces recorded from the RBCs of a healthy donor (C19), whose blood was delivered together with the blood of P19.1 **(Bc)** and of patient P19.1 **(Bd)** are presented. Capacitances were not any different either with the transportation control (0.66 pA/pF P19.1 vs. 0.58 pA/pF C19; $p > 0.05$) or with the general control (0.66 pA/pF patient vs. 0.69 pA/pF general control; $p > 0.05$). Significant differences are determined based on an unpaired t-test with * representing $p < 0.05$. Mutations below patients numbers are designated as amino acid substitutions in the respective protein. The label α^{LELY} next to the mutation stands for the presence of an α^{LELY} allele in the corresponding patient.

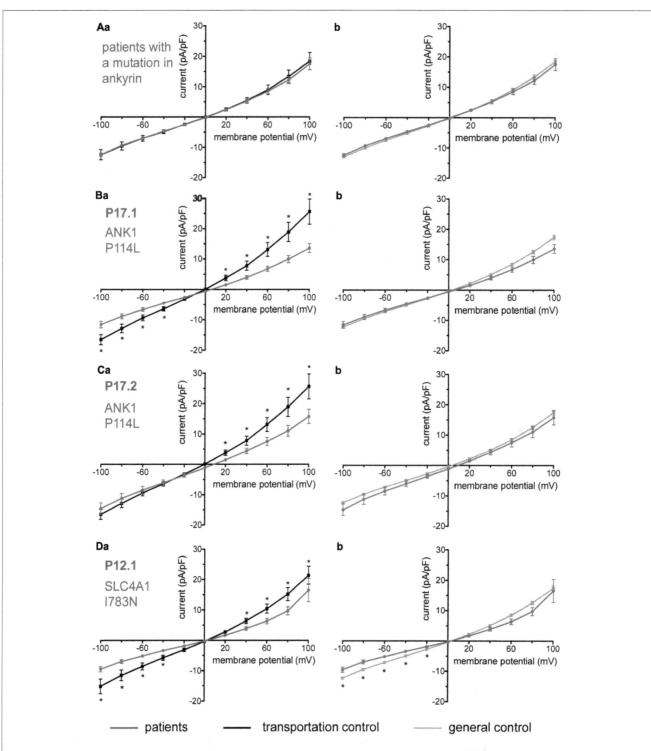

FIGURE 4 | Whole-cell recordings of ion currents from RBCs of healthy donors and HS patients. Whole-cell recordings of ion currents from RBCs of healthy donors and HS patients with ankyrin mutations **(A–C)**. Compared are the I/V-curves of all HS patients with ankyrin mutations (N = 6) with the I/V curves of their own transportation controls (N = 4) **(Aa)** and with the I/V curves of all healthy subjects delivered throughout the study (N = 27) **(Ab)**, where N denotes the number of healthy subjects or HS patients. No changes were observed in capacitance either with the transportation (0.67 pA/pF patients vs. 0.63 pA/pF transportation control; p > 0.05) or with the general control (0.67 pA/pF patients vs. 0.69 pA/pF general control; p > 0.05). Compared are the I/V curves of P17.1 (n = 13) and its own transportation control C17 (n = 6) **(Ba)** and the I/V curves of P17.2 (n = 11) with its own transportation control C17 (n = 6) **(Ca)**, where n denotes the number of cells from the patient or the control. **(Bb,Cb)** Compare the I/V curve of a general control based on currents recorded from all cells of all healthy subjects delivered throughout the study (n = 175) with the I/V curve of P17.1 (n = 13) **(Bb)** and P17.2 (n = 11) **(Cb)** (n denotes number of cells).

(Continued)

FIGURE 4 | Continued

Both patients 17.1 and 17.2 showed no differences in capacitance either with their transportation or with the general control (0.67 pA/pF P17.1 vs. 0.525 pA/pF C17, $p > 0.05$; 0.67 pA/pF P17.1 vs. 0.69 pA/pF general control, $p > 0.05$; 0.62 pA/pF P17.2 vs. 0.525 pA/pF C17, $p > 0.05$; 0.62 pA/pF P17.2 vs. 0.69 pA/pF general control, $p > 0.05$). However, a difference was uncovered between C17 and the general control (0.525 pA/pF C17 vs. 0.69 pA/pF general control; $p < 0.05$). Whole-cell recordings of ion currents from RBCs of a healthy donor and a HS patient with band 3 protein mutation **(D)**. Compared are the I/V curves of P12.1 ($n = 17$) with its own transportation control C12 ($n = 7$) **(Da)** as well as with a general control ($n = 175$) **(Db)**, where n is the number of cells of the patient or the controls. No changes were observed in capacitance either with the transportation (0.65 pA/pF P12.1 vs. 0.59 pA/pF C12; $p > 0.05$) or with the general control (0.65 pA/pF P12.1 vs. 0.69 pA/pF general control; $p > 0.05$). Currents were elicited by voltage steps from -100 to 100 mV for 500 ms in 20 mV increments at $V_h = -30$ mV. Data expressed as mean current density $\pm$ SEMs. Significant differences are determined based on an unpaired t-test with * representing $p < 0.05$. Mutations below patients numbers are designated as amino acid substitutions in the respective protein.

$p > 0.05$; 0.525 pA/pF C17 vs. 0.69 pA/pF general control; $p < 0.05$. Moreover a patient with a band 3 protein mutation [SLC4A1 (2348T > A, Ile783Asn), P12.1 showed a decreased current compared to its own, transportation, control (C12) and to a pooled general control (**Figures 4Da,b**, respectively)]. No difference was found when the capacitance of the patient was compared with that of the general or the transportation control (0.65 pA/pF P12.1 vs. 0.59 pA/pF C12, $p > 0.05$; 0.65 pA/pF P12.1 vs. 0.69 pA/pF general control, $p > 0.05$). Out of the two patients with SPTB mutations (P10.1 and P21.1) (**Figures 5A,Ba,b**) one patient, P10.1, showed a significantly different conductance compared to its transportation control C10 (**Figure 5Ba**). However, based on the fact that P10.1 showed no difference with the general control (**Figure 5Bb**) and that P21.1 showed no difference either with its transportation control (**Figure 5Aa**) or with the general control (**Figure 5Ab**) as well as on the fact that C10 is very different from the general, pooled control (an outlier according to the Grubbs' test) (**Figure 5Bc**), we conclude that patients with β-spectrin mutations show no changes in their current. Comparison of capacitances of P21.1 and P10.1 with their controls as well as the capacitance of C10 with the general control is as follows: 0.63 pA/pF P21.1 vs. 0.69 pA/pF C21, $p > 0.05$; 0.63 pA/pF P21.1 vs. 0.69 pA/pF general control, $p > 0.05$; 0.68 pA/pF P10.1 vs. 0.82 pA/pF C10, $p < 0.05$; 0.68 pA/pF P10.1 vs. 0.69 pA/pF general control, $p > 0.05$; 0.82 pA/pF C10 vs. 0.69 pA/pF general control; $p < 0.05$. C10 shows a significantly increased capacitance compared to P10.1 as well as to the general control.

Two additional patients P11.1 and P22.1, carriers of several mutations and a complex genotype (*SPTB* c.154delC; p.Arg52fs + *RHAG* c.808G > A; p.Val270Ile and *SPTA1* c.460_462dupTTG; p.Leu154dup + *PKLR* c.1687G > A; p.Gly563Ser + del3.7Kb *HBA*, respectively) show an increase in their currents (**Figures 6A,B**, respectively). The capacitances of none of the patients show any difference with their controls (0.59 pA/pF P11.1 vs. 0.66 pA/pF C11, $p > 0.05$; 0.59 pA/pF P11.1 vs. 0.69 pA/pF general control, $p > 0.05$; 0.61 pA/pF P22.1 vs. 0.64 pA/pF C22, $p > 0.05$; 0.61 pA/pF P22.1 vs. 0.69 pA/pF general control, $p > 0.05$).

Hereditary Xerocytosis

Considered were 4 families with mutations in the PIEZO1 gene (Family 1 with patients P51.3 and P51.4; Family 2 with P53.2 and P53.3; Family 3 with P50.2 and Family 4 with P52.1), whose blood was delivered and recorded from, together with the blood of a healthy subject (transportation control) (C51,

C53, C50, and C52, respectively). No changes in the membrane conductance or in the membrane capacitance were revealed with patients taken altogether (**Figure 7A**) as well as in two families (Family1 (P51.3 and P51.4) and Family 2 (P53.2 and P53.3) compared both to their transportation controls and to a general control (**Figures 7Ba,b,Ca,b**, respectively). However, P50.2 (Family 3), although showing no difference with its transportation control (**Figure 8Aa**), demonstrated increased conductance compared to the general, pooled, control (**Figure 8Ab**). There was also a family (Family 4 with P52.1) in which the Piezo1 mutation (c.7483_7488dupCTGGAG p.2495_2496dupLeuGlu) was associated with a decreased conductance compared both to the transportation and to the general, pooled, control (**Figures 8Ba,b**, respectively). Both Family 3 and Family 4 did not show a change in their capacitance compared to their transportation or to the general control.

Enzymopathies

Considered were 6 patients with enzymatic disorders as follows: 3 patients with glucose-6-phosphate dehydrogenase deficiency (P40.1, P41.1, and P42.1), 1 patient with pyruvate kinase deficiency (P45.1), 1 patient with glutamate-cysteine ligase deficiency (P43.1) and 1 patient with glutathione reductase deficiency (P44.1). None of the patients showed a difference in their membrane conductance or capacitance compared to a general or their own transportation control (**Figures 9, 10**).

Beta-Thalassemia

The patient (P60.1) with β-thalassemia showed no difference in its membrane conductance or membrane capacitance either compared to a general or to its own, transportation, control (**Figure 11**).

DISCUSSION

Hereditary Spherocytosis

Electrophysiological measurements revealed additional new characteristics for HS and confirmed the heterogeneity of the disease showing that changes in membrane conductance are not an overall feature of the disease but depend on the particular, specific mutation (Huisjes et al., unpublished).

Interesting is that out of the many patients with SPTA1 mutations it is the two patients carrying a *SPTA1* α^{LELY}

Diagnosis and Treatment of Anemia

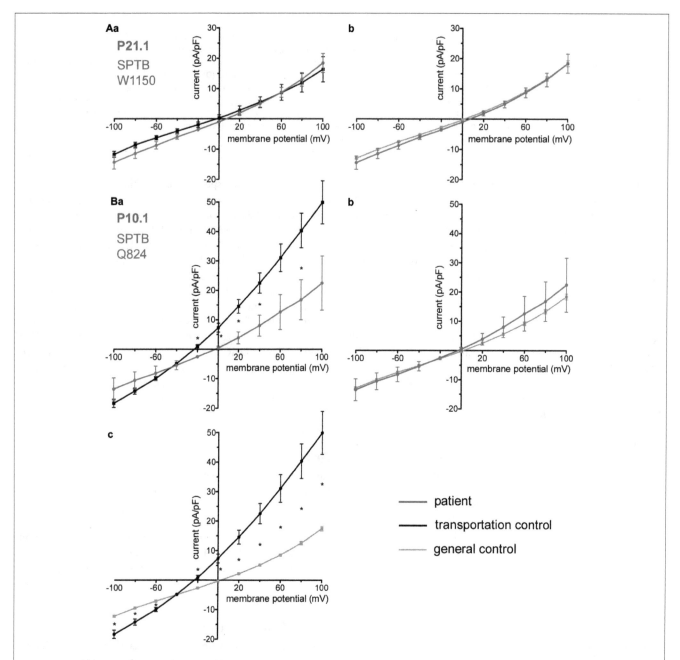

FIGURE 5 | Whole-cell recordings of ion currents from RBCs of healthy donors and HS patients. Whole-cell recordings of ion currents from RBCs of healthy donors and HS patients with β-spectrin mutations **(A,Ba,b)**. Compared are the I/V curves of P21.1 (n = 8) with its own transportation control C21 (n = 5) **(Aa)** as well as with a general control (n = 175) **(Ab)**. Compared are the I/V curves of P10.1 (n = 3) with its own transportation control C10 (n = 6) **(Ba)** as well as with a general control (n = 175) **(Bb)**. **(Bc)** Compares the I/V curve of the transportation control of P10.1, C10 (n = 6) with a general control (n = 175), where n denotes the number of cells. Currents were elicited by voltage steps from −100 to 100 mV for 500 ms in 20 mV increments at V_h = −30 mV. Data are expressed as mean current density ± SEMs. Significant differences are determined based on an unpaired t-test with * representing p < 0.05. Mutations below patients numbers are designated as amino acid substitutions in the respective protein.

allele that show a change in their membrane conductance: an increase in their inward current. This holds true for P18.1 vs. its own transportation control and vs. the general control of 175 cells and also for patient P19.1 vs. the pooled control. Although not reaching statistical significance the inward current of P19.1 compared to its own transportation control is also increased. Evident are the large variations within the cells of the patients for both patient P18.1 and P19.1 but especially for P19.1. This might explain why the difference in the inward current between P19.1 and its transportation control does not reach a statistical significance.

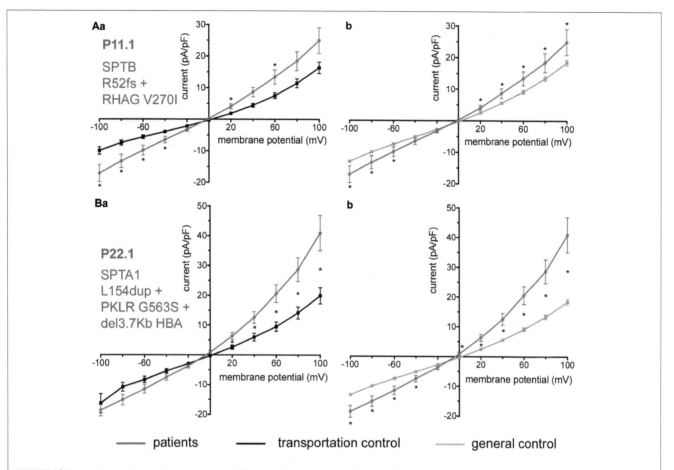

FIGURE 6 | Whole-cell recordings of ion currents from RBCs of healthy donors and patients, carriers of several mutations and a complex genotype. Compared are the I/V curves of P11.1 (*n* = 11) with its own transportation control C11 (*n* = 13) **(Aa)** as well as with a general control (*n* = 175) **(Ab)**. Compared are the I/V curves of P22.1 (*n* = 8) with its own transportation control C22 (*n* = 5) **(Ba)** as well as with a general control (*n* = 175) **(Bb)**, where *n* denotes the number of cells. Currents were elicited by voltage steps from −100 to 100 mV for 500 ms in 20 mV increments at V_h = −30 mV. Data are expressed as mean current density ± SEMs. Significant differences are determined based on an unpaired *t*-test with * representing $p < 0.05$. Mutations below patients numbers are designated as amino acid substitutions in the respective proteins. Additionally to having an α-spectrin mutation P22.1 is PK deficiency carrier as well as an α-thalassemia carrier.

Allele α^{LELY} is a common polymorphic allele and its presence in humans is by itself asymptomatic. The α^{LELY} allele, however, plays the role of an exacerbating factor when it occurs in trans to an α-spectrin mutation resulting in a disastrously weak spectrin network (Viel and Branton, 1996; Iolascon et al., 2003). This is because, due to their reduced ability to form dimers, α chains from α^{LELY} alleles are underrepresented in the mature RBC cytoskeleton. Accordingly underrepresented are any spectrin mutations found on the same allele and in turn overrepresented if found on the opposite allele (Wilmotte et al., 1997). How a destabilized cytoskeleton might have an effect on membrane conductance is a subject of speculations but as the RBC membrane has little structural integrity without the support of an intact and steady protein scaffold below, it might be that conformational changes influence the proper functioning of channels and lead to increased membrane conductance.

Noteworthy, in many cases, aggravating conditions such as an α^{LELY} allele or a superimposed erythrocytic defect lead to an enhanced membrane conductance and a leaky cell. Thus P11.1 with a mutation in β-spectrin as well as a mutation in RHAG and

P22.1 with a mutation in α-spectrin as well as being a pyruvate kinase deficiency and a thalassemia carrier show an increase both in their inward and outward current. While in the case of P22.1 such an increase cannot be straightforwardly explained as neither thalassemia nor pyruvate kinase deficiency alone give any change in conductance, P11.1 is particularly interesting. The Rh-associated glycoprotein (RhAG) coded by the RHAG gene, together with the RhD and RhCcEe proteins, is a major component of the Rh blood group system. It is essential for assembly of the Rh protein complex in the RBC membrane and for expression of the Rh antigens (Avent and Reid, 2000). The exact function of RhAG is not completely understood but it is suggested to be involved in RBC gas exchange as it promotes transmembrane NH_3 transport (additionally NH_4^+) (Bakouh et al., 2006) as well as facilitates CO_2 membrane permeation (Endeward et al., 2008). More interesting is, however, that RhAG can act as a pore for monovalent cations (Na^+, K^+, and Li^+) and RHAG point mutations leading to Ile61Arg and Phe65Ser substitutions result in massively increased permeabilities for K^+ and Na^+ and to overhydrated stomatocytosis (Bruce et al., 2009).

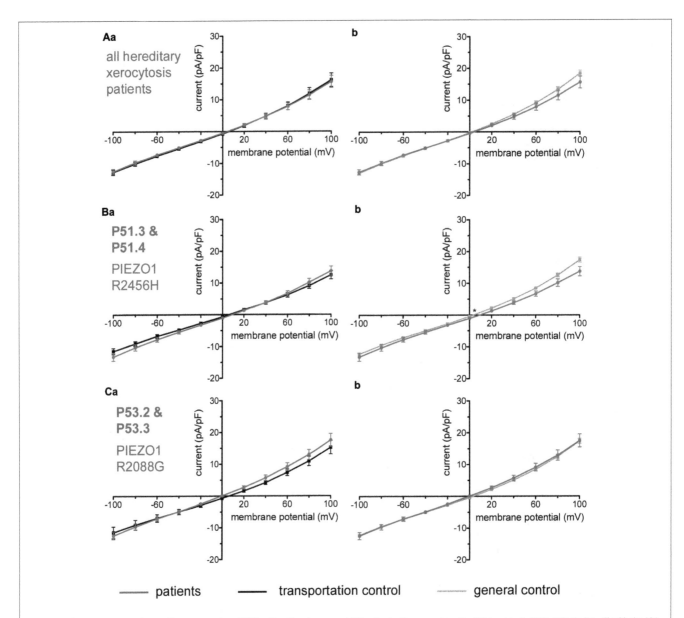

FIGURE 7 | Whole-cell recordings of ion currents from RBCs of healthy donors and HX patients. Compared are the I/V-curves of all HX patients (N = 6) with the I/V curves of their own transportation controls (N = 4) **(Aa)** and with the I/V curves of all healthy subjects delivered throughout the study (N = 27) **(Ab)**, where N denotes the number of healthy subjects or HX patients. No changes were observed in capacitance either with the transportation (0.725 pA/pF patients vs. 0.71 pA/pF transportation control; $p > 0.05$) or with the general control (0.725 pA/pF patients vs. 0.69 pA/pF general control; $p > 0.05$). Compared are the I/V curves of P51.3 and P51.4 pooled together (Family 1) (n = 22) with their own transportation control C51 (n = 7) **(Ba)** and the I/V curves of P53.2 and P53.3 pooled together (Family 2) (n = 27) with their own transportation control C53 (n = 9) **(Ca)**, where n denotes the number of cells from the patients or the controls. **(Bb,Cb)** Compare the I/V curve of a general control based on currents recorded from all cells of all healthy subjects delivered throughout the study (n = 175) with the I/V curve of P51.3 and P51.4 pooled together (n = 22) **(Bb)** and P53.2 and P53.3 pooled together (n = 27) **(Cb)** (n denotes number of cells). P51.3 and P51.4 pooled together (Family 1) and P53.2 and P53.3 pooled together (Family 2) did not show a difference in their capacitance compared to the general or transportation control (0.69 pA/pF P51.3 and P51.4 vs. 0.72 pA/pF C51, $p > 0.05$; 0.69 pA/pF P51.3 and P51.4 vs. 0.69 pA/pF general control, $p > 0.05$; 0.75 pA/pF P53.2 and P53.3 vs. 0.71 pA/pF P53, $p > 0.05$; 0.75 pA/pF P53.2 and P53.3 vs. 0.69 pA/pF general control, $p > 0.05$) Currents were elicited by voltage steps from −100 to 100 mV for 500 ms in 20 mV increments at V_h = −30 mV. Data are expressed as mean current density ± SEMs. Significant differences are determined based on an unpaired t-test with * representing $p < 0.05$. Mutations below patients numbers are designated as amino acid substitutions in the respective protein.

Expression of the mutated RhAGs in xenopus oocytes confirms the large monovalent leaks imposed by the mutations and modeling studies correlate those leaks with possibly widening the pore structures permitting passive diffusion of Na^+ and K^+ (Bruce et al., 2009). Mutation c.808G > A in P11.1 with a substitution Val270Ile residing in the 5th endoloop of RhAG (Huang et al., 1999) although not linked to overhydrated stomatocytosis relates to the Rh^{null} syndrome accordingly characterized by varying degrees of chronic haemolytic anemia and spherostomatocytosis (Nash and Shojania, 1987). Without

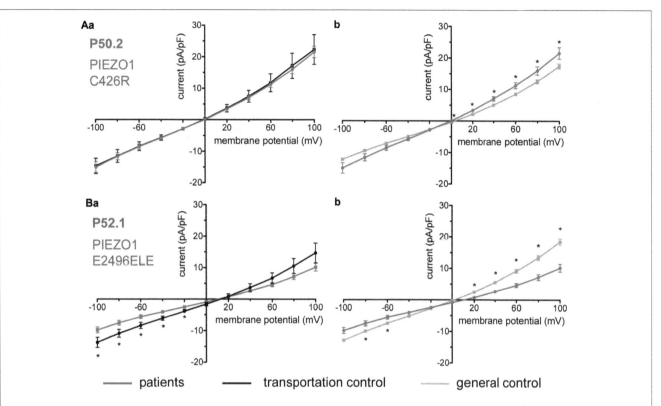

FIGURE 8 | Whole-cell recordings of ion currents from RBCs of healthy donors and HX patients. Compared are the I/V curves of P50.2 ($n = 14$) with its own transportation control C50 ($n = 7$) **(Aa)** as well as with a general control ($n = 175$) **(Ab)**. Comparison of capacitance of P50.2 with control capacitances gave no difference with the general or the transportation control (0.73 pA/pF P50.2 vs. 0.80 pA/pF transportation control; $p > 0.05$; 0.73 pA/pF P50.2 vs. 0.69 pA/pF general control; $p > 0.05$). Compared are the I/V curves of P52.1 ($n = 20$) with its own transportation control C52 ($n = 11$) **(Ba)** as well as with a general control ($n = 175$) **(Bb)**, where n denotes the number of cells. No changes were observed in capacitance either with the transportation (0.75 pA/pF P52.1 vs. 0.62 pA/pF C52; $p > 0.05$) or with the general control (0.75 pA/pF P52.1 vs. 0.69 pA/pF general control; $p > 0.05$). Currents were elicited by voltage steps from −100 to 100 mV for 500 ms in 20 mV increments at V_h = −30 mV. Data are expressed as mean current density ± SEMs. Significant differences are determined based on an unpaired t-test with * representing $p < 0.05$. Mutations below patients numbers are designated as amino acid substitutions in the respective protein.

knowing the mechanism that might relate mutation RHAG c.808G > A (or the complex defect c.808G > A+SPTB c.154delC) to changes in the RBC membrane conductance, P11.1 has been described with having less K^+ in the plasma than its transportation control yet more than a non-transported normal control and a much increased activity of its Na^+/K^+ pump (Huisjes et al., unpublished). Thus, it could well be that a possibly increased K^+ leak underlined by the detected increased membrane conductance triggers compensatory changes, namely enhanced ion pumping that might explain the partially compensated K^+ leak (i.e., that K^+ in the plasma of the patient is less than K^+ in the plasma of its transportation control). This is in line with observations that haemolytic diseases showing increased non-Na^+/K^+ pump and non-NaK2Cl cotransport, K^+ fluxes [ouabain- (an inhibitor of the Na^+/K^+ pump) and bumetanide-(an inhibitor of the NaK2Cl cotransport) resistant K^+ fluxes] are accompanied by increased Na^+/K^+ pump fluxes (ouabain- sensitive fluxes) (Stewart, 2004).

Not always, however, a resulting changed membrane conductance is manifested as an increase in current. A patient (P12.1) with a mutation in band 3 protein shows a decrease in

current and, although counterintuitive, also accompanied by a significant loss of K^+ from the RBC.

The major function of band 3 protein is of an anion transporter exchanging a bicarbonate for a chloride ion across the RBC plasma membrane thus ensuring efficient removal of CO_2 from tissues (Guyton and Hall, 2006). However, data in the literature show that point mutations resulting in single amino acid substitutions cause Na^+ and K^+ leaks with anion transport activity either maintained or abolished depending on the mutation (Bruce et al., 1993, 2005; Salhany et al., 1995; Stewart et al., 2010, 2011). Those mutations causing predominantly stomatocytosis but also spherocytosis (Arakawa et al., 2015) have been suggested to induce monovalent cation leaks in one of 3 possible ways: (i) converting the anion exchanger in a non-selective cation conductor, (ii) inducing cation conductance in a still functioning exchanger and (iii) causing the anion exchanger to stimulate endogenous cation transporters (Badens and Guizouarn, 2016). The latter has been shown in heterologous expression systems (Stewart et al., 2010) as well as in RBCs (H734R) (Bogdanova et al., 2009). It could indeed be that band 3 protein is engaged in complex interactions modulating cation permeability pathways (both

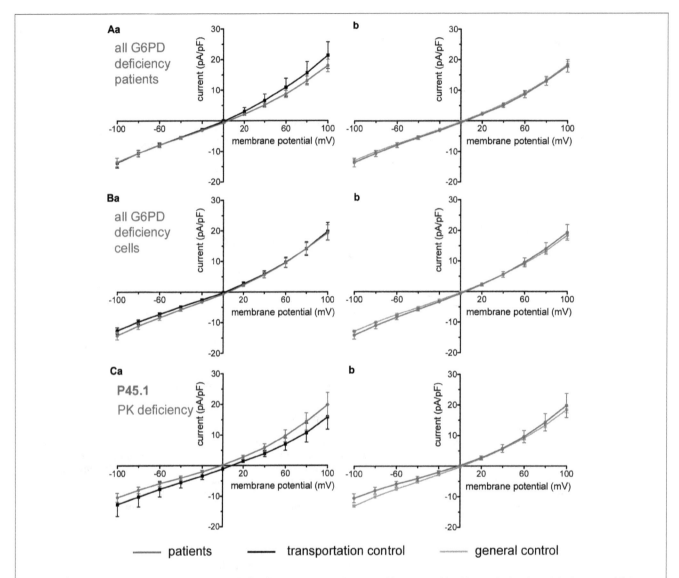

FIGURE 9 | Whole-cell recordings of ion currents from RBCs of healthy donors and patients with enzymopathies (glucose-6-phosphate dehydrogenase deficiency and pyruvate kinase deficiency). Compared are the I/V-curve of all glucose-6-phosphate dehydrogenase deficiency patients (N = 3) with the I/V curve of their own transportation controls (N = 3) **(Aa)** and with the I/V curve of all healthy subjects delivered throughout the study (N = 27) **(Ab)**, where N denotes the number of healthy subjects or patients. Capacitance of the three patients P40.1, P41.1, P42.1 was not any different from that of the controls (0.62 pA/pF P40.1 + P41.1 + P42.1 vs. 0.68 pA/pF C40 + C41 + C42, p > 0.05; 0.62 pA/pF P40.1 + P41.1 + P42.1 vs. 0.69 pA/pF general control, p > 0.05). Compared are the I/V-curve of all glucose-6-phosphate dehydrogenase deficiency patients cells (n = 27) with the I/V curve of all transportation control cells (n = 22) **(Ba)** as well as with a general control (n = 175) **(Bb)**, where n denotes the number of cells. Compared are the I/V curves of P45.1 ("PK" below the patient number stands for pyruvate kinase deficiency) (n = 15) with its own transportation control C45 (n = 5) **(Ca)** as well as with a general control (n = 175) **(Cb)**. No changes were observed in capacitance either with the transportation (0.72 pA/pF P45.1 vs. 0.68 pA/pF C45; p > 0.05) or with the general control (0.72 pA/pF P45.1 vs. 0.69 pA/pF general control; p > 0.05). Currents were elicited by voltage steps from −100 to 100 mV for 500 ms in 20 mV increments at V_h = −30 mV. Data are expressed as mean current density ± SEMs.

channels and transporters) and that mutations changing its conformation or its availability in the membrane might lead to multifaceted effects either increasing or decreasing membrane conductance (both of which with the detrimental result of disturbing RBC ion homeostasis). In line is a study showing kidney band 3 protein interaction with nephrin (Wu et al., 2010). The intracellular domain of nephrin interacts with TRPC6, believed to be present in erythrocytes (Foller et al., 2008; Danielczok J. et al., 2017) suggesting a possible functional link between band 3 protein and TRPC6 in erythrocytes as well. While no changes in cation channel activity (not an increase either, regardless of the reported substantially elevated cation leak) have been detected in band 3 protein R730C RBCs [as measured by on-cell patch-clamp, (Stewart et al., 2011)] as well as in band 3 protein H734R RBCs [as judged by membrane potential changes, (Bogdanova et al., 2009)], it could be that each mutation alters in a different way endogenous permeability pathways.

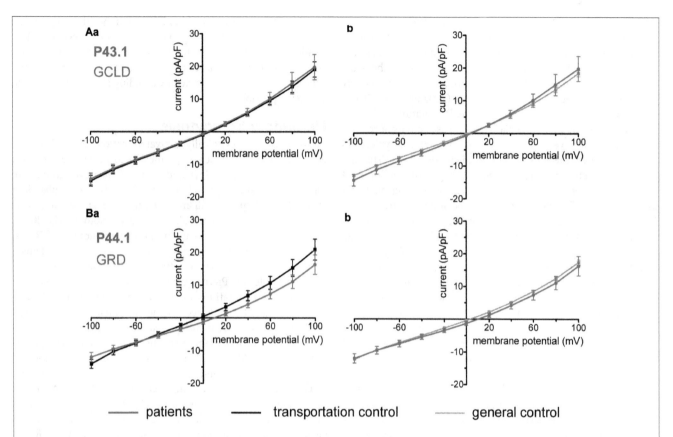

FIGURE 10 | Whole-cell recordings of ion currents from RBCs of healthy donors and patients with enzymopathies. Compared are the I/V curves of P43.1 (GCLD below the patient number stands for glutamate-cysteine ligase deficiency) (n = 6) with its own transportation control C43 (n = 5) **(Aa)** as well as with a general control (n = 175) **(Ab)**. No changes were observed in capacitance either with the transportation (0.64 pA/pF P43.1 vs. 0.65 pA/pF C43; $p > 0.05$) or with the general control (0.64 pA/pF P43.1 vs. 0.69 pA/pF general control; $p > 0.05$). Compared are the I/V curves of P44.1 (GRD below the patient number stands for glutathione reductase deficiency) (n = 9) with its own transportation control C44 (n = 5) **(Ba)** as well as with a general control (n = 175) **(Bb)**, where n denotes the number of cells. No changes were observed in capacitance either with the transportation (0.76 pA/pF P44.1 vs. 0.65pA/pF C44; $p > 0.05$) or with the general control (0.76 pA/pF P44.1 vs. 0.69 pA/pF general control; $p > 0.05$). Currents were elicited by voltage steps from −100 to 100 mV for 500 ms in 20 mV increments at V_h = −30 mV. Data are expressed as mean current density ± SEMs.

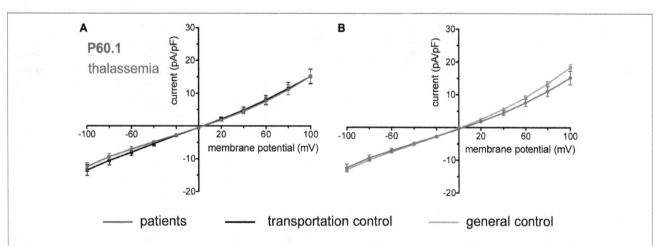

FIGURE 11 | Whole-cell recordings of ion currents from RBCs of healthy donors and a patient with β-thalassemia. Compared are the I/V curves of P60.1 (n = 12) with its own transportation control C60 (n = 5) **(A)** as well as with a general control (n = 175) **(B)**. No changes were observed in capacitance either with the transportation (0.72 pA/pF P60.1 vs. 0.64 pA/pF C60; $p > 0.05$) or with the general control (0.72 pA/pF P60.1 vs. 0.69 pA/pF general control; $p > 0.05$). Currents were elicited by voltage steps from −100 to 100 mV for 500 ms in 20 mV increments at V_h = −30 mV. Data are expressed as mean current density ± SEMs.

Regarding mutation Ile783Asn of patient P12.1, it is not in the cytoplasmic half of the core domain of band 3 protein, where most of the mutations causing stomatocytosis are (Arakawa et al., 2015), yet it is very close to and in the same transmembrane domain (TM 12) as another mutation, namely Gly796Arg, also triggering stomatocytosis (Arakawa et al., 2015). According to (Huisjes et al., unpublished) mutation Ile783Asn is accompanied by increased Na^+-K^+-ATPase activity, a referral to stomatocytosis, yet by an osmoscan curve with a typical HS pattern and extremely low eosin-5-maleimide (EMA) staining (61%), likely reflecting strongly reduced copy numbers of band 3 protein, a referral to spherocytosis. (EMA-binding on RBCs involves the ε-NH group of lysine at position 430 from band 3 protein (Nicolas et al., 2003) and is experimentally found to correlate with band 3 protein expression on RBCs (Huisjes et al., 2018). Thus the question whether it is the unavailability of band 3 protein or a possible structural and conformational change that causes the decreased outward current, remains open.

In our study, as outlined in the Results section, we have compared the currents measured from the RBCs of our patients once with their transportation control, i.e., currents measured from the RBCs of a healthy subject, whose blood was delivered together with the blood of the patient, and once with a general control, i.e., currents measured from the cells of all healthy subjects delivered throughout the study. Inevitably a question comes up, especially when there are differences in the comparisons with the two controls, which is the more appropriate one. Whereas, undoubtedly, considering the transportation control, allows us to take into account the particular transportation conditions such as temperature, vibration intensity and shipment duration, it has limitations. Such limitations are the low number of measured cells but mostly the fact that the control subject, although judged healthy, might not be a representative control. Thus in the case with C17, the control for patients P17.1 and P17.2, the averaged capacitance of C17 RBCs (0.53 pA/pF) is statistically significantly smaller than the averaged capacitance of the RBCs of the general control (0.69 pA/pF). This in turn results in an increased current density (current divided by capacitance) for the transportation control which might explain the observed difference of P17.1 and P17.2 compared to C17 but not to the general control (**Figures 4B,C**).

With C10, the control of P10.1, the situation is even more extreme, as, even though the averaged capacitance of the RBCs of the transportation control is higher compared to the averaged capacitance of the general control, which results in a lower current density, the current density still remains much higher than the one of the general control. The appearance of the I/V curve is also very different with the reversal potential being much shifted to the more negative values compared to the general control (**Figure 5Bc**). The above mentioned limitations could be avoided by considering the general control which, due to the high number of cells, is balancing (smoothing out) the effect of a healthy but unrepresentative subject and is close to an 'ideal' control. At the same time what is an advantage of the general control is simultaneously a disadvantage as it 'balances' also the specific transportation effects on the samples. A way out of accidentally coming across a non-representative

healthy subject is using the blood of several healthy subjects as a transportation control or, even better, the blood of several healthy relatives. A further problem, however, is that transportation could have different effects on the patient and on the control. This problem could be avoided by avoiding transportation itself, whenever possible.

Hereditary Xerocytosis

Piezo 1 is a mechanically activated cation channel (Coste et al., 2010, 2012), which is permeable to monovalent cations ($P_K > P_{Cs} \cong P_{Na} > P_{Li}$) and to most divalent cations like Ba^{2+}, Ca^{2+}, and Mg^{2+}, but not Mn^{2+} (Gnanasambandam et al., 2015). Expressed in many tissues like kidney, lung and urinary bladder (Coste et al., 2010; Miyamoto et al., 2014), Piezo 1 has been detected in the plasma membrane of RBCs, e.g., by mass spectroscopy and immunologically (Zarychanski et al., 2012; Andolfo et al., 2013; Kaestner and Egée, 2018). A major role of Piezo1 channels in RBCs is in volume regulation and mutations in the channel have been linked to HX, a dominantly inherited haemolytic anemia, characterized by decreased K^+ and increased Na^+ RBCs content, as well as dehydration resulting in increased mean corpuscular hemoglobin concentrations (MCHC), a leftward shift of the osmotic gradient ektacytometry curve and increased osmotic resistance of the RBCs (Gallagher, 2013; Shmukler et al., 2014; Glogowska and Gallagher, 2015; Andolfo et al., 2016). Disease clinical manifestations are variable and may include mild to moderate haemolysis, perinatal edema and non-immune hydrops fetalis that spontaneously resolve, thrombosis, pseudohyperkalemia and sometimes severe iron overload in the course of the disease (Gallagher, 2013; Glogowska and Gallagher, 2015; Andolfo et al., 2016). Out of the four mutations in our study [R2456H (P51.3 and P51.4), R2088G (P53.3 and P53.2), C426R (P50.2), and E2496ELE (P52.1)], three (R2456H, R2088G, and E2496ELE) are known and have been extensively characterized including expression of the mutant Piezo1 channel in heterologous systems and characterization of the channel activity (Zarychanski et al., 2012; Albuisson et al., 2013; Andolfo et al., 2013; Bae et al., 2013; Sandberg et al., 2014; Shmukler et al., 2014; Glogowska et al., 2017). Two of the mutations, R2456H and E2496ELE, among the most common ones found in typical HX patients (Zarychanski et al., 2012; Albuisson et al., 2013; Andolfo et al., 2013; Shmukler et al., 2014), are in the C-terminal region, part of the pore module of Piezo1 (Coste et al., 2015; Ge et al., 2015). Those mutations do not alter the sensitivity of the channel to mechanical stimulation but cause considerable increase in the inactivation time constant thus giving rise to an increased channel activity in response to a given mechanical stimulus (Albuisson et al., 2013; Glogowska et al., 2017). Could an increased channel activity lasting only for the duration of a short mechanical stimulus explain the ion disbalance observed in HX? A possible answer is that during their circulation in the vascular system RBCs are under constant mechanical stress squeezing in capillaries and in the tiny slits of the spleen undergoing numerous rounds of mechanical stimulation with Piezo1 activation (Danielczok J.G. et al., 2017) and, in the case of Piezo1 prolonged inactivation, not being capable of replenishing their ions. However, it is also likely that slowing of inactivation could potentially cause a slight increase in a basal Piezo1 activity (independent of mechanical stimulation) (Albuisson et al., 2013). This is supported by the study of (Andolfo et al., 2013), which demonstrates spontaneous ion channel activity in R2456H patient RBCs, blocked by GsMTx-4 and not observed in healthy cells. In addition are the on-cell patch recordings from the RBCs of another R2456H patient revealing once again an increased cation channel activity (independent of mechanical stimulation) without information on the identity of the channel (Shmukler et al., 2014). Consistent with Piezo 1 increased activity having direct or secondary effects on membrane conductance is the observed decrease in conductance in P52.1 (E2496ELE) RBCs. Also in P51.3 and P51.4 (R2456H) and P52.1 (E2496ELE) a rightward shift of the I/V curve is observed (**Figures 7Bb, 8Bb**) indicative of an upregulation/downregulation of a channel/channels. Whether the shift is pertinent to the mutations though is not explicitly clear as such a shift is not detected when patients' currents are compared with their transportation controls (**Figures 7Ba, 8Ba**). Concerning mutation C426R (P50.2) which shows an increase in current only with the general control but not with its transportation control we tend to disregard the difference shown with the general control as the transportation control was taken from a genetically related healthy subject and it indeed shows a remarkable similarity with the I/V curve of the patient (**Figure 8Aa**).

Enzymopathies and Beta-Thalassemia

Metabolic enzyme deficiencies (glucose-6-phosphate dehydrogenase deficiency, pyruvate kinase deficiency, glutamate-cysteine ligase deficiency and glutathione reductase deficiency) as well as β-thalassemia are not accompanied by changes in membrane conductance. The former is consistent with the lack of changes also in the K^+ and Na^+ content of 11 patients with congenital non-spherocytic haemolytic anemia including pyruvate kinase deficiency (Vives Corrons and Besson, 2001).

CONCLUSION

Trying to summarize and come up with a common channel increased activity/dysfunction or just an effect (decrease or increase in conductance) accompanying RBCs ion disbalance disorders, we stumble upon a great variability in results. Such a variability is of course reflecting the many triggers of the disbalance and for sure not lessened by the fact that not only between different mutations but also among members of a family with the same mutation there are distinct differences starting from the severity of the disease and extending down to the cellular level. Such a summary is even harder and certainly not helped by the great variability in healthy subjects reflected in control membrane conductance measurements as seen in our study. And last but not least answers are yet heavier without so far clearly knowing how an increased Na^+ and a decreased K^+ can lead to overhydration as in OHSt or to dehydration as in HX. Nevertheless based on our study we conclude that changes in conductance are incurred by certain α-spectrin [c.2755G > T (p.Glu919) and c.678G > A p.(Glu227fs) whenever an α^{LELY} allele is present], band 3 protein [c.2348T > A p.(Ile783Asn)] and Piezo1 (c.7483_7488dupCTGGAG p.2495_2496dupLeuGlu) mutations as a difference is observed with both the general and the transportation control. Identification of the channel/channels that underlie the changed conductances demands future studies.

AUTHOR CONTRIBUTIONS

All authors listed have made a substantial, direct and intellectual contribution to the work, and approved it for publication.

REFERENCES

Albuisson, J., Murthy, S. E., Bandell, M., Coste, B., Louis-Dit-Picard, H., Mathur, J., et al. (2013). Dehydrated hereditary stomatocytosis linked to gain-of-function mutations in mechanically activated PIEZO1 ion channels. *Nat. Commun.* 4:1884. doi: 10.1038/ncomms 2899

Andolfo, I., Alper, S. L., De Franceschi, L., Auriemma, C., Russo, R., De Falco, L., et al. (2013). Multiple clinical forms of dehydrated hereditary stomatocytosis arise from mutations in PIEZO1. *Blood* 121, 3925–3935. doi: 10.1182/blood-2013-02-482489

Andolfo, I., Russo, R., Gambale, A., and Iolascon, A. (2016). New insights on hereditary erythrocyte membrane defects. *Haematologica* 101, 1284–1294. doi: 10.3324/haematol.2016.142463

Arakawa, T., Kobayashi-Yurugi, T., Alguel, Y., Iwanari, H., Hatae, H., Iwata, M., et al. (2015). Crystal structure of the anion exchanger domain of human erythrocyte band 3. *Science* 350, 680–684. doi: 10.1126/science.aaa4335

Avent, N. D., and Reid, M. E. (2000). The Rh blood group system: a review. *Blood* 95, 375–387.

Badens, C., and Guizouarn, H. (2016). Advances in understanding the pathogenesis of the red cell volume disorders. *Br. J. Haematol.* 174, 674–685. doi: 10.1111/bjh. 14197

Bae, C., Gnanasambandam, R., Nicolai, C., Sachs, F., and Gottlieb, P. A. (2013). Xerocytosis is caused by mutations that alter the kinetics of the mechanosensitive channel PIEZO1. *Proc. Natl. Acad. Sci. U.S.A.* 110, E1162–E1168. doi: 10.1073/pnas.1219777110

Bakouh, N., Benjelloun, F., Cherif-Zahar, B., and Planelles, G. (2006). The challenge of understanding ammonium homeostasis and the role of the Rh glycoproteins. *Transfus. Clin. Biol.* 13, 139–146. doi: 10.1016/j.tracli.2006.02.008

Bogdanova, A. Y., Goede, J. S., Weiss, E., Bogdanov, N., Bennekou, P., Bernhardt, I., et al. (2009). Cryohydrocytosis: increased activity of cation carriers in red cells from a patient with a band 3 mutation. *Haematologica* 95, 189–198. doi: 10.3324/haematol.2009.010215

Bruce, L. J., Guizouarn, H., Burton, N. M., Gabillat, N., Poole, J., Flatt, J. F., et al. (2009). The monovalent cation leak in overhydrated stomatocytic red blood cells results from amino acid substitutions in the Rh-associated glycoprotein. *Blood* 113, 1350–1357. doi: 10.1182/blood-2008-07-171140

Bruce, L. J., Kay, M. M., Lawrence, C., and Tanner, M. J. (1993). Band 3 HT, a human red-cell variant associated with acanthocytosis and increased anion transport, carries the mutation Pro-868→Leu in the membrane domain of band 3. *Biochem. J.* 293, 317–320. doi: 10.1042/bj2930317

Bruce, L. J. L., Robinson, H. C. H., Guizouarn, H. H., Borgese, F. F., Harrison, P. P., King, M.-J. M., et al. (2005). Monovalent cation leaks in human red cells caused by single amino acid substitutions in the transport domain of the band 3 chloride-bicarbonate exchanger, AE1. *Nat. Genet.* 37, 1258–1263. doi: 10.1038/ng1656

Cao, A., and Galanello, R. (2010). Beta-thalassemia. *Genet. Med.* 12, 61–76. doi: 10.1097/GIM.0b013e3181cd68ed

Coste, B., Mathur, J., Schmidt, M., Earley, T. J., Ranade, S., Petrus, M. J., et al. (2010). Piezo1 and Piezo2 are essential components of distinct mechanically activated cation channels. *Science* 330, 55–60. doi: 10.1126/science.1193270

Coste, B., Murthy, S. E., Mathur, J., Schmidt, M., Mechioukhi, Y., Delmas, P., et al. (2015). Piezo1 ion channel pore properties are dictated by C-terminal region. *Nat. Commun.* 6:7223. doi: 10.1038/ncomms8223

Coste, B., Xiao, B., Santos, J. S., Syeda, R., Grandl, J., Spencer, K. S., et al. (2012). Piezo proteins are pore-forming subunits of mechanically activated channels. *Nature* 483, 176–181. doi: 10.1038/nature10812

Danielczok, J. G., Terriac, E., Hertz, L., Petkova-Kirova, P., Lautenschläger, F., Laschke, M. W., et al. (2017). Red blood cell passage of small capillaries is associated with transient Ca2+-mediated adaptations. *Front. Physiol.* 8:979. doi: 10.3389/fphys.2017.00979

Danielczok, J., Hertz, L., Ruppenthal, S., Kaiser, E., Petkova-Kirova, P., Bogdanova, A., et al. (2017). Does erythropoietin regulate TRPC channels in red blood cells? *Cell. Physiol. Biochem.* 41, 1219–1228. doi: 10.1159/000464384

Dhaliwal, G., Cornett, P. A., and Tierney, L. M. (2004). Hemolytic anemia. *Am. Fam. Physician* 69, 2599–2606.

Endeward, V., Cartron, J.-P., Ripoche, P., and Gros, G. (2008). RhAG protein of the Rhesus complex is a CO2 channel in the human red cell membrane. *FASEB J.* 22, 64–73. doi: 10.1096/fj.07-9097com

Fermo, E., Bogdanova, A., Petkova-Kirova, P., Zaninoni, A., Marcello, A. P., Makhro, A., et al. (2017). "Gardos Channelopathy": a variant of hereditary stomatocytosis with complex molecular regulation. *Sci. Rep.* 7:1744. doi: 10.1038/s41598-017-01591-w

Foller, M., Kasinathan, R. S., Koka, S., Lang, C., Shumilina, E. V., Birnbaumer, L., et al. (2008). TRPC6 contributes to the Ca(2+) leak of human erythrocytes. *Cell. Physiol. Biochem.* 21, 183–192. doi: 10.1159/000113760

Gallagher, P. G. (2013). Disorders of red cell volume regulation. *Curr. Opin. Hematol.* 20, 201–207. doi: 10.1097/MOH.0b013e32835f6870

Ge, J., Li, W., Zhao, Q., Li, N., Chen, M., Zhi, P., et al. (2015). Architecture of the mammalian mechanosensitive Piezo1 channel. *Nature* 527, 64–69. doi: 10.1038/nature15247

Glogowska, E., and Gallagher, P. G. (2015). Disorders of erythrocyte volume homeostasis. *Int. J. Lab. Hematol.* 37(Suppl. 1), 85–91. doi: 10.1111/ijlh.12357

Glogowska, E., Schneider, E. R., Maksimova, Y., Schulz, V. P., Lezon-Geyda, K., Wu, J., et al. (2017). Novel mechanisms of PIEZO1 dysfunction in hereditary xerocytosis. *Blood* 130, 1845–1856. doi: 10.1182/blood-2017-05-786004

Gnanasambandam, R., Bae, C., Gottlieb, P. A., and Sachs, F. (2015). Ionic selectivity and permeation properties of human PIEZO1 channels. *PLoS One* 10:e0125503. doi: 10.1371/journal.pone.0125503

Guyton, A. C., and Hall, J. E. (2006). *Medical Physiology*. Amsterdam: Elsevier Saunders.

Hertz, L., Huisjes, R., Llaudet-Planas, E., Petkova-Kirova, P., Makhro, A., Danielczok, J. G., et al. (2017). Is increased intracellular calcium in red blood cells a common component in the molecular mechanism causing anemia? *Front. Physiol.* 8:673. doi: 10.3389/fphys.2017.00673

Huang, C. H., Cheng, G., Liu, Z., Chen, Y., Reid, M. E., Halverson, G., et al. (1999). Molecular basis for Rh(null) syndrome: identification of three new missense mutations in the Rh50 glycoprotein gene. *Am. J. Hematol.* 62, 25–32. doi: 10.1002/(SICI)1096-8652(199909)62:1<25::AID-AJH5>3.0.CO;2-K

Huisjes, R., Satchwell, T. J., Verhagen, L. P., Schiffelers, R. M., van Solinge, W. W., Toye, A. M., et al. (2018). Quantitative measurement of red cell surface protein expression reveals new biomarkers for hereditary spherocytosis. *Int. J. Lab. Hematol.* 40, e74–e77. doi: 10.1111/ijlh.12841

Iolascon, A., Perrotta, S., and Stewart, G. W. (2003). Red blood cell membrane defects. *Rev. Clin. Exp. Hematol.* 7, 22–56.

Kaestner, L., and Egée, S. (2018). Commentary: voltage gating of mechanosensitive PIEZO channels. *Front. Physiol.* 9:1565. doi: 10.3389/fphys.2018.01565

Luzzatto, L., Nannelli, C., and Notaro, R. (2016). Glucose-6-phosphate dehydrogenase deficiency. *Hematol. Oncol. Clin. North Am.* 30, 373–393. doi: 10.1016/j.hoc.2015.11.006

Makhro, A., Huisjes, R., Verhagen, L. P., Mañú Pereira, M. D. M., Llaudet-Planas, E., Petkova-Kirova, P., et al. (2016). Red cell properties after different

modes of blood transportation. *Front. Physiol.* 7:288. doi: 10.3389/fphys.2016.00288

Miyamoto, T., Mochizuki, T., Nakagomi, H., Kira, S., Watanabe, M., Takayama, Y., et al. (2014). Functional role for Piezo1 in stretch-evoked Ca2+ influx and ATP release in urothelial cell cultures. *J. Biol. Chem.* 289, 16565–16575. doi: 10.1074/jbc.M113.528638

Nash, R., and Shojania, A. M. (1987). Hematological aspect of Rh deficiency syndrome: a case report and a review of the literature. *Am. J. Hematol.* 24, 267–275. doi: 10.1002/ajh.2830240306

Nicolas, V., Le Van Kim, C., Gane, P., Birkenmeier, C., Cartron, J.-P., Colin, Y., et al. (2003). Rh-RhAG/ankyrin-R, a new interaction site between the membrane bilayer and the red cell skeleton, is impaired by Rh(null)-associated mutation. *J. Biol. Chem.* 278, 25526–25533. doi: 10.1074/jbc.M302816200

Petkova-Kirova, P., Hertz, L., Makhro, A., Danielczok, J., Huisjes, R., Llaudet-Planas, E., et al. (2018). A previously unrecognized Ca2+-inhibited nonselective cation channel in red blood cells. *Hemasphere* 2:e146. doi: 10.1097/HS9.0000000000000146

Ristoff, E., and Larsson, A. (1998). Patients with genetic defects in the gamma-glutamyl cycle. *Chem. Biol. Interact.* 11, 113–121. doi: 10.1016/S0009-2797(97)00155-5

Rotordam, G. M., Fermo, E., Becker, N., Barcellini, W., Brüggemann, A., Fertig, N., et al. (2018). A novel gain-of-function mutation of Piezo1 is functionally affirmed in red blood cells by high-throughput patch clamp. *Haematologica* doi: 10.3324/haematol.2018.201160 [Epub ahead of print].

Salhany, J. M., Schopfer, L. M., Kay, M. M., Gamble, D. N., and Lawrence, C. (1995). Differential sensitivity of stilbenedisulfonates in their reaction with band 3 HT (Pro-868- > Leu). *Proc. Natl. Acad. Sci. U.S.A.* 92, 11844–11848. doi: 10.1073/pnas.92.25.11844

Sandberg, M. B., Nybo, M., Birgens, H., and Frederiksen, H. (2014). Hereditary xerocytosis and familial haemolysis due to mutation in the PIEZO1 gene: a simple diagnostic approach. *Int. J. Lab. Hematol.* 36, e62–e65. doi: 10.1111/ijlh.12172

Shmukler, B. E., Vandorpe, D. H., Rivera, A., Auerbach, M., Brugnara, C., and Alper, S. L. (2014). Dehydrated stomatocytic anemia due to the heterozygous mutation R2456H in the mechanosensitive cation channel PIEZO1: a case report. *Blood Cells Mol. Dis.* 52, 53–54. doi: 10.1016/j.bcmd.2013.07.015

Stewart, A. K., Kedar, P. S., Shmukler, B. E., Vandorpe, D. H., Hsu, A., Glader, B., et al. (2011). Functional characterization and modified rescue of novel AE1 mutation R730C associated with overhydrated cation leak stomatocytosis. *Am. J. Physiol. Cell Physiol.* 300, C1034–C1046. doi: 10.1152/ajpcell.00447.2010

Stewart, A. K., Vandorpe, D. H., Heneghan, J. F., Chebib, F., Stolpe, K., Akhavein, A., et al. (2010). The GPA-dependent, spherostomatocytosis mutant AE1 E758K induces GPA-independent, endogenous cation transport in amphibian oocytes. *Am. J. Physiol. Cell Physiol.* 298, C283–C297. doi: 10.1152/ajpcell.00444.2009

Stewart, G. W. (2004). Hemolytic disease due to membrane ion channel disorders. *Curr. Opin. Hematol.* 11, 244–250. doi: 10.1097/01.moh.0000132240.20671.33

van Zwieten, R., Verhoeven, A. J., and Roos, D. (2014). Inborn defects in the antioxidant systems of human red blood cells. *Free Radic. Biol. Med.* 67, 377–386. doi: 10.1016/j.freeradbiomed.2013.11.022

Viel, A., and Branton, D. (1996). Spectrin: on the path from structure to function. *Curr. Opin. Cell Biol.* 8, 49–55. doi: 10.1016/S0955-0674(96)80048-2

Vives Corrons, L., and Besson, I. (2001). Red cell membrane Na+ transport systems in hereditary spherocytosis: relevance to understanding the increased Na+ permeability. *Ann. Haematol.* 80, 535–539. doi: 10.1007/s002770100342

Ware, R. E., de Montalembert, M., Tshilolo, L., and Abboud, M. R. (2017). Sickle cell disease. *Lancet* 390, 311–323. doi: 10.1016/S0140-6736(17)30193-9

Wilmotte, R., Harper, S. L., Ursitti, J. A., Maréchal, J., Delaunay, J., and Speicher, D. W. (1997). The exon 46-encoded sequence is essential for stability of human erythroid alpha-spectrin and heterodimer formation. *Blood* 90, 4188–4196.

Wu, F., Saleem, M. A., Kampik, N. B., Satchwell, T. J., Williamson, R. C., Blattner, S. M., et al. (2010). Anion exchanger 1 interacts with nephrin in podocytes. *J. Am. Soc. Nephrol.* 21, 1456–1467. doi: 10.1681/ASN.2009090921

Zanella, A., Fermo, E., Bianchi, P., and Valentini, G. (2005). Red cell pyruvate kinase deficiency: molecular and clinical aspects. *Br. J. Haematol.* 130, 11–25. doi: 10.1111/j.1365-2141.2005.05527.x

13

Oral Vitamin B12 Replacement for the Treatment of Pernicious Anemia

Catherine Qiu Hua Chan[1]*, Lian Leng Low[1,2]* and Kheng Hock Lee[1,2]

[1]Department of Family Medicine and Continuing Care, Singapore General Hospital, Singapore, [2]Family Medicine, Duke-NUS Medical School, Singapore

*Correspondence:
Catherine Qiu Hua Chan
catherine.chan.q.h@sgh.com.sg;
Lian Leng Low
low.lian.leng@singhealth.com.sg

Many patients with pernicious anemia are treated with lifelong intramuscular (IM) vitamin B12 replacement. As early as the 1950s, there were studies suggesting that oral vitamin B12 replacement may provide adequate absorption. Nevertheless, oral vitamin B12 replacement in patients with pernicious anemia remains uncommon in clinical practice. The objective of this review is to provide an update on the effectiveness of oral vitamin B12 for the treatment of pernicious anemia, the recommended dosage, and the required frequency of laboratory test and clinical monitoring. Relevant articles were identified by PubMed search from January 1, 1980 to March 31, 2016 and through hand search of relevant reference articles. Two randomized controlled trials, three prospective papers, one systematic review, and three clinical reviews fulfilled our inclusion criteria. We found that oral vitamin B12 replacement at 1000 µg daily was adequate to replace vitamin B12 levels in patients with pernicious anemia. We conclude that oral vitamin B12 is an effective alternative to vitamin B12 IM injections. Patients should be offered this alternative after an informed discussion on the advantages and disadvantages of both treatment options.

Keywords: oral vitamin B12, pernicious anemia, mecobalamin, cobalamin, cyanocobalamin

INTRODUCTION

Vitamin B12 deficiency is a common condition, and many are undiagnosed. Absolute deficiency occur up to 6% of those aged 60 years and older, whereas marginal deficiency occur in close to 20% of patients in later life (1). The manifestation of Vitamin B12 deficiency ranges from subtle, non-specific clinical features to serious neurological and neuropsychiatric complication if left untreated. With an aging population, screening for vitamin B12 level as part of anemia and cognitive impairment workup is more common. More cases are diagnosed, resulting in rising incidence of patients with vitamin B12 deficiency. The common causes of vitamin B deficiency are food-cobalamin (vitamin B12) malabsorption and pernicious anemia.

Pernicious anemia is an autoimmune gastritis resulting from the destruction of gastric parietal cells and consequent impairment of intrinsic factors secretion to bind the ingested vitamin B12. Other autoimmune disorders, especially thyroid disease, diabetes mellitus, and vitiligo, are also commonly associated with pernicious anemia. The cost and availability of auto-antibodies testing, such as intrinsic factor and anti-parietal cell antibodies, can be a barrier to further investigation for vitamin B12 deficiency to exclude pernicious anemia. Therefore, the exact prevalence of pernicious anemia is difficult to ascertain. It has been estimated that the prevalence of pernicious anemia in European countries is approximately 4% of the population (2). It is also well acknowledged that the prevalence increase with age and therefore more common in the elderly

---

Abbreviation: RCT, randomized controlled trial.

For patients with pernicious anemia, lifelong vitamin B12 therapy is indicated. Vitamin B12 is absorbed in the terminal ileum. This absorption is almost entirely dependent on intrinsic factor binding to vitamin B12. This bound complex in turn binds to the cubam receptor in the terminal ileum and is internalized. The complex is eventually released from lysosomes and transported across the cell membrane bound to transcobalamin in the blood circulation. Traditionally, vitamin B12 replacement is administered intramuscularly. However, it is believed that oral vitamin B12 can be absorbed passively independent of intrinsic factors. Passive diffusion accounts for about 1% of total absorption, and this route of absorption is unaffected in patients with pernicious anemia (3).

There were studies in the 1950s and the1960s that showed that oral vitamin B12 could be absorbed by patients with pernicious anemia and could lead to resolution of the anemia (3–6). However, lifelong intramuscular (IM) injection for replacement is still a common practice. In 1991, a survey done on Minneapolis internists led one commentary to conclude that oral vitamin B12 replacement for pernicious anemia was one of "medicine's best kept secret" (7). In 1996, when the survey was repeated again in the same area, awareness and use of oral vitamin B12 for pernicious anemia had increased substantially (0–19%), but the majority of doctors still remain unaware of this treatment option (61%) (8).

The objective of our review is to inform clinicians on the effectiveness of oral vitamin B12 as adequate replacement in patients with pernicious anemia, as well as make recommendations on the dosing and frequency of clinical and laboratory monitoring.

METHODS

A PubMed search was conducted in April 2016 to identify suitable articles published from January 1, 1980 to March 31, 2016. The following search strategy was applied: "Administration, Oral" (MeSH term) AND "Vitamin B12" (MeSH term) AND "Anaemia, Pernicious" (MeSH term). Only studies evaluating the effectiveness of oral vitamin B12 replacement on pernicious anemia patients in entirety or as a subset were included for review. The search was limited to English articles.

The search strategy was summarized in the following flow chart.

Flowchart on Selection of Articles

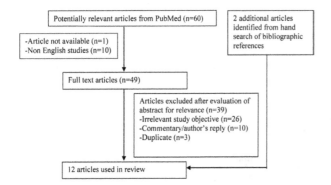

Grading of level of evidence and strength of recommendation was based on strength of recommendation taxonomy (SORT)

framework (9). The description and level of evidence of included studies are shown in **Table 1**.

RESULTS

Sixty articles were identified through the electronic database search. Non-English studies were excluded. The abstracts of the remaining 49 articles were evaluated for relevance. Articles that did not involve or discuss about patients with pernicious anemia treated with oral vitamin B12 replacement were excluded. Duplicated articles and commentary/author's reply were excluded. Another two articles were identified from hand search of bibliographic references of the shortlisted articles. A total of 12 articles [2 randomized controlled trials (RCTs) (10, 11), 3 prospective studies (12–14), 1 systematic review (15), and 6 clinical reviews (2, 16–20)] were obtained for the review.

Effectiveness of Oral Vitamin B12

The data given in the studies all supported the use of oral vitamin B12 as a valid and effective way of treating vitamin B12 deficiency, including pernicious anemia. The age range of the study population was 23–92 years old. The RCT by Kuzminski et al. (10) and prospective study by Delpre et al. (12) were done in America. The RCT by Bolaman et al. (11) was done in Turkey. The other two prospective studies by Nyholm et al. (13) and Andres et al. (14) were done in United Kingdom and France, respectively. The studies were conducted during the period of late 1990s to early 2000s.

In Kuzminski's study, serum vitamin B12 levels were significantly higher in the oral (vitamin B12 2000 µg) compared with IM (vitamin B12 1000 µg) group (643 ± 328 vs. 306 ± 118 pg/mL; $p < 0.001$) at 2 months. The difference was even greater at 4 months (1005 ± 595 vs. 325 ± 165 pg/mL). Five of the patients who had pernicious anemia in the oral vitamin B12 replacement group all had increase in serum vitamin B12 level. Four of the 18 in the oral group and 4 of the 15 in the IM group had a neurological response with a marked improvement or clearing of paresthesia, ataxia, or memory loss.

For Bolaman's study, there was also an increase in serum vitamin B12 levels in both groups (oral vitamin B12 1000 µg vs. IM vitamin B12 1000 µg) at 90 days (Oral group 213.8 pg/mL and IM group 225.5 pg/mL). There was a statistically significant difference between days 0 and 90 in both groups ($p < 0.0001$), but authors did not analyze difference between both groups. Both groups reported improvements of cognitive functions, sensory neuropathy, and vibration sense, but there was no statistical significant difference between both groups.

The systematic review by Butler et al. (15) done on these two RCTs concluded that high oral doses of vitamin B12 could be as effective as IM administration in achieving short-term hematological and neurological responses. However, the two RCTs were limited by their small sample size and short follow-up period.

The rest of studies also had small sample size but some had longer follow-up period (up to 18 months). Normalization of serum vitamin B12 levels was seen in all patients (inclusive of patients with pernicious anemia) in Delpre's study. An increase

TABLE 1 | Description and level of evidence for articles reviewed.

Study and study type	Participants, sample size, follow-up duration	Intervention, outcome measure	Results	Level of evidence (based on SORT)
Kuzminski et al. (10), randomized controlled trial (RCT), not blinded	Newly diagnosed vitamin B12-deficient patients	Oral vitamin B12 2000 µg daily for 120 days vs. intramuscular (IM) vitamin B12 1000 µg on days 1, 3, 7, 10, 14, 21, 30, 60, and 90	Serum vitamin B12 levels were significantly higher in the oral compared with IM group (643 ± 328 vs. 306 ± 118 pg/mL; $p < 0.001$) at 2 months. The difference was even greater at 4 months (1005 ± 595 vs. 325 ± 165 pg/mL)	2
	N (total number) = 33 Intervention = 18 (5 had pernicious anemia) Control = 15 (2 had pernicious anemia) 120 days	Primary outcomes: serum vitamin B12, methylmalonic acid, homocysteine neurologic responses	Four of the 18 in the oral group and 4 of the 15 in the IM group had a neurological response with a marked improvement or clearing of paresthesia, ataxia, or memory loss	
Bolaman et al. (11), RCT, not blinded	Megaloblastic anemia due to vitamin B12 deficiency	Oral vitamin B12 1000 µg daily for 90 days vs. IM vitamin B12 1000 µg daily for 10 days, then once weekly for 28 days and after that continued with once monthly	Serum vitamin B12 levels increased in both groups at 90 days (oral group 213.8 pg/mL and IM group 225.5 pg/mL). There was a statistically significant difference between day 0 and day 90 in both groups ($p < 0.0001$) but authors did not analyze difference between both groups	2
	N = 60 Intervention = 26 (8 had presence of anti-parietal call antibody) Control = 34 (3 had presence of anti-parietal call antibody) 90 days	Primary outcomes: serum vitamin B12, hemoglobin, platelet count, MCV, WBC, mini-mental state examination, neurological assessment	Both groups reported improvements of cognitive functions, sensory neuropathy, and vibration sense, but there was no statistical significant difference between both groups	
Delpre et al. (12), Prospective, open-label	Vitamin B12 deficiency N = 18 (inclusive of patients with pernicious anemia but did not state number) 7–12 days	Sublingual vitamin B12 1000 µg daily for 7–12 days Primary outcome: serum vitamin B12	Normalization of serum vitamin B12 levels was seen in all patients. An increase in vitamin B12 level was as much as fourfold compared with pretreatment in most patients. The mean change of 387.7 pg/mL was statistically significant ($p = 0.0001$, Student's t-test)	3
Nyholm et al. (13), Prospective, case series	Vitamin B12 deficiency	Loading dose of IM vitamin B12 till vitamin B12 level reached lower 25th centile (418 pg/mL) and then converted to oral vitamin B12 1000 µg daily	Oral vitamin B12 was effective in all the patients (no patients had to restart IM vitamin B12). At 3 months, the median serum vitamin B12 level was 1193 pg/mL	3
	N = 40 (10 patients had pernicious anemia) 3–18 months	Primary outcomes: serum vitamin B12, hemoglobin, MCV, homocysteine, and neurological assessment	Oral treatment did not result in any new neurological complications	
Andres et al. (14), Prospective, open-label	Pernicious anemia N = 10 3 months	Oral vitamin B12 1000 µg daily for 3 months Primary outcome: serum vitamin B12, secondary outcomes: hemoglobin, platelet count, and MCV	After 3 months, serum vitamin B12 levels were increased in all 9 patients (mean increase, 117.4 pg/mL; $p < 0.001$). One patient's result was not available due to technical problem	3

in vitamin B12 level was as much as fourfold compared with pretreatment in most patients. The mean change of 387.7 pg/mL was significant ($p = 0.0001$ in Student's t-test). Oral vitamin B12 was effective in all the patients (10 patients had pernicious anemia) in Nyholm's study with the median serum vitamin B12 level of 1193 pg/mL after 3 months of treatment. It was also reported that using oral treatment did not result in any new neurological complications. Andres's study was the only study done on patients with pernicious anemia in entirety. All nine patients' serum vitamin B12 levels improved (mean increase, 117.4 pg/mL; $p < 0.001$) after 3 months.

Dosage of Oral Vitamin B12 Replacement Required

In all the five studies, an oral (Delpre's study via sublingual route) dose of 1000 µg vitamin B12 was used with the exception of Kuzminski's study, whereby a higher dose of 2000 µg was used. It had been showed that oral vitamin B12 at 1000 µg was adequate replacement in pernicious anemia patients.

There was a dose-finding trial done by Eussen et al. (21), and the results indicated that the lowest dose of oral vitamin B12 required to normalize biochemical markers of mild vitamin B12 deficiency in older people was more than 200 times greater than the recommended dietary allowance for vitamin B12 of approximately 3 µg/day. However, this study did not distinguish the extent to which differences in individual responses were due to active as opposed to passive absorption of vitamin B12.

In some of the clinical reviews, it was stated that many do not use oral vitamin B12 replacement in view of concern on the unpredictable absorption at low doses of oral replacement. Daily vitamin B12 turnover rate is about 2 µg/day, so an oral dose of 100–250 µg/day is sufficient for normal patients. However, in view of the estimated 1% of total absorption *via* passive diffusion in patients with pernicious anemia, a 1000 µg daily dose is recommended.

Frequency of Monitoring

The outcome measurement of vitamin B12 level was done from a range of 1–3 months (exception of Delpre's study, which was done ranging from 9 to 14 days). Improvement in vitamin B12 was seen as early as within a month. Only in Nyholm's study, 11 of their patients were followed up until 18 months, whereby the vitamin B12 levels were maintained.

Close monitoring monthly is necessary at the start of oral replacement to verify normalization of lab results and monitoring for symptoms. Thereafter, annual monitoring should suffice. It should be carried out on a regular interval that is safe for patients and acceptable to both patients and doctors.

DISCUSSION

We summarized the level of evidence of using oral vitamin B12 replacement for patients with pernicious anemia (**Table 1**). The strength of clinical recommendations based on the SORT framework is provided in **Table 2**.

There is no "gold standard" in testing for vitamin B12 deficiency. It has been recommended that serum total homocysteine (Hcy) and methylmalonic acid (MMA) levels are more sensitive indicators of vitamin B12 status in pernicious anemia patients without any other disorders of vitamin B12 metabolism. In our review, some (10, 13), but not all, studies determine metabolite levels (Hcy and MMA) in pernicious anemia to assess effectiveness of therapy with vitamin B12. Most patients with pernicious

anemia are not screened genetically for confirmatory causes of the disease. There are genetic errors of metabolism where serum vitamin B12 levels are normal, but there is a functional (cellular) level deficiency of the micronutrient that is often overlooked unless Hcy and MMA levels are also measured. Both Hcy and MMA levels are elevated in patients with vitamin B12 deficiency. Elevated serum Hcy and MMA levels (>3 SDs above the mean in normal subjects) have a sensitivity of 95.9 and 98.4%, respectively, to diagnose vitamin B12 deficiency (22). The levels decrease immediately after treatment and repeat measurements have clinical utility to document adequate vitamin B12 replacement. However, considerations of using Hcy and MMA levels would include cost, availability of the test, as well as having standardized reference intervals.

Patients with vitamin B12 deficiency who are symptomatic have severe neurological deficits or have critically low blood levels of vitamin B12 should be treated with IM administration. This is to ensure rapid replenishment of body stores to prevent irreversible consequences of deficiency. Subsequently, patients may be able to convert to oral replacement with close monitoring. For long-term maintenance therapy, oral vitamin B12 replacement can be effective in patients with pernicious anemia. Patient preference should be taken into consideration in the choice of treatment options. Few studies had included surveying patients regarding preference of choice between oral vs. IM replacement of vitamin B12. In Delpre's study, 87% of them preferred tablets to injection (12). Eighty-seven percent found the tablets highly acceptable, while the remaining 13% agreed that tablets were acceptable. It must also be considered that adherence is likely to be better if the patient's preferred route of administration is taken into consideration.

Additional factors to consider when helping patient to make an informed choice are as follows.

Cost

In a study done in United Kingdom by Vidal-Alaball et al. (23), using oral vitamin B12 after diagnosis or switching from IM route could save resources in the medium and long term. The use of oral route results in significant reduction in manpower costs.

Reduction of Scheduled Visits to Clinics

Many patients with vitamin B12 deficiency are elderly and have multiple co-morbidities. They often have multiple appointments to attend various clinics and may have frequent hospitalization episodes. The need to schedule vitamin B12 injections is an avoidable addition to the cost and complexity of their care.

Adherence

In patients with non-compliance to oral medication, IM route may be a better option to ensure timely administration. On the other hand, oral replacement may improve adherence for patients who prefer oral medication to injections.

Discomfort/Pain

Oral replacement will be useful in patients who are averse to injection. For elderly patients with sarcopenia, injections can painful and difficult to administer.

TABLE 2 | SORT recommendations for clinical practice.

Clinical recommendation	Strength of recommendation
Oral vitamin B12 can be used for adequate replacement in patients with pernicious anemia	B
An oral vitamin B12 dose at 1000 µg is adequate replacement in patients with pernicious anemia	B
Close monitoring monthly is necessary at the start of oral replacement to verify normalization of lab results and monitoring for symptoms	C
Thereafter, annual monitoring should suffice	
Elevated serum homocysteine and methylmalonic acid levels should be included in future assessments of pernicious anemia and corrected to normal levels in patients with pernicious anemia	C

Risk Associated with IM Injection

In patients, whereby IM injections are contraindicated because of coagulopathy or the use anti-coagulation/anti-platelet medication. Oral replacement is the best option.

LIMITATIONS

1. The review was conducted only using PubMed and hand search.

2. Studies were mainly on patients with vitamin B12 deficiency with a subset of patients with pernicious anemia. Therefore, the actual sample size of pernicious anemia patients in each study may not reach statistical significance. We overcome this by triangulating our conclusions and recommendations based on the findings from multiple studies and the consistent oral vitamin B12 dosage of 1000 µg.

3. Many of the studies had small sample size and assessed only short-term outcomes. The long-term efficacy and side effects require further evaluation.

4. A few possible relevant articles were excluded due to language issues.

DIRECTION OF FUTURE RESEARCH

A multicenter randomized clinical trial is current in progress in Spain primary health-care setting called Project OB12 (24). This study aims to provide a more conclusive answer with a large sample size of 320 patients and longer follow-up period of 52 weeks. Further studies should include testing the efficacy of different dosages. It may be important to study the knowledge and practices of doctors/health-care workers with regard to oral replacement therapy with vitamin B12 for patients with pernicious anemia. Surveys on patients' preferences for oral or IM replacement would be informative to guide clinical decision-making.

CONCLUSION

Oral vitamin B12 replacement at 1000 µg daily is an adequate alternative to IM B12 injections. Close monitoring with clinical review and repeat vitamin B12 levels are required on a monthly basis to review symptoms and ensure normalization of B12 deficiency. Elevated serum Hcy and MMA levels should be included in future assessments of pernicious anemia and corrected with normal levels in patients with pernicious anemia.

AUTHOR CONTRIBUTIONS

Conceived and designed the study: CC, LL, and KL. Performed the study: CC and LL. Analyzed the data: CC and LL. Interpreted the results: CC and LL. Wrote the paper: CC, LL, and KL. Principal Investigator of this study and supervised this study: CC. Revised the paper critically and give final approval for publication: all authors.

REFERENCES

Allen LH. How common is vitamin B-12 deficiency? *Am J Clin Nutr* (2009) 89(2):693S–6S. doi:10.3945/ajcn.2008.26947A

Stabler SP. Clinical practice. Vitamin B12 deficiency. *N Engl J Med* (2013) 368(2):149–60. doi:10.1056/NEJMcp1113996

Berlin H, Berlin R, Brante G. Oral treatment of pernicious anemia with high doses of vitamin B12 without intrinsic factor. *Acta Med Scand* (1968) 184(4):247–58. doi:10.1111/j.0954-6820.1968.tb02452.x

Withey JL, Jones JH, Kilpatrick GS. Long-term trial of oral treatment of pernicious anaemia with vitamin-B12-peptide. *Br Med J* (1963) 1(5345):1583–5. doi:10.1136/bmj.1.5345.1583

Meyer LM, Sawitsky A, Cohen BS, Krim M, Fadem R. Oral treatment of pernicious anemia with vitamin B12. *Am J Med Sci* (1950) 220(6):604–9. doi:10.1097/00000441-195022060-00002

Ungley CC. Absorption of vitamin B12 in pernicious anaemia. I. Oral administration without a source of intrinsic factor. *Br Med J* (1950) 2(4685):905–8. doi:10.1136/bmj.2.4685.908

Lederle FA. Oral cobalamin for pernicious anemia. Medicine's best kept secret? *JAMA* (1991) 265(1):94–5. doi:10.1001/jama.265.1.94

Lederle FA. Oral cobalamin for pernicious anemia: back from the verge of extinction. *J Am Geriatr Soc* (1998) 46(9):1125–7. doi:10.1111/j.1532-5415.1998.tb06651.x

Ebell MH, Siwek J, Weiss BD, Woolf SH, Susman J, Ewigman B, et al. Strength of recommendation taxonomy (SORT): a patient-centered approach to grading evidence in the medical literature. *Am Fam Physician* (2004) 69(3):548–56.

Kuzminski AM, Del Giacco EJ, Allen RH, Stabler SP, Lindenbaum J. Effective treatment of cobalamin deficiency with oral cobalamin. *Blood* (1998) 92(4):1191–8.

Bolaman Z, Kadikoylu G, Yukselen V, Yavasoglu I, Barutca S, Senturk T. Oral versus intramuscular cobalamin treatment in megaloblastic anemia: a single-center, prospective, randomized, open-label study. *Clin Ther* (2003) 25(12):3124–34. doi:10.1016/S0149-2918(03)90096-8

Delpre G, Stark P, Niv Y. Sublingual therapy for cobalamin deficiency as an alternative to oral and parenteral cobalamin supplementation. *Lancet* (1999) 354(9180):740–1. doi:10.1016/S0140-6736(99)02479-4

Nyholm E, Turpin P, Swain D, Cunningham B, Daly S, Nightingale P, et al. Oral vitamin B12 can change our practice. *Postgrad Med J* (2003) 79(930):218–20. doi:10.1136/pmj.79.930.218

Andres E, Henoun Loukili N, Noel E, Maloisel F, Vinzio S, Kaltenbach G, et al. Effects of oral crystalline cyanocobalamin 1000 mug/d in the treatment of pernicious anemia: an open-label, prospective study in ten patients. *Curr Ther Res Clin Exp* (2005) 66(1):13–22. doi:10.1016/j.curtheres.2005.02.001

Butler CC, Vidal-Alaball J, Cannings-John R, McCaddon A, Hood K, Papaioannou A, et al. Oral vitamin B12 versus intramuscular vitamin B12 for vitamin B12 deficiency: a systematic review of randomized controlled trials. *Fam Pract* (2006) 23(3):279–85. doi:10.1093/fampra/cml008

Shipton MJ, Thachil J. Vitamin B12 deficiency – a 21st century perspective. *Clin Med (Lond)* (2015) 15(2):145–50. doi:10.7861/clinmedicine.15-2-145

Andres E, Serraj K. Optimal management of pernicious anemia. *J Blood Med* (2012) 3:97–103. doi:10.2147/JBM.S25620

Oh R, Brown DL. Vitamin B12 deficiency. *Am Fam Physician* (2003) 67(5):979–86.

Lane LA, Rojas-Fernandez C. Treatment of vitamin B(12)-deficiency anemia: oral versus parenteral therapy. *Ann Pharmacother* (2002) 36(7–8):1268–72. doi:10.1345/aph.1A122

Paauw DS. Did we learn evidence-based medicine in medical school? Some common medical mythology. *J Am Board Fam Pract* (1999) 12(2):143–9. doi:10.3122/jabfm.12.2.143

Eussen SJ, de Groot LC, Clarke R, Schneede J, Ueland PM, Hoefnagels WH, et al. Oral cyanocobalamin supplementation in older people with vitamin B12 deficiency: a dose-finding trial. *Arch Intern Med* (2005) 165(10):1167–72. doi:10.1001/archinte.165.10.1167

Savage DG, Lindenbaum J, Stabler SP, Allen RH. Sensitivity of serum methylmalonic acid and total homocysteine determinations for diagnos- ing cobalamin and folate deficiencies. *Am J Med* (1994) 96(3):239–46. doi:10.1016/0002-9343(94)90149-X

Vidal-Alaball J, Butler CC, Potter CC. Comparing costs of intramuscular and oral vitamin B12 administration in primary care: a cost-minimization anal- ysis. *Eur J Gen Pract* (2006) 12(4):169–73. doi:10.1080/14017430601049449

Sanz-Cuesta T, Gonzalez-Escobar P, Riesgo-Fuertes R, Garrido- Elustondo S, del Cura-Gonzalez I, Martin-Fernandez J, et al. Oral versus intramuscular administration of vitamin B12 for the treatment of patients with vitamin B12 deficiency: a pragmatic, randomised, multicentre, non-inferiority clinical trial undertaken in the primary healthcare setting (project OB12). *BMC Public Health* (2012) 12:394. doi:10.1186/1471-2458- 12-394

14

Predict Postoperative Anemia of Patients: Nomogram Construction and Validation

Yimin Dai[2†], Chang Han[1,2†] and Xisheng Weng[1]*

[1]Department of Orthopaedic Surgery, Peking Union Medical College Hospital, Chinese Academy of Medical Sciences & Peking Union Medical College, Beijing, China, [2]Peking Union Medical College, Eight-year MD program, Chinese Academy of Medical Sciences, Beijing, China

*Correspondence:
Xisheng Weng,
wengxshlc@163.com

†These authors have contributed equally to this work

Introduction: The loss of blood is a significant problem in Total Knee Arthroplasty (TKA). Anemia often occurs after such surgeries, leading to serious consequences, such as higher postoperative infection rates and longer hospital stays. Tools for predicting possible anemia can provide additional guidance in realizing better blood management of patients.

Methods: 2,165 patients who underwent TKA from 2015 to 2019 in the same medical center were divided into training and validation cohorts. Both univariate and multivariate logistic regression analyses were performed to identify independent preoperative risk factors for anemia. Based on these predictors, a nomogram was established using the area under the curve (AUC), calibration curve (AUC), and the area under the curve (AUC). The model was then applied to the validation cohort, and decision curve analyses (DCA) were also plotted.

Results: Through analysis of both univariate and multivariate logistic regression, five independent predictors were found in the training cohort: female, relatively low BMI, low levels of preoperative hemoglobin, abnormally high levels of ESR, and simultaneously two sides of TKA in the same surgery. The AUCs of the nomogram were 74.6% (95% CI, 71.35%–77.89%) and 68.8% (95% CI, 63.37%–74.14%) of training and the validation cohorts separately. Furthermore, the calibration curves of both cohorts illustrated the consistency of the nomogram with the actual condition of anemia of patients after TKA. The DCA curve was higher for both treat-none and treat-all, further indicating the relatively high practicality of the model.

Conclusion: Female, lower BMI, lower levels of preoperative Hb, simultaneous bilateral TKA, and high levels of preoperative ESR were figured out as five independent risk factors for postoperative anemia (<9.0 g/dL) in patients undergoing TKA. Based on the findings, a practical nomogram was constructed to predict risk of postoperative anemia. The evidence level should be level 4 according to guideline.

Keywords: anemia, predictors, nomogram, total knee arthroplasty, ESR

INTRODUCTION

Total knee arthroplasty (TKA) is widely performed to improve mobility and quality of life for symptomatic knee osteoarthritis patients. More than 500,000 knee replacements are performed annually in the USA (1). This number was projected to grow by 673% from 2005 to 2030 (2). Patients undergoing TKA are often elderly, suffer from comorbidities and poorer recovery ability. A significant proportion of these patients have preoperative anemia and the trauma caused by surgery is great. All these factors tend to cause or aggravate postoperative anemia. Postoperative anemia in itself is considered an independent risk factor predisposing to poor prognosis, including higher postoperative infection rates (3), longer hospital stays (4), higher mortality rates (5), longer durations of rehabilitation (4) and worse quality of life (6).

A significant number of frail older people with complex co-morbid conditions are currently receiving knee arthroplasty. High-risk patients must be recognized early so that measures may be implemented to reduce the risk of anemia. The treatment involves the treatment of underlying diseases, a balanced diet and the use of erythropoietin and iron. However, there is still no simple and easy method for evaluating the risk of postoperative anemia in clinical practice. Whether to use erythropoietin and iron for outpatients continues to perplex orthopedists.

We aimed to investigate the incidence and preoperative risk factors for postoperative anemia in patients following TKA and develop a cost-efficient dynamic nomogram to be implemented into clinical practice.

MATERIALS AND METHODS

From June 2016 to June 2019, 2,166 patients who received TKA in the same medical center were retrospectively reviewed. The inclusion criteria included: (1) diagnosed with osteoarthritis independently by two orthopedic doctors that met surgery indications; (2) received primary TKA that was performed by the same team; (3) accurate records of previous medical history; (4) received no extra iron supplements or blood transfusions prior to admission. All patients were given the same intraoperative blood management measures, such as tranexamic acid administration. Patients who met one of the following criteria were excluded: (1) revision arthroplasty; (2) coagulation disorders; (3) patients with preoperative Hb < 9.0 g/dL. This study was approved by the Ethics Committee of Peking Union Medical College Hospital. All patients signed informed consent forms before surgery.

Surgical Procedure

After being diagnosed with osteoarthritis in our hospital, patients who met the surgery indication would be given a booklet on perioperative information of knee surgery to make sure them were fully informed of their own illness. Once patients chose to receive TKA, preoperative evaluation would be performed about two weeks before surgery, including a necessary imaging examination, bone density test, serum hemoglobin (Hb), erythrocyte sedimentation rate (ESR), etc. Close monitoring will be required if Hb < 9.0 g/dL, and 1. ferralia and erythropoietin (EPO) 2. transfusion would be given if necessary.

All patients enrolled in this study underwent standard TKA performed in the supine position by two orthopedists from the same hospital with over 30-year experience. Tourniquets were commonly used during the operations, and the pressure was set to 60 mmHg. Posterior cruciate stabilizing (PS) prosthesis was used in the operation. Physical exercise and continuous passive motion exercise device (CPM) were applied on post-operative day 1 until discharge, which were performed twice daily according to standard guidelines (7).

Study Variable

We used a total of 24 variables for the modeling analysis in this study. Postoperative anemia is defined as Postoperative Hb < 9.0 g/dLl. The patient-related characteristics included sex, age, body mass index (BMI), smoking status and comorbidities. Smoking was defined as the number of times a patient reported smoking cigarettes in the year before admission for TKA. Comorbidities may have an important impact on survival, and comorbidity scores are often implemented in studies assessing prognosis.

This study used the Charlson-based ICD-10 co-morbidity instrument developed by the Royal College of Surgeons of England (8). It reflects current understanding of the prognostic impact of co-morbid disease and aims explicitly to avoid misclassifying surgical complications as co-morbidities. The comorbidities involved Myocardial infarction, Congestive cardiac failure, Peripheral vascular disease, Cerebrovascular disease, Dementia, Chronic pulmonary disease, Rheumatological disease, Liver disease, Diabetes mellitus, Hemiplegia or paraplegia, Renal disease, Any malignancy, Metastatic solid tumor and AIDS/HIV. All available information was collected before surgery.

Statistical Analysis

Patients were randomly divided into a training cohort and a validation cohort with a ratio of 7:3. Using the training cohort, the logistic regression models were constructed by incorporating these variables. Performance of the models in both the training cohort and validation cohort included discrimination and calibration. Discrimination is the predictive accuracy of distinguishing patients with anemia from those without anemia and can be measured by the area under the receiver operating characteristic (ROC) curve (AUC).

Calibration curves were plotted using 1,000 bootstrap resamples, which reflected the model's agreement between the predicted probability and the actual probability. Decision curve analysis (DCA) was used to assess the model's clinical usefulness. Based on the logistic regression model, a dynamic nomogram was developed, presenting a specific mechanism for calculating the risk of postoperative anemia.

Continuous data were expressed as median and interquartile (IQR). Statistical analysis was performed using IBM SPSS 25.0

(SPSS Inc; Chicago, IL, USA) and R software version 3.6.3. Pearson's Chi-square test was used for categorical data analysis (Fisher exact test was used if necessary), while Mann–Whitney U-test was used for comparing quantitative parameters. $P < 0.05$ were considered statistically significant. All statistical analyses were two-sided.

RESULTS

Basic Variables and Information of Patients

A total of 3,547 consecutive patients who underwent TKA at Peking Union Medical College from June 2015 to June 2019 were retrospected, while 2,165 of them met the inclusion criteria; in chronological order, 1,517 were included in the training group and the rest were in the validation group. The ages of patients varied between 20 and 94, while the mean age was 66.9; they were divided into five subgroups: younger than 60 years old, 60–65, 65–70, 70–75, and over 75 years old; while the patients aged 65–70 were the most, up to 27.8%. There were 1,795 females and 370 males. 159 and 79 patients had the habit of smoking and drinking separately, and 260 patients took drugs regularly. The average BMI was 27.01 kg/m^2, varied between 14.7–42.9 kg/m^2. The proportions of different constitutions from both cohorts were quite similar. Detailed information about the variables and patients is displayed in **Table 1**.

Possible Risk Factors for Postoperative Anemia

Anemia occurred in 253 patients in the training cohort within 3 days after TKA, accounting for 16.7% of the cohort. Several potential risk factors were identified for postoperative anemia by regression analyses. In the training cohort, sex, Body Mass Index (BMI), Erythrocyte Sedimentation Rate (ESR), Hemoglobin (Hb) and the sides of TKA were found to be associated with postoperative anemia by univariate logistic regression analysis. These variables were further analyzed by multivariable logistic regression; independent risk factors were ultimately identified as sex, BMI, hemoglobin and sides of TKA (**Table 2**). For sex of patients, females were more likely to suffer from anemia after operation (adjusted odds ratio: 0.458, 95% CI, 0.289–0.727, $p < 0.001$). BMI was another predictor; patients with lower BMI tended to have higher rates of postoperative anemia, considering the contrast between BMI < 24 kg/m^2 and BMI > 28 kg/m^2 (adjusted OR: 0.312, 95% CI, 0.206–0.473, $p < 0.001$). The ones with 24 < BMI < 28 kg/m^2 also had lower rates of postoperative anemia, though the results were not quite significant ($p > 0.01$). In addition, lower levels of preoperative Hb and both sides rather than one side of TKA suggested possible postoperative anemia separately (former adjusted OR: 5.671, 95% CI, 3.255, $p < 0.001$; latter adjusted OR: 4.247, 95% CI, 3.156–5.714, $p < 0.001$). Surprisingly, the influence of comorbidities was not as significant as people commonly think; patients with over one to two comorbidities didn't show higher rates of anemia, and though those with more than three comorbidities did suffer

from anemia more easily, the results weren't significant enough (OR: 1.162, 95% CI, 0.842–1.602, $p = 0.361$).

A similar analysis was performed in the validation group, as shown in **Table 3**. Sex, preoperative Hb levels and sides of TKA were still strong risk factors. However, BMI did not show comparable effects, while ESR did; in univariate analysis, high ESR was strongly associated with worse ending of anemia, though such associations slightly weakened in multivariable logistic regression (OR: 1.666, 95% CI, 1.043–2.66, $p = 0.033$).

Establishment and Validation of the Nomogram to Predict Anemia Ending

Based on the final results of multivariate analysis, the nomogram was established and displayed in **Figure 1**. The total point of every given patient could be calculated from the nomogram, which was the sum of each risk factor mentioned above. Possibility of postoperative anemia was predicted by the final score.

To ensure the feasibility and accuracy of the nomogram, we performed discrimination and calibration assessments for the model. For discrimination, the ROC curves of the nomogram applied to both training and validation cohorts were plotted to perform validation internally and externally, together with the AUC values (**Figures 2A,B**), which showed relatively high predictive accuracy (internal validation, AUC: 74.6%, 95% CI, 71.35%–77.89%; external validation, AUC: 68.8%, 95% CI, 63.37%–74.14%). Moreover, the calibration of both internal and external curves also demonstrated high consistency between the monogram and practicalities (**Figures 2C,D**). Though with a high AUC value, we further performed Decision Curve Analysis (DCA), which indicated that the nomogram did predict anemia outcome better than no model for predicting (**Figure 2E**).

DISCUSSION

A nomogram was established using five preoperative factors to predict postoperative anemia in patients who underwent TKA. Before and after TKA, it would probably be a useful tool for better blood management of individualized patients.

This study was based on previous predictive models with some improvements. First of all, at the level of method design, the endpoint was widened from transfusion to anemia, which differed from previous researches (9–13). Those who had postoperative Hb lower than 90 g/L but didn't meet the indications for transfusion were not usually included in previous researches, yet their relatively mild anemia had also been identified to adversely influence the recovery, discharge and life quality change after orthopedic surgeries (14); also, they could do damage to major organs such as kidney, heart, brain, etc. (15). Indeed, even no surgeries were performed, anemia that did not need transfusion was found to be associated with increased risk of hospitalization and mortality of any cause; and anemic elderly people tended to be in worse condition for cognition and mood (16). All in all, previous studies had strongly suggested long-term side effects of

TABLE 1 | Basic characteristics of patients from both training and validation cohort.

Variables	Training cohort		Validation cohort		p-value
	N **1,517**	**%** **70.1**	**N** **648**	**%** **29.9**	
Age (years)					0.948
<60	206	(13.6)	85	(13.1)	
60–65	293	(19.3)	135	(20.8)	
65–70	422	(27.8)	180	(27.8)	
70–75	302	(19.9)	125	(19.3)	
>75	294	(19.4)	123	(19.0)	
Sex					0.366
Male	1,395	(92.0)	611	(94.3)	
Female	122	(8.0)	37	(5.7)	
BMI (kg/m²)					0.136
<24	280	(18.5)	143	(22.1)	
24–28	655	(43.0)	273	(42.1)	
>28	584	(35.8)	232	(35.8)	
Smoking					0.069
Yes	122	(8.0)	37	(5.7)	
No	1,395	(92.0)	611	(94.3)	
Drinking					0.591
Yes	58	(3.8)	21	(3.2)	
No	1,459	(96.2)	627	(96.8)	
Drug					0.335
Yes	175	(11.5)	85	(13.1)	
No	1,342	(88.5)	563	(86.9)	
Infusion of protein					0.679
Yes	408	(26.9)	168	(25.9)	
No	1,109	(73.1)	480	(74.1)	
Abnormally high CRP levels					0.912
Yes	197	(13)	86	(13.3)	
No	1,320	(87)	562	(86.7)	
Abnormally high ESR levels					0.451
Yes	357	(23.5)	163	(25.2)	
No	1,160	(76.5)	485	(74.8)	
Hb < 12.0 g/dL (male) or <11.0 g/dL (female) (preoperative anemia or not)					0.861
Yes	66	(4.4)	30	(4.6)	
No	1,451	(95.6)	618	(95.4)	
Sides of TKA					0.058
One side	494	(32.6)	239	(36.9)	
Two sides	1,023	(67.4)	409	(63.1)	
Number of comorbidities					0.97
<2 kinds of comorbidities	732	(48.3)	313	(48.3)	
2 kinds of comorbidities	385	(25.4)	167	(25.8)	
>2 kinds of comorbidities	400	(26.4)	168	(25.9)	
Anemia in three days after operation					0.778
Yes	253	(16.7)	112	(17.3)	
No	1,264	(83.3)	536	(82.7)	

Data are n (%) or mean ± SD. Bold represents p-value of the variable is less than 0.05.

TABLE 2 | Postoperative anemia of TKA: univariate and multivariate analysis of possible risk factors in the training cohort.

Variables	Univariate analysis OR (95% CI)	p-value	Multivariate analysis Adjusted OR (95% CI)	p-value
Age (years)				
<60	1.000			
60–65	1.131 (0.709–1.804)	0.605		
65–70	0.955 (0.617–1.480)	0.838		
70–75	0.977 (0.655–1.459)	0.911		
>75	0.992 (0.644–1.527)	0.971		
Sex				
Female	1.000		1.000	
Male	0.440 (0.283–0.686)	**<0.001**	0.458 (0.289–0.727)	**<0.001**
Drug				
No	1.000			
Yes	0.732 (0.461–1.160)	0.732		
BMI (kg/m²)				
<24	1.000		1.000	
24–28	0.832 (0.591–1.169)	0.289	0.683 (0.471–0.991)	**0.045**
>28	0.417 (0.284–0.611)	**0**	0.312 (0.206–0.473)	**<0.001**
Infusion of protein				
No	1			
Yes	0.793 (0.590–1.065)	0.123		
Abnormally high CRP levels				
No	1			
Yes	0.880 (0.596–1.299)	0.520		
Hb < 12.0 g/dL (male) or <11.0 g/dL (female) (preoperative anemia or not)				
No	1			
Yes	4.903 (2.962–8.117)	**<0.001**	5.671 (3.156–5.714)	
Abnormally high ESR levels				
No	1.000		1.000	
Yes	1.537 (1.140–2.073)	**0.005**		
Sides of TKA				
One side	1			
Two sides	3.740 (2.829–4.943)	**<0.001**	4.247 (3.156–5.714)	**<0.001**
Number of comorbidities				
<2 kinds of comorbidities	1.000			
2 kinds of comorbidities	0.999 (0.714–1.397)	0.994		
>2 kinds of comorbidities	1.162 (0.942–1.602)	0.361		
Anemia in three days after operation				
No	1,264 (83.3%)			
Yes	253 (16.7%)			

anemia on patients who did not need transfusion. Thus, it is worth for surgeons to know that no need for transfusion does not mean no demand for blood management; and undoubtedly, this study provided a better predictive method for blood management of patients, including consideration of side effects of anemia which did not need transfusion. In contrast to models which simply included preoperative hemoglobin as the cut-off value for transfusion (17), the nomogram in this study consisting of multiple predictors is even more advantageous in comprehensively evaluating patients' conditions. In terms of participants, the nearly three thousand ones ensured the accuracy and feasibility of the nomogram to a certain extent; and investigating both unilateral and bilateral TKA provided more reasonable evidence in explaining postoperative anemia than simply covering unilateral ones (9, 11, 13). In addition, we ensured

TABLE 3 | Postoperative anemia of TKA: univariate and multivariate analysis of possible risk factors in the validation cohort.

Variables	Univariate analysis OR (95% CI)	p-value	Multivariate analysis Adjusted OR (95% CI)	p-value
Age (years)				
<60	1.000			
60–65	0.764 (0.385–1.520)	0.443		
65–70	0.836 (0.439–1.589)	0.584		
70–75	0.709 (0.350–1.437)	0.340		
>75	0.638 (0.310–1.313)	0.222		
Sex				
Female	1.000		1.000	
Male	0.306 (0.138–0.678)	**0.004**	0.399 (0.177–0.900)	**0.027**
Drug				
No	1.000			
Yes	0.846 (0.451–1.588)	0.603		
BMI (kg/m²)				
<24	1.000			
24–28	0.747 (0.440–1.266)	0.278		
>28	0.908 (0.534–1.544)	0.721		
Infusion of protein				
No	1.000			
Yes	0.697 (0.424–1.145)	0.154		
Abnormally high CRP levels				
No	1.000			
Yes	1.211 (0.682–2.152)	0.514		
Hb < 12.0 g/dL (male) or <11.0 g/dL (female) (preoperative anemia or not)				
No	1.000		1.000	
Yes	6.214 (2.937–13.15)	**<0.001**	6.152 (2.724–13.89)	**<0.001**
Abnormally high ESR levels				
No	1.000	1.000		
Yes	2.160 (1.403–3.326)	**0.000**	1.666 (1.043–2.66)	0.033
Sides of TKA				
One side	1.000			
Two sides	2.63 (1.737–3.981)	**<0.001**	2.90 (1.866–4.495)	**<0.001**
Number of comorbidities				
<2 kinds of comorbidities	1.000			
2 kinds of comorbidities	0.946 (0.570–1.571)	0.830		
>2 kinds of comorbidities	1.154 (0.710–1.875)	0.562		

that patients in both the training and validation cohorts received the operation in relatively the same period of time, thus preventing interference of changing with the operation and ensuring the stability of baseline.

After both univariate and multivariate regression analyses, a total of five risk factors were found to be associated with postoperative anemia: female sex, low BMI, low preoperative hemoglobin level, high levels of ESR, and simultaneous bilateral TKA. These predictors were in line with our perceived common sense, and were also mentioned in several previous studies. Females tended to have lower Hb levels before surgery;

Steuber et al. identified females accounting for 92% of patients with pre-operative iron deficiency anemia (18). Biboulet et.al found blood transfusion was more common in females through univariate analysis, though such significance disappeared in multivariate analysis (19). Another group of researchers obtained similar results that female patients were more likely to receive transfusion than males (20); thus, it's reasonable that we included sex as one of the predictors in our nomogram.

Low BMI quantifies underweight as reflecting malnutrition to a certain extent. There have already been multiple studies showing people with lower BMI were at higher risk of anemia,

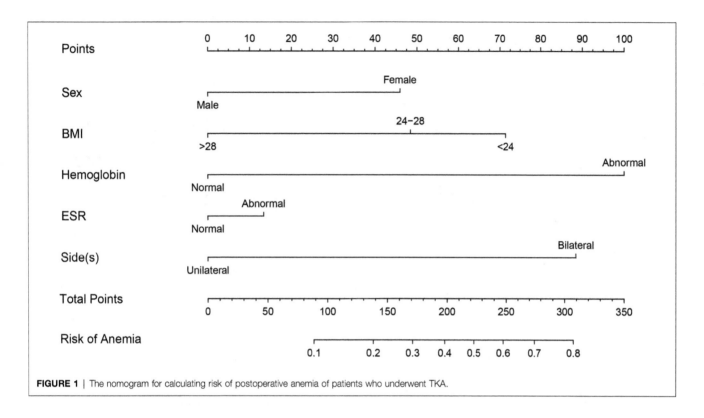

FIGURE 1 | The nomogram for calculating risk of postoperative anemia of patients who underwent TKA.

while in contrast, overweight and obesity were inversely correlated with anemia (21–23). In research specifically accessing in-hospital outcomes among underweight patients after operations, low BMI was particularly pointed out to be an important risk factor for poor clinical outcomes including postoperative anemia, considering that such patients were more prone to poorer nutritional reserves and more susceptible to other comorbidities (24). However, not all similar predictive models considered low BMI as a significant risk factor (9, 20); and those models covering BMI didn't agree on the same cut-off value with each other (11, 25, 26), neither of us. This was probably resulted from the differences among participants. In our study, we separated patients into 3 groups of different BMI ranges and identified their contributions to postoperative anemia, which were feasible in both training and validation cohorts.

Among the five, preoperative hemoglobin seems to be the most influential predictor; this has already been validated in multiple previous studies. Gu et.al revealed that preoperative mild anemia was significantly associated with a series of postoperative complications including anemia which required transfusion (27). Similar conclusions were also given by other group of researchers (13, 28), and predictive models included the factor as key predictor (10, 29). Specifically, in our research, we excluded those patients with moderate to severe anemia to prevent possible complex interferences, and set the observational endpoint as postoperative anemia rather than transfusion; even so, mild anemia before operation still had powerful influence. It's easy to understand that anemic patients themselves should have disorders in the production of hemoglobin; and TKA, a

blood-consuming operation undoubtedly could not correct such disorders but promote their exacerbation.

A relatively surprising finding turned out to be the effect of ESR; few studies and predictive models mentioned it. In our nomogram, this factor did not show as strong an effect as other factors, yet it remained significant after both univariate as well as multivariate regression analyses. Cathrin et.al pointed out that anemia frequently accompanied chronic diseases, which were related to systemic inflammation, as reflected by markers like ESR (30). Examples of possible chronic diseases include chronic obstructive pulmonary diseases (COPD), and anemia was found to be independently correlated with ESR in COPD patients (31). In our study, patients undergoing TKA were relatively elderly and had a relatively high probability of suffering from chronic diseases.

Finally, bilateral TKA in the same operation was a significant risk factor compared to unilateral one, and the effect was only secondary to preoperative anemia. Relevant researches were plenty, and above-mentioned effect could be understood easily. Many models contained sides of TKA (10, 25, 29); in bilateral TKA, time for operation tended to be longer, and more autologous blood could be lost, which could probably explain such effects.

Since the predictive model was constructed, indicating the clinical utility of the model seems to be quite significant, though high AUC values were received; thus, DCA was performed, showing that the nomogram presented a net benefit which was much higher than both the treat-none and treat-all lines. This is significant for developing countries, considering the possible economic burden from ferralia

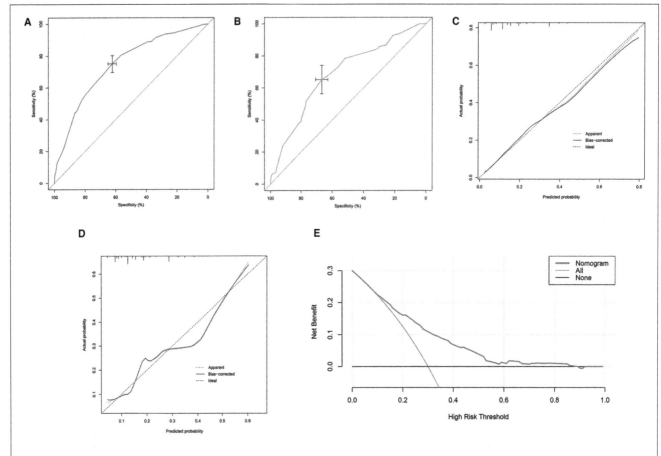

FIGURE 2 | The receiver operating characteristic (ROC) curve of training cohort (**A**) validation cohort (**B**), the calibration curve of training cohort (**C**) and validation cohort (**B**), and decision curve analysis (DCA) of training set (**E**).

consumption. Therefore, the nomogram could be a utilitarian tool for clinicians to better perform blood management in advanced and timely care to prevent severe endings of anemia.

Several factors were identified to be irrelevant for postoperative anemia, such as age, smoking, drinking, drug taking, high CRP levels, comorbidities, etc. In previous researches, predictors like age, comorbidities, etc showed significant results and were included in the predictive models in previous researches (10, 11, 32); unfortunately, such relevance was not identified in this study, along with other factors such as high CRP levels, smoking, drug taking. The varied results across studies could be explained by diverse composition of patients, different tyoes of surgeries as well as the varied design of the studies. Particularly, postoperative anemia was not found to be associated with comorbidities in this study. According to previous studies, diabetes, one of the classic chronic comorbidities, was identified to be related to anemia through functional erythropoietin deficiency (33); others also identified possible interactions between coronary heart diseases and anemia (34). However, those with serious comorbidities were not able to receive the operation and were excluded from the very beginning. As a selective operation, TKA was performed to improve the life quality of patients

who would otherwise not have received the operation, and to improve management of comorbidities. Thus, it is reasonable to believe that comorbidities may not be associated with postoperative anemia in such well-managed patients.

There are some limitations in this study. First of all, this is a single-center study without external validation in other medical centers. This weakened the feasibility of our model to a certain extent; we therefore welcome colleagues from all over the world to try the nomogram in perioperative blood management for patients undergoing TKA. Secondly, though more than 2,000 patients were included in the study, the sample size was still limited. More patients are expected to be studied to generate even better results in the future.

CONCLUSION

In this study, female, lower BMI, lower preoperative Hb levels, simultaneous bilateral TKA, and higher levels of preoperative ESR were identified as five independent risk factors for postoperative anemia (<9.0 g/dL) in patients undergoing TKA. This is a typical clinical study of level 4 of evidence. To better predict risk of such postoperative anemia, a nomogram integrating all of the factors was constructed which could greatly help to predict the risk of postoperative anemia requiring intervention.

and institutional requirements. The patients/participants provided their written informed consent to participate in this study.

ETHICS STATEMENT

Ethical review and approval was not required for the study on human participants in accordance with the local legislation and institutional requirements. The patients/participants provided their written informed consent to participate in this study.

Ethical review and approval was not required for the study on human participants in accordance with the local legislation

AUTHOR CONTRIBUTIONS

CH put forward the idea of the research and performed the statistics of the whole study. YMD integrated all of the results and wrote the most of the article. XSW provided guidance on design of the research and writing of the article. All authors contributed to the article and approved the submitted version.

REFERENCES

1. Kurtz S, Ong K, Lau E, Mowat F, Halpern M. Projections of primary and revision hip and knee arthroplasty in the United States from 2005 to 2030. *J Bone Joint Surg Am.* (2007) 89(4): 780–5. doi: 10.2106/00004623-200704000-00012
2. Lawrence RC, Felson DT, Helmick CG, Arnold LM, Choi H, Deyo RA. Estimates of the prevalence of arthritis and other rheumatic conditions in the United States. Part II. *Arthritis Rheum.* (2008) 58(1):26–35. doi: 10.1002/art.23176
3. Rasouli MR, Restrepo C, Maltenfort MG, Purtill JJ, Parvizi J. Risk factors for surgical site infection following total joint arthroplasty. *J Bone Joint Surg Am.* (2014) 96(18):e158. doi: 10.2106/JBJS.M.01363
4. Foss NB, Kristensen MT, Kehlet H. Anaemia impedes functional mobility after hip fracture surgery. *Age Ageing.* (2008) 37(2):173–8. doi: 10.1093/ageing/afm161
5. Spahn DR. Anemia and patient blood management in hip and knee surgery: a systematic review of the literature. *Anesthesiology.* (2010) 113(2):482–95. doi: 10.1097/ALN.0b013e3181e08e97
6. Conlon NP, Bale EP, Herbison GP, McCarroll M. Postoperative anemia and quality of life after primary hip arthroplasty in patients over 65 years old. *Anesth Analg.* (2008) 106(4): 1056–61. doi: 10.1213/ane.0b013e318164f114
7. Kristensen SD, Knuuti J, Saraste A, Anker S, Bøtker HE, De Hert S. 2014 ESC/ESA Guidelines on non-cardiac surgery: cardiovascular assessment and management: the Joint Task Force on non-cardiac surgery: cardiovascular assessment and management of the European Society of Cardiology (ESC) and the European Society of Anaesthesiology (ESA). *Eur Heart J.* (2014) 35 (35):2383–431. doi: 10.1093/eurheartj/ehu285
8. Armitage JN, van der Meulen JH, G. Royal College of Surgeons Co-morbidity Consensus. Identifying co-morbidity in surgical patients using administrative data with the Royal College of Surgeons Charlson Score. *Br J Surg.* (2010) 97(5): 772–81. doi: 10.1002/bjs.6930
9. Noticewala MS, Nyce JD, Wang W, Geller JA, Macaulay W. Predicting need for allogeneic transfusion after total knee arthroplasty. *J Arthroplasty.* (2012) 27(6):961–7. doi: 10.1016/j.arth.2011.10.008
10. Hu C, Wang Y-H, Shen R, Liu C, Sun K, Ye L. Development and validation of a nomogram to predict perioperative blood transfusion in patients undergoing total knee arthroplasty. *BMC Musculoskelet Disord.* (2020) 21 (1):315. doi: 10.1186/s12891-020-03328-9
11. Hart A, Khalil JA, Carli A, Huk O, Zukor D, Antoniou J. Blood transfusion in primary total hip and knee arthroplasty. Incidence, risk factors, and thirty-day complication rates. *J Bone Joint Surg Am.* (2014) 96(23):1945–51. doi: 10.2106/JBJS.N.00077
12. Jans Ø, Jørgensen C, Kehlet H, Johansson PI. Role of preoperative anemia for risk of transfusion and postoperative morbidity in fast-track hip and knee arthroplasty. *Transfusion.* (2014) 54(3):717–26. doi: 10.1111/trt.12332

13. Maempel JF, Wickramasinghe NR, Clement ND, Brenkel IJ, Walmsley PJ. The pre-operative levels of haemoglobin in the blood can be used to predict the risk of allogenic blood transfusion after total knee arthroplasty. *Bone Joint J.* (2016) 98-b(4):490–7. doi: 10.1302/0301-620X.98B4.36245
14. Jans Ø, Bandholm T, Kurbegovic S, Solgaard S, Kjaersgaard-Andersen P, Johansson PI. Postoperative anemia and early functional outcomes after fast-track hip arthroplasty: a prospective cohort study. *Transfusion.* (2016) 56(4): 917–25. doi: 10.1111/trf.13508
15. Choi YJ, Kim S-O, Sim JH, Hahm K-D. Postoperative anemia is associated with acute kidney injury in patients undergoing total hip replacement arthroplasty: a retrospective study. *Anesth Analg.* (2016) 122(6):1923–8. doi: 10.1213/ANE.0000000000001003
16. Lucca U, Tettamanti M, Mosconi P, Apolone G, Gandini F, Nobili A. Association of mild anemia with cognitive, functional, mood and quality of life outcomes in the elderly: the "Health and Anemia" study. *PLoS One.* (2008) 3(4):e1920. doi: 10.1371/journal.pone.0001920
17. Yeh JZY, Chen JY, Razak HRBA, Loh BHG, Hao Y, Yew AKS. Preoperative haemoglobin cut-off values for the prediction of post-operative transfusion in total knee arthroplasty. *Knee Surg Sports Traumatol Arthrosc.* (2016) 24 (10):3293–8. doi: 10.1007/s00167-016-4183-1
18. Steuber TD, Howard ML, Nisly SA. Strategies for the management of postoperative anemia in elective orthopedic surgery. *Ann Pharmacother.* (2016) 50(7):578–85. doi: 10.1177/1060028016647977
19. Biboulet P, Motais C, Pencole M, Karam O, Dangelser G, Smilevitch P. Preoperative erythropoietin within a patient blood management program decreases both blood transfusion and postoperative anemia: a prospective observational study. *Transfusion.* (2020) 60(8): 1732–40. doi: 10.1111/trf.15900
20. Klement MR, Peres-Da-Silva A, Nickel BT, Green CL, Wellman SS, Attarian DE. What should define preoperative anemia in primary THA? *Clin Orthop Relat Res.* (2017) 475(11):2683–91. doi: 10.1007/s11999-017-5469-4
21. Ghose B, Yaya S, Tang S. Anemia status in relation to body mass index among women of childbearing age in Bangladesh. *Asia Pac J Public Health.* (2016) 28(7):611–9. doi: 10.1177/1010539516660374
22. Kamruzzaman M. Is BMI associated with anemia and hemoglobin level of women and children in Bangladesh: a study with multiple statistical approaches. *PLoS One.* (2021) 16(10):e0259116. doi: 10.1371/journal.pone.0259116
23. Qin Y, Melse-Boonstra A, Pan X, Yuan B, Dai Y, Zhao J. Anemia in relation to body mass index and waist circumference among Chinese women. *Nutr J.* (2013) 12:10. doi: 10.1186/1475-2891-12-10
24. Anoushiravani AA, Sayeed Z, Chambers MC, Gilbert TJ, Scaife SL, El-Othmani MM. Assessing in-hospital outcomes and resource utilization after primary total joint arthroplasty among underweight patients. *J Arthroplasty.* (2016) 31(7):1407-12. doi: 10.1016/j.arth.2015.12.053
25. Mufarrih SH, Qureshi NQ, Ali A, Malik AT, Naim H, Noordin S. Total knee Arthroplasty: risk factors for allogeneic blood transfusions in the South Asian population. *BMC Musculoskelet Disord.* (2017) 18(1):359. doi: 10.1186/s12891-017-1728-5

Preoperative anaemia in primary hip and knee arthroplasty. *Z Orthop Unfall.* (2020) 158(2):194–200. doi: 10.1055/a-0974-4115

Jo C, Ko S, Shin WC, Han H-S, Lee MC, Ko T, Ro DH. Transfusion after total knee arthroplasty can be predicted using the machine learning algorithm. *Knee Surg Sports Traumatol Arthrosc.* (2020) 28(6):1757–64. doi: 10.1007/ s00167-019-05602-3

Nikolaisen C, Figenschau Y, Nossent JC. Anemia in early rheumatoid arthritis is associated with interleukin 6-mediated bone marrow suppression, but has no effect on disease course or mortality. *J Rheumatol* (2008) 35(3):380–6.

Corsonello A, Pedone C, Battaglia S, Paglino G, Bellia V, Incalzi RA. C-reactive protein (CRP) and erythrocyte sedimentation rate (ESR) as inflammation markers in elderly patients with stable chronic obstructive pulmonary disease (COPD). *Arch Gerontol Geriatr.* (2011) 53(2): 190–5. doi: 10.1016/j. archger.2010.10.015

Cao G, Yang X, Xu H, Yue C, Huang Z, Zhang S. Association between preoperative hemoglobin and postoperative moderate and severe anemia among patients undergoing primary total knee arthroplasty: a single-center retrospective study. *J Orthop Surg Res.* (2021) 16(1): 572. doi: 10.1186/ s13018-021-02727-5

Thomas MC. The high prevalence of anemia in diabetes is linked to functional erythropoietin deficiency. *Semin Nephrol.* (2006) 26(4):275–82. doi: 10.1016/j. semnephrol.2006.05.003

Rymer JA, Rao SV. Anemia and coronary artery disease: pathophysiology, prognosis, and treatment. *Coron Artery Dis.* (2018) 29(2):161–7. doi: 10. 1097/ MCA.0000000000000598

15

Type-I Interferon Signaling in Fanconi Anemia

Karima Landelouci [1,2], Shruti Sinha [3] and Geneviève Pépin [1,2]*

[1] Département de Biologie Médicale, Université du Québec à Trois-Rivières, Trois-Rivières, QC, Canada, [2] Groupe de Recherche en Signalisation Cellulaire, Université du Québec à Trois-Rivières, Trois-Rivières, QC, Canada, [3] Department of Biotechnology, GITAM Institute of Technology, GITAM deemed to be University, Visakhapatnam, India

*Correspondence:
Geneviève Pépin
Genevieve.pepin3@uqtr.ca

Fanconi Anemia (FA) is a genome instability syndrome caused by mutations in one of the 23 repair genes of the Fanconi pathway. This heterogenous disease is usually characterized by congenital abnormalities, premature ageing and bone marrow failure. FA patients also show a high predisposition to hematological and solid cancers. The Fanconi pathway ensures the repair of interstrand crosslinks (ICLs) DNA damage. Defect in one of its proteins prevents functional DNA repair, leading to the accumulation of DNA breaks and genome instability. Accumulating evidence has documented a close relationship between genome instability and inflammation, including the production of type-I Interferon. In this context, type-I Interferon is produced upon activation of pattern recognition receptors by nucleic acids including by the cyclic GMP-AMP synthase (cGAS) that detects DNA. In mouse models of diseases displaying genome instability, type-I Interferon response is responsible for an important part of the pathological symptoms, including premature aging, short stature, and neurodegeneration. This is illustrated in mouse models of Ataxia-telangiectasia and Aicardi-Goutières Syndrome in which genetic depletion of either Interferon Receptor IFNAR, cGAS or STING relieves pathological symptoms. FA is also a genetic instability syndrome with symptoms such as premature aging and predisposition to cancer. In this review we will focus on the different molecular mechanisms potentially leading to type-I Interferon activation. A better understanding of the molecular mechanisms engaging type-I Interferon signaling in FA may ultimately lead to the discovery of new therapeutic targets to rescue the pathological inflammation and premature aging associated with Fanconi Anemia.

Keywords: Fanconi anemia, interferon, inflammation, DNA damage, cytosolic DNA, cGAS/STING, RIG-I

INTRODUCTION

Fanconi anemia (FA) is a rare recessive disease characterized by genome instability that results from a defect in the Fanconi DNA repair pathway. FA patients present aplastic anemia, congenital defects and cancer predisposition (Rodriguez and D'Andrea, 2017). Mechanistically, the FA pathway contributes to DNA damage recognition and repair, thus mutations in genes encoding FA pathway proteins lead to DNA damage accumulation and chromosome instability. As of today, 23 Fanconi and Fanconi-like DNA repair genes encoding either core complex proteins (FANCA, FANCB, FANCC, FANCE, FANCF, FANCG, FANCL and FANCM), ID2 complex proteins (FANCD2 and FANCI), and downstream proteins (FANCD1 (BRCA2), FANCJ (BRIP1), FANCN (PALB2), FANCO (RAD51C), FANCP (SLX4), FANCQ (ERCC4), FANCR (RAD51), FANCS (BRCA1), FANCT (UBE2T), FANCU (XRXX2), FANCV (MAD2L2/REV7), FANCW (RFWD3) and FANCY) have been identified. Findings from the last decade have unambiguously improved the management of the disease and prolonged the life of patients, and the many FA mouse models developed along the years were invaluable in getting a better understanding of the underlying cause of FA (Guitton-Sert et al., 2021).

FA PROTEINS ARE INVOLVED IN DNA REPAIR PROCESSES

The primary role attributed to FA proteins is the repair of interstrand crosslinks (ICLs) DNA damage. ICLs, known to interfere with DNA replication and transcription, can be caused by exogenous sources such as chemotherapeutic agents like cisplatin and mitomycin C, or by endogenous cellular products like aldehydes. ICLs are repaired by the FA pathway (**Figure 1**), in the S-phase of the cell cycle (Knipscheer et al., 2009). The ICLs

are first recognized by the FANCM–MHF1–MHF2 complex (Singh et al., 2010), followed by the activation of FANCM, which allows the recruitment of the core complex composed of ten proteins (FANCA, FANCB, FANCC, FANCE, FANCF, FANCG, FANCL, FA associated protein 100 (FAAP100), FAAP20 and FAAP24). The core complex possesses an ubiquitin E3 ligase that upon detection of the ICLs will monoubiquitinate FANCI and FANCD2 (ID2 complex) to form a higher order structure that initiates DNA repair (Tan et al., 2020; Tan and Deans, 2021). This latter step is essential to recruit nucleases such as FANCP (SLX4) – FANCQ (XPF) and FAN1, and to activate downstream repair factors that belong to the Homologous Recombination (HR) DNA repair complex: FANCJ – FANCN (PALB2) – FANCD1 (BRCA2) – FANCO (RAD51C) (Tan et al., 2020; Tan and Deans, 2021).

Besides the repair of ICLs, FA proteins are involved in other aspects of genome stability maintenance (Rodriguez and D'Andrea, 2017). For instance, the FA pathway stabilizes the replication fork during DNA synthesis to prevent accumulation of ssDNA or DNA-RNA hybrids called R-loops (Garcia-Rubio et al., 2015; Schwab et al., 2015; Xu et al., 2021). FANCJ promotes

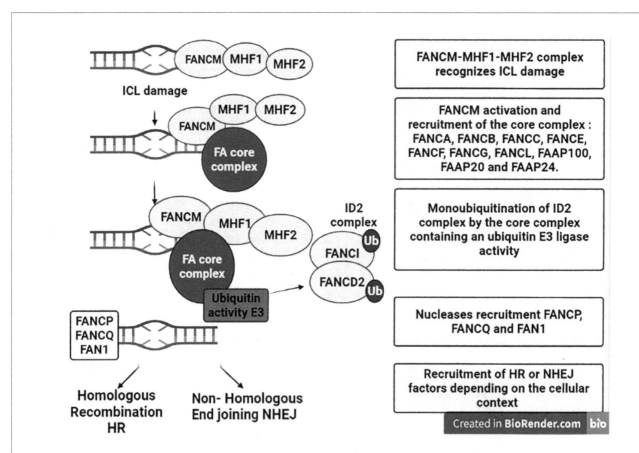

FIGURE 1 | Schematic representation of ICLs repair by the Fanconi Anemia pathway. The protein complex composed of FANCM-MHF1-MHF2 is recruited to the chromatin upon recognition of ICL damage. Then, FANCM is activated and allows the recruitment of the core complex of the FA pathway composed of: FANCA, FANCB, FANCC, FANCE, FANCF, FANCG, FANCL, FAAP100, FAAP20 and FAAP24. The core complex contains an ubiquitin E3 ligase activity and is responsible for the monoubiquitylation of the ID2 complex composed of FANCI and FANCD2 proteins. Monoubiquitinylation of ID2 complex promotes the recruitment of the nucleases FANP, FANCQ and FAN1 and end resection at the DNA damage site. Depending on the cellular context, recruitment of downstream factors belonging to either Homologous Recombination (HR) or to Non-homologous End Joining (NHEJ) will finalize the repair.

RPA phosphorylation during nucleotide excision repair (NER) and interacts with the mismatched repair (MMR) proteins MLH1 and MSH2 after UV irradiation to maintain genome stability (Guillemette et al., 2014). Furthermore, FANCC and FANCD2 cooperate with P53 to maintain the DNA damage-induced G2 checkpoint (Freie et al., 2004). FANCA and FANCB were both reported to catalyze single-strand annealing and strand exchange independently of their canonical role in the FA pathway (Benitez et al., 2018). The FA pathway is also linked to the maintenance of telomere integrity as FANCD2 mutated patient cells display several telomeric abnormalities (Joksic et al., 2012). How these different genome stabilization roles directly translate into all of the FA associated pathological symptoms, however, remains to be clarified. Interestingly, in previous studies FA-patients- or FA mouse models-derived cells with mutation in either FANCA, B, C or D, were shown to express higher levels of pro-inflammatory cytokines. In addition, FA cells (FANCA, B, C, D) were more susceptible to inflammatory stimulus (Rosselli et al., 1994; Dufour et al., 2003). These phenotypes were partly attributed to the dysregulated anti-oxidative response, as exemplified by the observation that FANCC knock-out cells express lower levels of anti-oxidative response genes and display higher levels of reactive oxygen species (ROS) (Zhang et al., 2007; Sejas et al., 2007).

During the last decade, a series of studies have demonstrated the complex intertwined relationship between DNA repair processes and immune responses. One key signaling axis involved in this association is the type-I Interferon (IFN-I) response known to play a critical role in the antiviral response (Taffoni et al., 2021). IFN-I response is essential to induce the transcription of genes involved in DNA repair and in nucleic acid degradation. Therefore, in the presence of defects in DNA repair processes or nucleic acid metabolism, cellular immune receptors can be activated by self-nucleic acids (Taffoni et al., 2021). Given that new evidence suggests that loss of function of FA proteins causes IFN-I production (Bregnard et al., 2016; Reislander et al., 2019; Heijink et al., 2019), this review explores how defect in the FA pathway might contribute to the accumulation of cytosolic nucleic acids and activation of IFN-I (**Figure 2**).

MICROBIAL NUCLEIC ACIDS ARE DETECTED BY CELLULAR RECEPTORS

During infections, cells rely on a complex system of cellular receptors called Pattern Recognition Receptors (PRRs) that recognize pathogen-associated molecular patterns (PAMPs) to elicit an immune response that will allow the cell to defend itself against the invaders and alert neighboring immune cells of the ongoing infection. Microbial nucleic acids are among these PAMPs and are detected by different families of PRRs including Toll-like receptors (TLR), RIG-I like receptors (RLR)

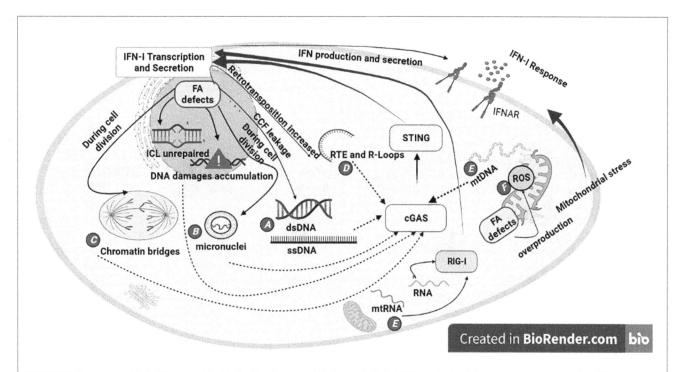

FIGURE 2 | Proposed model depicting how defect in the FA pathway could induce pathological IFN-I production. FA proteins prevent genome instability by repairing DNA damage, repressing retrotransposition and allowing accurate cell division. In addition, FA proteins modulate anti-oxidative response and participate in mitochondria clearance by autophagy and mitophagy processes. Mutations in FA genes or loss of FA proteins contribute to DNA damage accumulation, genome instability, reactive oxygen species (ROS) production and defect in mitochondria's clearance. Under these pathological conditions, many types of self-nucleic acids such as ssDNA and dsDNA **(A)**, micronuclei **(B)** chromatin bridges **(C)** retroelements (RTE) and R-loops **(D)**, mtDNA/RNA **(E)**, can activate type-I Interferon (IFN-I). This would occur by cGAS and RIG-I detection of cytosolic DNA and RNA molecules respectively and subsequent production of IFN-I. In addition, elevated levels of ROS might contribute to fuel the production of IFN-I by creating more DNA and mitochondria damage **(F)**.

and cyclic GMP-AMP synthase (cGAS) (Kretschmer and Lee-Kirsch, 2017). TLRs that detect nucleic acids (TLR3-7-8 detect RNA and TLR9 detects DNA) are found predominantly within endosomes and are mostly expressed in specialized immune cells (monocytes, macrophages, dendritic cells and B lymphocytes) (Schlee and Hartmann, 2016). On the contrary, RLR and cGAS are expressed ubiquitously and are located within the cytoplasm of cells. While RIG -I and MDA-5 activate IFN-I upon sensing short and long cytosolic dsRNA respectively (Reikine et al., 2014), cGAS detects dsDNA (or ssDNA fold into dsDNA) and DNA : RNA hybrids (Ablasser et al., 2013; Mankan et al., 2014; Schlee and Hartmann, 2016). Upon sensing their specific nucleic acids, these PRRs activate an immune response that leads to the production of inflammatory cytokines and type I-Interferons (IFN-I). Cells and organisms rely on this response to fight microbial infections.

SENSING OF NUCLEIC ACIDS BY CELLULAR RECEPTORS ACTIVATES THE TYPE-I INTERFERON RESPONSE

At the molecular level, RIG-I and MDA5 receptors signal through the Mitochondrial antiviral-signaling adaptor protein (MAVS) to allow the translocation and activation of Interferon Regulatory Factor 3 (IRF3) that binds to regulatory elements on IFN-I genes to induce their transcription and translation (Schlee and Hartmann, 2016). Binding of IFN-I in an autocrine or paracrine manner activates Janus Kinase 1 (JAK1) and Tyrosine Kinase 2 (TYK2), which then phosphorylate the Signal Transducer and Activator of Transcription 1 (STAT1) and 2 (STAT2) transcription factors to allow the transcription of thousands of genes collectively referred to as Interferon Stimulated Genes (ISGs) (Platanias, 2005; Rusinova et al., 2013). These genes are known to alter cellular metabolism, arrest the cell cycle, induce apoptosis and favor the clearance of damaged cells by immune cells (Rusinova et al., 2013).

Upon cytosolic DNA detection, cGAS catalyzes the production of the cyclic dinucleotide GMP-AMP (cGAMP) from ATP and GTP (Ablasser et al., 2013). Then, cGAMP acts as a secondary messenger to activate the Stimulator of Interferon Genes (STING), inducing its conformational change and subsequent activation (Ablasser et al., 2013; Wu et al., 2013; Sun et al., 2013). In its activated form, STING interacts with Tank-binding Kinase I (TBK1) and the IKK complex to activate them, which leads to STING phosphorylation by TBK1, then recruitment and activation of IRF3 followed by the release of Nuclear Factor-kappaB (NF-κB), ultimately promoting the production of IFN-I and other inflammatory cytokines (Balka and De Nardo, 2021). During acute immune responses, IFN-I activation is usually beneficial to the host by providing transcriptional changes that allow the orchestration of an efficient response. However, when this activation persists, it becomes detrimental and is associated with chronic diseases (Crow and Stetson, 2021).

CYTOSOLIC ACCUMULATION OF SELF-NUCLEIC ACIDS ALLOWS ACTIVATION OF RLRs AND cGAS

During the last decades, these PRRs were also shown to alert the host of the loss of cellular integrity. Indeed, RLRs and cGAS can also detect self-nucleic acids in non-infectious contexts (Ablasser and Hur, 2020). To prevent unwanted inflammation, nucleic acids are usually protected from recognition by PRRs by localizing inside organelles or by being coated with proteins. However, under certain cellular conditions, these barriers are broken and self-nucleic acids are released into the cytosol. Fortunately, to avoid persistent immune activation, the genome encodes many DNases and RNases to degrade cytosolic nucleic acids (Santa et al., 2021). Whether or not PRRs will get activated by self-nucleic acids is thus dependent on the balance between the activity of DNases and RNases versus the amount of nucleic acids released into the cytosol at a given point. Thus, defect in either of these processes can result in PRR activation. This model has been validated by in vitro experiment, mouse models and clinical data. Indeed, higher levels of circulating IFN-I in mouse models and in patients with mutations in gene encoding DNases and RNases were detected (Crow and Stetson, 2021). In addition to this, organelles and genome integrity also play a critical part in safeguard mechanisms. For instance, the nuclear envelope (NE) protects the genome inside the nucleus, maintains its dynamic shapes and regulates nuclear exchanges with the cytosol. Mutations in NE gene's structure result in the loss of NE integrity and promote genome instability and the release of nucleic acids into the cytosol (Gauthier and Comaills, 2021). Similarly, loss of mitochondria integrity causes mitochondrial (mt) DNA release into the cytosol and immune activation (Lepelley et al., 2021).

CONSTITUTIVE ACTIVATION OF IFN-I IN DNA REPAIR AND DNA METABOLISM RELATED-DISEASES

Constitutive IFN-I activation is detected in different autoinflammatory syndromes such as Aicardi-Goutières syndrome (AGS) and Ataxia-telangiectasia (AT) syndrome. AGS is caused by mutations in genes involved in nucleic acid metabolism such as those encoding the Three Prime Repair Exonuclease 1 (TREX1) (Rice et al., 2007), the RNASEH2 (Crow et al., 2006) and the triphosphohydrolase SAMHD1 (Coquel et al., 2018). In mouse models of AGS, cytosolic DNA accumulation activates IFN-I. Notably, genetic depletion of cgas (Gray et al., 2015), sting (Gall et al., 2012), irf3 or ifnar (Stetson et al., 2008) inhibits the IFN-I response and relieves autoinflammatory symptoms, confirming the important contribution of IFN-I to AGS pathology. AT syndrome is, on the other hand, more closely related to FA pathophysiology and also relies on chronic STING activation (Hartlova et al., 2015; Aguado et al., 2021). AT is caused by mutations in the Ataxia-

Telangiectasia-Mutated kinase (ATM), a master regulator of DNA repair. In fact, loss of ATM activity results in cytosolic DNA accumulation due to genomic instability (Hartlova et al., 2015). This can be explained by the crucial role of ATM in coordinating the cellular response to double-strand DNA breaks (DSBs). AT patients-derived cells and cells isolated from Atm[-/-] mice harbor single-strand (ss)DNA in their cytoplasm and an elevated IFN-I signature. Genetic depletion of sting inhibits the pathological IFN-I response in those cells (Hartlova et al., 2015). As AT shares redundant phenotypes with FA, including high genomic instability, dysregulated immune responses, neurodegeneration, premature aging and predisposition to cancers and leukemias, and considering the preponderant role of IFN-I in AT, it is reasonable to suspect that IFN-I also contributes to the pathophysiology of FA.

FA DEFICIENT CELLS DISPLAY CYTOSOLIC DNA ACCUMULATION

FA is a genome instability syndrome. The literature suggests that FA deficient cells display accumulation of cytosolic DNA, loss of nuclear integrity and a defect in mitochondria clearance (Naim and Rosselli, 2009; Bregnard et al., 2016; Shyamsunder et al., 2016; Sumpter et al., 2016; Reislander et al., 2019; Heijink et al., 2019). As mentioned above, these processes contribute to tipping the scale toward PRR activation and IFN-I production. Indeed, with their reported roles in DNA repair and cell division processes, FA proteins prevent genome instability and cytosolic DNA accumulation. In other genome instability syndromes, higher levels of IFN-I have been linked to neurological disorders, growth delays, premature ageing and skin pathologies among others.

ACCUMULATION OF CYTOSOLIC ssDNA IN CELLS WITH DEFECT IN DNA REPAIR MECHANISMS

Following the elucidation of how ATM deficiency activates the IFN-I response (Hartlova et al., 2015), several other examples of how DNA-repair defects trigger unwanted immune activation through the release of cytosolic ssDNA were reported (Bregnard et al., 2016; Chen et al., 2017; Erdal et al., 2017; Coquel et al., 2018; Gratia et al., 2019; Heijink et al., 2019; Guan et al., 2021). During repair, the ubiquitylated ID2 complex recruits the scaffold protein FANCP/SLX4 which serves as a docking site for the endonucleases that cleave the damaged DNA to create a DSB that will be repaired by homologous recombination (HR). These endonucleases generate ssDNA overhangs that are coated and protected from degradation by the replication protein A (RPA) and the recombinase RAD51. Notably, mutations in proteins controlling long-range DNA resection following double-strand break repair, like the endonuclease MUS81, the Bloom syndrome helicase (BLM) and the exonuclease 1 (EXO1)

result in cytosolic ssDNA accumulation and cGAS-STING-IFN-I activation - a phenotype negatively controlled by the TREX1 exonuclease, which degrades these ssDNA (Ho et al., 2016; Erdal et al., 2017; Guan et al., 2021). Furthermore, knockdown of RPA or RAD51 leads to unprotected ssDNA which favors IFN-I production by the cGAS-STING pathway (Wolf et al., 2016). This phenomenon is seen in at least one other DNA repair mechanism. Indeed, defects in the mismatch repair pathway (MMR) have recently been shown to induce an uncontrolled activity of the EXO1 nuclease, leading to ssDNA release and RPA exhaustion causing cGAS-STING activation (Guan et al., 2021). Given that FA proteins (FANCJ, FANCD2 and BRCA1) were suggested to interact with the MHL1 MMR factor during mismatch repair (Peng et al., 2014), this could be another mechanism that leads to IFN-I production in FA. Together, these data suggest that many factors like nucleases or signaling proteins are implicated in the amount of ssDNA released into the cytosol and thus in the activation of IFN-I. Indeed, in lymphomas, cytosolic DNA presence is dependent on the downstream signaling of Ataxia Telangiectasia and Rad3-related protein (ATR) and to a lesser extent on ATM (Lam et al., 2014). Given that FA deficient cells have defect in DNA repair mechanisms, cytosolic DNA could accumulate and be detected by cGAS to activate the production of IFN-I, as schematized in **Figure 2A**.

THE PRESENCE OF MICRONUCLEI CORRELATES WITH cGAS SELF-DNA SENSING

In addition to ssDNA fragments release, cGAS-STING-dependent IFN-I response correlates with micronuclei generation upon chromosomes mis-segregation (Harding et al., 2017; Mackenzie et al., 2017; Gratia et al., 2019), as represented in **Figure 2B**. In a seminal study, Harding et al. demonstrated that micronuclei formation requires cell division and a functional Non-Homologous End Joining (NHEJ) DNA repair pathway. Hence, inhibition of either NHEJ or cell cycle progression prevents cGAS activation (Harding et al., 2017). However, how the DNA packaged in micronuclei activates cGAS is still under debate. Some plausible explanations include nuclear envelope rupture and then cGAS detection of the released cytosolic DNA (Mackenzie et al., 2017). Alternatively, if nuclear cGAS is packaged within micronuclei, cGAS activation after the nuclear envelope ruptures would require its reactivation because nuclear cGAS displays reduced enzymatic activity (Harding et al., 2017; Gentili et al., 2019; Volkman et al., 2019). There might also be a threshold that needs to be reached/crossed since a recent study suggested that cGAS itself contributes to autophagic clearance of micronuclei (Zhao et al., 2021). Nonetheless, other less-visible DNA structures in cells displaying micronuclei could also contribute to the IFN-I activation. This hypothesis is supported by a new study in which the authors claim that DNA bridges and not micronuclei are responsible for cGAS activation (Flynn and

P.D. and Mitchison, 2021). However, whether cGAS is directly located along DNA bridges and how this positioning would allow cGAS activation remains to be elucidated. New data also proposes that the inclusion of cGAS in micronuclei can be modulated by the end-resection machinery, as pharmaceutical inhibition of end-resection or depletion of its components NBS1 and the DNA endonuclease CtlP favor cGAS localization in micronuclei (Abdisalaam et al., 2020). Of interest, micronuclei were also observed in cancer cells in which FANCD1 (BRCA2) expression was abrogated (Heijink et al., 2019; Reislander et al., 2019). Interestingly, depletion of BRCA2 renders the cells more sensitive to Poly [ADP-ribose] polymerase (PARP) inhibitors (Reislander et al., 2019) and to TNFα cytotoxicity in a cGAS dependent manner (Heijink et al., 2019). Given that cancer cells have already accumulated mutations, whether this would occur in FA patients-derived cells remains to be investigated.

THE cGAS-STING-IFN-I AXIS MIGHT CONTRIBUTE TO THE HR-NHEJ DNA REPAIR SWITCH

FA cells are characterized by a propension to repair their DSBs using the more error-prone and mutagenic NHEJ rather than HR, which utilizes end-resection during the process (Adamo et al., 2010; Eccles et al., 2018). Accordingly, FA proteins cooperate with the kinase ATM to stimulate end-resection repair (Cai et al., 2020). Thus, loss of either ATM or FA proteins shifts the repair mechanism toward NHEJ. Surprisingly, cGAS and STING were both reported to inhibit HR DNA repair, albeit using different mechanisms (Liu et al., 2018; McLaughlin et al., 2020). STING-driven IFN-I production negatively regulates the transcription of genes implicated in HR repair like FANCD2 and other BRCA genes (including FANCC and FANCE). Importantly, treatment with the Jak 1/2 inhibitor, Ruxolitinib, was sufficient to rescue the HR defect, suggesting that their transcriptional repression is a result of IFN-I signaling (McLaughlin et al., 2020). Additionally, cGAS also prevents HR repair by a distinct mechanism. cGAS was shown to translocate to the nuclear compartment upon treatment with DNA damage agents, where cGAS inhibits HR by preventing the formation of PARP1-Timeless complex. However, it is not clear what the contribution of cGAS catalytic activity is in this model since the experiments were performed in U2OS cells which lack expression of the downstream signalling STING protein (Deschamps and Kalamvoki, 2017). Given this newly discovered relationship, it would be of interest to determine if the depletion of cGAS-STING or IFNAR in FA deficient cells would redirect DNA repair toward HR.

cGAS INDEPENDENT ACTIVATION OF IFN-I RESPONSE

As discussed above, cGAS detection of cytosolic DNA is a major route to produce IFN-I upon DNA damage. However, it is worth noting that several other mechanisms were also described. For instance, studies showed that DNA damage induced by etoposide or by doxorubicin instigates an ATM-dependent but cGAS-independent immune response (Luthra et al., 2017; Dunphy et al., 2018). In addition, DNA-dependent protein kinase (DNA-PK) was characterized as another DNA sensor contributing to IFN-I (Ferguson et al., 2012), and more recently, DNA-PK has been suggested to induce a cGAS-STING-independent IFN-I induction upon DNA damage in humans but not in mice, highlighting species differences in immune activation following DNA breaks (Burleigh et al., 2020). Further, DNA-PK antagonizes cGAS activation through inhibition of its catalytic activity. In accordance with a role as a negative regulator of cGAS, cells lacking DNA-PK display an abnormal antiviral response and patients with mutations in the gene encoding DNA-PK suffer from autoimmunity (Sun et al., 2020). Given that cGAS expression itself is induced by IFN-I, cGAS-independent activation of IFN-I is expected to sensitize cells to cGAS detection of cytosolic DNA including R-loops, which are also released in the context of FA (Mankan et al., 2014; Chatzidoukaki et al., 2021). This positive loop might explain why healthy cells do not necessarily engage cGAS upon DNA damage while cells with defect in DNA repair with a basal IFN-I activation have a lower threshold for cGAS engagement (Pepin et al., 2017a; Pepin et al., 2017b).

MICRONUCLEI FORMATION AND CHROMATIN BRIDGES ARE A HALLMARK OF CELLS WITH DEFECTIVE CELL DIVISION

Unrepaired DNA damage during cell division can result in chromatin bridges (**Figure 2C**) and micronuclei formation (**Figure 2B**) and thus cause aneuploidy and genome instability. As mentioned in the previous section, these structures containing genomic DNA can activate cGAS (Harding et al., 2017; Mackenzie et al., 2017; Gratia et al., 2019; Flynn and P.D. and Mitchison, 2021). Besides their roles in DNA repair, evidence suggests that the FA proteins (FANCA, C, D2, D1, G, I, M) also regulate chromosome separation and cytokinesis (Nakanishi et al., 2007; Naim and Rosselli, 2009; Vinciguerra et al., 2010; Kim et al., 2013; Nalepa et al., 2013; Zou et al., 2013). As such, an RNAi screen targeting 16 members of the FA complex showed that FA proteins prevent multinucleation of Taxol-treated cells. The relevance of this finding was confirmed by the fact that multinucleation was only observed in FA patients-derived fibroblast cells treated with Taxol but not in healthy patient cells (Nalepa et al., 2013). In line with their role in cell division, many FA proteins, including FANCA and FANCG, localize to the centrosome or elsewhere on mitotic chromosomes to prevent the formation of ultrafine chromatin bridges (Nakanishi et al., 2007; Naim and Rosselli, 2009; Vinciguerra et al., 2010; Nalepa et al., 2013; Zou et al., 2013). Accordingly, FANCA interacts with the spindle assembly checkpoint to prevent premature anaphase onset and sister chromatids segregation (Nalepa et al., 2013). FANCA is also responsible for centrosome integrity since overexpression of a mutant form leads to an aberrant number of centrosomes (Kim et al., 2013). As micronuclei and chromatin bridges activate cGAS, the defects in chromosome segregation and cytokinesis, observed in FA cells, are logically expected to result in IFN-I production (**Figures 2B, C**).

DEREPRESSION OF RETROELEMENTS RESULTS IN CYTOSOLIC SELF-NUCLEIC ACIDS ACCUMULATION

Retroelements (RTE) such as LINE1 are ancient sequences that occupy around 40% of the genome. They can be transcribed into RNA and retrotranscribed into DNA forming RNA : DNA hybrids. Because of their retrotransposition activity, RTE contributes to genome instability and their expression correlates with ageing and induces IFN-I. Repressing RTE is another function of FA proteins. BRCA1 and the proteins of the FA core complex contribute to the broad repression of RTE, albeit using distinct mechanisms (Mita et al., 2020) (**Figure 2D**). In addition, Laguette's group showed that a mutation in SLX4 (FANCP) or loss of FANCD2 or MUS81 increases retrotransposition and IFN-I activation (Bregnard et al., 2016). Accordingly, treatment of their cells with the retro-transcriptase inhibitor (RTi) Tenofovir abrogates both retrotransposition and IFN-I response. They went on to show that IFN-I production was dependent on the cGAS-STING pathway using specific shRNAs (Bregnard et al., 2016). In cells derived from AGS mouse models, RTE induce both the cGAS-STING (Achleitner et al., 2017) and the RIG-I signaling axes (Zhao et al., 2018). However, the use of RTi *in vivo* did not impact the systemic IFN-I response observed in AGS mouse models while still preventing retrotransposition in the animal cells (Achleitner et al., 2017). Lack of therapeutic effect of RTi in AGS mouse models might be attributed to the difference in the cell population studied *in vitro* vs the cell populations implicated in the pathophysiology of the disease. Thus, the relevance of RTE-driven IFN-I response in FANCP (SLX4) mutated cells to FA pathophysiology warrants further investigation.

FA DEFICIENT CELLS DISPLAY SENESCENT FEATURES

Cellular senescence is defined as a stable cell-cycle arrest. It occurs naturally during embryogenesis and can be triggered in different contexts such as replicative senescence, oncogene-induced senescence or following cellular stress. Apart from developmental senescence, the other senescence categories usually rely on the p53/p21 axis and the pRB/p16 axis, the former usually triggered by DNA damage and genome instability. During senescence, cells undergo major phenotypic and molecular changes including structural changes as well as

secretion of inflammatory molecules, proteases and signalling molecules that are collectively referred to as the senescence associated secretory phenotype (SASP). FA was recently suggested to be a premature ageing disease based on the several senescence characteristics observed in FA cells and patients (Helbling-Leclerc et al., 2021). In many FA mouse models, including Fancd2$^{-/-}$, Fancc$^{-/-}$ and Fanca$^{-/-}$, an exacerbated p53/p21 axis has been documented, contributing to bone marrow failure (Ceccaldi et al., 2012). This hyperactive p53/p21 axis has also been observed in FA patient-derived cells (Ceccaldi et al., 2012). Mechanistically, activation of the p53/p21 axis induces high levels of S-phase inhibitors which stop FA cell's growth leading them to arrest in G0/G1 due to replicative stress (Ceccaldi et al., 2012). Another study reported that FANCD2 proteins prevent the progression of oncogene-induced senescence, meaning that its depletion favors premature senescence (Helbling-Leclerc et al., 2019). In parallel, Tumor Growth Factor β1 (TGFβ1), a known inducer of the cyclin-dependent kinase (CDK) inhibitor p21, is overproduced in cells isolated from the bone marrow of Fancd2$^{-/-}$ mice (Zhang et al., 2016), thus inhibiting hematopoietic stem cell (HSC) cycling and precipitating bone marrow failure by incapacitating the HSC to repopulate progenitor and differentiated blood cells. Notably, specific deletion of either TGFβ1 or p53 rescues bone marrow failure by stimulating HSC cycling (Ceccaldi et al., 2012; Zhang et al., 2016). To overcome this cycling blockade, FA cells overexpressed the transcription factor MYC, which causes proliferative pressure and more DNA damage (Rodriguez et al., 2021). However, HSC cycling stimulation in FA mouse models leads to HSC exhaustion and bone marrow aplasia, indicating that the search for a better target in FA should continue. In this context, IFN-I signalling also promotes HSC cycling at the cost of more DNA damage in Fanca$^{-/-}$ mice (Walter et al., 2015). These studies confirm the close relationship between FA and cell cycle arrest, but whether it is best characterized by senescence remains to be demonstrated. This idea is however supported by the fact that overexpression of SIRT6 histone deacetylases, previously reported to inhibit RTE transcription in Fanca$^{-/-}$ or Fancd2$^{-/-}$ mouse models, rescues stem cell exhaustion by reducing pathological inflammation (Li et al., 2018; Simon et al., 2019). Interestingly, a study showed that RTE are derepressed in late senescence, allowing them to be detected by the cGAS-STING pathway, thus contributing to the IFN-I response (De Cecco et al., 2019).

ACCUMULATION OF CYTOSOLIC DNA DURING SENESCENCE DRIVES IFN-I ACTIVATION

Several reports have established that the cGAS-STING axis is activated in stress-induced senescence (e.g., replicative, oxidative and oncogene-induced senescence). The groups of Chen (Yang et al., 2017), Berger (Dou et al., 2017) and Hornung (Gluck et al., 2017) demonstrated that cytosolic DNA detection by cGAS is a critical step in the amplification of the SASP. The faster spontaneous immortalization of mouse embryonic fibroblast (MEF) cells deficient in cGAS was the first hint to its role in senescence (Yang et al., 2017). Initially associated to its role in SASP production, it was later discovered that cGAS also has a role in slowing down the replication fork and thus cell replication (Chen et al., 2020). Nonetheless, cGAS engagement clearly contributes to the SASP. Micronuclei, cytosolic chromatin fragments (CCF) and RTE are all suggested to be a source of cGAS activation in this context (**Figures 2A, B, D**). Similar to what was found for the role of NBS1 in controlling cGAS localization in micronuclei, cGAS detection of CCF has been suggested to depend on HMGB2 and topoisomerase 1-DNA covalent cleavage complex (TOP1cc) (Zhao et al., 2020). Activation of cGAS in a senescent context might also result from an imbalance between the production of CCF and the cell capacity to degrade these CCF. Accordingly, DNASE2 and TREX1 usually prevent CCF accumulation; however, during senescence, their expression is reduced and CCF accumulates and activates cGAS (Takahashi et al., 2018). In the disease context of AT syndrome, which presents striking phenotypic similarities to FA, cGAS is engaged during the senescence of AT patients olfactory neurosphere-derived cells and brain organoids, which display micronuclei. Importantly, cGAS and STING inhibition in this model prevents astrocyte senescence and protects brain organoids from neurodegeneration (Aguado et al., 2021). Given that FA syndrome was recently described as a 'senescence syndrome' (Helbling-Leclerc et al., 2021), the premature ageing observed in FA might also be an important source of IFN-I production.

CONSTITUTIVE REACTIVE OXYGEN SPECIES PRODUCTION IN FA FUELS DNA DAMAGE

Reactive oxygen species (ROS), mainly but not exclusively produced by mitochondria, have many functions in cells. They serve as signalling molecules and they oxidize biological molecules. The discovery that lymphocytes from FA patients grew better and generated less DNA breaks in low oxygen concentration was the first hint that the oxidative response was aberrant in these cells (Joenje et al., 1981; Schindler and Hoehn, 1988). This was later confirmed by the observation that cells isolated form $Fancc^{-/-}$ mice overproduced ROS upon inflammatory stimulation (Sejas et al., 2007). ROS are indeed produced upon stimulation with TNFα, a pro-inflammatory cytokine overproduced by FA cells *in vitro* and *in vivo* (Rosselli et al., 1994; Dufour et al., 2003; Zhang et al., 2007). ROS overproduction has many effects on cells, one of which is the generation of DNA damage through the oxidation of DNA bases. Guanines are hypersensitive to oxidation and result in 8-oxoguanine (8-oxoG), the most abundant DNA lesion formed after oxidative exposure. Accordingly, unrepaired 8-oxoG lesions have been observed in the peripheral tissues of FA patients harboring mutations in FANCA, FANCC and FANCD2 genes (Du et al., 2012). These lesions correlate with a lower expression

of antioxidant genes, contributing to the excessive oxidation detected in cells from FA patients (Du et al., 2012). $Fancc^{-/-}$ mice also display higher levels of 8-oxoG DNA and yH2AX positive cells basally compare to wt mice. Interestingly, 8-oxoG DNA is resistant to degradation by TREX1 exonuclease (Gehrke et al., 2013). ROS can also cause mtDNA damage, and a new study suggests that mtRNA is released and then detected by RIG-I, a potent activator of IFN-I, upon mtDNA double-strand breaks (Tigano et al., 2021) as illustrated in **Figure 2E**. To our knowledge, RLR receptors have not been implicated in FA yet. In addition to mtRNA release, the RAD51C (FANCO) protein was recently shown to protect mitochondrial replication fork from degradation by the MRE11 mitochondrial nuclease during oxidative stress. In FA-derived patient cells with RAD51C mutation, this protection is lost and thus cytosolic mtDNA, derived from nascent mtDNA cleaved by MRE11, activates the cGAS-STING pathway (Luzwick et al., 2021). Importantly, this process has been reported to rely on FANCD2 and downstream FANC factors but to be independent of the FA core complex, highlighting the importance of understanding the specific roles of FA proteins (Luzwick et al., 2021). Thus, high levels of ROS might contribute to the creation of a pathological feedback loop by creating more DNA damage, ssDNA and mtDNA/RNA release and micronuclei formation that will induce IFN-I production which in turn would stimulate the production of more ROS (**Figure 2F**).

CONSTITUTIVE IFN-I SIGNALING IN CELLS WITH DEFECTS IN MITOCHONDRIA CLEARANCE

Damaged mitochondria can be removed from the cell by classical autophagy, during which a membrane is formed around it and then it is fused to a lysosome, or by mitophagy, a process based on the specific recognition of mitochondrial factors by mitophagy receptors. Many FA proteins, including FANCC, FANCA and BRCA2, are required for two types of selective autophagy, the selective clearance of viruses (virophagy) and mitophagy. Consequently, a lack of these FA proteins impairs mitochondria clearance resulting in cellular accumulation of damaged mitochondria (**Figures 2E, F**) (Shyamsunder et al., 2016; Sumpter et al., 2016). FANCC directly interacts with PARKIN, which is involved in the clearance of damaged mitochondria and the reduction of ROS production. Importantly, using a specific variant of FANCC, c.67delG, it was shown that the DNA repair function and the mitophagy clearance function of FANCC are uncoupled, which suggests that the role of FANCC in mitophagy is relevant to FA pathophysiology (Sumpter et al., 2016). Damaged mitochondria release Danger Associated Molecular Patterns (DAMPs), including mtDNA, that are detected by innate immune receptors. Accordingly, mitochondrial stress arising from ATM inhibitor treatment, deletion of the nucleoid protein TFAM or Herpesvirus infection, causes mtDNA release and IFN-I response (West et al., 2015; Hu et al., 2021). The underlying mechanism of DNA release is not fully understood, although it was demonstrated that mitochondrial herniation mediated by BAK and BAX could be responsible for the DNA release (McArthur et al., 2018).

The fact that FA mouse models do not recapitulate the full spectrum of FA pathophysiology has hampered our understanding of this disease for a long time. However, the discovery that FA mice subjected to environmental stress such as tail bleeding or inflammatory stimulus undergo complete bone marrow failure (Walter et al., 2015) changed our understanding of the disease. It became clear that FA mice, in their highly controlled living conditions, did not reflect the complexity of a human life. Researchers working on Parkinson's using mice genetically deficient in PINK1/Parkin faced the same challenge. In a seminal paper, Slitter and colleagues elegantly showed that if you submit these mice to exercise training, they developed cGAS-STING dependent symptoms highly resembling Parkinson's disease. They went on to characterize the underlying molecular mechanism and demonstrated that faulty mitophagy was causing mtDNA release and cGAS activation (Sliter et al., 2018). Critically, genetic depletion of Sting in their model abolishes the pathological inflammation and prevents dopaminergic neuron death. Damaged mitochondria and STING-dependent neuronal cell death were also observed in Amyotrophic lateral sclerosis, suggesting that STING activation is a recurrent cause of neurodegeneration (Yu et al., 2020). Altogether, these findings highlight the complex interplay between DNA damage, immune response and cellular homeostasis.

TARGETING IFN-I IN FA AND OTHER GENOME INSTABILITY SYNDROMES

To our knowledge, there are currently no clinical trials involving the use of Jak 1,2 inhibitors or IFN-I receptor blocking antibodies in FA's closely-related syndromes such as AT. However, medical benefits were observed in diseases involving gain-of-function of STING and STAT1 (Forbes et al., 2018; Crow et al., 2021). In these syndromes, patients usually display measurably high levels of IFN-I. In AGS, treatment with the Janus kinase inhibitor Baricitinib confers a significant reduction in skin lesions and a possible improvement in neurologic symptoms (Vanderver et al., 2020). Although these data are encouraging, it is worth noting that IFN-I signaling could still be measured in the blood of patients suggesting that these inhibitors have limited efficacy (Crow et al., 2021). This lack of efficacy might be explained by the possibilities that the dosage needed to reach a stronger inhibition is prevented by the toxicity-associated side-effects of the drug or that the drug does not reach all cell populations equally. Nonetheless, these results suggest that IFN-I inhibition could relieve central nervous system (CNS) abnormalities in FA patients (Stivaros et al., 2015; Aksu et al., 2020).

Bone marrow failure is one of the most frequent symptoms for FA patients. IFN-I signalling is linked to bone marrow (BM) suppression. For instance, treatment of HCV patients with PEG- IFNα2a mediates BM suppression (King et al., 2015).

Interestingly, BM failure has also been documented in case of chronic viral infection suggesting that persistent low levels of IFN-I might be sufficient to promote BM failure (Binder et al., 1997). In line with what is observed in FA, major suppressive impact of IFN-I on bone marrow will often occur following secondary stress (de Bruin et al., 2013). While worth testing, long-term treatment to inhibit IFN-I might also worsen cytopenia as observed upon treatment with Jak inhibitor for patients with myelofibrosis (Bose and Verstovsek, 2020). Whether this side-effect would be observed in FA patients needs further investigation.

FA patients display a high prevalence of many types of cancer. Given the opposing roles of IFN-I in cancer, the use of Jak inhibitor might worsen FA patient's prevalence to cancer. On one side, IFN-I has critical role in cancer anti-tumor immunity, meaning it stimulates the ability of immune cells to destroy cancer cells. On the other side, prolonged IFN-I signaling can contribute to immune exhaustion and stimulates tumor growth (Boukhaled et al., 2021).

DISCUSSION

The last decade of research has recognized the crosstalk between DNA damage responses and inflammation, and emphasized its relevance in the study of syndromes caused by mutations in genes that maintain genome stability. The first demonstration of the implication of IFN-I in FA cells by Laguette's group opened new and exciting avenues to determine its importance in FA pathophysiology. Currently, a strong correlation between IFN-I signaling and defect in BRCA2 related genes has been made in several cancer cell lines (Heijink et al., 2019; Reislander et al., 2019). An important question arising from these studies is how transposable to primary cells are the findings obtained using cancer cells? We previously reported that primary cells were more refractory to IFN-I induction upon DNA damage than their immortalized counterparts (Pepin et al., 2017a; Pepin et al., 2017b). In primary cells, prolonged cell cycle arrest following checkpoint activation prevents accumulation of self-nucleic acids (Chen et al., 2020). To investigate this question, it would be important to analyze primary tissues and a diversity of cell population from FA patients when possible and mouse models. However, when analyzing tissue from mouse models, non-canonical roles of proteins will need to be considered. Recent studies indicating that cGAS promotes genome instability (Liu et al., 2018; Jiang et al., 2019; Banerjee et al., 2021) and that STING modulates ROS metabolism (Hayman et al., 2021) add new layers of complexity to the molecular mechanism underlying this already complex disease. Indeed, in future studies it might be recognized that the depletion of these proteins will not only affect IFN-I production but potentially genome stability itself, which will need to be considered.

Evidence suggesting that IFN-I in FA arises from the cGAS-STING pathway is accumulating. However, given the findings on mtRNA released after mtDNA damage (Ghosh et al., 2018), and the accumulation of RTE (Zhao et al., 2018) and R-loops in FA deficient cells (Garcia-Rubio et al., 2015), it is possible that RLRs also contribute to IFN-I production in FA. In such cases, both self-DNA and self-RNA would have the capacity to further induce the expression of RLRs and cGAS, since these PRRs are themselves IFN-stimulated genes (Rusinova et al., 2013). Elevated levels of these PRRs could then sensitize the cells even further to self-nucleic acids sensing, which would create a pathological feedback loop. However, similar to the role of cGAS in inhibiting HR, RIG-I has recently been shown to suppress NHEJ (Guo et al., 2021). Given that FA deficient cells are more prone to repair their DNA using the NHEJ pathway rather than the HR pathway, these data suggest that in the context of FA, RIG-I would not play this NHEJ inhibitory role. These findings reflect the complex integration of immune signalling and DNA repair pathway. Thus, it is expected that RLRs and cGAS might have different roles and be differently regulated depending on the cellular context promoted by specific FA gene mutations.

Another important question is whether defect in each one of the 23 FA proteins have similar consequences on IFN-I. Research suggests that FA genes downstream of ID2 complex have a crucial role in orchestrating the HR response through the recruitment of endonucleases and other factors that will allow strand invasion and recombination. Loss of BRCA related genes contributes to a switch from HR to NHEJ and consequently facilitates cytosolic self-DNA accumulation and thus cGAS activation. Nonetheless, whether FA proteins upstream of ID2 complex will have the same consequences remains to be demonstrated specifically in cells with functional cell cycle checkpoint. In fact, in the case of the structure-specific endonuclease MUS81, a study shows that its activity was critical to the accumulation of cytosolic DNA. Consequently, if defects in specific FA genes prevent the action of endonucleases, inflammatory signals will not be produced.

FA is a phenotypically heterogenous disease, and while we can easily expect a role for IFN-I in bone marrow failure and cancer, its importance in congenital abnormalities is less clear. Contrary to AGS, IFN-I in FA is not expected to be produced at high levels and may be restricted to specific cell populations. In AGS, degradation of nucleic acids is impaired and, thus, self-nucleic acids accumulate without the need for cells to display high levels of DNA damage. In FA however, only cells that proliferate in the presence of DNA damage or with high demands in mitochondria clearance for instance are expected to display high levels of cytosolic DNA. As we report in this review, IFN-I in FA could be produced by distinct molecular mechanisms. As such, it would be of interest to investigate what the predominant mechanism in different cell populations is.

FUTURE PERSPECTIVES

Many questions warrant further investigations that will necessitate the generation of new mouse models. Generation of complete knock-out and subsequently tissue-specific knock-out for the different players implicated in IFN-I signaling in FA (IFNAR, cGAS, STING and RIG-I). These new models should reveal not only if IFN-I is implicated in the pathophysiology of FA, but also in which cell population the production of IFN-I originates. Given the challenge associated with a complete inhibition of the IFN-I signaling, it is difficult to predict how Jak inhibitor would work in FA patients since we expect IFN-I levels to be lower than in AGS. To achieve better clinical results, other therapeutic targets, such as cGAS or STING, might need to be considered. On a positive note, these future researches have the potential to uncover new therapeutic opportunities for FA patients and hence contribute to expand their life expectancy.

AUTHOR CONTRIBUTIONS

KL wrote sections of the first draft and edited the manuscript. SS designed, drew the schematic and edited the manuscript. GP designed, wrote and edited the manuscript. All authors approved the final version of the manuscript.

FUNDING

Fonds de Recherche du Québec (FRSQ) – Santé (35071 to GP); Chaire de Recherche Junior UQTR (GP); CERMO-FC (GP); the Canadian Foundation for Innovation (CFI-40780 to GP); MITACS Globalink scholarship (UQTR-97834 to SS).

ACKNOWLEDGMENTS

We would like to thank Mélodie B. Plourde for editing; Dr Laure Guitton-Sert, Dr Sofiane Y. Mersaoui, Dr Jean-Yves Masson and Dr Patrick Narbonne for critical reading of this manuscript.

REFERENCES

Abdisalaam, S. M., Bhattacharya, S., Sinha, D., Kumari, S., Sadek, H. A., Ortega, J., et al. (2020). NBS1-CtIP–Mediated DNA End Resection Regulates cGAS Binding to Micronuclei. *bioRxiv.* 2020.07.27.222380. doi: 10.1101/2020.07.27.222380

Ablasser, A., Goldeck, M., Cavlar, T., Deimling, T., Witte, G., Rohl, I., et al. (2013). cGAS Produces a 2'-5'-Linked Cyclic Dinucleotide Second Messenger That Activates STING. *Nature* 498, 380–384. doi: 10.1038/nature12306

Ablasser, A., Hur, S. (2020). Regulation of cGAS- and RLR-Mediated Immunity to Nucleic Acids. *Nat. Immunol.* 21, 17–29. doi: 10.1038/s41590-019-0556-1

Achleitner, M., Kleefisch, M., Hennig, A., Peschke, K., Polikarpova, A., Oertel, R., et al. (2017). Lack of Trex1 Causes Systemic Autoimmunity Despite the Presence of Antiretroviral Drugs. *J. Immunol.* 199, 2261–2269. doi: 10.4049/jimmunol.1700714

Adamo, A., Collis, S. J., Adelman, C. A., Silva, N., Horejsi, Z., Ward, J. D., et al. (2010). Preventing Nonhomologous End Joining Suppresses DNA Repair Defects of Fanconi Anemia. *Mol. Cell* 39, 25–35. doi: 10.1016/j.molcel.2010.06.026

Aguado, J., Chaggar, H. K., Gomez-Inclan, C., Shaker, M. R., Leeson, H. C., Mackay-Sim, A., et al. (2021). Inhibition of the cGAS-STING Pathway Ameliorates the Premature Senescence Hallmarks of Ataxia-Telangiectasia Brain Organoids. *Aging Cell* 20, e13468. doi: 10.1111/acel.13468

Aksu, T., Gumruk, F., Bayhan, T., Coskun, C., Oguz, K. K., Unal, S. (2020). Central Nervous System Lesions in Fanconi Anemia: Experience From a Research

Center for Fanconi Anemia Patients. *Pediatr. Blood Cancer* 67, e28722. doi: 10.1002/pbc.28722

Balka, K. R., De Nardo, D. (2021). Molecular and Spatial Mechanisms Governing STING Signalling. *FEBS J.* 288, 5504–5529. doi: 10.1111/febs.15640

Banerjee, D., Langberg, K., Abbas, S., Odermatt, E., Yerramothu, P., Volaric, M., et al. (2021). A Non-Canonical, Interferon-Independent Signaling Activity of cGAMP Triggers DNA Damage Response Signaling. *Nat. Commun.* 12, 6207. doi: 10.1038/s41467-021-26240-9

Benitez, A., Liu, W., Palovcak, A., Wang, G., Moon, J., An, K., et al. (2018). FANCA Promotes DNA Double-Strand Break Repair by Catalyzing Single-Strand Annealing and Strand Exchange. *Mol. Cell* 71, 621–628.e4. doi: 10.1016/j.molcel.2018.06.030

Binder, D., Fehr, J., Hengartner, H., Zinkernagel, R. M. (1997). Virus-Induced Transient Bone Marrow Aplasia: Major Role of Interferon-Alpha/Beta During Acute Infection With the Noncytopathic Lymphocytic Choriomeningitis Virus. *J. Exp. Med.* 185, 517–530. doi: 10.1084/jem.185.3.517

Bose, P., Verstovsek, S. (2020). JAK Inhibition for the Treatment of Myelofibrosis: Limitations and Future Perspectives. *Hemasphere* 4, e424. doi: 10.1097/HS9.0000000000000424

Boukhaled, G. M., Harding, S., Brooks, D. G. (2021). Opposing Roles of Type I Interferons in Cancer Immunity. *Annu. Rev. Pathol.* 16, 167–198. doi: 10.1146/annurev-pathol-031920-093932

Bregnard, C., Guerra, J., Dejardin, S., Passalacqua, F., Benkirane, M., Laguette, N. (2016). Upregulated LINE-1 Activity in the Fanconi Anemia Cancer Susceptibility Syndrome Leads to Spontaneous Pro-Inflammatory Cytokine Production. *EBioMedicine* 8, 184–194. doi: 10.1016/j.ebiom.2016.05.005

Burleigh, K., Maltbaek, J. H., Cambier, S., Green, R., Gale, M.Jr., James, R. C., et al. (2020). Human DNA-PK Activates a STING-Independent DNA Sensing Pathway. *Sci. Immunol.* 5 (43), eaba4219. doi: 10.1126/sciimmunol.aba4219

Cai, M. Y., Dunn, C. E., Chen, W., Kochupurakkal, B. S., Nguyen, H., Moreau, L. A., et al. (2020). Cooperation of the ATM and Fanconi Anemia/BRCA Pathways in Double-Strand Break End Resection. *Cell Rep.* 30, 2402–2415 e5. doi: 10.1016/j.celrep.2020.01.052

Ceccaldi, R., Parmar, K., Mouly, E., Delord, M., Kim, J. M., Regairaz, M., et al. (2012). Bone Marrow Failure in Fanconi Anemia is Triggered by an Exacerbated P53/P21 DNA Damage Response That Impairs Hematopoietic Stem and Progenitor Cells. *Cell Stem Cell* 11, 36–49. doi: 10.1016/j.stem.2012.05.013

Chatzidoukaki, O., Stratigi, K., Goulielmaki, E., Niotis, G., Akalestou-Clocher, A., Gkirtzimanaki, K., et al. (2021). R-Loops Trigger the Release of Cytoplasmic ssDNAs Leading to Chronic Inflammation Upon DNA Damage. *Sci. Adv.* 7, eabj5769. doi: 10.1126/sciadv.abj5769

Chen, H., Chen, H., Zhang, J., Wang, Y., Simoneau, A., Yang, H., et al. (2020). cGAS Suppresses Genomic Instability as a Decelerator of Replication Forks. *Sci. Adv.* 6 (42), eabb8941. doi: 10.1126/sciadv.abb8941

Chen, J., Harding, S. M., Natesan, R., Tian, L., Benci, J. L., Li, W., et al. (2020). Cell Cycle Checkpoints Cooperate to Suppress DNA- and RNA-Associated Molecular Pattern Recognition and Anti-Tumor Immune Responses. *Cell Rep.* 32, 108080. doi: 10.1016/j.celrep.2020.108080

Chen, Y. A., Shen, Y. L., Hsia, H. Y., Tiang, Y. P., Sung, T. L., Chen, L. Y. (2017). Extrachromosomal Telomere Repeat DNA Is Linked to ALT Development *via* cGAS-STING DNA Sensing Pathway. *Nat. Struct. Mol. Biol.* 24, 1124–1131. doi: 10.1038/nsmb.3498

Coquel, F., Silva, M. J., Techer, H., Zadorozhny, K., Sharma, S., Nieminuszczy, J., et al. (2018). SAMHD1 Acts at Stalled Replication Forks to Prevent Interferon Induction. *Nature* 557, 57–61. doi: 10.1038/s41586-018-0050-1

Crow, Y. J., Leitch, A., Hayward, B. E., Garner, A., Parmar, R., Griffith, E., et al. (2006). Mutations in Genes Encoding Ribonuclease H2 Subunits Cause Aicardi-Goutieres Syndrome and Mimic Congenital Viral Brain Infection. *Nat. Genet.* 38, 910–916. doi: 10.1038/ng1842

Crow, Y. J., Neven, B., Fremond, M. L. (2021). JAK Inhibition in the Type I Interferonopathies. *J. Allergy Clin. Immunol.* 148, 991–993. doi: 10.1016/j.jaci.2021.07.028

Crow, Y. J., Stetson, D. B. (2021). The Type I Interferonopathies: 10 Years on. *Nat. Rev. Immunol.* doi: 10.1038/s41577-021-00633-9

de Bruin, A. M., Demirel, O., Hooibrink, B., Brandts, C. H., Nolte, M. A. (2013). Interferon-Gamma Impairs Proliferation of Hematopoietic Stem Cells in Mice. *Blood* 121, 3578–3585. doi: 10.1182/blood-2012-05-432906

De Cecco, M., Ito, T., Petrashen, A. P., Elias, A. E., Skvir, N. J., Criscione, S. W., et al. (2019). L1 Drives IFN in Senescent Cells and Promotes Age Associated Inflammation. *Nature* 566, 73–78. doi: 10.1038/s41586-018-0784-9

Deschamps, T., Kalamvoki, M. (2017). Impaired STING Pathway in Human Osteosarcoma U2OS Cells Contributes to the Growth of ICP0-Null Mutant Herpes Simplex Virus. *J. Virol.* 91 (9), e00006-17. doi: 10.1128/JVI.00006-17

Dou, Z., Ghosh, K., Vizioli, M. G., Zhu, J., Sen, P., Wangensteen, K. J., et al. (2017). Cytoplasmic Chromatin Triggers Inflammation in Senescence and Cancer. *Nature* 550, 402–406. doi: 10.1038/nature24050

Dufour, C., Corcione, A., Svahn, J., Haupt, R., Poggi, V., Beka'ssy, A. N., et al. (2003). TNF-Alpha and IFN-Gamma are Overexpressed in the Bone Marrow of Fanconi Anemia Patients and TNF-Alpha Suppresses Erythropoiesis In Vitro. *Blood* 102, 2053–2059. doi: 10.1182/blood-2003-01-0114

Dunphy, G., Flannery, S. M., Almine, J. F., Connolly, D. J., Paulus, C., Jonsson, K. L., et al. (2018). Non-Canonical Activation of the DNA Sensing Adaptor STING by ATM and IFI16 Mediates NF-kappaB Signaling After Nuclear DNA Damage. *Mol. Cell* 71, 745–760.e5. doi: 10.1016/j.molcel.2018.07.034

Du, W., Rani, R., Sipple, J., Schick, J., Myers, K. C., Mehta, P., et al. (2012). The FA Pathway Counteracts Oxidative Stress Through Selective Protection of Antioxidant Defense Gene Promoters. *Blood* 119, 4142–4151. doi: 10.1182/blood-2011-09-381970

Eccles, L. J., Bell, A. C., Powell, S. N. (2018). Inhibition of Non-Homologous End Joining in Fanconi Anemia Cells Results in Rescue of Survival After Interstrand Crosslinks But Sensitization to Replication Associated Double-Strand Breaks. *DNA Repair (Amst.)* 64, 1–9. doi: 10.1016/j.dnarep.2018.02.003

Erdal, E., Haider, S., Rehwinkel, J., Harris, A. L., McHugh, P. J. (2017). A Prosurvival DNA Damage-Induced Cytoplasmic Interferon Response Is Mediated by End Resection Factors and Iis Limited by Trex1. *Genes Dev.* 31, 353–369. doi: 10.1101/gad.289769.116

Ferguson, B. J., Mansur, D. S., Peters, N. E., Ren, H., Smith, G. L. (2012). DNA-PK is a DNA Sensor for IRF-3-Dependent Innate Immunity. *Elife* 1, e00047. doi: 10.7554/eLife.00047.012

Flynn, P. J., Koch, P. D., Mitchison, T. J. (2021). Chromatin Bridges, Not Micronuclei, Activate cGAS After Drug-Induced Mitotic Errors in Human Cells. *Proc. Natl. Acad. Sci. U. S. A.* 118 (48), e2103585118. doi: 10.1073/pnas.2103585118

Forbes, L. R., Vogel, T. P., Cooper, M. A., Castro-Wagner, J., Schussler, E., Weinacht, K. G., et al. (2018). Jakinibs for the Treatment of Immune Dysregulation in Patients With Gain-of-Function Signal Transducer and Activator of Transcription 1 (STAT1) or STAT3 Mutations. *J. Allergy Clin. Immunol.* 142, 1665–1669. doi: 10.1016/j.jaci.2018.07.020

Freie, B. W., Ciccone, S. L., Li, X., Plett, P. A., Orschell, C. M., Srour, E. F., et al. (2004). A Role for the Fanconi Anemia C Protein in Maintaining the DNA Damage-Induced G2 Checkpoint. *J. Biol. Chem.* 279, 50986–50993. doi: 10.1074/jbc.M407160200

Gall, A., Treuting, P., Elkon, K. B., Loo, Y. M., Gale, M.Jr., Barber, G. N., et al. (2012). Autoimmunity Initiates in Nonhematopoietic Cells and Progresses *via* Lymphocytes in an Interferon-Dependent Autoimmune Disease. *Immunity* 36, 120–131. doi: 10.1016/j.immuni.2011.11.018

Garcia-Rubio, M. L., Perez-Calero, C., Barroso, S. I., Tumini, E., Herrera-Moyano, E., Rosado, I. V., et al. (2015). The Fanconi Anemia Pathway Protects Genome Integrity From R-Loops. *PloS Genet.* 11, e1005674. doi: 10.1371/journal.pgen.1005674

Gauthier, B. R., Comaills, V. (2021). Nuclear Envelope Integrity in Health and Disease: Consequences on Genome Instability and Inflammation. *Int. J. Mol. Sci.* 22 (14), 7281. doi: 10.3390/ijms22147281

Gehrke, N., Mertens, C., Zillinger, T., Wenzel, J., Bald, T., Zahn, S., et al. (2013). Oxidative Damage of DNA Confers Resistance to Cytosolic Nuclease TREX1 Degradation and Potentiates STING-Dependent Immune Sensing. *Immunity* 39, 482–495. doi: 10.1016/j.immuni.2013.08.004

Gentili, M., Lahaye, X., Nadalin, F., Nader, G. P. F., Puig Lombardi, E., Herve, S., et al. (2019). The N-Terminal Domain of cGAS Determines Preferential Association With Centromeric DNA and Innate Immune Activation in the Nucleus. *Cell Rep.* 26, 2377–2393.e13. doi: 10.1016/j.celrep.2019.03.049

Ghosh, R., Roy, S., Franco, S. (2018). PARP1 Depletion Induces RIG-I-Dependent Signaling in Human Cancer Cells. *PloS One* 13, e0194611. doi: 10.1371/journal.pone.0194611

Gluck, S., Guey, B., Gulen, M. F., Wolter, K., Kang, T. W., Schmacke, N. A., et al. (2017). Innate Immune Sensing of Cytosolic Chromatin Fragments Through cGAS Promotes Senescence. *Nat. Cell Biol.* 19, 1061–1070. doi: 10.1038/ncb3586

Gratia, M., Rodero, M. P., Conrad, C., Bou Samra, E., Maurin, M., Rice, G. I., et al. (2019). Bloom Syndrome Protein Restrains Innate Immune Sensing of Micronuclei by cGAS. *J. Exp. Med.* 216, 1199–1213. doi: 10.1084/jem.20181329

Gray, E. E., Treuting, P. M., Woodward, J. J., Stetson, D. B. (2015). Cutting Edge: cGAS Is Required for Lethal Autoimmune Disease in the Trex1-Deficient Mouse Model of Aicardi-Goutieres Syndrome. *J. Immunol.* 195, 1939–1943. doi: 10.4049/jimmunol.1500969

Guan, J., Lu, C., Jin, Q., Lu, H., Chen, X., Tian, L., et al. (2021). MLH1 Deficiency-Triggered DNA Hyperexcision by Exonuclease 1 Activates the cGAS-STING Pathway. *Cancer Cell* 39, 109–121.e5. doi: 10.1016/j.ccell.2020.11.004

Guillemette, S., Branagan, A., Peng, M., Dhruva, A., Scharer, O. D., Cantor, S. B. (2014). FANCJ Localization by Mismatch Repair is Vital to Maintain Genomic Integrity After UV Irradiation. *Cancer Res.* 74, 932–944. doi: 10.1158/0008-5472.CAN-13-2474

Guitton-Sert, L., Gao, Y., Masson, J. Y. (2021). Animal Models of Fanconi Anemia: A Developmental and Therapeutic Perspective on a Multifaceted Disease. *Semin. Cell Dev. Biol.* 113, 113–131. doi: 10.1016/j.semcdb.2020.11.010

Guo, G., Gao, M., Gao, X., Zhu, B., Huang, J., Tu, X., et al. (2021). Reciprocal Regulation of RIG-I and XRCC4 Connects DNA Repair With RIG-I Immune Signaling. *Nat. Commun.* 12, 2187. doi: 10.1038/s41467-021-22484-7

Harding, S. M., Benci, J. L., Irianto, J., Discher, D. E., Minn, A. J., Greenberg, R. A. (2017). Mitotic Progression Following DNA Damage Enables Pattern Recognition Within Micronuclei. *Nature* 548, 466–470. doi: 10.1038/nature23470

Hartlova, A., Erttmann, S. F., Raffi, F. A., Schmalz, A. M., Resch, U., Anugula, S., et al. (2015). DNA Damage Primes the Type I Interferon System *via* the Cytosolic DNA Sensor STING to Promote Anti-Microbial Innate Immunity. *Immunity* 42, 332–343. doi: 10.1016/j.immuni.2015.01.012

Hayman, T. J., Baro, M., MacNeil, T., Phoomak, C., Aung, T. N., Cui, W., et al. (2021). STING Enhances Cell Death Through Regulation of Reactive Oxygen Species and DNA Damage. *Nat. Commun.* 12, 2327. doi: 10.1038/s41467-021-22572-8

Heijink, A. M., Talens, F., Jae, L. T., van Gijn, S. E., Fehrmann, R. S. N., Brummelkamp, T. R., et al. (2019). BRCA2 Deficiency Instigates cGAS-Mediated Inflammatory Signaling and Confers Sensitivity to Tumor Necrosis Factor-Alpha-Mediated Cytotoxicity. *Nat. Commun.* 10, 100. doi: 10.1038/s41467-018-07927-y

Helbling-Leclerc, A., Dessarps-Freichey, F., Evrard, C., Rosselli, F. (2019). Fanconi Anemia Proteins Counteract the Implementation of the Oncogene-Induced Senescence Program. *Sci. Rep.* 9, 17024. doi: 10.1038/s41598-019-53502-w

Helbling-Leclerc, A., Garcin, C., Rosselli, F. (2021). Beyond DNA Repair and Chromosome Instability-Fanconi Anaemia as a Cellular Senescence-Associated Syndrome. *Cell Death Differ.* 28, 1159–1173. doi: 10.1038/s41418-021-00764-5

Ho, S. S., Zhang, W. Y., Tan, N. Y., Khatoo, M., Suter, M. A., Tripathi, S., et al. (2016). The DNA Structure-Specific Endonuclease MUS81 Mediates DNA Sensor STING-Dependent Host Rejection of Prostate Cancer Cells. *Immunity* 44, 1177–1189. doi: 10.1016/j.immuni.2016.04.010

Hu, M., Zhou, M., Bao, X., Pan, D., Jiao, M., Liu, X., et al. (2021). ATM Inhibition Enhances Cancer Immunotherapy by Promoting mtDNA Leakage and cGAS/STING Activation. *J. Clin. Invest.* 131 (3), e139333. doi: 10.1172/JCI139333

Jiang, H., Xue, X., Panda, S., Kawale, A., Hooy, R. M., Liang, F., et al. (2019). Chromatin-Bound cGAS is an Inhibitor of DNA Repair and Hence Accelerates Genome Destabilization and Cell Death. *EMBO J.* 38, e102718. doi: 10.15252/embj.2019102718

Joenje, H., Arwert, F., Eriksson, A. W., de Koning, H., Oostra, A. B. (1981). Oxygen-Dependence of Chromosomal Aberrations in Fanconi's Anaemia. *Nature* 290, 142–143. doi: 10.1038/290142a0

Joksic, I., Vujic, D., Guc-Scekic, M., Leskovac, A., Petrovic, S., Ojani, M., et al. (2012). Dysfunctional Telomeres in Primary Cells From Fanconi Anemia FANCD2 Patients. *Genome Integr.* 3, 6. doi: 10.1186/2041-9414-3-6

Kim, S., Hwang, S. K., Lee, M., Kwak, H., Son, K., Yang, J., et al. (2013). Fanconi Anemia Complementation Group A (FANCA) Localizes to Centrosomes and Functions in the Maintenance of Centrosome Integrity. *Int. J. Biochem. Cell Biol.* 45, 1953–1961. doi: 10.1016/j.biocel.2013.06.012

King, K. Y., Matatall, K. A., Shen, C. C., Goodell, M. A., Swierczek, S. I., Prchal, J. T. (2015). Comparative Long-Term Effects of Interferon Alpha and

Hydroxyurea on Human Hematopoietic Progenitor Cells. *Exp. Hematol.* 43, 912–918.e2. doi: 10.1016/j.exphem.2015.05.013

Knipscheer, P., Raschle, M., Smogorzewska, A., Enoiu, M., Ho, T. V., Scharer, O. D., et al. (2009). The Fanconi Anemia Pathway Promotes Replication-Dependent DNA Interstrand Cross-Link Repair. *Science* 326, 1698–1701. doi: 10.1126/science.1182372

Kretschmer, S., Lee-Kirsch, M. A. (2017). Type I Interferon-Mediated Autoinflammation and Autoimmunity. *Curr. Opin. Immunol.* 49, 96–102. doi: 10.1016/j.coi.2017.09.003

Lam, A. R., Bert, N. L., Ho, S. S., Shen, Y. J., Tang, L. F., Xiong, G. M., et al. (2014). RAE1 Ligands for the NKG2D Receptor are Regulated by STING-Dependent DNA Sensor Pathways in Lymphoma. *Cancer Res.* 74, 2193–2203. doi: 10.1158/0008-5472.CAN-13-1703

Lepelley, A., Wai, T., Crow, Y. J. (2021). Mitochondrial Nucleic Acid as a Driver of Pathogenic Type I Interferon Induction in Mendelian Disease. *Front. Immunol.* 12, 729763. doi: 10.3389/fimmu.2021.729763

Li, Y., Li, X., Cole, A., McLaughlin, S., Du, W. (2018). Icariin Improves Fanconi Anemia Hematopoietic Stem Cell Function Through SIRT6-Mediated NF-Kappa B Inhibition. *Cell Cycle* 17, 367–376. doi: 10.1080/15384101.2018.1426413

Liu, H., Zhang, H., Wu, X., Ma, D., Wu, J., Wang, L., et al. (2018). Nuclear cGAS Suppresses DNA Repair and Promotes Tumorigenesis. *Nature* 563, 131–136. doi: 10.1038/s41586-018-0629-6

Luthra, P., Aguirre, S., Yen, B. C., Pietzsch, C. A., Sanchez-Aparicio, M. T., Tigabu, B., et al. (2017). Topoisomerase II Inhibitors Induce DNA Damage-Dependent Interferon Responses Circumventing Ebola Virus Immune Evasion. *mBio* 8 (2), e00368–17. doi: 10.1128/mBio.00368-17

Luzwick, J. W., Dombi, E., Boisvert, R. A., Roy, S., Park, S., Kunnimalaiyaan, S., et al. (2021). MRE11-Dependent Instability in Mitochondrial DNA Fork Protection Activates a cGAS Immune Signaling Pathway. *Sci. Adv.* 7, eabf9441. doi: 10.1126/sciadv.abf9441

Mackenzie, K. J., Carroll, P., Martin, C. A., Murina, O., Fluteau, A., Simpson, D. J., et al. (2017). cGAS Surveillance of Micronuclei Links Genome Instability to Innate Immunity. *Nature* 548, 461–465. doi: 10.1038/nature23449

Mankan, A. K., Schmidt, T., Chauhan, D., Goldeck, M., Honing, K., Gaidt, M., et al. (2014). Cytosolic RNA : DNA Hybrids Activate the cGAS-STING Axis. *EMBO J.* 33, 2937–2946. doi: 10.15252/embj.201488726

McArthur, K., Whitehead, L. W., Heddleston, J. M., Li, L., Padman, B. S., Oorschot, V., et al. (2018). BAK/BAX Macropores Facilitate Mitochondrial Herniation and mtDNA Efflux During Apoptosis. *Science* 359 (6378), eaao6047. doi: 10.1126/science.aao6047

McLaughlin, L. J., Stojanovic, L., Kogan, A. A., Rutherford, J. L., Choi, E. Y., Yen, R. C., et al. (2020). Pharmacologic Induction of Innate Immune Signaling Directly Drives Homologous Recombination Deficiency. *Proc. Natl. Acad. Sci. U. S. A.* 117, 17785–17795. doi: 10.1073/pnas.2003499117

Mita, P., Sun, X., Fenyo, D., Kahler, D. J., Li, D., Agmon, N., et al. (2020). BRCA1 and S Phase DNA Repair Pathways Restrict LINE-1 Retrotransposition in Human Cells. *Nat. Struct. Mol. Biol.* 27, 179–191. doi: 10.1038/s41594-020-0374-z

Naim, V., Rosselli, F. (2009). The FANC Pathway and BLM Collaborate During Mitosis to Prevent Micro-Nucleation and Chromosome Abnormalities. *Nat. Cell Biol.* 11, 761–768. doi: 10.1038/ncb1883

Nakanishi, A., Han, X., Saito, H., Taguchi, K., Ohta, Y., Imajoh-Ohmi, S., et al. (2007). Interference With BRCA2, Which Localizes to the Centrosome During S and Early M Phase, Leads to Abnormal Nuclear Division. *Biochem. Biophys. Res. Commun.* 355, 34–40. doi: 10.1016/j.bbrc.2007.01.100

Nalepa, G., Enzor, R., Sun, Z., Marchal, C., Park, S. J., Yang, Y., et al. (2013). Fanconi Anemia Signaling Network Regulates the Spindle Assembly Checkpoint. *J. Clin. Invest.* 123, 3839–3847. doi: 10.1172/JCI67364

Peng, M., Xie, J., Ucher, A., Stavnezer, J., Cantor, S. B. (2014). Crosstalk Between BRCA-Fanconi Anemia and Mismatch Repair Pathways Prevents MSH2-Dependent Aberrant DNA Damage Responses. *EMBO J.* 33, 1698–1712. doi: 10.15252/embj.201387530

Pepin, G., Nejad, C., Ferrand, J., Thomas, B. J., Stunden, H. J., Sanij, E., et al. (2017a). Topoisomerase 1 Inhibition Promotes Cyclic GMP-AMP Synthase-Dependent Antiviral Responses. *mBio* 8 (5), e01611–17. doi: 10.1128/mBio.01611-17

Pepin, G., Nejad, C., Thomas, B. J., Ferrand, J., McArthur, K., Bardin, P. G., et al. (2017b). Activation of cGAS-Dependent Antiviral Responses by DNA Intercalating Agents. *Nucleic Acids Res.* 45, 198–205. doi: 10.1093/nar/gkw878

Platanias, L. C. (2005). Mechanisms of Type-I- and Type-II-Interferon-Mediated Signalling. *Nat. Rev. Immunol.* 5, 375–386. doi: 10.1038/nri1604

Reikine, S., Nguyen, J. B., Modis, Y. (2014). Pattern Recognition and Signaling Mechanisms of RIG-I and MDA5. *Front. Immunol.* 5, 342. doi: 10.3389/fimmu.2014.00342

Reislander, T., Lombardi, E. P., Groelly, F. J., Miar, A., Porru, M., Di Vito, S., et al. (2019). BRCA2 Abrogation Triggers Innate Immune Responses Potentiated by Treatment With PARP Inhibitors. *Nat. Commun.* 10, 3143. doi: 10.1038/s41467-019-11048-5

Rice, G., Newman, W. G., Dean, J., Patrick, T., Parmar, R., Flintoff, K., et al. (2007). Heterozygous Mutations in TREX1 Cause Familial Chilblain Lupus and Dominant Aicardi-Goutieres Syndrome. *Am. J. Hum. Genet.* 80, 811–815. doi: 10.1086/513443

Rodriguez, A., D'Andrea, A. (2017). Fanconi Anemia Pathway. *Curr. Biol.* 27, R986–R988. doi: 10.1016/j.cub.2017.07.043

Rodriguez, A., Zhang, K., Farkkila, A., Filiatrault, J., Yang, C., Velazquez, M., et al. (2021). MYC Promotes Bone Marrow Stem Cell Dysfunction in Fanconi Anemia. *Cell Stem Cell* 28, 33–47.e8. doi: 10.1016/j.stem.2020.09.004

Rosselli, F., Sanceau, J., Gluckman, E., Wietzerbin, J., Moustacchi, E. (1994). Abnormal Lymphokine Production: A Novel Feature of the Genetic Disease Fanconi Anemia. II. *In Vitro* and *In Vivo* Spontaneous Overproduction of Tumor Necrosis Factor Alpha. *Blood* 83, 1216–1225. doi: 10.1182/blood.V83.5.1216.1216

Rusinova, I., Forster, S., Yu, S., Kannan, A., Masse, M., Cumming, H., et al. (2013). Interferome V2.0: An Updated Database of Annotated Interferon-Regulated Genes. *Nucleic Acids Res.* 41, D1040–D1046. doi: 10.1093/nar/gks1215

Santa, P., Garreau, A., Serpas, L., Ferriere, A., Blanco, P., Soni, C., et al. (2021). The Role of Nucleases and Nucleic Acid Editing Enzymes in the Regulation of Self-Nucleic Acid Sensing. *Front. Immunol.* 12, 629922. doi: 10.3389/fimmu.2021.629922

Schindler, D., Hoehn, H. (1988). Fanconi Anemia Mutation Causes Cellular Susceptibility to Ambient Oxygen. *Am. J. Hum. Genet.* 43, 429–435.

Schlee, M., Hartmann, G. (2016). Discriminating Self From non-Self in Nucleic Acid Sensing. *Nat. Rev. Immunol.* 16, 566–580. doi: 10.1038/nri.2016.78

Schwab, R. A., Nieminuszczy, J., Shah, F., Langton, J., Lopez Martinez, D., Liang, C. C., et al. (2015). The Fanconi Anemia Pathway Maintains Genome Stability by Coordinating Replication and Transcription. *Mol. Cell* 60, 351–361. doi: 10.1016/j.molcel.2015.09.012

Sejas, D. P., Rani, R., Qiu, Y., Zhang, X., Fagerlie, S. R., Nakano, H., et al. (2007). Inflammatory Reactive Oxygen Species-Mediated Hemopoietic Suppression in Fancc-Deficient Mice. *J. Immunol.* 178, 5277–5287. doi: 10.4049/jimmunol.178.8.5277

Shyamsunder, P., Esner, M., Barvalia, M., Wu, Y. J., Loja, T., Boon, H. B., et al. (2016). Impaired Mitophagy in Fanconi Anemia Is Dependent on Mitochondrial Fission. *Oncotarget* 7, 58065–58074. doi: 10.18632/oncotarget.11161

Simon, M., Van Meter, M., Ablaeva, J., Ke, Z., Gonzalez, R. S., Taguchi, T., et al. (2019). LINE1 Derepression in Aged Wild-Type and SIRT6-Deficient Mice Drives Inflammation. *Cell Metab.* 29, 871–885.e5. doi: 10.1016/j.cmet.2019.02.014

Singh, T. R., Saro, D., Ali, A. M., Zheng, X. F., Du, C. H., Killen, M. W., et al. (2010). MHF1-MHF2, a Histone-Fold-Containing Protein Complex, Participates in the Fanconi Anemia Pathway *via* FANCM. *Mol. Cell* 37, 879–886. doi: 10.1016/j.molcel.2010.01.036

Sliter, D. A., Martinez, J., Hao, L., Chen, X., Sun, N., Fischer, T. D., et al. (2018). Parkin and PINK1 Mitigate STING-Induced Inflammation. *Nature* 561, 258–262. doi: 10.1038/s41586-018-0448-9

Stetson, D. B., Ko, J. S., Heidmann, T., Medzhitov, R. (2008). Trex1 Prevents Cell-Intrinsic Initiation of Autoimmunity. *Cell* 134, 587–598. doi: 10.1016/j.cell.2008.06.032

Stivaros, S. M., Alston, R., Wright, N. B., Chandler, K., Bonney, D., Wynn, R. F., et al. (2015). Central Nervous System Abnormalities in Fanconi Anaemia: Patterns and Frequency on Magnetic Resonance Imaging. *Br. J. Radiol.* 88, 20150088. doi: 10.1259/bjr.20150088

Sumpter, R.Jr., Sirasanagandla, S., Fernandez, A. F., Wei, Y., Dong, X., Franco, L., et al. (2016). Fanconi Anemia Proteins Function in Mitophagy and Immunity. *Cell* 165, 867–881. doi: 10.1016/j.cell.2016.04.006

Sun, X., Liu, T., Zhao, J., Xia, H., Xie, J., Guo, Y., et al. (2020). DNA-PK Deficiency Potentiates cGAS-Mediated Antiviral Innate Immunity. *Nat. Commun.* 11, 6182. doi: 10.1038/s41467-020-19941-0

Sun, L., Wu, J., Du, F., Chen, X., Chen, Z. J. (2013). Cyclic GMP-AMP Synthase Is a Cytosolic DNA Sensor That Activates the Type I Interferon Pathway. *Science* 339, 786–791. doi: 10.1126/science.1232458

Taffoni, C., Steer, A., Marines, J., Chamma, H., Vila, I. K., Laguette, N. (2021). Nucleic Acid Immunity and DNA Damage Response: New Friends and Old Foes. *Front. Immunol.* 12, 660560. doi: 10.3389/fimmu.2021.660560

Takahashi, A., Loo, T. M., Okada, R., Kamachi, F., Watanabe, Y., Wakita, M., et al. (2018). Downregulation of Cytoplasmic DNases Is Implicated in Cytoplasmic DNA Accumulation and SASP in Senescent Cells. *Nat. Commun.* 9, 1249. doi: 10.1038/s41467-018-03555-8

Tan, W., Deans, A. J. (2021). The Ubiquitination Machinery of the Fanconi Anemia DNA Repair Pathway. *Prog. Biophys. Mol. Biol.* 163, 5–13. doi: 10.1016/j.pbiomolbio.2020.09.009

Tan, W., van Twest, S., Leis, A., Bythell-Douglas, R., Murphy, V. J., Sharp, M., et al. (2020). Monoubiquitination by the Human Fanconi Anemia Core Complex Clamps FANCI : FANCD2 on DNA in Filamentous Arrays. *Elife* 9, e54128. doi: 10.7554/eLife.54128.sa2

Tigano, M., Vargas, D. C., Tremblay-Belzile, S., Fu, Y., Sfeir, A. (2021). Nuclear Sensing of Breaks in Mitochondrial DNA Enhances Immune Surveillance. *Nature* 591, 477–481. doi: 10.1038/s41586-021-03269-w

Vanderver, A., Adang, L., Gavazzi, F., McDonald, K., Helman, G., Frank, D. B., et al. (2020). Janus Kinase Inhibition in the Aicardi-Goutieres Syndrome. *N. Engl. J. Med.* 383, 986–989. doi: 10.1056/NEJMc2001362

Vinciguerra, P., Godinho, S. A., Parmar, K., Pellman, D., D'Andrea, A. D. (2010). Cytokinesis Failure Occurs in Fanconi Anemia Pathway-Deficient Murine and Human Bone Marrow Hematopoietic Cells. *J. Clin. Invest.* 120, 3834–3842. doi: 10.1172/JCI43391

Volkman, H. E., Cambier, S., Gray, E. E., Stetson, D. B. (2019). Tight Nuclear Tethering of cGAS is Essential for Preventing Autoreactivity. *Elife* 8, e47491. doi: 10.7554/eLife.47491.sa2

Walter, D., Lier, A., Geiselhart, A., Thalheimer, F. B., Huntscha, S., Sobotta, M. C., et al. (2015). Exit From Dormancy Provokes DNA-Damage-Induced Attrition in Haematopoietic Stem Cells. *Nature* 520, 549–552. doi: 10.1038/nature14131

West, A. P., Khoury-Hanold, W., Staron, M., Tal, M. C., Pineda, C. M., Lang, S. M., et al. (2015). Mitochondrial DNA Stress Primes the Antiviral Innate Immune Response. *Nature* 520, 553–557. doi: 10.1038/nature14156

Wolf, C., Rapp, A., Berndt, N., Staroske, W., Schuster, M., Dobrick-Mattheuer, M., et al. (2016). RPA and Rad51 Constitute a Cell Intrinsic Mechanism to Protect the Cytosol From Self DNA. *Nat. Commun.* 7, 11752. doi: 10.1038/ncomms11752

Wu, J., Sun, L., Chen, X., Du, F., Shi, H., Chen, C., et al. (2013). Cyclic GMP-AMP Is an Endogenous Second Messenger in Innate Immune Signaling by Cytosolic DNA. *Science* 339, 826–830. doi: 10.1126/science.1229963

Xu, X., Xu, Y., Guo, R., Xu, R., Fu, C., Xing, M., et al. (2021). Fanconi Anemia Proteins Participate in a Break-Induced-Replication-Like Pathway to Counter Replication Stress. *Nat. Struct. Mol. Biol.* 28, 487–500. doi: 10.1038/s41594-021-00602-9

Yang, H., Wang, H., Ren, J., Chen, Q., Chen, Z. J. (2017). cGAS is Essential for Cellular Senescence. *Proc. Natl. Acad. Sci. U. S. A.* 114, E4612–E4620. doi: 10.1073/pnas.1705499114

Yu, C. H., Davidson, S., Harapas, C. R., Hilton, J. B., Mlodzianoski, M. J., Laohamonthonkul, P., et al. (2020). TDP-43 Triggers Mitochondrial DNA Release *via* mPTP to Activate cGAS/STING in ALS. *Cell* 183, 636–649.e18. doi: 10.1016/j.cell.2020.09.020

Zhang, H., Kozono, D. E., O'Connor, K. W., Vidal-Cardenas, S., Rousseau, A., Hamilton, A., et al. (2016). TGF-Beta Inhibition Rescues Hematopoietic Stem Cell Defects and Bone Marrow Failure in Fanconi Anemia. *Cell Stem Cell* 18, 668–681. doi: 10.1016/j.stem.2016.03.002

Zhang, X., Sejas, D. P., Qiu, Y., Williams, D. A., Pang, Q. (2007). Inflammatory ROS Promote and Cooperate With the Fanconi Anemia Mutation for Hematopoietic Senescence. *J. Cell Sci.* 120, 1572–1583. doi: 10.1242/jcs.003152

Zhao, K., Du, J., Peng, Y., Li, P., Wang, S., Wang, Y., et al. (2018). LINE1 Contributes to Autoimmunity Through Both RIG-I- and MDA5 Mediated RNA Sensing Pathways. *J. Autoimmun.* 90, 105–115. doi: 10.1016/j.jaut.2018.02.007

Zhao, B., Liu, P., Fukumoto, T., Nacarelli, T., Fatkhutdinov, N., Wu, S., et al. (2020). Topoisomerase 1 Cleavage Complex Enables Pattern Recognition and Inflammation During Senescence. *Nat. Commun.* 11, 908. doi: 10.1038/s41467-020-14652-y

Zhao, M., Wang, F., Wu, J., Cheng, Y., Cao, Y., Wu, X., et al. (2021). CGAS Is a Micronucleophagy Receptor for the Clearance of Micronuclei. *Autophagy* 17 (12), 3976–3991. doi: 10.1080/15548627.2021.1963155

Zou, J., Tian, F., Li, J., Pickner, W., Long, M., Rezvani, K., et al. (2013). FancJ Regulates Interstrand Crosslinker Induced Centrosome Amplification Through the Activation of Polo-Like Kinase 1. *Biol. Open* 2, 1022–1031. doi: 10.1242/bio.20135801

16

Prevalence of Anemia and its Associated Risk Factors Among 6-Months-Old Infants in Beijing

Qinrui Li, Furong Liang, Weilan Liang, Wanjun Shi and Ying Han*

Department of Pediatrics, Peking University First Hospital, Beijing, China

*Correspondence:
Ying Han
hanying1568@126.com

Objective: The worldwide prevalence of anemia is $\sim$24.8%. Iron deficiency anemia is common in children and women and associated with sensory, motor, cognitive, language, and socioemotional deficits. Therefore, detection and early intervention strategies for anemia in infants are urgently needed. To prevent the occurrence of iron deficiency anemia, we aimed to identify risk factors associated with anemia in infants.

Methods: This investigation involved a cross-sectional study of 6-months-old infants discharged between April 2014 and September 2017 from Peking University First Hospital. We assessed birth information, maternal age, and maternal educational level as well as data on feeding style, complementary foods and primary caregivers. The infants were assessed with the Denver Developmental Screening Test (DDST).

Results: A total of 1,127 6-months-old infants were enrolled at the hospital. We found that the prevalence of anemia among infants in Beijing was $\sim$11.8%. Premature infants had a higher rate of anemia than full-term infants ($\chi^2 = 40.103$, $P < 0.001$). Infants born in autumn or winter were at an elevated risk of developing anemia ($\chi^2 = 22.949$, $P < 0.001$). Birth weight had no effect on the rate of anemia in infants ($\chi^2 = 0.023$, $P = 0.568$). Infants who were exclusively breastfeeding had higher anemia rates than those who were fed formula ($\chi^2 = 38.466$, $P < 0.001$). Infants whose caregivers added no complementary foods had higher anemia rates (24.7%) than those whose caregivers added more than two kinds of complementary food (8.2%). The type of caregiver had no effect on the anemia rate in infants ($\chi^2 = 0.031$, $P = 1.000$).

Conclusions: The following factors resulted in a higher prevalence of anemia in our study a gestational age at birth of <37 weeks, exclusive breastfeeding, a lack of supplementation with complementary foods and a spring birth date. No significant differences in DDST pass rates were evident between infants with and without anemia.

Keywords: iron deficiency anemia, growth and development, infants, Denver Development Screen Test (DDST), feeding style

BACKGROUND

Anemia is a common disease that affects ~1.6 billion people worldwide, especially infants and women. The World Health Organization (WHO) has estimated that the global prevalence of anemia to be ~24.8% (1). Anemia is defined as a hemoglobin (Hb) concentration that is two standard deviations below the mean for the patient's age. The factors associated with anemia may include genetics, chronic infections, and nutritional deficiencies, such as hemoglobinopathies, iron deficiency, folate deficiency, and vitamin B12 deficiency. Iron deficiency anemia is common in children, and iron deficiency has a very important influence on infant neurological development. Iron is an essential factor in neuronal myelination, metabolism, neurotransmission and neurogenesis, and it affects behavior, memory, learning and sensory systems (2, 3). In rodents, iron deficiency alters the metabolome in the striatum and delays behavioral development (4). Iron deficiency also alters the neurochemical profile associated with cognitive function in the developing hippocampus (5). Iron deficiency in infancy is associated with impaired mental and motor development, especially in language capabilities, bodily balance and ordination skills (6, 7). Morath and Mayer-Proschel (8) found that iron deficiency during pregnancy affected the function of glial precursor cells in rats. Iron is essential for multiple enzymes associated with the synthesis of neurotransmitters, including dopamine and norepinephrine, which are associated with learning and memory function (9). Iron is important for multiple electron transfer reactions associated with brain energy metabolism (10). Perinatal iron deficiency reduces neuronal activity, especially in the hippocampal region, which is associated with memory function (11).

Infants aged 6–12 months are at an elevated risk of anemia because they are developing and growing rapidly and because the stored iron from the mother may be deficient. The addition of complementary food during this period is important. Complementary foods influence the overall nutritional status of the infant. The risk of iron deficiency increases in later infancy if infants are exclusively breastfeeding (12). A study of infants in poor rural areas of China showed that complementary food supplements could reduce the prevalence of anemia (13). Moreover, home food fortification with iron increased Hb levels and decreased anemia rates (14). Hong et al. (15) showed that the combination of prolonged breastfeeding and an inadequate supply of red meat results in iron deficiency and iron deficiency anemia. Insufficient complementary feeding behavior is associated with undernutrition, which results in poor growth and cognitive development. Baye et al. (16) found that positive, responsive maternal feeding behavior was positively associated with Hb concentrations. Other factors also influence the iron status of infants; one example is the maternal iron status, which is associated with anemia in children. In this case, anemia occurs because an infant cannot obtain enough iron from the stored iron transferred from the mother or from breast milk (17). The educational level of the mother or caregiver is also associated with the anemia rate (18, 19).

Rapid economic development and the acceleration of industrialization in China have led to major changes in Chinese lifestyles, especially for new parents. As the capital city of China, Beijing is more representative of such changes than other cities. Infants in Beijing consume increasingly rich diets, and their developmental health is better now than in the past. As the education level of the mother increases, her knowledge of how to feed her children improves. In the present study, we aimed to investigate the factors currently associated with infant anemia in Beijing, with the goal of improving the health of these infants.

METHODS

Participants

This investigation involved a cross-sectional study conducted at Peking University First Hospital. The participants were enrolled between April 2014 and September 2017. The infants included in this study were 6 months old and did not have severe disease or any abnormality at birth. The exclusion criteria were as follows: younger or older than 6 months old, a history of asphyxia at birth, and a history of severe disease. Children who met the inclusion criteria and did not meet the exclusion criteria were enrolled in our study. For each infant, we collected data regarding sex (male or female), maternal education level (less than undergraduate, undergraduate, or more than undergraduate), birth weight, birth season, caregivers (parent, grandparent, or babysitter), feeding style (exclusive breastfeeding, mixed feeding or formula feeding), and complementary food usage (none, one kind of complementary food or two or more kinds of complementary food). We defined the four seasons as follows: winter (December, January, and February), spring (March, April, and May), summer (June, July, and August), and autumn (September, October, and November).

Diagnostic Criteria and Classification

Anemia is defined as an Hb concentration <110 g/L according to the WHO diagnostic criteria. Mild anemia is defined as an Hb concentration between 90 and 110 g/L, moderate anemia is defined as an Hb concentration between 60 and 90 g/L, and severe anemia is defined as an Hb concentration <60 g/L. Iron deficiency anemia is defined as a mean cell volume (MCV) <80 fl, mean cell hemoglobin (MCH) <27 pg, and mean corpuscular Hb concentration (MCHC) <310 g/L.

Assessment of Ability Development

The development of the infants' intelligence was assessed with the Denver Developmental Screening Test (DDST). The DDST was standardized for Chinese use in 1982 and has been utilized worldwide to assess the intelligence development of children aged 1 month to 6 years. The standardized DDST consists of 104 items and covers four areas of development: (a) personal/social, (b) fine motor/adaptive, (c) language, and (d) gross motor. In the present study, three trained professionals examined the children. The response options for the items were "passes," "fails," "refuses," and "has not had the opportunity." The results of the DDST could be normal (no delays), suspect (2 or more caution items and/or 1 or more delays), abnormal (2 or more delays) or untestable (refusal

TABLE 1 | Infant birth information.

Sex	N	Birth weight (kg)	Birth length (cm)	Hemoglobin (g/L)
Male	591	3.38 ± 0.42	50.6 ± 2.1	117.9 ± 8.5
Female	536	3.26 ± 0.45	50.2 ± 1.8	118.4 ± 7.8

of one or more items completely to the left of the age line or more than one item intersected by the age line in the 75–90% area). The children with suspect or abnormal results were retested 2 or 3 weeks later.

Statistical Analysis

The data were analyzed with SPSS 18.0. Numerical variables are presented as the mean ± standard deviation (SD) (birth weight). Enumeration data and ranked data are presented as percentages. ANOVA, the χ^2 test and non-parametric tests were used to assess the differences in child development between the three groups. A P-value <0.05 was considered statistically significant.

Ethics

The study was carried out in accordance with recommendations of the Clinical Research Ethics Committee of Peking University First Hospital (Permit Number: 2017 [1375]). All parents provided written informed consent before the start of the study.

RESULTS

A total of 1,127 infants (591 male and 536 female) aged 6 months were included in this study. The average birth weights of the infants were 3.38 ± 0.42 kg for males and 3.26 ± 0.45 kg for females. The average birth lengths were 50.6 ± 2.1 cm for males and 50.2 ± 1.8 cm for females. The average Hb levels were 117.9 ± 8.5 g/L in males and 118.4 ± 7.8 g/L in females (**Table 1**). The mean maternal age was ~31.8 ± 3.5 years.

Table 2 contains the demographic information (e.g., maternal educational level, maternal age, gestational age at birth, and birth season) and Hb levels of the included infants. The mean Hb value was 118.2 ± 8.1 g/L (range 80.0–146.0 g/L). A total of 133 (11.8%) infants had microcytic hypochromic anemia (MCV <80 fl, MCH <27 pg, and MCHC <310 g/L), including 126 (11.2%) with mild anemia (104.6 ± 4.7 g/L) and 7 (0.6%) with moderate anemia (85.3 ± 3.1 g/L). No infants displayed severe anemia. The mean Hb level in the non-anemia group was 120.1 ± 6.1 g/L. The mean Hb values of the groups with maternal educational levels of less than undergraduate, undergraduate and more than undergraduate were 118.0 ± 8.9, 118.7 ± 7.5, and 117.4 ± 8.5 g/L, respectively. The ages of the mothers ranged from 22 to 45 years old. The effects of maternal age on the Hb levels of the infants are shown in **Table 2**. The study group contained 65 premature infants, whose mean Hb level was 113.3 ± 10.3 g/L. The study group contained 1,062 full-term infants, whose mean Hb level was 118.5 ± 7.9 g/L. **Table 2** also shows the effects of birth season and birth weight on Hb levels.

As shown in **Table 3**, feeding practices affected the infants' Hb levels. A total of 197 (17.5%) infants were fed formula and had a mean Hb level of 120.7 ± 7.3 g/L. A total of 634 (56.3%)

TABLE 2 | Demographic information and hemoglobin levels.

Characteristics	n	Percent (%)	Hemoglobin (g/L)
Hemoglobin (g/L)			
Normal (>110)	994	88.2%	120.1 ± 6.1
Mild (90–109)	126	11.2%	104.6 ± 4.7
Moderate (60–89)	7	0.6%	85.3 ± 3.1
Severe (<59)	0	0	–
Maternal educational level			
Less than undergraduate	185	17.6%	118.0 ± 8.9
Undergraduate	580	55.2%	118.7 ± 7.5
More than undergraduate	285	27.1%	117.4 ± 8.5
Maternal age			
<25 years	8	0.7%	114.9 ± 6.6
25–29 years	289	26.9%	118.3 ± 8.1
30–34 years	556	51.8%	118.6 ± 7.8
35–39 years	187	17.4%	117 5 ± 8.4
>39 years	33	3.1%	116.8 ± 8.7
Gestational age at birth			
<37 weeks	65	5.8%	113.3 ± 10.3
>37 weeks	1,062	94.2%	118.5 ± 7.9
Birth season			
Spring	220	19.5%	117.1 ± 7.4
Summer	292	25.9%	118.1 ± 5.3
Autumn	336	29.8%	118.3 ± 9.5
Winter	279	24.8%	119.0 ± 9.2
Birth weight			
<2,500 g	36	3.3%	118.5 ± 9.5
>2,500 g	1,063	96.7%	118.1 ± 8.1

infants were exclusively fed breast milk and had a mean Hb level of 116.6 ± 8.5 g/L. A total of 296 (26.3%) infants received mixed feeding and had a mean Hb level of 119.9 ± 7.0 g/L. Most infants (96.3%) had diets containing complementary foods as follows: one type of complementary food (rice flour) or two or more types of complementary foods (rice flour, yolk or liver paste). A total of 202 (41.6%) infants, 253 (52.1%) infants, and 31 (6.4%) infants were cared for by their parents, grandparents and babysitters, respectively, and the mean Hb levels of these infants were 117.3 ± 7.6, 117.7 ± 8.2, and 118.3 ± 9.7 g/L, respectively.

The factors that affected infant anemia are shown in **Table 4**. Gestational age at birth, birth season, feeding style and complementary food supplementation had clear effects on infant anemia. Premature infants had higher rates of anemia than full-term infants ($\chi^2 = 40.103$, $P < 0.001$). The infants born in autumn or winter were at an increased risk of developing anemia ($\chi^2 = 22.949$, $P < 0.001$). Birth weight had no effect on the rate of anemia in infants ($\chi^2 = 0.023$, $P = 0.568$). Infants who were exclusively breastfeeding had higher anemia rates than infants who were fed formula ($\chi^2 = 38.466$, $P < 0.001$). Infants whose caregivers added no complementary foods had higher anemia rates (24.7%) than infants whose caregivers added two or more types of complementary food (8.2%). The type of caregiver had no effect on infant anemia rates ($\chi^2 = 0.031$, $P = 1.000$). **Table 5** shows the multivariate logistic regression analysis results of the

TABLE 3 | Infant feeding practices.

Feeding practice	n	Percent (%)	Hemoglobin (g/L)
Feeding style			
Exclusive breastfeeding	634	56.3%	116.6 ± 8.5
Mixed feeding	296	26.3%	119.9 ± 7.0
Artificial feeding	197	17.5%	120.7 ± 7.3
Complementary foods			
None	85	3.7%	115.7 ± 11.7
One kind	390	32.3%	119.0 ± 8.9
More than two kinds	478	64.0%	119.1 ± 7.0
Caregivers			
Parents	202	41.6%	117.3 ± 7.6
Grandparents	253	52.1%	117.7 ± 8.2
Babysitters	31	6.4%	118.3 ± 9.7

TABLE 4 | Factors associated with infant anemia.

Factors	Anemia N (%)	Non-anemia N (%)	χ^2	P
			1.799	0.196
Male	77 (13%)	514 (87%)		
Female	56 (10.4%)	480 (89.6%)		
Maternal educational level			2.132	0.352
Less than undergraduate	24 (13%)	161 (87%)		
Undergraduate	61 (10.5%)	519 (89.5%)		
More than undergraduate	39 (13.7%)	246 (86.3%)		
Maternal age			3.147	0.672[a]
<25 years	1 (12.5%)	7 (87.5%)		
25–29 years	38 (13.1%)	251 (86.9%)		
30–34 years	58 (10.4%)	498 (89.6%)		
35–39 years	22 (11.8%)	165 (88.2%)		
40–44 years	5 (15.6%)	27 (84.4%)		
>44 years	0 (0%)	1 (100%)		
Gestational age at birth			40.103	0.000*
<37 weeks	25 (38.5%)	40 (61.5%)		
>37 weeks	108 (10.2%)	954 (89.8%)		
Birth season			22.949	0.000*
Spring	13 (5.9%)	207 (94.1%)		
Summer	22 (7.5%)	270 (92.5%)		
Autumn	51 (15.2%)	285 (84.8%)		
Winter	47 (16.8%)	232 (83.2%)		
Birth weight			0.023	0.568
<2,500 g	4 (11.1%)	32 (88.9%)		
>2,500 g	127 (11.9%)	936 (88.1%)		
Feeding style			38.466	0.000*
Exclusive breastfeeding	108 (17%)	526 (83%)		
Mixed feeding	13 (4.4%)	283 (95.6%)		
Artificial feeding	12 (6.1%)	185 (93.9%)		
Complementary foods			21.509	0.000*
None	21 (24.7%)	64 (75.3%)		
One kind	51 (13.1%)	339 (86.9%)		
More than two kinds	44 (8.2%)	495 (91.8%)		
Caregivers			0.031	1.000
Parents	27 (13.4%)	175 (86.6%)		
Grandparents	34 (13.4%)	219 (86.6%)		
Babysitters	4 (12.9%)	27 (87.1%)		

[a]Fisher's exact test.
*P < 0.001.

risk factors for infant anemia. Gestational age at birth, birth season, feeding style and complementary food supplementation significantly affected infant anemia rates ($P < 0.05$).

As shown in **Table 6**, anemia had no significant effect on the DDST pass rates ($\chi^2 = 5.600$, $P = 0.051$).

DISCUSSION

The present study examined information associated with 1,127 6-months-old infants and revealed an anemia prevalence of 11.8%. In our study, the risk factors associated with anemia were gestational age at birth, birth season, feeding style and complementary food supplementation. No significant difference in the DDST pass rate was evident between infants with and without anemia.

The anemia rate in our study was lower than the global anemia rate (24.8%) (1). The WHO has estimated that anemia affects 1.62 billion people globally, including 293 million preschool-aged children, 56 million pregnant women and 468 million non-pregnant women. A total of 54.3% of infants aged 6–11 months are reportedly anemic, and 24.3% of infants in rural China suffer from moderate or severe anemia (20). Although the prevalence of anemia in China has gradually decreased, the adverse impacts of anemia on infants and society are profound. The most common form of anemia is iron deficiency anemia (21). Iron deficiency in children <3 years of age negatively affects their physical and intellectual development (22). Additionally, the prevalence of anemia is highest at the ages of 6–12 months, a period that is critical for psychomotor development. Some studies have shown that infants with iron deficiency have lower auditory brainstem response (ABR) responses than those with normal iron levels, representing the iron deficiency anemia infants with delayed central nervous system (CNS) myelination (23). Therefore, we aimed to identify the risk factors associated with anemia.

In our study, we found that premature infants had an increased risk of developing anemia at 6 months of age, which was consistent with other studies (24, 25). Halliday et al. (26) found that 26% of premature infants had iron deficiency during the first year of life. Preterm infants are at high risk

of nutritional deficiency because they have low stores of iron, zinc and vitamin A (27). Preterm infants can experience blood loss at birth, inadequate erythropoiesis, blood sampling, rapid growth, hemorrhage and hemolysis. Therefore, most premature infants have smaller blood volumes and experience more profound anemia than full-term infants (28). The effects of iron deficiency include poor physical growth, gastrointestinal disturbances, neurodevelopmental impairments and altered immunity (29, 30). Therefore, premature infants should receive iron supplementation from sources, such as fortified human milk, iron-fortified formula or medicinal elemental iron (e.g., 2–4 mg/kg/d).

TABLE 5 | Univariate analysis of factors influencing infant anemia.

Factors	B	SE	P	OR	95% CI for Exp (B)
Gestational age at birth	−1.979	0.303	0.000*	0.138	0.076–0.250
Birth season	−0.473	0.098	0.000*	0.623	0.515–0.755
Feeding style	0.847	0.169	0.000*	2.332	1.675–3.247
Complementary foods	0.254	0.096	0.008*	1.289	1.068–1.554

B, coefficient; SE, standard error; OR, odds ratio, which equals to the power of the coefficient B; 95% CI for Exp (B), 95% confidence interval of the exponentiation of the coefficient B.
*P < 0.001.

TABLE 6 | Effect of anemia on DDST pass rates.

	Pass	Suspect	Abnormal	χ^2	P
Anemia	121 (91.0%)	8 (6.0%)	4 (3.0%)	5.600	0.051
Non-anemia	910 (91.5%)	77 (7.7%)	7 (0.7%)		

We showed that infants born in spring had lower Hb levels than infants born in winter. A previous study also showed that the incidence of anemia in infants aged 5–7 months who were born in spring and summer was higher than that in infants aged 5–7 months who were born in autumn or winter (31). This difference is probably due to seasonal variations in the folate and vitamin B6 statuses among women who may be attempting to become pregnant (32, 33).

In our study, we found that feeding style and complementary foods affected the prevalence of anemia in infants. Infants who were exclusively breastfeeding (17%) had a higher prevalence of anemia than infants whose diets were mixed or infants who were fed formula (4.4 and 6.1%). The formula consumed by the infants contained iron; therefore, the infants whose diets were mixed and the infants who were fed formula were unlikely to develop anemia. The addition of two or more types of complementary foods was associated with the lowest prevalence of anemia among the three groups (8.2 vs. 24.7% and 13.1%). The WHO recommends exclusive breastfeeding without the introduction of any nutritious complementary foods for the first 6 months (34). The concentration of iron in human milk is relatively low. In China, some parents do not add complementary foods or iron supplementation during the first 6 months, which has become an important cause of infant anemia. As the infant grows, iron from human milk becomes insufficient to meet the increasing needs of the body tissue and circulation (35). Therefore, complementary foods containing iron should be given to infants at the proper time to avoid anemia (36). In our study, the infants who were fed one type of food were always fed rice flour, and the infants who were fed two or more types of complementary foods were always fed liver paste, yolk or meat paste, which contain high levels of iron. Wang et al. (37) found that the introduction of complementary foods comprising rice cereal, porridge, and bread was more likely to result in the development of anemia than the introduction of animal-based

foods. Rice cereal, porridge, and bread contain low amounts of bioavailable iron and have phytates that inhibit iron absorption (38). One study showed that deficiencies in vitamin A, vitamin C, zinc and iron were associated with the late introduction of complementary food (39). Thus, the addition of complementary foods should begin when maternal milk no longer meets the nutritional needs of the infant. Complementary foods not only provide nutrition to infants but also shape their future eating habits (40). However, some studies have shown that the early introduction of complementary foods is associated with allergies (41). Conversely, the late introduction of complementary foods is associated with developmental delays, such as motor skill deficits (42). In subsequent studies, we intend to identify a suitable time for the introduction of complementary foods.

In our study, we found that anemia was not associated with the DDST pass rates. This lack of association was probably because the duration of anemia in the infants was not sufficient to influence the DDST results. Iron requirements are most likely to exceed iron intake during the first 6–18 months of life because infants' growth and blood volume expansion proceed rapidly during this time (43). In our study, we investigated 6-months-old infants with anemia; thus, anemia had not been present for long. Lozoff et al. (44) showed that infants with iron deficiency anemia processed information slower at 12 months of age than infants with a good iron status. Infants with iron deficiency anemia have reduced dopamine function at 9 months, and this condition worsens at 12 months (45). Shafir et al. (46) found that 12- to 23-months-old infants with iron deficiency anemia did not catch up in motor development, although iron therapy during infancy corrected their anemia. In summary, anemia in infants should be detected as soon as possible. We examined Hb levels at the age of 6 months to select anemic infants and provide therapy early, thus preventing unfavorable outcomes caused by iron deficiency. Some studies have shown that at 6–8 weeks after birth, infants should receive iron supplementation (2–3 mg/kg per day) or formula containing iron (12 mg/L) to prevent iron deficiency anemia. Infants with birth weights below 1,000 g require additional iron (47).

Our study showed that the gestational age at birth, birth season, feeding style and complementary food supplementation affected anemia in infants aged 6 months. Early detection is of utmost importance to prevent adverse outcomes caused by infant anemia. Next, the caregiver should add iron-containing complementary foods, such as liver paste, yolk and meat paste, at a suitable time, especially in infants whose gestational age at birth is <37 weeks. In addition, infants born during different seasons should be supplied with nutrition accordingly. For example, infants born during spring should be provided with more iron than those born during winter.

Nevertheless, our study had several limitations. First, China is an expansive country that contains individuals of different ethnicities who inhabit different geographic locations and have various dietary traditions. These factors are probably associated with the prevalence of anemia. However, our study was limited to the population in Beijing. Further studies should focus on low income and middle-income provinces in China. Second, we also lacked information regarding maternal anemia. Maternal anemia has been associated with infant anemia (48). In future studies, we will examine data on maternal anemia.

CONCLUSIONS

Anemia is a global public health problem that influences infant development, resulting in poor outcomes in adulthood. The risk factors identified in our study, such as a gestational age at birth of <37 weeks, exclusive breastfeeding, a lack of supplementation with complementary foods and a spring birth date, may be meaningful for the early detection of infant anemia and the prompt delivery of interventions.

ETHICS STATEMENT

The study was carried out in accordance with the recommendations of the Clinical Research Ethics Committee of Peking University First Hospital. All subjects gave written informed consent in accordance with the Declaration of Helsinki.

The protocol was approved by the Ethics Committee of Peking University First Hospital, China.

AUTHOR CONTRIBUTIONS

QL conducted the experiments, analyzed the data, wrote the manuscript, and approved the final version to be published. YH contributed to the conception and design of the experiment, acquired the data, revised the manuscript, approved the final version to be published, and agreed to be accountable for all aspects of the work. FL and WL contributed to the conception and design of the experiment, acquired the data, critically revised the manuscript, and approved the final version to be published. WS contributed to the conception and design of the experiment and approved the final version to be published.

ACKNOWLEDGMENTS

We are grateful to the caregivers and infants who participated in this study.

REFERENCES

McLean E, Cogswell M, Egli I, Wojdyla D, de Benoist B. Worldwide prevalence of anaemia, WHO Vitamin and mineral nutrition information system, 1993–2005. *Public Health Nutr.* (2009) 12:444–54. doi: 10.1017/S1368980008002401

Ortiz E, Pasquini JM, Thompson K, Felt B, Butkus G, Beard J, et al. Effect of manipulation of iron storage, transport, or availability on myelin composition and brain iron content in three different animal models. *J Neurosci Res.* (2004) 77:681–9. doi: 10.1002/jnr.20207

Lozoff B. Iron deficiency and child development. *Food Nutr Bull.* (2007) 28:S560–71. doi: 10.1177/15648265070284S409

Ward KL, Tkac I, Jing Y, Felt B, Beard J, Connor J, et al. Gestational and lactational iron deficiency alters the developing striatal metabolome and associated behaviors in young rats. *J Nutr.* (2007) 137:1043–9. doi: 10.1093/jn/137.4.1043

Rao R, Tkac I, Townsend EL, Gruetter R, Georgieff MK. Perinatal iron deficiency alters the neurochemical profile of the developing rat hippocampus. *J Nutr.* (2003) 133:3215–21. doi: 10.1093/jn/133.10.3215

Walter T, Kovalskys J, Stekel A. Effect of mild iron deficiency on infant mental development scores. *J Pediatr.* (1983) 102:519–22.

Lozoff B, Brittenham GM, Wolf AW, McClish DK, Kuhnert PM, Jimenez E, et al. Iron deficiency anemia and iron therapy effects on infant developmental test performance. *Pediatrics.* (1987) 79:981–95.

Morath DJ, Mayer-Proschel M. Iron deficiency during embryogenesis and consequences for oligodendrocyte generation *in vivo. Dev Neurosci.* (2002) 24:197–207. doi: 10.1159/000065688

Lozoff B, Beard J, Connor J, Barbara F, Georgieff M, Schallert T. Long-lasting neural and behavioral effects of iron deficiency in infancy. *Nutr Rev.* (2006) 64:S34–43; discussion S72–91. doi: 10.1301/nr.2006.may.s34-s43

Beard J. Iron deficiency alters brain development and functioning. *J Nutr.* (2003) 133:1468S–72S. doi: 10.1093/jn/133.5.1468S

de Deungria M, Rao R, Wobken JD, Luciana M, Nelson CA, Georgieff MK. Perinatal iron deficiency decreases cytochrome c oxidase (CytOx) activity in selected regions of neonatal rat brain. *Pediatric Res.* (2000) 48:169–76. doi: 10.1203/00006450-200008000-00009

Clark KM, Li M, Zhu B, Liang F, Shao J, Zhang Y, et al. Breastfeeding, mixed, or formula feeding at 9 months of age and the prevalence of iron deficiency and iron deficiency anemia in two cohorts of infants in China. *J Pediatric.* (2017)

181:56–61. doi: 10.1016/j.jpeds.2016.10.041

Zhang Y, Wu Q, Wang W, van Velthoven MH, Chang S, Han H, et al. Effectiveness of complementary food supplements and dietary counselling on anaemia and stunting in children aged 6-23 months in poor areas of Qinghai Province, China: a controlled interventional study. *BMJ Open.* (2016) 6:e011234. doi: 10.1136/bmjopen-2016-011234

Huo J, Sun J, Fang Z, Chang S, Zhao L, Fu P, et al. Effect of home- based complementary food fortification on prevalence of anemia among infants and young children aged 6 to 23 months in poor rural regions of China. *Food Nutr Bull.* (2015) 36:405–14. doi: 10.1177/0379572115 616001

Hong J, Chang JY, Shin S, Oh S. Breastfeeding and red meat intake are associated with iron status in healthy Korean weaning-age infants. *J Korean Med Sci.* (2017) 32:974–84. doi: 10.3346/jkms.2017.32.6.974

Baye K, Tariku A, Mouquet-Rivier C. Caregiver-infant's feeding behaviours are associated with energy intake of 9–11 month-old infants in rural Ethiopia. *Matern Child Nutr.* (2018) 14:e12487. doi: 10.1111/mcn.12487

Zhao A, Zhang Y, Peng Y, Li J, Yang T, Liu Z, et al. Prevalence of anemia and its risk factors among children 6–36 months old in Burma. *Am J Trop Med Hyg.* (2012) 87:306–11. doi: 10.4269/ajtmh.2012.11-0660

Abubakar A, Uriyo J, Msuya SE, Swai M, Stray-Pedersen B. Prevalence and risk factors for poor nutritional status among children in the Kilimanjaro region of Tanzania. *Int J Environ Res Public Health.* (2012) 9:3506–18. doi: 10.3390/ijerph9103506

Ayoya MA, Ngnie-Teta I, Seraphin MN, Mamadoultaibou A, Boldon E, Saint- Fleur JE, et al. Prevalence and risk factors of anemia among children 6–59 months old in Haiti. *Anemia.* (2013) 2013:502968. doi: 10.1155/2013/502968

Luo R, Shi Y, Zhou H, Yue A, Zhang L, Sylvia S, et al. Anemia and feeding practices among infants in rural Shaanxi Province in China. *Nutrients.* (2014) 6:5975–91. doi: 10.3390/nu6125975

Martorell R, Ascencio M, Tacsan L, Alfaro T, Young MF, Addo OY, et al. Effectiveness evaluation of the food fortification program of Costa Rica: impact on anemia prevalence and hemoglobin concentrations in women and children. *Am J Clin Nutr.* (2015) 101:210–7. doi: 10.3945/ajcn.114.097709

Black RE, Victora CG, Walker SP, Bhutta ZA, Christian P, de Onis M, et al. Maternal and child undernutrition and overweight in low- income and middle-income countries. *Lancet.* (2013) 382:427–51. doi: 10.1016/S0140-6736(13)60937-X

Amin SB, Orlando M, Eddins A, MacDonald M, Monczynski C, Wang H. *In utero* iron status and auditory neural maturation in premature infants as evaluated by auditory brainstem response. *J Pediatr.* (2010) 156:377–81. doi: 10.1016/j.jpeds.2009.09.049

Shaw JC. Iron absorption by the premature infant. The effect of transfusion and iron supplements on the serum ferritin levels. *Acta Paediatr Scand Suppl.* (1982) 299:83–9.

Rao R, Georgieff MK. Iron therapy for preterm infants. *Clin Perinatol.* (2009) 36:27–42. doi: 10.1016/j.clp.2008.09.013

Halliday HL, Lappin TR, McClure G. Iron status of the preterm infant during the first year of life. *Biol Neonate.* (1984) 45:228–35.

Shah MD, Shah SR. Nutrient deficiencies in the premature infant. *Pediatr Clin North Am.* (2009) 56:1069–83. doi: 10.1016/j.pcl.2009.08.001

Jeon GW, Sin JB. Risk factors of transfusion in anemia of very low birth weight infants. *Yonsei Med J.* (2013) 54:366–73. doi: 10.3349/ymj.2013.54.2.366

Aggett PJ. Trace elements of the micropremie. *Clin Perinatol.* (2000) 27:119–29, vi. doi: 10.1016/S0095-5108(05)70009-9

Lozoff B, Georgieff MK. Iron deficiency and brain development. *Semin Pediatr Neurol.* (2006) 13:158–65. doi: 10.1016/j.spen.2006.08.004

Yalcin SS, Dut R, Yurdakok K, Ozmert E. Seasonal and gender differences in hemoglobin value in infants at 5–7 months of age. *Turk J Pediatr.* (2009) 51:572–7.

Zhang J, Cai WW, Chen H. Perinatal mortality in Shanghai: 1986–1987. *Int J Epidemiol.* (1991) 20:958–63.

Ronnenberg AG, Goldman MB, Aitken IW, Xu X. Anemia and deficiencies of folate and vitamin B-6 are common and vary with season in Chinese women of childbearing age. *J Nutr.* (2000) 130:2703–10. doi: 10.1093/jn/130.11.2703

Ye F, Chen ZH, Chen J, Liu F, Zhang Y, Fan QY, et al. Chi-squared automatic interaction detection decision tree analysis of risk factors for infant anemia in Beijing, China. *Chin Med J (Engl).* (2016) 129:1193–9. doi: 10.4103/0366-6999.181955

Tsai SF, Chen SJ, Yen HJ, Hung GY, Tsao PC, Jeng MJ, et al. Iron deficiency anemia in predominantly breastfed young children. *Pediatr Neonatol.* (2014) 55:466–9. doi: 10.1016/j.pedneo.2014.02.005

Krebs NF, Hambidge KM. Complementary feeding: clinically relevant factors affecting timing and composition. *Am J Clin Nutr.* (2007) 85:639S–45S. doi: 10.1093/ajcn/85.2.639S

Wang F, Liu H, Wan Y, Li J, Chen Y, Zheng J, et al. Age of complementary foods introduction and risk of anemia in children aged 4–6 years: a prospective birth cohort in China. *Sci Rep.* (2017) 7:44726. doi: 10.1038/srep44726

Zimmermann MB, Chaouki N, Hurrell RF. Iron deficiency due to consumption of a habitual diet low in bioavailable iron: a longitudinal cohort study in Moroccan children. *Am J Clin Nutr.* (2005) 81:115–21. doi: 10.1093/ajcn/81.1.115

Wutich A, McCarty C. Social networks and infant feeding in Oaxaca, Mexico. *Matern Child Nutr.* (2008) 4:121–35. doi: 10.1111/j.1740-8709.2007. 00122.x

Pantoja-Mendoza IY, Melendez G, Guevara-Cruz M, Serralde-Zuniga AE. Review of complementary feeding practices in Mexican children. *Nutr Hosp.* (2014) 31:552–8. doi: 10.3305/nh.2015.31.2.7668

Grimshaw KE, Maskell J, Oliver EM, Morris RC, Foote KD, Mills EN, et al. Introduction of complementary foods and the relationship to food allergy. *Pediatrics.* (2013) 132:e1529–38. doi: 10.1542/peds.2012-3692

Lutter CK. Macrolevel approaches to improve the availability of complementary foods. *Food Nutr Bull.* (2003) 24:83–103. doi: 10.1177/156482650302400105

Beard JL. Why iron deficiency is important in infant development. *J Nutr.* (2008) 138:2534–6. doi: 10.1093/jn/138.12.2534

Lozoff B, De Andraca I, Castillo M, Smith JB, Walter T, Pino P. Behavioral and developmental effects of preventing iron deficiency anemia in healthy full-term infants. *Pediatrics.* (2003) 112:846–54.

Lozoff B, Armony-Sivan R, Kaciroti N, Jing Y, Golub M, Jacobson SW. Eye- blinking rates are slower in infants with iron deficiency anemia than in nonanemic iron-deficient or iron-sufficient infants. *J Nutr.* (2010) 140:1057– 61. doi: 10.3945/jn.110.120964

Shafir T, Angulo-Barroso R, Calatroni A, Jimenez E, Lozoff B. Effects of iron deficiency in infancy on patterns of motor development over time. *Hum Mov Sci.* (2006) 25:821–38. doi: 10.1016/j.humov.2006.06.006

Siimes MA. Iron requirement in low birthweight infants. *Acta Paediatr Scand Suppl.* (1982) 296:101–3.

Meinzen-Derr JK, Guerrero ML, Altaye M, Ortega-Gallegos H, Ruiz-Palacios GM, Morrow AL. Risk of infant anemia is associated with exclusive breast- feeding and maternal anemia in a Mexican cohort. *J Nutr.* (2006) 136:452–8. doi: 10.1093/jn/136.2.452

17

Mild Anemia May Affect Thyroid Function in Pregnant Chinese Women During the First Trimester

Guan-ying Nie[1], Rui Wang[2], Peng Liu[1], Ming Li[1*] and Dian-jun Sun[1*]

[1] Key Lab of Etiology and Epidemiology, National Health Commission & Education Bureau of Heilongjiang Province (23618504), Key Laboratory of Trace Elements and Human Health, Center for Endemic Disease Control, Chinese Center for Disease Control and Prevention, Harbin Medical University, Harbin, China, [2] Examination Department, Central Hospital Affiliated to Shenyang Medical College, Shenyang, China

Correspondence:
Ming Li
liming@hrbmu.edu.cn
Dian-jun Sun
hrbmusdj@163.com

Background: Pregnant women are often susceptible to anemia, which can damage the thyroid gland. However, compared with moderate and severe anemia, less attention has been paid to mild anemia. The purpose of this study was to evaluate the effect of mild anemia on the thyroid function in pregnant women during the first trimester.

Methods: A total of 1,761 women in the first trimester of their pregnancy were enrolled from Shenyang, China, and divided into mild anemia and normal control groups based on their hemoglobin levels. Thyroid-stimulating hormone (TSH), free thyroxine (FT4), and free triiodothyronine (FT3) levels were compared between the two groups.

Results: The TSH levels of pregnant women with mild anemia were higher than those of pregnant women without mild anemia (p < 0.05). Normal control women were selected to set new reference intervals for TSH, FT3, and FT4 levels during the first trimester, which were 0.11–4.13 mIU/l, 3.45–5.47 pmol/l, and 7.96–16.54 pmol/l, respectively. The upper limit of TSH 4.13 mU/l is close to the upper limit 4.0 mU/l recommended in the 2017 American Thyroid Association (ATA) guidelines, indicating that exclusion of mild anemia may reduce the difference in reference values from different regions. Mild anemia was related to 4.40 times odds of abnormally TSH levels (95% CI: 2.84, 6.76) and 5.87 increased odds of abnormal FT3 (95% CI: 3.89, 8.85). The proportion of hypothyroidism and subclinical hypothyroidism in patients with mild anemia was higher than that in those without anemia (0.6% vs. 0, p = 0.009; 12.1% vs. 1.9%, p < 0.001). Mild anemia was related to 7.61 times increased odds of subclinical hypothyroidism (95% CI: 4.53, 12.90).

Conclusions: Mild anemia may affect thyroid function during the first trimester, which highlights the importance of excluding mild anemia confounding when establishing a locally derived specific reference interval for early pregnancy.

Keywords: the first trimester, mild anemia, FT4, TSH, reference values, subclinical hypothyroidism

INTRODUCTION

Thyroid dysfunction during pregnancy increases the risk of miscarriage, premature birth, fetal malformation, and even fetal death (1, 2). Therefore, to maintain maternal and child health, thyroid function should be actively advocated for all pregnant women.

Anemia is defined as a hemoglobin level of 120 g/l or less in women, and 110 g/l or less in pregnant women (3–5). The World Health Organization (WHO) has reported that 23% of pregnant women in industrialized countries and 52% in non-industrialized countries suffer from anemia (6). Iron deficiency (ID) is the main cause of anemia (7). Other causes include lack of vitamin A, B12, or folic acid; infectious diseases such as malaria and AIDS; and other hereditary anemias such as sickle cell disease (8). Anemia and thyroid function studies carried out in animal models have verified that low iron intake significantly decreases hemoglobin (Hb) levels, thyroid peroxidase (TPO) activity (9, 10), and serum concentrations of T3 and T4 (11), while increasing TSH levels (12). In 2007, Zimmermann et al. first reported that ID was associated with higher TSH and lower T4 levels in Swiss pregnant women (13). In recent years, studies in China have shown that ID can also be associated with abnormal thyroid function of pregnant women (14–17). Additionally, hypothyroidism occurs in patients with chronic hemolytic anemia, and its incidence is positively correlated with age and the severity of anemia (18).

Nevertheless, insufficient attention has been directed toward the relationship between mild anemia and thyroid function in pregnant women. Mild, moderate, and severe anemia in women was defined as a hemoglobin level of 110–119, 80–109, and <80 g/l, while that in pregnant women was defined as 100–109, 70–99, and <70 g/l (3–5). A study has revealed that pregnant women with mild, moderate, or severe anemia are related to infant anemia (19). Compared to those of moderate and severe anemia, the symptoms of mild anemia are non-specific and are only clinically detectable, which might explain why little attention is paid to mild anemia. A study has reported the prevalence of anemia among Chinese women before pregnancy to be 21. 64% (mild: 14.10%, moderate: 7.17%, and severe: 0.37%) in 2017 (20). According to the results monitored from 2010 to 2012, the anemia rate in pregnant women in China was 17.2%, while mild anemia accounted for approximately 61.0% (21). Mild anemia accounted for the highest proportion of overall anemia. Therefore, this study aimed to explore the effect of mild anemia in early pregnancy on the thyroid function of pregnant women in Shenyang, a city in northeast of China.

MATERIALS AND METHODS

Study Population

The study was approved by the Ethics Committee of Harbin Medical University. We extracted the first routine evaluation results of pregnant women in the obstetric outpatient department of the Affiliated Central Hospital of Shenyang Medical College from September 2011 to December 2018. Prior to enrollment into the study, the pregnant women underwent routine blood and thyroid function examination (n = 2,902). Women with a pregnancy of 10–12 weeks of gestation were included in the study. Those women with a pregnancy of less than 10 weeks or more than 12 weeks of gestation were not eligible to participate (n = 712). Pregnant women with moderate anemia, severe anemia, self-reported blood diseases, infections, fever, drug treatment, or supplement treatment (n = 129) were also excluded. Pregnant women with self-reported thyroid disease (n = 154) or positive thyroid autoantibodies (TPOAb, TgAb, or TMAb) (n = 146) were also considered to be ineligible. Based on the abovementioned criteria, a total of 1,761 pregnant women were selected, including 314 pregnant women with mild anemia and 1,447 pregnant women without anemia as the control group (**Figure 1**).

Method

Venous blood samples were collected in the morning after overnight fasting for more than 8 h. Blood samples were centrifuged to obtain serum, which was sent to the clinical laboratory for testing. The levels TSH, FT4, and FT3 were determined in all subjects on the same day of sampling, using a commercial electrochemiluminescence immunoassay kit (Beckman UniCel DxI800 automatic chemiluminescence analyzer, USA). Hemoglobin (Hb) levels were measured using an automated hematology analyzer XE-2100 (Sysmex Diagnostics, Japan). The women were considered to have mild anemic if their Hb was determined to be in the range 100–109 g/l.

Statistical Analysis

Statistical analysis was performed using the Statistical Product and Service Solutions (SPSS) software (version 17.0, Chicago, IL). The Kolmogorov–Smirnov test was performed to confirm normality. Normally distributed FT4 were represented as mean

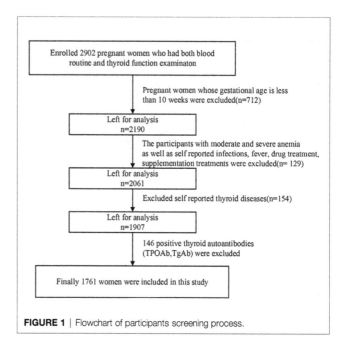

FIGURE 1 | Flowchart of participants screening process.

± standard deviation (SD), while FT3 and TSH did not follow a Gaussian distribution which were represented by a median (minimum–maximum). For normally distributed data, a t-test was applied to compare groups. For non-normal data, a Kruskal–Wallis test and subsequent Mann–Whitney test were used to compare groups. When comparing the rates between groups, we use the chi-square test. We used univariable and multivariate logistic regression to examine the significant influence factors for thyroid function. A two-tailed p-value < 0.05 was considered statistically significant. Statistical power analyses were done using G*Power 3.1 (22). According to NCCLS C28-A2, the 2.5th and 97.5th percentiles were considered as the lower and upper limits, respectively, of the reference intervals (23). The 95% confidence interval (CI) of the two limits was obtained through bootstrap by R 4.0.2.

RESULTS

Subject Characterization

In total, 1,761 individuals with a mean age of 29.37 ± 3.84 years participated in this study. The average gestation age was 11 ± 1 week. The median TSH level was 1.6 mIU/l (range 0.01, 9.67 mIU/l), the median FT4 level was 12.57 pmol/l (range 1.15, 23.06 pmol/l), and the median FT3 level was 4.26 pmol/l (range 2.67, 13.15 pmol/l). The prevalence of mild anemia among all women was 17.8% (314/1761).

Different Distribution of Thyroid Hormones During the First Trimester Between Women With Mild Anemic and Control Pregnant Women

We compared the thyroid function values between pregnant women with mild anemia and the control group and found that there was no difference in the levels of FT3 and FT4 between the two groups. The TSH levels in pregnant women with mild anemia were higher than those in pregnant women without anemia (p < 0.001), as shown in **Table 1**.

Reference Range for Thyroid Hormones During the First Trimester in Pregnant Women

We choose pregnant women in the control group to set a new reference interval. As shown in **Table 2**, the TSH ranges from 0.11 to 4.13 mIU/l, FT3 from 3.45 to 5.47 pmol/l, and FT4 from 7.96 to

16.54 pmol/l. The standard reference ranges provided by manufacturers are as follows: TSH ranges from 0.68 to 5.59 mIU/l, FT3 from 3.28 to 6.47 pmol/l, and FT4 from 7.64 to 16.03 pmol/l. We selected pregnant women from both the control group and the group comprising women with mild anemia to calculate a reference interval, wherein the range of TSH was considered to be from 0.13 to 4.65 mIU/l, FT3 from 3.43 to 5.91 pmol/l, and FT4 from 7.98 to 16.54 pmol/l.

On comparing our new reference with the standard references, serum TSH levels were decreased in the first trimester, with the upper limit declining by 26.2% and the lower limit declining by 83.4%. The upper limit of serum FT3 declined by 15.5%, and the lower limit increased by 5.2%. Serum FT4 showed an increase too, with the upper and lower limits raised by 3.2% and 4.2%, respectively.

Comparison between the new reference with the references including mild anemia demonstrated the following changes. Serum TSH levels decreased in the first trimester, with the upper limit declining by 11.1% and the lower limit declining by 15.4%, while the serum FT3 upper limit declined by 7.5%.

TSH and FT3 but Not FT4 May Be Affected by Mild Anemia in Early Pregnancy

Based on the reference range of healthy control pregnant women, we compared the indicators of thyroid function between pregnant women with mild anemia and the control group. As shown in **Table 3**, the rate of TSH values above the upper limit in pregnant women with mild anemia was notably higher than that in the control (12.7% vs. 1.9%, $p < 0.0001$). The percent of FT3 values under the lower limit or above the upper limit in pregnant women with mild anemia was greater than that in the control (3.8% vs. 1. 9%, 15.0% vs. 1.9%, $p < 0.0001$). In addition, there was no significant difference between the FT4 values.

As shown in **Table 5**, mild anemia [OR 4.26 (95% CI: 2.82, 6.43); p < 0.001)] was independently associated with a higher risk for abnormal TSH levels. After adjustment for confounding variables in the final step forward logistic regression, mild anemia (OR 4.40 (95% CI: 2.84, 6.76); p < 0.001) was independently associated with a higher risk for abnormal TSH levels. Mild anemia (OR 5.86 (95% CI: 3.96, 8.67); p < 0.001) was independently associated with a higher risk for FT3 abnormality risk. In addition, age >35 years (OR 2.45 (95% CI: 1.30, 4.33); p < 0.001) was associated with a higher FT3 abnormality risk. After adjustment for confounding variables in the final step forward logistic regression, mild anemia (OR 5.87 (95% CI: 3.89, 8.85);

TABLE 1 | Comparison of thyroid functions between pregnant women with mild anemia and control group.

Thyroid function	Pregnant women		p value
	Control (n = 1447)	Mild anemia (n = 314)	
FT3 (pmol/L), median [min, max]	4.24 [2.67, 5.94]	4.35 [3.11, 13.15]	0.05[a]
FT4 (pmol/L), mean ± SD	12.43 ± 2.29	12.49 ± 2.34	0.655[b]
TSH (mIU/L), median [min, max]	1.58 [0.01, 6.47]	1.72 [0.01, 9.67]	<0.001[a]*

[a]Mann–Whitney U-test was used to compare the groups.
[b]T-test was used to compare the groups.
*Statistical significance was assumed when the p-value was < 0.05.

TABLE 2 | Reference ranges of thyroid function.

Thyroid function	n	P2.5	95% CI (P 2.5)	P 97.5	95% CI (P 97.5)
FT3 (pmol/L)					
Standard		3.28		6.47	
Pregnant women	1761	3.43	3.39–3.46	5.91	5.81–6.36
New	1447	3.45	3.41–3.49	5.47	5.42–5.56
FT4 (pmol/L)					
Standard		7.64		16.03	
Pregnant women	1761	7.98	7.85–8.16	16.54	16.27–16.90
New	1447	7.96	7.79–8.09	16.54	16.28–16.86
TSH (mIU/L)					
Standard		0.68		5.59	
Pregnant women	1761	0.13	0.06–0.44	4.65	4.56–5.03
New	1447	0.11	0.07–0.18	4.13	3.98–4.26

Standard, the reference ranges provided by manufacturers.
Pregnant women, pregnant women from both the control group as well as the group comprising women with mild anemia were selected to calculate a reference interval.
New, only chose control pregnant women to set the new reference interval.

TABLE 3 | Comparison of thyroid functions abnormal between pregnant women with mild anemia and control group.

	Pregnant women		Chi-square χ2	p value
	Control (n = 1447) n (%)	Mild anemia (n = 314) n (%)		
FT3			84.240	<0.0001*
Low	27 (1.9%)	12 (3.8%)		
Normal	1392 (96.2%)	255 (81.2%)		
High	28 (1.9%)	47 (15.0%)		
FT4			0.617	0.734
Low	28 (1.9%)	5 (1.6%)		
Normal	1391 (96.1%)	301 (95.9%)		
High	28 (1.9%)	8 (2.5%)		
TSH			60.064	<0.0001*
Low	28 (1.9%)	6 (1.9%)		
Normal	1391 (96.1%)	268 (85.4%)		
High	28 (1.9%)	40 (12.7%)		

Statistical significance was assumed when the p-value was < 0.05.

$p < 0.001$) was independently associated with a higher FT3 abnormality risk. Age >35 years was no longer associated with a higher risk for FT3 abnormal.

Mild Anemia May Be Related to Subclinical Hypothyroidism in Early Pregnancy

As shown in **Table 4**, the prevalence of subclinical hypothyroidism was markedly higher in pregnant women with mild anemia than in the control group (12.1% vs. 1.9%, $p < 0.001$). Moreover, there were two (0.64%) overt hypothyroidism cases in pregnant women with mild anemia, but none was found in the control group. These differences were significant ($p = 0.009$). In contrast, there was no significant difference in the prevalence of subclinical hyperthyroidism and hyperthyroidism between the pregnant women with mild anemia and the controls. As shown in **Table 5**, mild anemia (OR 6.98 (95% CI: 4.23, 11.65); p < 0.001)) was independently associated with a higher risk for subclinical hypothyroidism. After adjustment for confounding variables in the final step forward logistic regression, mild anemia (OR 7.61 (95% CI: 4.53, 12.90); p < 0.001) was independently associated with a higher risk for subclinical hypothyroidism.

DISCUSSION

Anemia is a common disease that may occur during pregnancy. A meta-analysis study from China demonstrated that the prevalence of anemia in pregnant women during the first trimester was found to be 10.1% (95% CI 6.2%–14%) during the period from 2012 to 2016 (24). The monitoring results from 2011 to 2012 showed that the anemia rate of pregnant women in small and medium-sized Chinese cities is 18.0% (25). A study has also proven that the risk of anemia in pregnant women in the north is higher than that in the south region of China (21). Mild anemia accounted for the highest proportion of overall anemia. Our study comprised data from women in early pregnancy from February 2012 to December 2018 in Tiexi District of Shenyang and found a mild anemia rate of 17.8% in pregnant women during their first trimester. Our study found that the high incidence of mild anemia was closely related to higher maternal age (older than 35 years) [OR 10.88 (95% CI: 7.02, 17.12)] (data not shown). This finding is similar to that reported by Lin et al. Their study surveyed 43,403 pregnant women in Beijing, Chengdu, and Guangzhou and found that maternal anemia was significantly related to maternal age 35 years and older (AOR =

TABLE 4 | Prevalence of thyroid diseases in pregnant women with mild anemia compared to the control group.

	Pregnant women		Chi-square χ2	p value
	Control (n = 1447) n (%)	Mild anemia (n = 314) n (%)		
Overt hypothyroidism, n (%)			6.907	**0.009***
Yes	0 (0.0)	2 (0.6)		
No	1447 (100.0)	312 (99.4)		
Subclinical hypothyroidism, n (%)			54.903	**<0.0001***
Yes	28 (1.9)	38 (12.1)		
No	1419 (98.1)	276 (87.9)		
Overt hyperthyroidism, n (%)			0.416	**0.519**
Yes	2 (0.1)	1 (0.3)		
No	1445 (99.9)	313 (99.7)		
Subclinical hyperthyroidism, n (%)			0.064	**0.800**
Yes	26 (1.8)	5 (1.6)		
No	1421 (98.2)	309 (98.4)		

*Statistical significance was assumed when the p-value was < 0.05.

TABLE 5 | Results from the univariable and multivariable logistic regression analysis.

Dependent/independent variables	Univariable analysis		Multivariable analysis	
	Rough OR (95% CI)	p value	Adjust OR[a] (95% CI)	p value
Outcome: abnormal FT3 levels (logistic regression)				
Mild anemia	5.86 (3.96,8.67)	**<0.0001***	5.87 (3.89,8.85)	**<0.0001***
Age group (>35)	2.45 (1.30,4.33)	**<0.0001***		
Outcome: abnormal FT4 levels (logistic regression)				
Age group (>35)	0.72 (0.17,1.99)	**0.589**		
Mild anemia	1.07 (0.55,1.92)	**0.823**		
Outcome: abnormal TSH levels (logistic regression)				
Mild anemia	4.26 (2.82,6.43)	**<0.0001***	4.40 (2.84,6.76)	**<0.0001***
Age group (>35)	1.83 (0.87,3.47)	**0.08**		
Outcome: subclinical hypothyroidism (logistic regression)				
Mild anemia	6.98 (4.23,11.65)	**<0.0001***	7.61 (4.53,12.90)	**<0.0001***
Age group (>35)	1.65 (0.62,3.62)	**0.25**		

*Statistical significance was assumed when the p-value was < 0.05.
[a]Adjust for age.

1.386) (26). Pregnancies at an advanced reproductive age are common now. Therefore, it is essential to give additional importance to the influence of mild anemia as well as anemia on health of pregnant women and fetus.

Fifty percent of overall anemia cases in populations is caused by ID (8). ID is frequent during the first trimester of pregnancy and is often related to a higher prevalence of thyroid autoimmunity, increased TSH, and lower FT3 levels (27). A study in Wuxi also confirmed that low iron stores showed a trend toward higher TSH, lower FT3, and lower FT4 levels during the first trimester of pregnancy (15). A study in Suzhou revealed that pregnant women with mild ID and ID anemia have higher TSH and lower FT4 status (16). These studies on TSH and FT3 are consistent with our study. In our study, we found that TSH levels were higher in pregnant women with mild anemia than in those without anemia (p < 0.001). According to our new intervals, we observed that mild anemia was independently associated with a higher risk for abnormal TSH and FT3 levels. In this study, we also found that the prevalence of subclinical hypothyroidism and overt hypothyroidism was markedly higher in women with mild anemia than in those without.

However, no differences were observed in FT4 values between pregnant women with mild anemia and those without it. The first reason may be that we excluded pregnant women with self-reported thyroid disease or positive thyroid autoantibodies during sample screening. These patients are the main contributors to the abnormal FT4 levels, which was standard for diagnosis of the thyroid disease. The second reason may be that previous studies focus on ID which includes not only mild anemia but also moderate and severe anemia. However, we just focus on mild anemia. Thirdly, lower FT4 levels may also be related to other factors such as iodine nutrition, age, and gestational weeks, which need to be further elucidated. Ipek et al. found no difference in FT4 levels between ID anemia children and normal children (28). Tienboon and Unachak found that there was no difference in T4, T3, fT4, fT3, thyroxine-binding globulin (TBG), and TSH levels before and after iron treatment in ID anemia children (29). Ravanbod et al. reported the absence of significant differences in Hb and TSH levels before and after 90 days of iron treatment in non-pregnant patients with ID anemia and subclinical hypothyroidism (SCH), which suggested that iron alone does not change the TSH level in non-pregnant patients with ID anemia and SCH (30). Infusion of concentrated red blood cells can increase Hb, thyroxine (T3), and free-T3 (FT3) levels in patients with thalassemia who possessed normal thyroid function before puberty, but it has no effect on patients with delayed puberty (31). Therefore, mild anemia might not be the only determining factor affecting thyroid function.

In our study, the temporality of the association between anemia and abnormal thyroid function could not be assessed because exposure and outcome were measured simultaneously. Nevertheless, anemia and thyroid function animal studies have demonstrated that low-iron food significantly decreased the Hb levels and TPO activity (9, 10), as well as serum concentrations of T3 and T4 (11), while a rise in TSH levels was observed (12). ID anemia resulted in maternal hypothyroxinemia from midgestation to the end of the pregnancy in pregnant rats (32). Interestingly, in Nepalese children, ID was also found to decrease the activity of TPO, an iron-containing enzyme involved in the synthesis of thyroid hormones (33). Iron therapy studies have implied that in ID adolescent girls, improvement in iron status was accompanied by an improvement in some indices of thyroid hormones (34). After treatment with iron, FT4 levels significantly increased in patients with ID anemia (35). Beard et al. reported that in women with ID anemia, iron supplementation corrected the anemia significantly (p = 0.03) improved the rectal temperature, and partially normalized the plasma thyroid hormone concentrations (36). Studies have emphasized that adding iron to thyroxine therapy improves both conditions compared to thyroxine therapy alone (30, 37). In addition, patients with chronic hemolytic anemia requiring repeated blood transfusion have a high prevalence of the hypothalamic–pituitary thyroid axis. Proper blood transfusion appears to prevent deterioration of thyroid function and, in many cases, can reverse thyroid pathology (18). Therefore, the significant auxiliary effect of mild anemia on thyroid function should not be ignored.

For the evaluation of thyroid function in pregnant women, there have been several studies and guidelines indicating that non-pregnant reference intervals for thyroid hormones are not applicable for pregnancy. There are many challenges in reference value formulation for thyroid function in pregnant women. Maternal human chorionic gonadotrophin (hCG) directly stimulates the TSH receptor, increasing thyroid hormone production by nearly 50%, resulting in a subsequent reduction in serum TSH concentration (38). The levels of thyroid hormones vary according to the gestational age (39). Moreover, the pregnancy reference intervals could be affected by race, kits, and test methods (40–42). It has been reported that the formulation of gestational reference ranges is always given to be inconsistent. The 2011 ATA guidelines suggested a specific upper limit cutoff (2.5 mU/l) for serum TSH levels in the first trimester of pregnancy (43). Nonetheless, the TSH upper limits given by studies worldwide are higher than 2.5 mU/l. Then, the 2017 ATA guidelines suggested an upper reference limit of 4.0 mU/l (1). Nevertheless, a series of studies have demonstrated that compared to the European and American population, or the

reference value suggested by ATA, the Chinese pregnant population has a higher upper TSH limit (43–45).

As described above, our study implied that pregnant women with mild anemia had abnormally high TSH levels. According to ATA recommendation, making thyroid function reference ranges should only include pregnant women with no known thyroid disease, optimal iodine intake, and negative thyroid peroxidase antibody (TPOAb) status (1). Conversely, they did not consider excluding pregnant women with mild anemia by clinically Hb detection. In our study, we excluded mild anemia and established a new first trimester-specific reference interval for pregnant women. Interestingly, the upper limit of 4.13 mU/l obtained was almost equal to the upper limit of 4.0 mU/l given by the 2017 ATA guideline (1). Therefore, inconsistent reference ranges worldwide may not only be due to race and iodine nutrition but also be due to the diverse degrees of mild anemia rate among different countries. Pregnant women with mild anemia are easily overlooked due to their symptoms which are non-specific and obscure. In addition, pregnant women with mild anemia during the first trimester may be healthy before pregnancy, and some symptoms of mild anemia are similar to general pregnancy symptoms. Therefore, mild anemia cannot be ruled out without routine blood examinations.

After excluding mild anemia, the upper and lower limits of serum TSH decreased. Therefore, if the reference interval is calculated with anemia confounding, the diagnosis of high TSH levels related to hypothyroidism in pregnant women will be missed, and the diagnosis of lower TSH levels related to hyperthyroidism in pregnant women will be misdiagnosed. After excluding mild anemia, the serum FT3 upper reference limit declined by 7.5%. Thus, if reference values were calculated with mild anemia included, the diagnosis of high FT3 levels related to thyroid function in pregnant women would be missed.

In addition, according to the 2017 ATA guidelines, the upper TSH limit of 4.0 mU/l represents a reduction of approximately 0.5 mU/l from the non-pregnant upper limit (1). The new reference value of 4.13 mU/l from our study represents a relatively decent rate of reduction (26%) from the non-pregnant TSH upper reference limit (5.59 mIU/l) rather than a reduction of 0.5 mU/l. A systematic review by Gao et al. also emphasized that pregnant women had a 22% reduction in the serum TSH upper limit from the non-pregnant value (42). This can be used as a suboptimal method to determine the threshold value for pregnant women in the first trimester.

It should be mentioned that the present study has several limitations, which need to be improved in further studies. First, certain parameters such as serum ferritin (SF), soluble transferrin receptor (sTfR), and total body iron (TBI) were not measured; the mild anemia status assessment would be more accurate with the measurement of these parameters. Secondly, this hospital-based study prevented us from obtaining detailed information on lifestyle factors and dietary habits, which may have a critical effect on the causal relationship between maternal thyroid function and mild anemia. Thirdly, pregnant women analyzed in the present study were not randomly selected, and the sample sizes of control and mild anemia groups were not equal, possibly introducing a selection bias. Although there is sufficient statistical power to investigate the association between abnormal thyroid function risk and anemia (see in **Supplementary Table 1**), larger prospective and different phases of pregnancy trials based on multicenters or community to replicate these findings are needed in the future. Fourth, the cross-sectional design of measuring exposure and results at the same time is the main limitation of this study; hence, it is impossible to assess the timeliness of the association between anemia and abnormal thyroid function. Therefore, in order to better understand the impact of mild anemia on thyroid function, the molecular mechanism should be studied based on animal models with different degrees of anemia during pregnancy and cell experiments in the future.

In conclusion, this study suggested a possible association between mild anemia and abnormal thyroid function in pregnant women during the first trimester; therefore, physicians should be aware of mild anemia during the first trimester to avoid adverse pregnancy outcomes. Moreover, the interval made by pregnant women without mild anemia is closer to the 2017 ATA reference, which indicated that the difference in TSH value in pregnant women globally might be partly due to the different incidence rates of mild anemia in pregnant women around the world. Therefore, formulation of thyroid hormones reference for pregnant women should exclude those with mild anemia, which need further study.

ETHICS STATEMENT

The studies involving human participants were reviewed and approved by the Ethics Committee of Harbin Medical University. The patients/participants provided their written informed consent to participate in this study.

AUTHOR CONTRIBUTIONS

ML and D-jS were involved in conception and design of the research. ML drafted the manuscript. G-yN and RW performed the experiments and analyzed the data. G-yN and ML prepared the figures and tables. ML interpreted the results of the experiments. G-yN, RW, PL, ML, and D-jS edited and revised the manuscript and approved the final version of the manuscript.

REFERENCES

Alexander EK, Pearce EN, Brent GA, Brown RS, Chen H, Dosiou C, et al. 2017 Guidelines of the American Thyroid Association for the Diagnosis and Management of Thyroid Disease During Pregnancy and the Postpartum. *Thyroid* (2017) 27:315–89. doi: 10.1089/thy.2016.0457

Nazarpour S, Ramezani TF, Simbar M, Azizi F. Thyroid Dysfunction and Pregnancy Outcomes. *Iranian J Reprod Med* (2015) 13:387–96.

Organization WH. Haemoglobin Concentrations for the Diagnosis of Anaemia and Assessment of Severity. (2011). Available at: https://www. who.int/vmnis/ indicators/haemoglobin.pdf.

Cappellini M, Motta I. Anemia in Clinical Practice-Definition and Classification: Does Hemoglobin Change With Aging? *Semin Hematol* (2015) 52:261–9. doi: 10.1053/j.seminhematol.2015.07.006

Method for Anemia Screen WS/T 441-2013. In: *N.H.C.o.t.P.s.R.o. China*.

Lopez A, Cacoub P, Macdougall IC, Peyrin-Biroulet L. Iron Deficiency Anaemia. *Lancet* (2016) 387:907–16. doi: 10.1016/S0140-6736(15)60865-0

WHO/UNICEF/UNU. *Iron Ddeficiency Anemia: Assessment, Prevention and Control-a Guide for Program Managers.* Geneva Switzerland: Who (2001). p. 1–132.

Yip R. Iron Deficiency: Contemporary Scientific Issues and International Programmatic Approaches. *J Nutr* (1994) 124:1479S–90S. doi: 10.1093/jn/ 124. suppl_8.1479S

Hess SY, Zimmermann MB, Arnold M, Langhans W, Hurrell RF. Iron Deficiency Anemia Reduces Thyroid Peroxidase Activity in Rats. *J Nutr* (2002) 132:1951–5. doi: 10.1093/jn/132.7.1951

Dillman E, Gale C, Green W, Johnson DG, Mackler B, Finch C. Hypothermia in Iron Deficiency Due to Altered Triiodothyronine Metabolism. *Am J Physiol* (1980) 239:377–81. doi: 10.1152/ajpregu.1980.239.5.R377

Smith SM, Johnson PE, Lukaski HC. *In Vitro* Hepatic Thyroid Hormone Deiodination in Iron-Deficient Rats: Effect of Dietary Fat. *Life Sci* (1993) 53:603–9. doi: 10.1016/0024-3205(93)90268-8

Mathur N, Joshi SC, Mathur S. Effect of Dietary Iron Deficiency Anaemia on TSH and Peripartum Thyroid Function. *BioScientifica* (2006) 12:123. doi: 10.5005/ jp/books/10766_74

Zimmermann MB, Hans B, Hurrell RF. Iron Deficiency Predicts Poor Maternal Thyroid Status During Pregnancy. *J Clin Endocrinol Metab* (2007) 3436–40. doi: 10.1210/jc.2007-1082

Teng X, Shan Z, Li C, Yu X, Mao J, Wang W, et al. Iron Deficiency May Predict Greater Risk for Hypothyroxinemia: A Retrospective Cohort Study of Pregnant Women in China. *Thyroid* (2018) 28:968–75. doi: 10.1089/ thy.2017.0491

Fu J, Yang A, Zhao J, Zhu Y, Chen D. The Relationship Between Iron Level and Thyroid Function During the First Trimester of Pregnancy: A Cross-Sectional Study in Wuxi, China. *J Trace Elements Med Biol* (2017) 43:148–52. doi: 10.1016/j.jtemb.2017.01.004

Li S, Xin G, Wei Y, Zhu G, Yang C. The Relationship Between Iron Deficiency and Thyroid Function in Chinese Women During Early Pregnancy. *J Nutr Sci Vitaminol* (2017) 62:397–401. doi: 10.3177/jnsv.62.397

Yu X, Shan Z, Li C, Mao J, Wang W, Xie X, et al. Iron Deficiency, an Independent Risk Factor for Isolated Hypothyroxinemia in Pregnant and Nonpregnant Women of Childbearing Age in China. *J Clin Endocrinol Metab* (2015) 100:1594–601. doi: 10.1210/jc.2014-3887

Soliman AT, De Sanctis V, Yassin M, Wagdy M, Soliman N. Chronic Anemia and Thyroid Function. *Acta BioMed* (2017) 88:119–27. doi: 10.23750/ abm. v88i1.6048

Leslie MS, Park J, Briggs LA, El-Banna MM, Greene J. Is Anemia in Low Income Pregnant Women Related to Their Infants' Having Anemia? A Cohort Study of Pregnant Women-Infant Pairs in the United States. *Matern Child Health J* (2020) 24:764–76. doi: 10.1007/s10995-020-02912-8

Zhao J, Zhu X, Dai Q, Hong X, Zhang H, Huang K, et al. The Prevalence and Influencing Factors of Anaemia Among Pre-Pregnant Women in Mainland China: A Large Population-Based, Cross-Sectional Study. *Br J Nutr* (2021) 5:1-12. doi: 10.1017/S0007114521001148

Jiang S, Pang XH, Duan YF, Bi Y, Wang J, Yin SA, et al. The Influencing Factors of Anemia for Pregnant Women Between 2010-2012 in China. *Zhonghua Yu Fang Yi Xue Za Zhi* (2018) 52:21-25. Chinese. doi: 10.3760/ cma.j.is sn.0253-9624.2018.01.005

Faul F, Erdfelder E, Lang AG, Buchner A. G*Power 3: A Flexible Statistical Power Analysis Program for the Social, Behavioral, and Biomedical Sciences. *Behav Res Methods* (2007) 39:175–91. doi: 10.3758/BF03193146

National Committee for Clinical Laboratory Standards (NCCLS). *NCCLS Proposed Guideline: How to define, determine, and utilize reference intervals in the clinical laboratory Second Edition[J]*. NCCLS Document C. (2000) 28–A2.

Zhao SY, Jing WZ, Liu J, Liu M. Prevalence of Anemia During Pregnancy in China,

2012-2016: a Meta-analysis. *Zhonghua Yu Fang Yi Xue Za Zhi* (2018) 52:951–7. doi: 10.3760/cma.j.issn.0253-9624.2018.09.016

Hu Y, Li M, Chen J, Wang R, Li W, Yang Y, et al. The Anemia and Vitamin A, Vitamin D Nutritional Status of Chinese Rural Pregnant Women in 2010- 2012. *Wei Sheng Yan Jiu* (2017) 46:361–72.

Lin L, Wei Y, Zhu W, Wang C, Su R, Feng H, et al. Prevalence, Risk Factors and Associated Adverse Pregnancy Outcomes of Anaemia in Chinese Pregnant Women: A Multicentre Retrospective Study. *BMC Pregnancy Childbirth* (2018) 18:111. doi: 10.1186/s12884-018-1739-8

Veltri F, Decaillet S, Kleynen P, Grabczan L, Belhomme J, Rozenberg S, et al. Prevalence of Thyroid Autoimmunity and Dysfunction in Women With Iron Deficiency During Early Pregnancy: Is it Altered? *Eur J Endocrinol* (2016) 175:191–9. doi: 10.1530/EJE-16-0288

Pek LZ, Ka?Maz E, Bozaykut A, Sezer R. The Effect of Iron Deficiency Anemia on Plasma Thyroid Hormone Levels in Childhood. *Turk Pediatri Arivi* (2011) 46:129–32.

Tienboon P, Unachak K. Iron Deficiency Anaemia in Childhood and Thyroid Function. *Asia Pacific J Clin Nutr* (2003) 12:198–202.

Ravanbod M, Asadipooya K, Kalantarhormozi M, Nabipour I, Omrani GR. Treatment of Iron-Deficiency Anemia in Patients With Subclinical Hypothyroidism. *Am J Med* (2013) 126:420–4. doi: 10.1016/j.amjmed. 2012.12.009

Gauger M, Mohr W. A Rise in Haemoglobin Levels may Enhance Serum Triiodothyronine (T3). Concentrations in Prepubertal Patients With Beta-Thalassaemia Major. *Exp Clin Endocrinol* (1990) 96:169–76. doi: 10.1055/s-0029-1211006

Hu X, Teng X, Zheng H, Shan Z, Li J, Jin T, et al. Iron Deficiency Without Anemia Causes Maternal Hypothyroxinemia in Pregnant Rats. *Nutr Res* (2014) 34:604–12. doi: 10.1016/j.nutres.2014.06.007

Khatiwada S, Gelal B, Baral N, Lamsal M. Association Between Iron Status and Thyroid Function in Nepalese Children. *Thyroid Res* (2016) 9:2. doi: 10.1186/s13044-016-0031-0

Eftekhari MH, Simondon KB, Jalali M, Keshavarz SA, Saadat N. Effects of Administration of Iron, Iodine and Simultaneous Iron-Plus-Iodine on the Thyroid Hormone Profile in Iron-Deficient Adolescent Iranian Girls. *Eur J Clin Nutr* (2006) 60:545–52. doi: 10.1038/sj.ejcn.1602349

Erdem G, Cengiz D, Imdat D. The Effects of Iron Deficiency Anemia on the

Thyroid Functions. *J Clin Exp Investigations* (2010) 1:1–5. doi: 10.5799/ahinjs.01.2010.03.0033

Beard JL, Borel MJ, Derr J. Impaired Thermoregulation and Thyroid Function in Iron-Deficiency Anemia. *Am J Clin Nutr* (1990) 52:813. doi: 10.1093/ajcn/52.5.813

Hakan C, Cemil B, Feyzi G, Talat B. Hematologic Effects of Levothyroxine in Iron-Deficient Subclinical Hypothyroid Patients: A Randomized, Double- Blind, Controlled Study. *J Clin Endocrinol Metab* (2009) 94:151–6. doi: 10.1210/jc.2008-1440

Kennedy RL, Darne J. The Role of hCG in Regulation of the Thyroid Gland in Normal and Abnormal Pregnancy. *Obstetrics Gynecol* (1991) 78:298–307.

Weeke J, Dybkjaer L, Granlie K, Jensen SE, Magnusson B. A Longitudinal Study of Serum TSH, and Total and Free Iodothyronines During Normal Pregnancy. *Acta Endocrinol* (1982) 101:531. doi:10.1530/acta.0.1010531

Boucai L, Surks MI. Reference Limits of Serum TSH and Free T4 are Significantly Influenced by Race and Age in an Urban Outpatient Medical Practice. *Clin Endocrinol* (2009) 70:788–93. doi: 10.1111/j.1365-2265.2008.03390.x

Han L, Zheng W, Zhai Y, Xie X, Zhang J, Zhang S, et al. Reference Intervals of Trimester-Specific Thyroid Stimulating Hormone and Free Thyroxine in Chinese Women Established by Experimental and Statistical Methods. *J Clin Lab Anal* (2018) 32:e22344. doi: 10.1002/jcla.22344

Gao X, Li Y, Li J, Liu A, Wei S, Teng W, et al. Gestational TSH and FT4 Reference Intervals in Chinese Women: A Systematic Review and Meta- Analysis. *Front Endocrinol* (2018) 9:432. doi: 10.3389/fendo.2018.00432

Stagnaro-Green A, Abalovich M, Alexander E, Azizi F, Mestman J, Negro R, et al. Guidelines of the American Thyroid Association for the Diagnosis and Management of Thyroid Disease During Pregnancy and Postpartum. *Thyroidol* (2011) 21:1081–125. doi: 10.1089/thy.2011.0087

Yan YQ, Dong ZL, Dong L, Wang FR, Yang XM, Jin XY, et al. Trimester- and Method-Specific Reference Intervals for Thyroid Tests in Pregnant Chinese Women: Methodology, Euthyroid Definition and Iodine Status can Influence the Setting of Reference Intervals. *Clin Endocrinol* (2011) 74:262–9. doi: 10.1111/j.1365-2265.2010.03910.x

Li C, Shan Z, Mao J, Wang W, Xie X, Zhou W, et al. Assessment of Thyroid Function During First-Trimester Pregnancy: What is the Rational Upper Limit of Serum TSH During the First Trimester in Chinese Pregnant Women? *J Clin Endocrinol Metab* (2014) 99:73–9. doi: 10.1210/jc.2013-1674

18

Hepcidin and Anemia: A Tight Relationship

Alessia Pagani[1], Antonella Nai[1,2], Laura Silvestri[1,2] and Clara Camaschella[1]*

[1]Division of Genetics and Cell Biology, San Raffaele Scientific Institute, Milan, Italy, [2]Vita-Salute San Raffaele University, Milan, Italy

*Correspondence:
Clara Camaschella
camaschella.clara@hsr.it

Hepcidin, the master regulator of systemic iron homeostasis, tightly influences erythrocyte production. High hepcidin levels block intestinal iron absorption and macrophage iron recycling, causing iron restricted erythropoiesis and anemia. Low hepcidin levels favor bone marrow iron supply for hemoglobin synthesis and red blood cells production. Expanded erythropoiesis, as after hemorrhage or erythropoietin treatment, blocks hepcidin through an acute reduction of transferrin saturation and the release of the erythroblast hormone and hepcidin inhibitor erythroferrone. Quantitatively reduced erythropoiesis, limiting iron consumption, increases transferrin saturation and stimulates hepcidin transcription. Deregulation of hepcidin synthesis is associated with anemia in three conditions: iron refractory iron deficiency anemia (IRIDA), the common anemia of acute and chronic inflammatory disorders, and the extremely rare hepcidin-producing adenomas that may develop in the liver of children with an inborn error of glucose metabolism. Inappropriately high levels of hepcidin cause iron-restricted or even iron-deficient erythropoiesis in all these conditions. Patients with IRIDA or anemia of inflammation do not respond to oral iron supplementation and show a delayed or partial response to intravenous iron. In hepcidin-producing adenomas, anemia is reverted by surgery. Other hepcidin-related anemias are the "iron loading anemias" characterized by ineffective erythropoiesis and hepcidin suppression. This group of anemias includes thalassemia syndromes, congenital dyserythropoietic anemias, congenital sideroblastic anemias, and some forms of hemolytic anemias as pyruvate kinase deficiency. The paradigm is non-transfusion-dependent thalassemia where the release of erythroferrone from the expanded pool of immature erythroid cells results in hepcidin suppression and secondary iron overload that in turn worsens ineffective erythropoiesis and anemia. In thalassemia murine models, approaches that induce iron restriction ameliorate both anemia and the iron phenotype. Manipulations of hepcidin might benefit all the above-described anemias. Compounds that antagonize hepcidin or its effect may be useful in inflammation and IRIDA, while hepcidin agonists may improve ineffective erythropoiesis. Correcting ineffective erythropoiesis in animal models ameliorates not only anemia but also iron homeostasis by reducing hepcidin inhibition. Some targeted approaches are now in clinical trials: hopefully they will result in novel treatments for a variety of anemias.

Keywords: anemia, iron, hepcidin, erythropoiesis, inflammation

INTRODUCTION

Anemia is one of the most common disorders worldwide and anemia due to iron deficiency is the prevalent form according to multiple analyses (review in Camaschella, 2019). This type of anemia results from the total body iron deficiency and the inability to supply the large amount of iron that the bone marrow consumes to produce an adequate number of red blood cells in order to maintain tissue oxygenation.

The iron availability is controlled by the liver peptide hormone hepcidin. The body iron increase causes the production of hepcidin, which is released in the circulation and acts on its receptor ferroportin, a transmembrane iron exporter protein highly expressed on enterocyte, macrophages, and hepatocytes. Hepcidin reduces the iron entry to plasma from absorptive duodenal cells and iron recycling macrophages by blocking iron export (Aschemeyer et al., 2018) and by degrading the iron exporter ferroportin (Nemeth et al., 2004). By regulating plasma iron and systemic iron homeostasis, the hepcidin/ferroportin axis strongly affects erythropoiesis, hence the possible development of anemia.

THE IRON-ERYTHROPOIESIS CONNECTION

The process of red blood cells production consumes approximately 80% of circulating iron for hemoglobin synthesis of maturing erythroblasts. Most iron (20–25 mg/daily) is recycled by macrophages, while a limited amount (1–2 mg daily) derives from intestinal absorption. The kidney hormone erythropoietin (EPO) controls the proliferation of erythroid progenitors, especially of CFU-e and at a lower degree of BFU-e, and the early phase of terminal erythropoiesis, while iron needs are increased in the late differentiation stages from proerythroblasts to reticulocyte, for the synthesis of heme incorporated into hemoglobin (Muckenthaler et al., 2017).

Hepcidin regulation requires a crosstalk between liver endothelial sinusoidal cells (LSEC) that produce the bone morphogenetic proteins (BMPs) to activate the BMP-SMAD pathway and hepatocytes that produce and release hepcidin (Babitt et al., 2006; Rausa et al., 2015). BMP6 and BMP2 are the most important BMPs that upregulate hepcidin, while BMP6 expression is iron dependent (Andriopoulos et al., 2009; Meynard et al., 2009) BMP2 appears less iron-responsive (Canali et al., 2017; Koch et al., 2017).

Hepcidin levels are low in absolute iron deficiency and iron deficiency anemia. In these conditions, the iron stores are exhausted and the BMP-SMAD signaling is switched off at multiple levels. First, BMP6 expression is suppressed; next, the activity of TMPRSS6, a protease that cleaves the BMP co-receptor hemojuvelin (Silvestri et al., 2008), is strongly increased (Lakhal et al., 2011); and third, histone deacetylase3 (HDAC3) suppresses the hepcidin locus (Pasricha et al., 2017). In conditions of iron deficiency, the reduction of hepcidin production is an adaptation mechanism that facilitates dietary and pharmacological iron absorption (Camaschella and Pagani, 2018).

When anemia is severe, the coexisting hypoxia stimulates erythropoiesis through increased kidney synthesis and release of EPO. This leads to suppression of hepcidin transcription by erythroferrone (ERFE), an EPO target gene produced by erythroblasts (Kautz et al., 2014), by molecules (e.g., PDGF-BB) released by other tissues (Sonnweber et al., 2014), and likely by soluble components of transferrin receptors (TFR), sTFR1 (Beguin, 2003), and sTFR2 (Pagani et al., 2015). The final aim is to supply enough iron for the needs of an expanded erythropoiesis.

ANEMIAS WITH ABNORMAL HEPCIDIN LEVELS

Anemias may be classified on the basis of hepcidin levels as anemias with high and low hepcidin. It is intuitive that persistently high hepcidin levels, by blocking iron absorption, cause iron deficiency anemia because of decreased iron supply to erythropoiesis. Conversely, ineffective erythropoiesis characterizes the so-called *iron-loading anemias* that have low hepcidin levels and iron overload. These two groups of anemias are the outcome of opposite pathophysiology mechanisms (**Figure 1**). In the first group, anemia is due to the inhibitory effect exerted by hepcidin on iron absorption and recycling that leads to systemic iron deficiency; in the second group, anemia is due to hepcidin suppression by an expanded abnormal erythropoiesis (Camaschella and Nai, 2016).

Anemia Associated With High Hepcidin Levels

This group includes two inherited rare disorders (iron refractory iron deficiency anemia and hepcidin-producing adenomas in an inborn error of glucose metabolism) and an acquired common condition: anemia of inflammation (**Table 1**).

Iron Refractory Iron Deficiency Anemia

Iron refractory iron deficiency anemia (IRIDA) is a rare recessive disorder characterized by hypochromic microcytic anemia, low transferrin saturation, and inappropriately normal/high hepcidin levels. It is caused by mutations of *TMPRSS6* (Finberg et al., 2008), a gene that encodes the type II serine protease, matriptase-2 (Du et al., 2008). Mutations of *TMPRSS6* are spread along the gene and may affect different domains especially the catalytic domain (De Falco et al., 2014). This transmembrane protease, highly expressed in the liver, inhibits hepcidin transcription by cleaving the cell surface BMP co-receptor hemojuvelin, thus attenuating the BMP signaling and hepcidin synthesis (Silvestri et al., 2008). TMPRSS6 function is essential in iron deficiency to allow the compensatory mechanism of increased iron absorption.

IRIDA is present since birth and usually diagnosed in childhood. Compared with classic iron deficiency, iron parameters are atypical and raise the suspicion of the disease. The percent saturation of transferrin is strongly reduced (less than 10%) as in other forms of iron deficiency; however, at variance with iron deficiency, levels of serum ferritin are normal/increased (Camaschella, 2013; De Falco et al., 2013) This reflects an increased ferritin accumulation in macrophages, due to the high hepcidin levels that induce store iron sequestration.

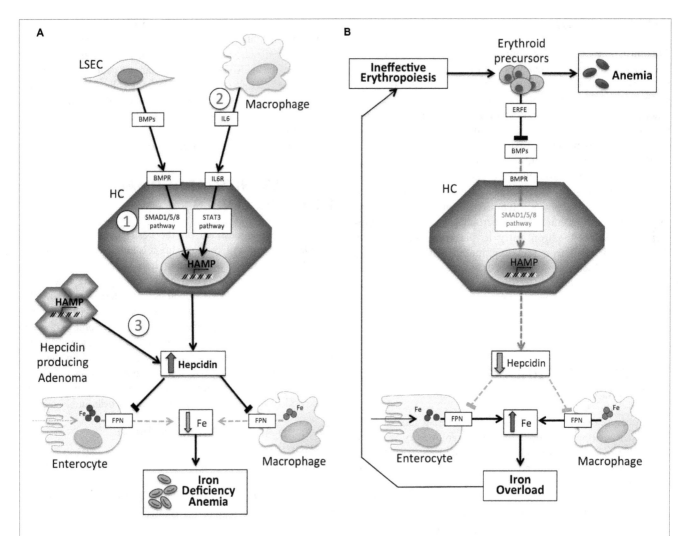

FIGURE 1 | Schematic representation of mechanisms of anemias with high (left panel) and low hepcidin (right panel). Panel **(A)**. Molecular pathogenesis of anemia associated with high hepcidin levels. LSEC, liver sinusoidal endothelial cells producing bone morphogenetic proteins (BMPs); BMPRs, BMP receptors; IL6, interleukin 6; HC, hepatocytes; HAMP, hepcidin gene. Fe, iron; FPN, ferroportin; 1, IRIDA; 2, Anemia of inflammation; 3, hepcidin producing adenoma. Panel **(B)**. Molecular pathogenesis of hepcidin variation in anemias due to ineffective erythropoiesis. ERFE, erythroferrone sequestering BMPs. Other mechanisms inhibiting hepcidin in this type of anemia, as decrease of transferrin saturation and hypoxia, are not shown. See text for details.

None of the tests proposed for IRIDA diagnosis covers 100% of the cases. The genetic test identifies that *TMPRSS6* mutations, that in some cases (non-sense, frame-shift, and splicing mutations), are clearly causal. In other cases, as for previously unreported missense mutations, functional studies are needed to demonstrate causality (Silvestri et al., 2013). However, these tests are scarcely available. Serum hepcidin levels are usually increased/normal, independently of iron deficiency, and consistent with high/normal ferritin. It is important to exclude inflammation by concomitantly dosing C-reactive protein.

Some patients with a phenotype of refractory iron deficiency have been reported to have a single *TMPRSS6* mutated allele; here, the debate is whether they should be considered IRIDA or not. A spectrum of conditions can be envisaged ranging from classic severe IRIDA due to homozygous or compound heterozygous *TMPRSS6* mutations to increased susceptibility to iron deficiency conferred by single mutations/polymorphic changes.

One approach proposed to predict classic IRIDA is hepcidin normalization on other iron parameters, as ratios transferrin saturation (Tsat)/log hepcidin or Tsat/log Ferritin (Donker et al., 2016). According to other authors, most patients with a severe IRIDA phenotype have biallelic *TMPRSS6* mutations and, when unidentified, the second allele may be genetically occult (Heeney et al., 2018). In general terms, subjects with a single allele have a milder phenotype than those with two mutations and respond better to iron treatment (Donker et al., 2016). Interestingly, several *TMPRSS6* SNPs have been shown to provide susceptibility to iron deficiency in some populations (An et al., 2012) and in blood donors (Sorensen et al., 2019).

A digenic inheritance has been reported in a 5-year-old female originally found to have an atypical IRIDA genotype with one *TMPRSS6* (I212T) causal and one (R271Q) silent mutation (De Falco et al., 2014). She was later diagnosed *Fibrodysplasia ossificans progressiva* (FOP), a rare dominant

TABLE 1 | Anemias classified according to hepcidin levels.

High-hepcidin anemias		
Hereditary	OMIM n.	Prevalence
Iron refractory iron deficiency anemia (IRIDA)	#206200	Rare
Hepcidin-producing adenomas*	#232200	Rare
Acquired		
Anemia of acute inflammation		Common**
Anemia of chronic inflammation		Common
(anemia of chronic disease)		
Low-hepcidin anemias		
Hereditary – iron loading anemias	OMIM n.	
β-thalassemia	#613985	Common***
Congenital dyserythropoietic anemia	#224100	Rare
Sideroblastic anemias	#300751	Rare
Acquired		
Low risk MDS with ringed sideroblasts		Rare

*OMIM, online Mendelian Inheritance In Man; MDS, myelodysplastic syndromes.*Described in glycogen-storage-disease 1a.*
**In hospitalized patients and in intensive care units.
***In people of Mediterranean or southern-east Asian origin.

disorder with ectopic bone formation in soft tissues due to mutated BMP type I receptor gene *ACVR1*, encoding ALK2 (Shore et al., 2006). The pathological allele *ALK2^{R258S}* is constitutively active since the mutation affects the glycine-serine-rich domain of the gene and renders the BMP/SMAD pathway overactive being unable to bind its specific inhibitor FKBP12 (Pagani et al., 2017).

This rare case is especially illustrative. First, since the ALK2 glycine-serine-rich domain interacts with FKBP12 and the mutation destabilizes the binding, it has revealed a previously unsuspected role for FKBP12 as a modulator of liver ALK2 and hepcidin (Colucci et al., 2017). Second, it has led to identify a link between activation of bone and liver BMP type I receptors. Third, the case strengthens the relevance of intact TMPRSS6 in controlling the hepatic BMP/SMAD signaling, since no IRIDA was identified among other FOP patients with the same *ACVR1* mutation and presumably normal *TMPRSS6* (Pagani et al., 2017). Finally, this case is consistent with the concept that *TMPRSS6* haploinsufficiency cannot cause classic IRIDA.

The optimal treatment of IRIDA is undefined. Oral iron is ineffective, since it is not absorbed. The addition of vitamin C allows sporadic response. Intravenous iron induces a partial response usually at a slower rate in comparison with patients with acquired iron deficiency. EPO is ineffective in classic cases (De Falco et al., 2013; Heeney and Finberg, 2014).

Anemia of Hepcidin-Producing Adenomas

This is an extremely rare condition in adult patients affected by *glycogen storage disease 1a*, a recessive disorder due to deficiency of glucose-6 phosphatase, which catalyzes a reaction involved in both glycogenolysis and gluconeogenesis. A common dangerous disease symptom is hypoglycemia. The current treatment leads to prolonged survival of affected children up to adult age with the occurrence of several complications, such as anemia and liver adenomas. Anemia is microcytic and hypochromic, iron deficient, and refractory to oral iron treatment

Anemia reverted after surgical adenoma resection. Adenoma tissue was found positive for hepcidin mRNA, while normal surrounding tissue showed hepcidin suppression, as expected because of the ectopic uncontrolled hepcidin production (Weinstein et al., 2002). The hematological features of patients resemble those of IRIDA as they share high hepcidin levels as a common mechanism of anemia.

Anemia of Inflammation

Anemia of inflammation (AI), previously known as anemia of chronic diseases, is a moderate normochromic-normocytic anemia that develops in conditions of systemic inflammation and immune activation. It occurs in several common disorders, including chronic infections, autoimmune diseases, advanced cancer, chronic kidney disease, congestive heart failure, chronic obstructive pulmonary disease, anemia of the elderly (at least partly), and graft versus host disease. AI is one of the most common anemias worldwide and the most frequent anemia in hospitalized patients. Acute inflammation contributes to the severity of anemia in intensive care units. Molecular mechanisms underlying AI are multiple and complex. Overproduction of cytokines such as IL1-β, TNF-α, and IL-6 by macrophages and INF-γ by lymphocytes blunts EPO production, impairs the erythropoiesis response, increases hepcidin levels, and may activate erythrophagocytosis, especially in the acute forms (Weiss and Goodnough, 2005; Ganz, 2019).

Hepcidin is activated by IL-6 through IL-6 receptor (IL-6R) and JAK2-STAT3 signaling. Full hepcidin activation requires an active BMP-SMAD pathway because inactivation of BMP signaling decreases hepcidin in animal models of inflammation (Theurl et al., 2011). The deregulation of systemic iron homeostasis causes macrophage iron sequestration and reduced absorption and recycling that leads to low saturation of transferrin and iron restriction of erythropoiesis and other tissues.

Traditional treatment of AI is based on reversibility/control of the underlying disease, whenever possible. If the disease is untreatable and anemia is mild, a careful evaluation of risks-benefits is needed to avoid side effects of any treatment. Pathophysiology-based treatments are limited to erythropoietin-like compounds and iron. The use of erythropoiesis stimulating agents (ESA) suppresses hepcidin by inducing erythropoiesis expansion. This approach is widely used in patients with chronic kidney disease, low-risk myelodysplastic syndromes, and cancer undergoing chemotherapy. However, a careful clinical control is necessary because high doses have cardiovascular side effects. The administration of intravenous iron may relieve iron restriction, caused by ESA-dependent expansion of erythropoiesis. Oral iron is usually ineffective since the high hepcidin levels counteract its intestinal absorption. Inhibitors of prolyl hydroxylase (hypoxia inducible factor, HIF stabilizers) are experimental in chronic kidney disease, to the aim of increasing endogenous EPO. Chronic treatment with red blood cells transfusions is not recommended because of transient effect and adverse reactions; it is limited to severe refractory anemia (Camaschella, 2019; Weiss et al., 2019).

Anemias Associated With Low Hepcidin Levels

Ineffective erythropoiesis and low or inappropriately normal hepcidin levels, with consequent iron overload, are typical features of the *"iron-loading anemias."* The prototype is β-thalassemia, a genetic recessive disease due to β-globin gene mutations that cause anemia and excess α-globin chain production. The latter precipitates as hemichromes in the bone marrow, damaging maturing erythroid precursors and leading to ineffective erythropoiesis. This occurs in non-transfusion-dependent thalassemia or thalassemia intermedia, whose erythropoiesis is characterized by the prevalence of immature cells that release erythroferrone to inhibit liver hepcidin expression. Hepcidin levels are usually greater in transfusion-dependent thalassemia, where endogenous ineffective erythropoiesis is at least partially suppressed by transfusions (Camaschella and Nai, 2016).

Hepcidin suppression is mediated by the increased cytokine erythroferrone (ERFE), a member of the TNF-α family encoded by *ERFE* gene, synthesized by erythroblasts upon EPO stimulation (Kautz et al., 2014). ERFE is released into the circulation and sequesters BMPs, especially BMP6 (Arezes et al., 2018), attenuating the hepcidin signaling in response to iron. In addition, an epigenetic suppression occurs at the hepcidin locus by histone deacetylase HDAC3 (Pasricha et al., 2017). When anemia causes hypoxia, other mediators such as PDGF-BB (Sonnweber et al., 2014), which is released by different cell types, suppress hepcidin.

Hepcidin levels are decreased by a special mechanism in low-risk myelodysplasia with ringed sideroblasts, a clonal disorder due to mutations of the spliceosome gene *SF3B1*. Iron accumulates in mitochondria, leading to ineffective erythropoiesis and systemic iron overload. An abnormally spliced, elongated ERFE protein is more powerful than wild type ERFE in suppressing hepcidin (Bondu et al., 2019) and causing transfusion-independent iron loading.

TARGETED THERAPIES FOR HEPCIDIN-RELATED ANEMIAS

The identification of molecular mechanisms responsible of the previously discussed anemias has stimulated research in developing targeted therapies to replace current symptomatic treatment (Sebastiani et al., 2016; Crielaard et al., 2017). Approaches differ according to the type of anemia and the aim of decreasing or increasing hepcidin levels or their effects (**Table 2**).

Experimental Therapies to Decrease Hepcidin Levels/Increase Ferroportin Function

Except for hepcidin producing tumors, which have to be surgically removed, compounds that antagonize hepcidin or its effects may be useful in all anemias characterized by high hepcidin levels. Their main application would be in chronic inflammatory diseases in order to reverse hypoferremia and anemia. Several experimental therapies aimed at manipulating the hepcidin

TABLE 2 | Experimental therapies targeting the hepcidin-ferroportin axis.

	Mechanism	Compounds
Compounds that decrease hepcidin or increase ferroportin function		
Class I	Reduction of the signaling pathway stimulating hepcidin	Anti IL6-R, anti IL-6
		Anti-BMP6 MoAb*
		BMPR inhibitors
		Anti-HJV MoAb
Class II	Hepcidin binders	Non anticoagulant heparins
		Anti-HAMP MoAb
		Oligonucleotides aptamers
Class III	Interfering with hepcidin-FPN interaction	Anti-FPN MoAb, GDP
Compounds that increase hepcidin or decrease ferroportin function		
Class I	Hepcidin mimics	Hepcidin analogues*
		Minihepcidin
Class II	Activating hepcidin	BMPs (preclinical studies)
	Blocking the hepcidin inhibitor	Anti-*TMPRSS6* (siRNA, ASO*)
	Blocking the hepcidin receptor	FPN Inhibitors*
Class III	Others	Human transferrin infusions
		Protoporphyrin IX (inhibition of HO)
		Bone marrow TFR2 inactivation

*BMPR, BMP receptor; HAMP, hepcidin gene; HJV, hemojuvelin; MoAb, monoclonal antibody; FPN, ferroportin; siRNA, small interfering RNA; ASO, antisense oligonucleotides; GDP, guanosine 5' diphosphate; HO, heme oxygenase; TFR2, transferrin receptor 2. Compounds indicated by * are in clinical trials.*

pathway and its function have been investigated in preclinical studies. Hepcidin antagonists are inhibitors of hepcidin synthesis/regulators (Ganz, 2019), hepcidin binders that block its function, and compounds that interfere with hepcidin-ferroportin interaction (**Table 2**). Some compounds are in clinical trials especially in chronic kidney disease (Sheetz et al., 2019). In IRIDA, manipulation of the hepcidin pathway has been proposed in preclinical studies with the use of anti-HJV MoAb (Kovac et al., 2016).

Experimental Therapies to Increase Hepcidin Levels/Decrease Ferroportin Function

Increasing hepcidin levels may not only reduce iron overload but also partially control ineffective erythropoiesis in *iron loading anemias*. β-thalassemia is the most studied among these conditions (Casu et al., 2018; Gupta et al., 2018). Proposed drugs are hepcidin analogs (some in clinical trials), hepcidin modulators, especially TMPRSS6 inhibitors, or compounds that interfere with hepcidin-ferroportin interaction decreasing iron export (**Table 2**).

While compounds that increase hepcidin reduce ineffective erythropoiesis due to the vicious cycle between ineffective erythropoiesis and iron loading (Camaschella and Nai, 2016), drugs that favor erythroid precursor maturation, as the activin receptor IIB ligand trap, luspatercept, not only improve anemia but also ameliorate iron homeostasis by reducing hepcidin inhibition (Piga et al., 2019).

Some targeted approaches now in clinical trials will hopefully result in novel treatments for a variety of anemias.

CONCLUSION

The spectacular advances in understanding the regulation of iron metabolism and hepcidin allowed a better understanding of erythropoiesis control, since together with erythropoietin iron is a fundamental factor for erythroid cells maturation. Conditions that lead to anemia can be associated with high and low hepcidin levels. In both instances, contrasting hepcidin deregulation may ameliorate/correct anemia in preclinical models, offering new tools that are already or will be soon clinically explored for the treatment of specific anemias.

AUTHOR CONTRIBUTIONS

AP drafted the paper. CC developed the final version. AN and LS contributed to writing and to critical review the manuscript. All the authors approved the final version.

REFERENCES

An, P., Wu, Q., Wang, H., Guan, Y., Mu, M., Liao, Y., et al. (2012). TMPRSS6, but not TF, TFR2 or BMP2 variants are associated with increased risk of iron-deficiency anemia. *Hum. Mol. Genet.* 21, 2124–2131. doi: 10.1093/hmg/dds028

Andriopoulos, B. Jr., Corradini, E., Xia, Y., Faasse, S. A., Chen, S., Grgurevic, L., et al. (2009). BMP6 is a key endogenous regulator of hepcidin expression and iron metabolism. *Nat. Genet.* 41, 482–487. doi: 10.1038/ng.335

Arezes, J., Foy, N., McHugh, K., Sawant, A., Quinkert, D., Terraube, V., et al. (2018). Erythroferrone inhibits the induction of hepcidin by BMP6. *Blood* 132, 1473–1477. doi: 10.1182/blood-2018-06-857995

Aschemeyer, S., Qiao, B., Stefanova, D., Valore, E. V., Sek, A. C., Ruwe, T. A., et al. (2018). Structure-function analysis of ferroportin defines the binding site and an alternative mechanism of action of hepcidin. *Blood.* 131, 899–910. doi: 10.1182/blood-2017-05-786590

Babitt, J. L., Huang, F. W., Wrighting, D. M., Xia, Y., Sidis, Y., Samad, T. A., et al. (2006). Bone morphogenetic protein signaling by hemojuvelin regulates hepcidin expression. *Nat. Genet.* 38, 531–539. doi: 10.1038/ng1777

Beguin, Y. (2003). Soluble transferrin receptor for the evaluation of erythropoiesis and iron status. *Clin. Chim. Acta* 329, 9–22. doi: 10.1016/S0009-8981(03)00005-6

Bondu, S., Alary, A. S., Lefevre, C., Houy, A., Jung, G., Lefebvre, T., et al. (2019). A variant erythroferrone disrupts iron homeostasis in SF3B1-mutated myelodysplastic syndrome. *Sci. Transl. Med.* 11:pii:eaav5467. doi: 10.1126/scitranslmed.aav5467

Camaschella, C. (2013). How I manage patients with atypical microcytic anaemia. *Br. J. Haematol.* 160, 12–24. doi: 10.1111/bjh.12081

Camaschella, C. (2019). Iron deficiency. *Blood* 133, 30–39. doi: 10.1182/blood-2018-05-815944

Camaschella, C., and Nai, A. (2016). Ineffective erythropoiesis and regulation of iron status in iron loading anaemias. *Br. J. Haematol.* 172, 512–523. doi: 10.1111/bjh.13820

Camaschella, C., and Pagani, A. (2018). Advances in understanding iron metabolism and its crosstalk with erythropoiesis. *Br. J. Haematol.* 182, 481–494. doi: 10.1111/bjh.15403

Canali, S., Wang, C. Y., Zumbrennen-Bullough, K. B., Bayer, A., and Babitt, J. L. (2017). Bone morphogenetic protein 2 controls iron homeostasis in mice independent of Bmp6. *Am. J. Hematol.* 92, 1204–1213. doi: 10.1002/ajh.24888

Casu, C., Nemeth, E., and Rivella, S. (2018). Hepcidin agonists as therapeutic tools. *Blood* 131, 1790–1794. doi: 10.1182/blood-2017-11-737411

Colucci, S., Pagani, A., Pettinato, M., Artuso, I., Nai, A., Camaschella, C., et al. (2017). The immunophilin FKBP12 inhibits hepcidin expression by binding the BMP type I receptor ALK2 in hepatocytes. *Blood* 130, 2111–2120. doi: 10.1182/blood-2017-04-780692

Crielaard, B. J., Lammers, T., and Rivella, S. (2017). Targeting iron metabolism in drug discovery and delivery. *Nat. Rev. Drug Discov.* 16, 400–423. doi: 10.1038/nrd.2016.248

De Falco, L., Sanchez, M., Silvestri, L., Kannengiesser, C., Muckenthaler, M. U., Iolascon, A., et al. (2013). Iron refractory iron deficiency anemia. *Haematologica* 98, 845–853. doi: 10.3324/haematol.2012.075515

De Falco, L., Silvestri, L., Kannengiesser, C., Moran, E., Oudin, C., Rausa, M., et al. (2014). Functional and clinical impact of novel TMPRSS6 variants in iron-refractory iron-deficiency anemia patients and genotype-phenotype studies. *Hum. Mutat.* 35, 1321–1329. doi: 10.1002/humu.22632

Donker, A. E., Schaap, C. C., Novotny, V. M., Smeets, R., Peters, T. M., van den Heuvel, B. L., et al. (2016). Iron refractory iron deficiency anemia: a heterogeneous disease that is not always iron refractory. *Am. J. Hematol.* 91, E482–E490. doi: 10.1002/ajh.24561

Du, X., She, E., Gelbart, T., Truksa, J., Lee, P., Xia, Y., et al. (2008). The serine protease TMPRSS6 is required to sense iron deficiency. *Science* 320, 1088–1092. doi: 10.1126/science.1157121

Finberg, K. E., Heeney, M. M., Campagna, D. R., Aydinok, Y., Pearson, H. A., Hartman, K. R., et al. (2008). Mutations in TMPRSS6 cause iron-refractory iron deficiency anemia (IRIDA). *Nat. Genet.* 40, 569–571. doi: 10.1038/ng.130

Ganz, T. (2019). Anemia of inflammation. *N. Engl. J. Med.* 381, 1148–1157. doi: 10.1056/NEJMra1804281

Gupta, R., Musallam, K. M., Taher, A. T., and Rivella, S. (2018). Ineffective erythropoiesis: anemia and iron overload. *Hematol. Oncol. Clin. North Am.* 32, 213–221. doi: 10.1016/j.hoc.2017.11.009

Heeney, M. M., and Finberg, K. E. (2014). Iron-refractory iron deficiency anemia (IRIDA). *Hematol. Oncol. Clin. North Am.* 28, 637–652. doi: 10.1016/j.hoc.2014.04.009

Heeney, M. M., Guo, D., De Falco, L., Campagna, D. R., Olbina, G., Kao, P. P., et al. (2018). Normalizing hepcidin predicts TMPRSS6 mutation status in patients with chronic iron deficiency. *Blood* 132, 448–452. doi: 10.1182/blood-2017-03-773028

Kautz, L., Jung, G., Valore, E. V., Rivella, S., Nemeth, E., and Ganz, T. (2014). Identification of erythroferrone as an erythroid regulator of iron metabolism. *Nat. Genet.* 46, 678–684. doi: 10.1038/ng.2996

Koch, P. S., Olsavszky, V., Ulbrich, F., Sticht, C., Demory, A., Leibing, T., et al. (2017). Angiocrine Bmp2 signaling in murine liver controls normal iron homeostasis. *Blood* 129, 415–419. doi: 10.1182/blood-2016-07-729822

Kovac, S., Boser, P., Cui, Y., Ferring-Appel, D., Casarrubea, D., Huang, L., et al. (2016). Anti-hemojuvelin antibody corrects anemia caused by inappropriately high hepcidin levels. *Haematologica* 101, e173–e176. doi: 10.3324/haematol.2015.140772

Lakhal, S., Schodel, J., Townsend, A. R., Pugh, C. W., Ratcliffe, P. J., and Mole, D. R. (2011). Regulation of type II transmembrane serine proteinase TMPRSS6 by hypoxia-inducible factors: new link between hypoxia signaling and iron homeostasis. *J. Biol. Chem.* 286, 4090–4097. doi: 10.1074/jbc.M110.173096

Meynard, D., Kautz, L., Darnaud, V., Canonne-Hergaux, F., Coppin, H., and Roth, M. P. (2009). Lack of the bone morphogenetic protein BMP6 induces massive iron overload. *Nat. Genet.* 41, 478–481. doi: 10.1038/ng.320

Muckenthaler, M. U., Rivella, S., Hentze, M. W., and Galy, B. (2017). A red carpet for iron metabolism. *Cell* 168, 344–361. doi: 10.1016/j.cell.2016.12.034

Nemeth, E., Tuttle, M. S., Powelson, J., Vaughn, M. B., Donovan, A., Ward, D. M., et al. (2004). Hepcidin regulates cellular iron efflux by binding to ferroportin and inducing its internalization. *Science* 306, 2090–2093. doi: 10.1126/science.1104742

Pagani, A., Colucci, S., Bocciardi, R., Bertamino, M., Dufour, C., Ravazzolo, R., et al. (2017). A new form of IRIDA due to combined heterozygous mutations of TMPRSS6 and ACVR1A encoding the BMP receptor ALK2. *Blood* 129, 3392–3395. doi: 10.1182/blood-2017-03-773481

Pagani, A., Vieillevoye, M., Nai, A., Rausa, M., Ladli, M., Lacombe, C., et al. (2015). Regulation of cell surface transferrin receptor-2 by iron-dependent cleavage and release of a soluble form. *Haematologica* 100, 458–465. doi: 10.3324/haematol.2014.118521

Pasricha, S. R., Lim, P. J., Duarte, T. L., Casu, C., Oosterhuis, D., Mleczko-Sanecka, K., et al. (2017). Hepcidin is regulated by promoter-associated histone acetylation and HDAC3. *Nat. Commun.* 8:403. doi: 10.1038/s41467-017-00500-z

Piga, A., Perrotta, S., Gamberini, M. R., Voskaridou, E., Melpignano, A., Filosa, A., et al. (2019). Luspatercept improves hemoglobin levels and blood transfusion requirements in a study of patients with beta-thalassemia. *Blood* 133, 1279–1289. doi: 10.1182/blood-2018-10-879247

Rausa, M., Pagani, A., Nai, A., Campanella, A., Gilberti, M. E., Apostoli, P., et al. (2015). Bmp6 expression in murine liver non parenchymal cells: a mechanism to control their high iron exporter activity and protect hepatocytes from iron overload? *PLoS One* 10:e0122696. doi: 10.1371/journal.pone.0122696

Sebastiani, G., Wilkinson, N., and Pantopoulos, K. (2016). Pharmacological targeting of the hepcidin/ferroportin axis. *Front. Pharmacol.* 7:160. doi: 10.3389/fphar.2016.00160

Sheetz, M., Barrington, P., Callies, S., Berg, P. H., McColm, J., Marbury, T., et al. (2019). Targeting the hepcidin-ferroportin pathway in anaemia of chronic kidney disease. *Br. J. Clin. Pharmacol.* 85, 935–948. doi: 10.1111/bcp.13877

Shore, E. M., Xu, M., Feldman, G. J., Fenstermacher, D. A., Cho, T. J., Choi, I. H., et al. (2006). A recurrent mutation in the BMP type I receptor ACVR1 causes inherited and sporadic fibrodysplasia ossificans progressiva. *Nat. Genet.* 38, 525–527. doi: 10.1038/ng1783

Silvestri, L., Pagani, A., Nai, A., De Domenico, I., Kaplan, J., and Camaschella, C. (2008). The serine protease matriptase-2 (TMPRSS6) inhibits hepcidin activation by cleaving membrane hemojuvelin. *Cell Metab.* 8, 502–511. doi: 10.1016/j.cmet.2008.09.012

Silvestri, L., Rausa, M., Pagani, A., Nai, A., and Camaschella, C. (2013). How to assess causality of TMPRSS6 mutations? *Hum. Mutat.* 34, 1043–1045. doi: 10.1002/humu.22321

Sonnweber, T., Nachbaur, D., Schroll, A., Nairz, M., Seifert, M., Demetz, E., et al. (2014). Hypoxia induced downregulation of hepcidin is mediated by platelet derived growth factor BB. *Gut* 63, 1951–1959. doi: 10.1136/gutjnl-2013-305317

Sorensen, E., Rigas, A. S., Didriksen, M., Burgdorf, K. S., Thorner, L. W., Pedersen, O. B., et al. (2019). Genetic factors influencing hemoglobin levels in 15,567 blood donors: results from the Danish blood donor study. *Transfusion* 59, 226–231. doi: 10.1111/trf.15075

Theurl, I., Schroll, A., Sonnweber, T., Nairz, M., Theurl, M., Willenbacher, W., et al. (2011). Pharmacologic inhibition of hepcidin expression reverses anemia of chronic inflammation in rats. *Blood* 118, 4977–4984. doi: 10.1182/blood-2011-03-345066

Weinstein, D. A., Roy, C. N., Fleming, M. D., Loda, M. F., Wolfsdorf, J. I., and Andrews, N. C. (2002). Inappropriate expression of hepcidin is associated with iron refractory anemia: implications for the anemia of chronic disease. *Blood* 100, 3776–3781. doi: 10.1182/blood-2002-04-1260

Weiss, G., Ganz, T., and Goodnough, L. T. (2019). Anemia of inflammation. *Blood* 133, 40–50. doi: 10.1182/blood-2018-06-856500

Weiss, G., and Goodnough, L. T. (2005). Anemia of chronic disease. *N. Engl. J. Med.* 352, 1011–1023. doi: 10.1056/NEJMra041809

19

Anemia in Chronic Kidney Disease: From Pathophysiology and Current Treatments, to Future Agents

Jose Portolés[1,2], Leyre Martín[1,2]*, José Jesús Broseta[3] and Aleix Cases[2,3]

[1] Department of Nephrology, Puerta de Hierro Majadahonda University Hospital, Madrid, Spain, [2] Anemia Working Group Spanish Society of Nephrology, Madrid, Spain, [3] Instituto de Investigaciones Biomédicas August Pi i Sunyer (IDIBAPS), Universitat de Barcelona, Barcelona, Spain

*Correspondence:
Leyre Martín
leyremaria.martin@salud.madrid.org
orcid.org/0000-0001-5854-0577

Anemia is a common complication in chronic kidney disease (CKD), and is associated with a reduced quality of life, and an increased morbidity and mortality. The mechanisms involved in anemia associated to CKD are diverse and complex. They include a decrease in endogenous erythropoietin (EPO) production, absolute and/or functional iron deficiency, and inflammation with increased hepcidin levels, among others. Patients are most commonly managed with oral or intravenous iron supplements and with erythropoiesis stimulating agents (ESA). However, these treatments have associated risks, and sometimes are insufficiently effective. Nonetheless, in the last years, there have been some remarkable advances in the treatment of CKD-related anemia, which have raised great expectations. On the one hand, a novel family of drugs has been developed: the hypoxia-inducible factor prolyl hydroxylase inhibitors (HIF-PHIs). These agents induce, among other effects, an increase in the production of endogenous EPO, improve iron availability and reduce hepcidin levels. Some of them have already received marketing authorization. On the other hand, recent clinical trials have elucidated important aspects of iron supplementation, which may change the treatment targets in the future. This article reviews the current knowledge of the pathophysiology CKD-related anemia, current and future therapies, the trends in patient management and the unmet goals.

Keywords: anemia, chronic kidney disease, erythropoiesis-stimulating agents, iron, HIF stabilizer, HIF prolyl-hydroxylase inhibitor, hepcidin, COVID 19

EPIDEMIOLOGY OF ANEMIA OF CKD

Anemia is a common complication in chronic kidney disease (CKD), and is associated with a reduced quality of life (1, 2), a worse renal survival (3), an increase in morbidity and mortality (4, 5), and higher costs (6). Several studies focused on prevalence of anemia on CKD non-dialysis dependent (NDD) report variable anemia rates up to 60%.

Anemia is more prevalent and severe as the estimated glomerular filtration rate (eGFR) declines. An analysis of the cross-sectional data from the National Health and Nutrition Examination Survey (NHANES) in 2007–2008 and 2009–2010 (7) revealed that anemia was twice as prevalent in patients with CKD as in the general population (15.4% vs. 7.6). The prevalence of anemia raised with the progression of CKD: 8.4% at stage 1 to 53.4% at stage 5. Similar data was observed in a more recent paper by the CKD Prognosis Consortium (8). In addition, they observed an increased prevalence of anemia among diabetic patients, independent of eGFR and albuminuria.

Regarding new onset of anemia, the observational study NADIR-3 followed CKD stage 3 patients without anemia during 3 years. The authors estimated an annual rate of onset of anemia of 11% in the first year, 20% in the second year and 26% in the third year. In addition, the study revealed that those that had developed anemia significantly progressed more rapidly to CKD stages 4–5, had higher rates of hospitalizations (31.4 vs. 16.1%), major cardiovascular events (16.4 vs. 7.2%) and mortality (10.3 vs. 6.6%) (9).

With regards to the *"real-world"* management of anemia in CKD, considerable controversies and variability exist in the context of guideline recommendations. However, few studies have evaluated this issue. An Italian observational study evaluated anemia management in two visits, among 755 prevalent NDD-CKD patients. Mean eGFR was 27.5 ± 10 mL/min/ 1.73 m^2. The prevalence of severe and mild anemia was 18 and 44%, and remained unchanged at month 6 (19.3 and 43.2%). Clinical inertia to ESA was similar at baseline and at month 6 (39.6 and 34.2%, respectively, $P = 0.487$) and it was less frequent than clinical inertia to iron therapy (75.7 and 72.0%, respectively) (10). A recent observational analysis from the Swedish Renal Registry evaluated the epidemiology and treatment patterns of all nephrology-referred adult CKD patients during 2015. Among 14 415 patients [Non-Dialysis Dependent (NDD), 11,370; Dialysis-Dependent (DD), 3,045] anemia occurred in 60% of NDD and 93% of DD patients. DD patients used more erythropoiesis-stimulating agents (ESAs; 82 vs. 24%) and iron (62 vs. 21%) than NDD patients. The prescribed ESA doses were low to moderate [median 48.2 IU/kg/week (NDD), 78.6 IU/kg/week (DD)]. Among ESA-treated patients, 6–21% had hemoglobin (Hb) >13 g/dL and 2–6% had Hb <9 mg/L. Inflammation (C-reactive protein >5 mg/L) was highly prevalent and associated with ESA resistance and higher ESA doses, but not with iron use. Further, higher ESA doses (>88 IU/kg/week) were associated with an increased risk of major adverse cardiovascular events. Despite the recommendations of guidelines, the use of iron was unexpectedly low, particularly in ESA-treated NDD patients, while a fifth of the dialysis patients receiving ESA had a hemoglobin above the recommended targets (11). A multicenter cross-sectional study conducted at specialist nephrology clinics in Ireland also showed an evident variability in the implementation of different guidelines, the high rates of anemia (from 21 to 63%; $p < 0.001$, depending on the CKD Stage), the low testing rates for iron deficiency (only 45% of anemic patients), and the low use of treatment (86 % of patients with confirmed iron deficiency were not on treatment) (12).

PHYSIOPATHOLOGY OF ANEMIA IN CKD

The mechanisms of anemia in CKD are multifactorial. The progressive reduction of endogenous erythropoietin (EPO) levels has classically been considered to play a preeminent role. However, other factors have also been described to contribute to anemia in CKD patients, such as an absolute iron deficiency due to blood losses or an impaired iron absorption, an ineffective use of iron stores due to increased hepcidin levels, systemic inflammation due to CKD and associated comorbidities, a reduced bone marrow response to EPO due to uremic toxins, a reduced red cell life span, or vitamin B12 or folic acid deficiencies (13).

Hypoxia Inducible Factor System

EPO is a glycoprotein (30.4 kDa) that binds to its receptor on the surface of erythroid progenitor cells mainly in the bone marrow, and serves as a key stimulus for red cell survival, proliferation and differentiation. EPO is produced predominantly by the fibroblast-like interstitial peritubular cells of the kidneys, and in a much lesser proportion, by the perisinusoidal cells in the liver, in response to changes in tissue oxygen tension (14). The production of EPO is controlled at the level of the EPO gene transcription. One of the most important factors that regulate its expression is the hypoxia-inducible factor (HIF) system, whose activity depends on the tissue oxygen levels.

In more detail, under hypoxia or anemic stress, the HIF1 binds to the EPO gene, and activates its expression. HIF1 is composed of two subunits, HIF1α and HIF1β. HIF1β is constitutively expressed whereas HIF1α is virtually absent under normoxic conditions. However, in low oxygen tension settings, HIF1α accumulates and translocates to the nucleus, where it binds to HIF1 β. The HIF1 α-β heterodimer binds to DNA sequences called hypoxia response elements (HRE), regulating the expression of various hypoxia-sensitive genes, either downregulating or upregulating them. The purpose of this rapid adaptive response is to protect against cellular damage, by improving oxygen delivery and by decreasing oxygen consumption. Among these hypoxia-sensitive genes is the EPO gene, which is activated, leading to an increased EPO production. Other genes that are transcriptionally upregulated by the HIF complex are those encoding EPO receptor, transferrin and transferrin receptor, vascular endothelial growth factor (VEGF) or endothelin-1 (15). Recent work has shown that the HIF transcription factors are key elements in the control of cell metabolism and function (16–18). An effect of HIF on total and LDL-cholesterol levels has also been described (19), probably in part by the effects of HIF on degradation of the rate-limiting enzyme, 3-hydroxy-3-methylglutaryl-CoA reductase (20), similar to what has been observed in high altitude settings (21).

Under normoxic conditions, HIF1α is degraded. For this purpose, HIF1α is hydroxylated at two proline residues. This hydroxylation is performed by specific HIF prolyl-hydroxylase enzymes called prolyl hydroxylase domain (PHD) enzymes that need the presence of oxygen, iron, and 2-oxoglutarate as co-factors. Three forms have been described: PHD1, PHD2, PHD3. PHD2 is the main isoform regulating HIF activity (22). Once HIF1α is hydroxylated, the E3 ubiquitin ligase von Hippel-Lindau (pVHL) binds HIF1α, and is targeted for proteasomal degradation. In contrast, under low oxygen tension the action of PHDs is prevented, allowing for HIF1α stabilization and translocation to the nucleus (23, 24). This pathway is the target of the new so-called hypoxia-inducible factor prolyl hydroxylase inhibitors (HIF-PHIs) (**Figure 1**).

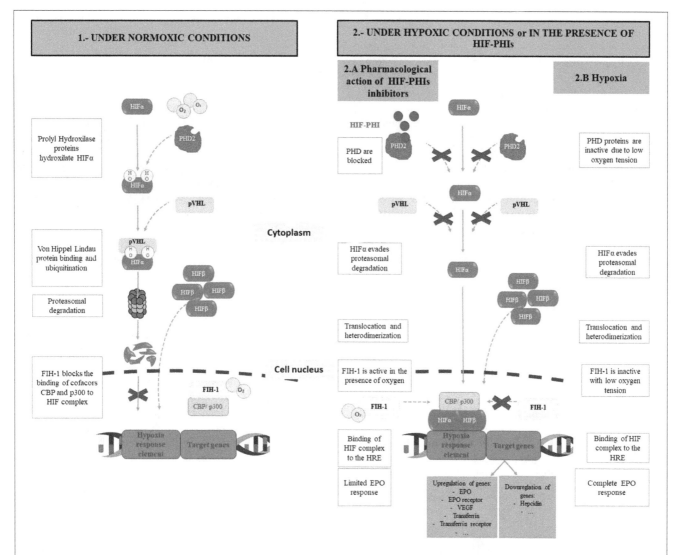

FIGURE 1 | Regulation of HIF under normoxic conditions, pharmacological effects of hypoxia-inducible factor prolyl hydroxylase inhibitors (HIF-PHIs) and under hypoxic conditions. HIF, hypoxia-inducible factor; O₂, oxygen; OH, hydroxyl; PHD, prolyl hydroxylase domain protein; HIF-PHI, hypoxia inducible factor prolyl hydroxylase inhibitor; pVHL, Von Hippel Lindau protein; FIH-1, Factor inhibiting HIF; CBP, CREB-binding protein.

HIF activity is also regulated through the hydroxylation at a carboxy-terminal asparagine residue of HIF1α by factor-inhibiting HIF (FIH) (25). This hydroxylation of HIF1α occurs with normal oxygen levels and reduces its transcriptional activity. Indeed, it prevents HIF from recruiting transcriptional coactivators such as p300 or CBP, that are needed for the transactivation of hypoxia-responsive genes (26, 27). Furthermore, angiotensin II, which is often found to be increased in CKD patients, raises the production of reactive oxygen species, leading to an inhibition of PHD enzymes, and therefore, a rise in EPO levels (28–30).

Nonetheless, recent animal studies have described important roles to other components of the HIF system. Three isoforms of HIFα have been described, that share similarities regarding oxygen-dependent hydroxylation: HIF1α, HIF2α, and HIF3α. All of them can bind to the HIFβ subunit. However, there may

be some differences amongst them: while HIF1α and HIF2α activate gene transcription, HIF3α downregulates HIF1α and HIF2α activity. Moreover, their effect on the expression of some genes may also vary. HIF2α may play a more important role than HIF1α in the regulation of EPO production, as it is specifically required for renal and hepatic production of EPO. The direct role of HIF3α on erythropoiesis has not been fully described. Finally, the expression of HIF2α and HIF3α is limited to several tissues, while HIF1α is ubiquitous (31).

EPO Production in CKD

In CKD patients, EPO levels are inadequately low with respect to the degree of anemia. EPO deficiency starts early in the course of CKD, but it appears that when eGFR falls below 30 ml/min per 1.73 m² this deficiency becomes more severe (32). This absolute EPO deficiency can be caused by a decrease in the EPO production and/or by errors in EPO-sensing. CKD associates an alteration in oxygen delivery to the kidneys due to a reduced blood flow. This results in an adaptation of renal tissue to consume less oxygen and the subsequent maintenance of a normal tissue oxygen gradient. As a consequence, PHD enzymes remain active, the HIF heterodimer is not formed and the EPO gene is not activated (33).

Furthermore, it has been demonstrated experimentally that hypoxia-induced EPO production is inhibited by some inflammatory cytokines such as interleukin-la (IL-la), IL-l beta, transforming growth factor-beta (TGF-beta), and tumor necrosis factor-a (TNF-a) (34, 35). It is well-known that CKD itself leads to an increase of inflammation and immune activation molecules, which would inhibit hypoxia-induced EPO production (36, 37). However, this mechanism of EPO production seems to be blunted rather than abolished in some CKD patients, as they are able to produce additional endogenous EPO in their kidneys and liver under certain circumstances. For instance, when exposed to high altitude or bleeding. Apparently, augmentation of HIF signaling can revert quiescent EPO-producing and oxygen-sensing (REPOS) cells back to EPO production (38). This has been confirmed in observational studies, where hemodialysis patients living in higher altitude require lower doses of recombinant human EPO (rhuEPO) (39).

Some CKD patients may also present with a functional EPO deficiency or EPO resistance, where normal range EPO levels coexist with low hemoglobin (Hb) levels (40), indicating that the bone marrow response to endogenous and exogenous EPO is blunted in patients with CKD. The mechanisms that have been hypothesized for the EPO resistance are various: Proinflammatory cytokines are thought to induce apoptosis as well as a to have a direct toxic effect *via* the induction of labile free radical nitric oxide on erythroid progenitor cells (41, 42). Proinflammatory cytokines are thought to downregulate the expression of EPO receptor on their surface too. It has also been shown that cytokines can induce the production of antagonistic peptides that bind to the EPO receptor, and inhibit the EPO-dependent proliferation (43–46). Moreover, hepcidin (whose production is enhanced by inflammation) might also contribute to EPO resistance, by directly inhibiting erythroid progenitor proliferation and survival (47). Lastly, neocytolysis is a homeostatic physiological process that leads to selective hemolysis of young circulating red blood cells, that has been found to contribute to resistance in CKD patients receiving exogenous EPO (48).

The search for new therapeutic options for these patients is essential. In this sense, some molecules of the HIF system have already been studied as new targets for anemia treatment with a view to increase endogenous EPO production and presumably improve the utilization of iron stores (**Figure 2**).

Iron Metabolism

Iron is required for an adequate erythropoietic response to EPO, and in anemic conditions having iron deficiency corrected allows lower exogenous EPO supplies (49).

Furthermore, iron is required in other essential non-erythropoietic effects that may help explain symptoms such as impaired exercise performance, cognitive impairment or decreased quality of life, and an increased risk in hospitalization or death in patients with heart failure and reduced ejection fraction, independent of anemia. Thus, these advocate for the need to correct iron deficiencies independent of Hb status (50). Iron is an essential component of myoglobin, which transports oxygen in the muscle cells. Iron also plays a substantive role in several oxidative reactions affecting intracellular metabolism, such as the electron transport chain or oxidative phosphorylation. Iron is involved in different mechanisms of DNA synthesis, degradation and repair. Finally, iron is an important component of cytochrome P450 family (51). In fact, there is an increasing evidence from observational studies that iron deficiency is associated with worse outcomes in CKD patients (52–54).

Most of the iron requirements are provided by recycling the iron present in senescent erythrocytes and the release of iron from storage sites (**Figure 2**). The proportion of iron that comes from the dietary uptake is much smaller. In addition, there is no physiological mechanism to regulate iron excretion. It is lost from the desquamation of intestinal epithelial cells, skin cells and blood loses and dietary iron absorption, which is regulated by hepcidin, compensate these loses.

The iron content of macrophages from the phagocytosis of senescent red blood cells, hepatocytes or enterocytes (dietary iron absorbed in the duodenum) is released into the circulation by ferroportin, the only iron exporter known. Iron is then transported through the circulation by transferrin, and delivered into target cells by transferrin binding to transferrin receptor (55). Transferrin receptors are regulated by intracellular iron quantity and cell growth. A circulating acute-phase protein produced in the liver, hepcidin, is the key regulator of iron metabolism. Its purpose is to maintain adequate systemic iron levels. Hepcidin is thought to decrease the absorption of iron in the doudenum by downregulating the expression of apical divalent metal transporter 1 (DMT1) in the enterocyte. Besides absorption, hepcidin also plays a role in iron storage. Indeed, hepcidin promotes the internalization of ferroportin into the cell for its degradation, and thus preventing iron form exiting into the circulation from enterocytes, macrophages or other iron stores. Iron overload increases hepcidin levels, whereas iron deficiency reduces its concentrations (55).

Absolute and relative iron deficiency are frequent conditions in CKD patients. Blood losses, for instance, due to blood left in the hemodialysis circuit are common. In addition, the "uremic" state and other comorbidities causing inflammation prevent from an adequate intestinal iron absorption and from the release of iron from the body stores. Proinflammatory cytokines contribute to a functional iron deficiency in several ways: They stimulate the hepatic synthesis of hepcidin, they induce the expression of DMT1 in macrophages, and induce the expression of ferritin, and inhibit that of ferroportin. They also promote the uptake of iron bound to transferrin into macrophages, *via* the transferrin receptor (56). Moreover, hepcidin is eliminated by kidney and its clearance is reduced as eGFR declines. All these mechanisms favor intracellular iron storage, limiting the availability of iron in CKD.

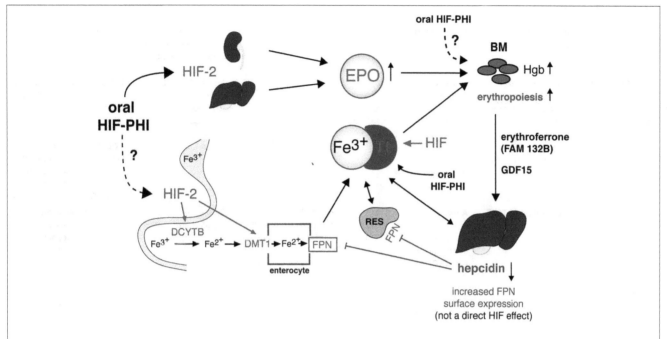

FIGURE 2 | Integrated model for CKD-anemia physiology and actual and potential treatments. HIF, hypoxia-inducible factor; Fe, iron; HIF-PHI, hypoxia inducible factor prolyl hydroxylase inhibitor; EPO, Erytrhopoietin; Tf, transferrin; DCYTB, duodenal cytochromeb; DMT1, divalent metal transporter 1; BM, Bone marrow; FPN, ferroportin; GDF15, Growth differentiation factor 15; Hgb, hemoglobin; RES, Reticuloendothelial system; FAM132B, Gene that codes for erythroferrone.

Under stress erythropoiesis, EPO suppresses hepcidin synthesis *via* erythroferrone (ERFE). ERFE is a hormone produced by erythroblasts in response to EPO (57). Also, HIF 1α and probably HIF2α regulates hepcidin production by directly binding to and repressing its promoter (58), while HIF-2α enhances iron availability through the activation of genes encoding DMT1 and duodenal cytochrome b (DCYTB) required for transport of dietary iron from the intestinal lumen and for the import of lysosomal iron arising from the circulation (59).

CURRENT CLINICAL PRACTICE GUIDELINES OF ANEMIA IN CKD

Anemia management in CKD has evolved dramatically: from the first oral iron supplements introduced in 1830s (ferrous sulfate), the use of red blood cell transfusions along the XX century, the appearance of the first rhuEPO use in late 1980s followed by long-acting ESAs, to finally, the widespread use of intravenous iron supplements in recent years. However, the actual management of anemia in patients with CKD varies among different countries and medical units (60, 61). Indeed, current guidelines KDIGO (13)—ERBP (62)—NICE (63) do not fully coincide with each other. Some controversies exist about the optimal Hb and iron targets. **Table 1** summarizes the main differences.

Further, these guidelines do not include more recent studies assessing the efficacy and safety of IV iron, as well as different strategies of iron repletion, which will probably change the clinical practice in the future. They demonstrate that in ND-CKD, renal transplant and PD patients IV iron is more efficacious

and safe. In addition, a high-dose low frequency administration strategy in dialysis dependent chronic kidney disease (DD-CKD) patents is safe and improves outcomes in patients (63).

CKD ANEMIA TREATMENT
Erythropoiesis-Stimulating Agents (ESAs)

The first EPO analog available was epoetin α and short time later epoetin β. It is produced by recombinant DNA technology in cell cultures. Darbepoetin alfa (DA) and methoxy polyethylene glycol-epoetin beta where developed thereafter and presented a prolonged half-life. More recently, biosimilars of the original epoetin have been introduced in the market.

Not all ESAs are equal. They have different pharmacokinetic and pharmacodynamic properties, such as different half-lives and EPO receptor affinity, allowing a less frequent dosing and ease of administration for NDD CKD patients with long-acting ESAs. In addition, it is important to point out the fact that the conversion factor between short-acting and long-acting ESAs is likely not linear. In fact, at higher doses, long-acting ESAs are more dose-effective (64). However, based on efficacy and safety data, various Cochrane metaanalysis advocate for insufficient evidence to suggest the superiority of any ESA formulation or any ESA administration pattern (65, 66).

Some observational studies have shown conflicting results regarding such outcomes. For instance, the Study of the Japanese Registry of Dialysis that showed a 20% higher risk of mortality from any cause in patients treated with long-acting ESAs compared to those treated with short-acting ESAs (67). On the contrary, an Italian observational study in ND-CKD that

TABLE 1 | Summary of the key recommendations of the most recent anemia guidelines.

	Diagnosis of iron deficiency	Treatment initiation	Hb target under treatment with ESAs	SF and TSAT objectives in patients under treatment	FE oral vs. IV
NICE (2015)	**Test every 3 months (1–3 m in HD)** - Use %HRC > 6%, only if blood processing within 6 h. - if not possible, use CHr < 29 pg - If not, use a combi-nation SF < 100 ng/mL and TSAT < 20%	**Correct iron deficiency before ESA therapy.** - Patient-centered: discuss risks benefits of treatment options. Take into account the person's choice. Avoid Hb < 10 g/dL.	Hb 10–12 g/dl	**Avoid SF > 800 ng/mL** To prevent this, review iron dose if SF > 500 ng/mL	**ND-CKD with anemia and iron deficiency:** - offer a 3 months trial of oral iron therapy. - If it fails, offer IV iron therapy. - **DD-CKD:** Preference for IV iron - **If IV iron, consider high dose, low frequency** formulations for ND and DD-CKD patients.
KDIGO (2012)	**SF ≤ 100 ng/mL and TSAT ≤ 20%.**	**A trial with IV iron** if Hb increase or ESA dose reduction is desired and SF≤ 500 ng/mL and TSAT ≤ 30% **ND-CKD: When Hb < 10 g/dL:** Individualize decision based on the rate of fall of Hb, risks and symptoms. **DD-CKD:** When Hb 9-10 g/dL. Avoid Hb < 9 g/dl.	Hb ≤ 11.5 g/dl - **Target to Hb > 11.5 g/dl if QoL improve** is foreseen and patient accepts risks. Avoid Hb >13 g/dL	**Stop iron supplements** if SF > 500 ng/mL	**ND-CKD: Select route based on severity of ID, prior response, side effects, costs,** A trial of iv iron, or a 1–3 month trial of oral iron therapy. - **DD- CKD:** Preference for IV iron
ERBP (2009)	**SF < 100 ng/mL and TSAT <20% if ESA naïve. SF ≤ 300 ng/mL and TSAT ≤ 30% if ESA treated**	**Avoid Hb < 10 g/dL.** - If low risk patients or a benefit in QoL foreseen ESA could start at ↑ Hb (avoid Hb >12 g/dL) - In high risk patients with worsening heart disease, treatment initiation at Hb9-10 g/dL.	Hb 10–12 g/dl - High risk patients with asymptomatic disease: target Hb around 10 g/dL	**Avoid SF > 500 ng/ml and TSAT > 30%.**	**ND-CKD and mild-moderate anemia:** Oral iron as first line therapy for > 3 months. **ND-CKD and severe anemia or when oral iron ineffective:** IV iron as first choice.

SF, serum ferritin; TSAT, Transferrin saturation; %HRC, percentage of hypochromic red blood cells; CHr, hemoglobin content in reticulocytes; Hob, Hemoglobin; ND-CKD, Non dialysis dependent Chronic kidney disease; DD-CKD, dialysis dependent CKD; QoL, quality of life; IV, intravenous ESA erythropoiesis stimulating agent; Fe, iron.

showed a higher risk of progression to ESKD and mortality in patients receiving short-acting ESAs at high doses (68). These results should be taken cautiously due to the study design and the risk of bias. In contrast, a recent randomized controlled trial (RCT) comparing monthly administration of CERA with reference shorter-acting agents epoetin alfa/beta and DA, showed non-inferiority regarding Hb target achievement, major adverse cardiovascular events or all-cause mortality in NDD and DD-CKD. It was however observed that patients who did not achieve levels of Hb above 10 g/dL or those at the highest quartile of ESA dose, had a higher risk of CV events or death, independent of the assigned treatment (69). More RCTs are needed to assess the differences between different ESA formulations and administration patterns, particularly in patients requiring higher doses of ESA.

Individualizing Hb Target According to the Patient Profile

The target Hb concentration during ESA therapy is still controversial. Studies early after the appearance of rhuEPO demonstrated its efficacy in reducing the need for blood transfusions, the symptoms related to anemia and an improved quality of life (70, 71). Various landmark trials have dwelt on the convenience of a complete correction of anemia. Indeed, in the CHOIR trial the use of a target Hb level of 13,5 g/dl was associated with increased risk of suffering a composite of death, myocardial infarction, hospitalization for congestive heart failure and stroke, and no incremental improvement in the quality of life. CREATE trial did not observe an increase of the risk of cardiovascular events, but showed an increase in the necessity of dialysis among the group that targeted Hb in normal range (13–15 g/dl) The TREAT trial compared the use of darbepoetin alfa targeting Hb level of 13 g/dl vs. a rescue therapy when Hb level dropped below 9 g/dl in patients with diabetes, NDD-CKD and moderate anemia. The use of darbepoetin alfa did not reduce the risk of either of the two primary composite outcomes (either death or a cardiovascular event or death or a renal event), and was associated with an increased risk of stroke (65, 72–75). Yet, it is still unclear whether this increased risk is due to the higher ESA doses and the possible non-erythropoietic effects, whether it is due to the underlying systemic inflammation in patients with ESA-hyporresponsiveness, rather than due to the high Hb level itself (76).

Conversely, although some trials have demonstrated significant improvements in quality of life (QoL) in patients targeted to normal Hb levels (73, 75, 77) the clinical relevance of these findings are questioned. The results of these trials were highly influential in changing the guidelines and clinical practice of anemia in NDD-CKD.

Current evidence, then, demonstrates a clear benefit in correcting Hb levels if they are below 10 g/dL, but also an increased risk when exceeding Hb 13 g/dl. The Hb target, then, appears to be somewhere in between 10 and 12 g/dl. Individualizing the Hb target relative to the patient's risks, basal conditions and preferences is advisable.

Iron Supplementation for Anemia in CKD

Guidelines acknowledge that the optimal strategy to manage iron metabolism remains unclear, and advocate for balancing the potential benefits and risks of iron supplementation (13, 62, 63). **Table 1** summarizes the principles and targets of the management of iron supplements of the KDIGO (13)—ERBP (62)—NICE (63) guidelines. In recent years some good quality pre-clinical studies, clinical trials and epidemiological studies have shed some light on the therapeutic approach regarding iron deficiency in CKD and will surely change clinical practice.

Intravenous (IV) iron has shown benefits both in DD-CKD and more recently in NDD-CKD, as it has proved to be more efficacious in rising ferritin and Hb levels, while reducing ESA and transfusion requirements. Specifically, in hemodialysis patients, oral preparations seem to be useless, maybe except for the phosphate binder ferric citrate (78). In addition, gastrointestinal intolerance and constipation reduce tolerance and compliance of oral iron formulations (79).

However, some concerns raised about IV iron formulation such as enhanced oxidative stress, endothelial dysfunction or the potential role in favoring infection. Further, IV iron administration has been associated with an increased risk of hypotension, headaches or hypersensitivity reactions. Labile iron, which is the iron that is freed into the circulation after administration and non-bound to transferrin, is an important cause of such adverse reactions.

IV iron supplements are non-biologic complex drugs. An iron core, covered by a complex structure of polysaccharides forms them. Indeed, the differences in the structure of the molecule among different IV iron formulations may be responsible for the differences in outcomes of each IV iron formulation. Some studies have even demonstrated differences in the attainment of Hb levels between the "original" brand and its generic form of iron sucrose (80).

On the other hand, there is growing evidence that oral compound can have a deleterious effect on gut microbiota which may worsen uremic dysbiosis (81, 82). Whether oral iron induced changes in gut microbiota, increases uremic toxins production and/or inflammation in CKD remain to be elucidated.

Dosing Patterns: The "Iron First-Approach" and the "High Dose-Low Frequency Approach"

As mentioned before, iron is essential for an adequate erythropoesis. In this sense, several trials have demonstrated that the correction of iron deficiency lessens the need for ESA in CKD

patients (FIND:CKD) (49). Hence, results from TREAT study demonstrate that control group receiving only IV iron but no ESAs may increase Hb by 1 g/dl. The so called "iron fist approach" suggested by guidelines (CITA) is based in his efficacy for anemia correction. Unfortunately, we have no evidence of the effect on hard end-points. Moreover, the risk of Hb overshooting depends on high levels of EPO but no IV iron use, since iron is not a growth factor.

In addition, various studies carried out in patients with heart failure (HF) with reduced ejection fraction and iron deficiency demonstrated that IV iron supplementation [but not oral iron, (83)] have shown an improvement outcomes, HF symptoms, functional class and quality of life, (FAIR-HF, CONFIRM-HF, EFFECT-HF) (84–86). Further, a meta-analysis demonstrated that these benefits of IV iron therapy were independent of the presence of anemia. More recently, a reduction of hospitalizations for HF has also been demonstrated in a study among patients with acute heart failure and iron deficiency (AFFIRM_AHF) (87). Likewise, an improvement in renal function has been observed with IV ferric carboximaltose in a subanalysis of the FAIR-HF study (88). In a small study in patients with HF, CKD and anemia with iron deficiency, IV iron was associated with an improvement of myocardial function and of cardiac dimensions (89), similar to the observations in another pilot study (90). There is a considerable correlation between heart failure, iron deficiency and renal failure and each comorbidity reduces the survival of these patients (91). Large registry data show that CKD is present in 12 to 74% of HF cases (92) and that its prevalence increases as renal function declines.

The Anemia Working Group of the Spanish Society of Nephrology published a review advocating for this "iron first-approach" and recommending the administration of IV ferric carboxymaltose in patients with CKD, HF with reduced ejection fraction and iron deficiency, even in the absence of anemia, extrapolating the recommendations of the Heart Failure Guidelines of the European Society of Cardiology (93, 94).

Moreover, newer IV iron formulations are more stable and have safer profiles that allows the administration of higher doses of iron per session (95, 96). The recent PIVOTAL trial has confirmed the efficacy and safety of high-dose IV iron sucrose: it is a UK open label, randomized controlled trial among 2,141 incident hemodialysis patients, that compared a proactively administered high-dose IV iron regimen with a reactively administered low-dose regimen. The trial demonstrated that a proactive high-dose schema reduced the death of all causes or an aggregated of non-fatal cardiovascular events [HR de 0.85: IC 95% (0.73–1.0); $p < 0.001$ for non-inferiority and $p = 0.04$ for superiority]. In addition, the high-dose regimen was not associated with higher risks of death, major adverse cardiovascular events, or infection (97). These findings should lead to a change in clinical guidelines.

Iron Targets: How Much Iron Is Too Much Iron?

Iron overload is a condition of elevated body iron content associated with signs of organ dysfunction that is presumably caused by excess iron. Some studies have demonstrated an increase in the liver iron content in hemodialysis patients, and an association between hepatic iron overload and hepatic steatosis has been recently described (98). However, its clinical relevance is still not known, and no deposits have been observed in other territories, such as cardiac or pancreatic (99–101). A metaanalysis of clinical trials and observational studies in the setting of hemodialysis suggests that patients that received higher doses of IV iron did not show a higher risk of mortality, infections or cardiovascular events (102). Nonetheless, the strength of the findings is limited by the small number of patients and of events in the clinical trials, and by the statistical heterogeneity in the observational studies included.

A recent epidemiological study has shown a slight higher mortality risk in patients with NDD-CKD and ferritin levels above 500 ng/ml, compared to patients with no iron deficiency, and patients with absolute or relative iron deficiency (40). These findings should be taken cautiously due to the presence of possible confounding factors. On the contrary, incident hemodialysis patients in the proactive high dose iron regimen in the PIVOTAL study showed a reduced risk in the primary end point (composite of death, MI, stroke, hospitalization and HF), as mentioned above in this article, and achieved higher mean ferritin levels (without exceeding 700 ng/ml, as per protocol). The upper limits of iron targets and the long-term safety of high doses of IV iron supplementation, specially of the accumulated high iron doses in hemodialysis patients, still needs to be clarified.

There has long been a concern whether iron supplements increased the risk of infections. A sub-analysis of PIVOTAL study did not show differences in infection episodes, hospitalization or death for infection between the proactive high dose regimen and reactive low dose-iron groups of patients (103).

Hypoxia-Inducible Factor Prolyl Hydroxylase Inhibitors

In recent years, new drugs have been developed for the treatment of anemia. These are the so called HIF-prolyl-hydroxylase inhibitors (HIF-PHIs). These drugs inhibit the action of prolyl-hydroxylase, which leads to an increase in the levels of HIF, and therefore, to an increase in endogenous EPO (24).There are currently four HIF-PHIs undergoing phase III clinical trials: roxadustat, daprodustat, vadadustat and molidustat. All of them are administered orally. However, they have differences in pharmacodynamics and pharmacokinetics, which probably determine differences in their interaction with the HIF system, and thus lead to differences in efficacy and safety profiles (104) (**Table 2**).

Other compounds such as desidustat (Zyan1; Cadila Healthcare), JNJ-42905343 (Janssen) or enarodustat (JTZ-951; Japan Tobacco/Akros Pharma), have completed phase II studies or are in early stages of development.

Efficacy of HIF Prolyl Hydroxylase Inhibitors

Roxadustat is the most advanced HIF-PHI under clinical development, which has already been approved in China and

Japan. Two phase 3 studies were published in 2019 comparing roxadustat with placebo in NDD, and with epoetin alfa in DD-CKD patients in China. These studies had a relative small sample size a study population and of short duration. The former compared roxadustat with placebo, without adjuvant iron supplements, and demonstrated its efficacy in rising hemoglobin levels after 9 weeks (105). The latter compared roxadustat with epoetin alfa, with iron supplement only as a rescue therapy. After 26 weeks of follow up, the attained hemoglobin levels in the roxadustat group were non-inferior to those in the epoetin alfa-arm, and both groups had a similar safety profile (106). These results were similar to those found by a phase 3 study comparing roxadustat to ESAs in hemodialysis and peritoneal dialysis patients in Japan (107, 108).

The results of several phase III clinical trials were presented in the past 2019 and 2020 Annual Meetings of the American Association of Nephrology. The ROCKIES, PYRENES and SIERRAS studies compared roxadustat vs. epoetin alpha in prevalent HD patients (109–111). The HIMALAYAS study compared roxadustat vs. epoetin alpha in incident HD patients (112). In a pooled analysis ($n = 3.917$) roxadustat was significantly superior to EPO in anemia correction and the roxadustat group received fewer transfusions 9.5 vs. 12.8%; HR (95% CI) =0.82 (0.689, 0.99). In prevalent DD patients the risk of major cardiovascular events (MACE) was comparable between the two treatment arms, whereas there was a 16% reduction in the risk of MACE plus [HR = 0.84 (0.73, 0.97); $p = 0.02$] in the roxadustat group. (MACE+: Mace plus heart failure and thromboembolic events). Interestingly, patients receiving roxadustat had reduced iron needs, and those on roxadustat and an elevated C-reactive protein were able to increase Hb levels. Among 1.526 incident DD patients, there was a 30% reduction in the risk of MACE and a 34% reduction in the risk of MACE+: [HR (95% CI) = 0.70 (0.51, 0.97); $p = 0.03$] and [HR 0.66 (0.50, 0.89); $p = 0.005$] respectively, among patients receiving roxadustat (113).

The OLYMPUS, ALPS, and ANDES trials evaluated roxadustat vs. placebo in NDD-CKD patients (110, 114, 115). An integrated analysis ($n = 4.270$) showed that roxadustat was efficacious in achieving and maintaining Hb levels, with lower risk of rescue therapy. Regarding adverse events, both arms of treatment had comparable safety profiles regarding cardiovascular events and all-cause mortality (113).

The results of the DOLOMITES trial were presented i in the past ERA-EDTA congress in June 2020 (116) and in the 2020 ASN Annual Meeting (117). This phase 3, randomized, open-label, active-controlled study evaluated the efficacy and safety of roxadustat compared to DA in the treatment of anemia in NDD- CKD patients. The median time of follow up was 104 weeks and the study enrolled 616 adult anemic patients with CKD stages 3–5. Roxadustat was non-inferior to DA in the primary endpoint, which was the achievement of Hb response during the first 24 weeks of treatment. Regarding secondary efficacy endpoints, roxadustat was superior in decreasing low-density lipoprotein cholesterol and in time to first IV iron use. Roxadustat was non-inferior in blood pressure control and time to first occurrence of hypertension, in changes in Quality of life

TABLE 2 | Pharmacological characteristics and current knowledge status of different Hypoxia-inducible factor prolyl hydroxylase inhibitors.

	Roxadustat (FBG-4592)	Vadadustat (AKB-6548)	Daprodustat (GSK 1278863)	Molidustat (BAY-3934)
Affinity IC50 (uM)	0.027	0.029	0.067	0.007
PHD Isoform Selectivity	PHD 1-3	PHD 3>2	PHD 2-3	PHD 2< 1 and 3
HIFα selectivity	HIF1α and 2α	HIF2α > 1α	HIF1α and 2α	HIF1α and 2α
Inhibitory concen-tration IC 50 (μM)	>100	29	21	65
Half life humans (h)	12	4.5	4	Not available
Current status of development	2019 approval in Japan and China Phase III reported at ASN 2019	Ongoing phase III Preliminary report at ASN 2020	Ongoing phase III	Completed phase II
Phase III clinical trials	DD (HD/DP) and NDD Correction and maintenance	DD (HD/DP) and NDD Correction and maintenance	DD (HD/DP) and NDD Correction and maintenance	Not available

IC50, half maximal receptor inhibitory concentration; PHD, prolyl hydroxylase domain protein; HIF, hypoxia-inducible factor; ASN, American Society of Nephrology; DD, Dialysis Dependent; HD, Hemodialysis; DP, Peritoneal dialysis; NDD, Non-dialysis dependent.

scores, and in Hb change. The occurrence of treatment-emergent adverse events (TEAEs) was similar between the two groups, and the TEAEs leading to withdrawal of treatment were more frequent in the roxadustat group. They reported no significant differences between groups in adjudicated cardiovascular events. In all the Roxadustat studies the roxadustat patients presented an early and sustained LDL-reduction as a pleiotropic effect.

Another compound, vadadustat has also been approved in Japan in 2020. The results of two phase III trials comparing vadadustat vs. DA in Japanese HD and non-dialysis dependent patients were presented in past 2019 ASN annual meeting (NCT03439137 and NCT03329196, respectively). Over 300 patients were followed for 52 weeks in each study. In both trials, vadadustat showed non-inferiority in maintaining Hb levels within the target range and a similar safety profile. Additionally, vadadustat was associated with an increase in total iron binding capacity and a decrease in hepcidin in DD and NDD-CKD (118, 119). Furthermore, the results of the PRO2TECT study (NCT02648347) were presented at the 2020 ASN annual meeting. It consists of two randomized, phase 3, global, open-label, sponsor-blind, parallel-group, active-controlled non-inferiority trials comparing oral daily vadadustat to parenteral DA in NDD-CKD patients, already treated for anemia and non-previously treated (naïve), respectively. Vadadustat did not meet the pre-specified non-inferiority criterion compared to DA with regards to cardiovascular safety. Interestingly, cardiovascular safety was similar between the two arms of treatment in the regions were the Hb target was 10–11 g/dL, but the cardiovascular risk was higher in patients randomized to vadadustat in regions with a Hb target of 10–12 g/dL.

Daprodustat has also been approved recently for use in Japan, and various phase III clinical trials are currently ongoing: ASCEND-D (NCT02879305), ASCEND-ID (NCT03029208), ASCEND-TD (NCT03400033), ASCEND-ND (NCT02876835), and ASCENDNHQ (NCT03409107). Daprodustat has already demonstrated its efficacy in managing anemia of CKD both in DD and NDD-CKD patients in phase II studies.

Lastly, molidustat, which is structurally different to the other study drugs mentioned before, is currently being evaluated in small phase III studies (NCT03351166, NCT03543657, NCT03418168, NCT03350321, NCT03350347). Several phase II studies, which are part of the DIALOGUE program, compared molidustat with either placebo or ESA therapy in CKD patients, demonstrating the efficacy, safety and tolerability of the drug (120).

By the time of elaboration of the present manuscript, the Cochrane Kidney and Transplant Group

Has published the protocol for a systematic review on HIF-PHIs for the treatment of anemia of chronic kidney disease (121).

Safety of HIF Prolyl Hydroxylase Inhibitors

From a mechanistic point of view, the inhibition of prolyl-hydroxylases prevents HIF from degradation, leading to an increase of endogenous EPO within the physiological range, rather than the pharmacological levels achieved by current ESAs. Therefore, the rate of adverse events related to the high EPO levels should be expected to be lower than with ESAs. However, as mentioned before, HIF also modulates many other non-erythropoietic genes. This activity would explain the potential beneficial effects seen in pre-clinical and early clinical studies such as an improved iron utilization, HDL and LDL lowering effect, ischemia protection and a protective effect on CKD progression, improved neo-vascularization or better blood pressure control (122).

Nonetheless, potential deleterious side effects due to the modulation of other genes with this new class of drugs have also been postulated, notably tumor progression, enhanced vascular calcification, enhanced growth of renal cysts, worsening of retinopathy, or an increase in pulmonary artery pressure. In addition, whether these prolyl-hydroxylase inhibitors inhibit other di-oxygenases beyond HIF-PHIs and thus other pathways is unknown. Data from large phase III studies are still to be published and will surely help to answer these open questions.

In conclusion, in light of this evidence, HIF-PHIs, can be a viable alternative for the treatment of NDD and DD anemic CKD patients. However, more data is required regarding their long-term safety and their possible non-erythropoietic effects. In addition, the subset of patients that may benefit from these new agents still needs to be elucidated.

ANEMIA MANAGEMENT, ESAs AND COVID 19

Infection with severe acute respiratory syndrome coronavirus 2 (SARS-COV-2) has become a worldwide pandemic during 2020 and millions of cases have been reported worldwide. The coronavirus disease can lead to sepsis, acute kidney injury (AKI), multiple organ dysfunction and an atypical form of the acute distress respiratory syndrome. Anemia and a disturbed iron metabolism are common in COVID 19 patients. In an observational study Among 11,265 patients across 13 New York hospitals admitted between March 1 and April 27 2020, an elevation in D-dimer level was associated with a lesser median hemoglobin level and a greater serum ferritin level. And so are they in patients with COVID 19 suffering an AKI and in maintenance dialysis patients (123, 124). The exact mechanisms of COVID 19 are not completely known, but patients with a severe COVID 19 often present with an intense inflammatory phase and with a prothrombotic state. In these cases, the efficacy of ESAs is limited and they could even be potentially harmful. Fishbane et al. in a recent editorial article suggest avoiding ESA therapy (124). In the case of maintenance dialysis if the patient was already on that treatment, the authors recommend the continuation of ESA at the same dose but targeting a lower Hb targets (Hb 8–9 g/dL). Some other authors speculate on the potential role of HIF –PHDs as a protective agents against COVID. Indeed, the activation of the HIF1α pathway would decrease angiotensin convertase enzyme 2 (ACE2), which is the bound for COVID 19 membrane spike protein to enter the host cell, and therefore, decrease the invasiveness of SARS-CoV-2 (125).

Regarding iron supplementation, systemic inflammatory processes as happens with severe COVID 19 decrease the availability of iron. Furthermore, iron is also essential for viral replication (126). In addition, patients with viral infections and iron overload have a poor prognosis. Therefore, limiting iron supplements could be beneficial for patients with severe COVID 19 although more studies are need to shed light into this subject (127).

Anemia in CKD-Key Points

- The pathophysiology of CKD-anemia is multifactorial, thus requiring a holistic approach

- Not all ESA are equal and whether their different pharmacokinetics and pharmacodynamics is associated with different outcomes in CKD patients remains to be elucidated.

- Iron is essential for other physiologic process beyond erythropoiesis. Observational studies in NDD-CKD patients suggest that iron deficiency is associated with worse outcomes, paving the way to randomized controlled trials that demonstrate the benefit of correcting iron deficiency beyond anemia.

- The upper limits of ferritin and TSAT indicating iron overload and risk of developing adverse events are still not clear, especially in the long-term.

- HIF prolyl hydroxylase inhibitors are new drugs under clinical evaluation. The available data suggest that they are efficacious and safe alternatives to ESA for the treatment of anemia in NDD and DD-CKD patients with several potential advantages over current therapies. However, more data is required to confirm these findings.

AUTHOR CONTRIBUTIONS

All authors contributed to the writing article and approved the submitted version.

ACKNOWLEDGMENTS

The authors gratefully acknowledge the cooperation Ms. Cristina Escudero Gómez for the bibliographic assistance.

REFERENCES

Moreno F, Gomez JML, Jofre R, Valderrabano F, Gonzalez L, Gorriz JL, et al. Nephrology dialysis transplantation quality of life in dialysis patients. A Spanish multicentre study. *NDT.* (1996) 11(Suppl 2):125–9. doi: 10.1093/ndt/11.supp2.125

Lefebvre P, Vekeman F, Sarokhan B, Enny C, Provenzano RCP. Relationship between hemoglobin level and quality of life in anemic patients with chronic kidney disease receiving epoetin alfa. *Curr Med Res Opin.* (2006) 22:1929–37. doi: 10.1185/030079906X132541

Minutolo R, Conte G, Cianciaruso B, Bellizzi V, Camocardi A, De Paola L DNL. Hyporesponsiveness to erythropoiesis-stimulating agents and renal survival in non-dialysis CKD patients. *Nephrol Dial Transplant.* (2012) 27:2880–6. doi: 10.1093/ndt/gfs007

Astor BC, Coresh J, Heiss G, Pettitt D. Kidney function and anemia as risk factors for coronary heart disease and mortality: the atherosclerosis risk in communities (ARIC) study. *Am Hear J.* (2006) 151:492–500. doi: 10.1016/j.ahj.2005.03.055

Kovesdy CP, Trivedi BK, Kalantar-Zadeh K, Anderson JE. Association of anemia with outcomes in men with moderate and severe chronic kidney disease. *Kidney Int.* (2006) 69:560–4. doi: 10.1038/sj.ki.5000105

Nissenson AR, Wade S, Goodnough T, Knight K, Dubois RW. Economic burden of anemia in an insured population. *J Manag Care Pharm.* (2005) 11:565–74. doi: 10.18553/jmcp.2005.11.7.565

Stauffer ME, Fan T. Prevalence of anemia in chronic kidney disease in the United States. *PLoS ONE.* (2014) 9:2–5. doi: 10.1371/journal.pone.0084943

Inker LA, Grams ME, Levey AS, Coresh J, Cirillo M, Collins JF, et al. Relationship of estimated GFR and albuminuria to concurrent laboratory abnormalities: an individual participant data meta-analysis in a global consortium. *Am J Kidney Dis.* (2019) 73:206–17. doi: 10.1053/j.ajkd.2018.08.013

Portolés J, Gorriz JL, Rubio E, De Alvaro F, García F, Alvarez-Chivas V, et al. The development of anemia is associated to poor prognosis in NKF/KDOQI stage 3 chronic kidney disease. *BMC Nephrol.* (2013) 14:2. doi: 10.1186/1471-2369-14-2

Minutolo R, Locatelli F, Gallieni M, Bonofiglio R, Fuiano G, Oldrizzi L, et al. Anaemia management in non-dialysis chronic kidney disease (CKD) patients: a multicentre prospective study in renal clinics. *Nephrol Dial Transplant.* (2013) 28:3035–45. doi: 10.1093/ndt/gft338

Evans M, Bower H, Cockburn E, Jacobson SH, Barany P, Carrero J- Contemporary management of anaemia, erythropoietin resistance and cardiovascular risk in patients with advanced chronic kidney disease: a nationwide analysis. *Clin Kidney J.* (2020) 13:821–7. doi: 10.1093/ckj/sfaa054

Stack AG, Alghali A, Li X, Ferguson JP, Casserly LF, Cronin CJ, et al. Quality of care and practice patterns in anaemia management at specialist kidney clinics in Ireland: a national study. *Clin Kidney J.* (2018) 11:99–107. doi: 10.1093/ckj/sfx060

KDIGO Anemia Working Group. KDIGO clinical practice guideline for anemia in chronic kidney disease. *Kidney Int.* (2012) 2:279–335. doi: 10.1038/kisup.2012.38

Pan X, Suzuki N, Hirano I, Yamazaki S, Minegishi N, Yamamoto M. Isolation and characterization of renal erythropoietin- producing cells from genetically produced anemia mice. *PLoS ONE.* (2011) 6:e0025839. doi: 10.1371/journal.pone.0025839

Carmeliet P, Dor Y, Herbert JM, Fukumura D, Brusselmans K, Dewerchin M, et al. Role of HIF-1 in hypoxia- mediated apoptosis, cell proliferationand tumourangiogenesis Peter. *Nature.* (1998) 394:485–90. doi: 10.1038/28867

Rankin EB, Rha J, Selak MA, Unger TL, Keith B, Liu Q HV. Hypoxia-inducible factor 2 regulates hepatic lipid metabolism. *Mol Cell Biol.* (2009) 29:4527–38. doi: 10.1128/MCB.00200-09

Marsch E, Demandt JA, Theelen TL, Tullemans BM, Wouters K, Boon MR, et al. Deficiency of the oxygen sensor prolyl hydroxylase 1 attenuates hypercholesterolaemia, atherosclerosis, and hyperglycaemia. *Eur Heart J.* (2016) 37:2993–7.

Palazon A, Goldrath AW, Nizet V, Johnson RS. HIF transcription factors, inflammation, and immunity. *Immunity.* (2014) 41:e008. doi: 10.1016/j.immuni.2014.09.008

Provenzano R, Besarab A, Sun CH, Diamond SA, Durham JH, Cangiano JL, et al. Oral hypoxia-inducible factor prolyl hydroxylase inhibitor roxadustat (FG-4592) for the treatment of anemia in patients with CKD. *Clin J Am Soc Nephrol.* (2016) 11:982–91. doi: 10.2215/CJN.06890615

Nguyen AD, McDonald JG, Bruick RK D-BR. Hypoxia stimulates degradation of 3-hydroxy-3-methylglutaryl-coenzyme A reductase through accumulation of lanosterol and hypoxia-inducible factor-mediated induction of insigs. *J Biol Chem.* (2007) 282:27436–46. doi: 10.1074/jbc.M704 976200

Férézou J, Richalet JP, Coste T, Rathat C. Changes in plasma lipids and lipoprotein cholesterol during a high altitude mountaineering expedition (4800 m). *Eur J Appl Physiol Occup Physiol.* (1988) 57:740–5. doi: 10.1007/BF01075997

Vogel S, Wottawa M, Farhat K, Zieseniss A, Schnelle M, Le-huu S, et al. Prolyl hydroxylase domain (PHD) 2 affects cell migration and F-actin formation *via* RhoA/Rho-associated kinase-dependent cofilin phosphorylation. *J Biol Chem.* (2010) 285:33756–63. doi: 10.1074/jbc.M110.132985

West JB. Physiological effects of chronic hypoxia. *NEJM.* (2017) 376:1965–71. doi: 10.1056/NEJMra1612008

Eckardt K-U. The noblesse of kidney physiology. *Kidney Int.* (2019) 96:1250–3. doi: 10.1016/j.kint.2019.10.007

Lando D, Peet DJ, Whelan DA, Gorman JJ, Whitelaw ML. Asparagine hydroxylation of the HIF transactivation domain: a hypoxic switch. *Science.* (2002) 295:858–61. doi: 10.1126/science 1068592

Freedman SJ, Sun ZJ, Poy F, Kung AL, Livingston DM, Wagner G, et al. Structural basis for recruitment of CBP p300 by hypoxia-inducible

factor-1. *PNAS.* (2002) 99:5367–72. doi: 10.1073/pnas.082117899

Chan MC, Ilott NE, Schödel J, Sims D, Tumber A, Lippl K, et al. Tuning the transcriptional response to hypoxia by inhibiting hypoxia-inducible factor (HIF) prolyl and asparaginyl. *J Biol Chem.* (2016) 291:20661–73. doi: 10.1074/jbc.M116.749291

Pagé EL, Chan DA, Giaccia AJ, Levine M, Richard DE. Hypoxia- inducible factor-1 stabilization in nonhypoxic conditions: role of oxidation and intracellular ascorbate depletion. *Mol Biol Cell.* (2008) 19:86–94. doi: 10.1091/mbc.e07-06-0612

Freudenthaler S, Lucht I, Schenk T, Brink M, Gleiter CH. Dose-dependent effect of angiotensin II on human erythropoietin production. *Pflügers Arch Eur J Physiol.* (2000) 439:838–44. doi: 10.1007/s004249900238

Pratt MC, Lewis-Barned NJ, Walker RJ, Bailey RR, Shand BI, Livesey Effect of angiotensin converting enzyme inhibitors on erythropoietin concentrations in healthy volunteers. *Br J Clin Pharmacol.* (1992) 34:363–5. doi: 10.1111/j.1365-2125.1992.tb05644.x

Kaplan JM, Sharma N, Dikdan S. Hypoxia-inducible factor and its role in the management of anemia in chronic kidney disease. *Int J Mol Sci.* (2018) 19:389. doi: 10.3390/ijms19020389

Fehr T, Ammann P, Garzon D, Korte W, Fierz W, Rickli H, et al. Interpretation of erythropoietin levels in patients with various degrees of renal insufficiency and anemia. *Kidney Int.* (2004) 66:1206–11. doi: 10.1111/j.1523-1755.2004.00880.x

Wenger RH, Hoogewijs D. Regulated oxygen sensing by protein hydroxylation in renal erythropoietin-producing cells. *Am J Physiol Ren Physiol.* (2010) 298:F1287–96. doi: 10.1152/ajprenal.00736.2009

Faquin WC, Schneider TJ, Goldberg MA. Effect of inflammatory cytokines on hypoxia-induced erythropoietin production. *Blood.* (1992) 79:1987–94. doi: 10.1182/blood.V79.8.1987.1987

Fandrey J, Jelmann WE. Interleukin-1 and tumor necrosis factor-alpha inhibit erythropoietin production *in vitro. Ann N Y Acad Sci.* (1991) 628:250–5. doi: 10.1111/j.1749-6632.1991.tb17252.x

Rao M, Wong C, Kanetsky P, Girndt M, Stenvinkel P, Reilly M, et al. Cytokine gene polymorphism and progression of renal and cardiovascular diseases. *Kidney Int.* (2007) 72:549–56. doi: 10.1038/sj.ki.5002391

Amdur RL, Feldman HI, Gupta J, Yang W, Kanetsky P, Shlipak M, et al. Inflammation and progression of CKD: the CRIC study. *Clin J Am Soc Nephrol.* (2016) 11:1546–56. doi: 10.2215/CJN.13121215

Souma T, Nezu M, Nakano D, Yamazaki S, Hirano I. Erythropoietin synthesis in renal myo fi broblasts is restored by activation of hypoxia signaling. *JASN.* (2016) 27:428–38. doi: 10.1681/ASN.2014121184

Brookhart MA, Schneeweiss S, Avorn J, Bradbury BD, Rothman KJ, Fischer M, et al. The effect of altitude on dosing and response to erythropoietin in ESRD. *J Am Soc Nephrol.* (2008) 19:1389–95. doi: 10.1681/ASN.2007111181

Wagner M, Alam A, Zimmermann J, Rauh K, Koljaja-Batzner A, Raff U, et al. Endogenous erythropoietin and the association with inflammation and mortality in diabetic chronic kidney disease. *Clin J Am Soc Nephrol.* (2011) 6:1573–9. doi: 10.2215/CJN.00380111

Libregts SF, Gutiérrez L, de Bruin AM, Wensveen FM, Papadopoulos P, van Ijcken W, et al. Chronic IFN-γ production in mice induces anemia by reducing erythrocyte life span and inhibiting erythropoiesis through an IRF- 1/PU.1 axis. *Blood.* (2011) 118:2578–88. doi: 10.1182/blood-2010-10-315218

Ganz T. Anemia of inflammation. *N Engl J Med.* (2019) 381:1148–57. doi: 10.1056/NEJMra1804281

Sasaki A, Yasukawa H, Shouda T, Kitamura T, Dikic I, Yoshimura CIS3/SOCS-3 suppresses erythropoietin (EPO) signaling by binding the EPO receptor and JAK2. *J Biol Chem.* (2000) 275:29338–47. doi: 10.1074/jbc.M003456200

Macdougall IC, Cooper AC. Erythropoietin resistance: the role of inflammation and pro-inflammatory cytokines. *Nephrol Dial Transpl.* (2002) 17:39–43. doi: 10.1093/ndt/17.suppl_11.39

Taniguchi S, Dai C-H, James O. Price and SBK, interferon. interferon g downregulates stem cell factor and erythropoietin receptors but not insulin- like growth factor-i receptors in human erythroid colony-forming cells. *Blood.* (1997) 90:2244–52. doi: 10.1182/blood.V90.6.2244

Van Der PK, Braam B, Jie KE, Gaillard CAJM. Mechanisms of Disease : erythropoietin resistance in patients with both heart and kidney failure. *Nature.* (2008) 4:47–57. doi: 10.1038/ncpneph0655

Dallalio G, Law E, Means RT, Jr. Hepcidin inhibits *in vitro* erythroid colony formation at reduced erythropoietin concentrations. *Blood.* (2006) 107:2792–04. doi: 10.1182/blood-2005-07-2854

Rice L, Alfrey CP, Driscoll T, Whitley CE, Hachey DL, Suki W. Neocytolysis contributes to the anemia of renal disease. *AJKD*. (1999) 33:59–62. doi: 10.1016/S0272-6386(99)70258-1

Macdougall IC, Bock A, Carrera F, Eckardt KU, Gaillard C, Van Wyck D, et al. The FIND-CKD study—A randomized controlled trial of intravenous iron versus oral iron in non-dialysis chronic kidney disease patients: background and rationale. *Nephrol Dial Transplant*. (2014) 29:843–50. doi: 10.1093/ndt/gft424

Jankowska EA, Tkaczyszyn M, Suchocki T, Drozd M, Von Haehling S, Doehner W, et al. Effects of intravenous iron therapy in iron-deficient patients with systolic heart failure : a meta-analysis of randomized controlled trials. *Eur J Heart Fail*. (2016) 18:786–95. doi: 10.1002/ejhf.473

Agarwal R. Nonhematological benefits of iron. *Am J Nephrol*. (2007) 46202:565–71. doi: 10.1159/000107927

Eisenga MF, Nolte IM, Van Der MP, Bakker SJL, Gaillard CAJM. Association of different iron deficiency cutoffs with adverse outcomes in chronic kidney disease. *BMC Nephrol*. (2018) 19:225. doi: 10.1186/s12882-018-1021-3

Cho ME, Hansen JL, Peters CB, Cheung AK, Greene T, Sauer BC. An increased mortality risk is associated with abnormal iron status in diabetic and non-diabetic Veterans with predialysis chronic kidney disease. *Kidney Int*. (2019) 96:750–60. doi: 10.1016/j.kint.2019.04.029

Awan AA, Walther CP, Richardson PA, Shah M, Winkelmayer WC, Navaneethan SD. Prevalence, correlates and outcomes of absolute and functional iron deficiency anemia in nondialysis-dependent chronic kidney disease. *Nephrol Dial Transplant*. (2021) 36:129–36. doi: 10.1093/ndt/gfz192

van Swelm RPL, Wetzels JFM, Swinkels DW. The multifaceted role of iron in renal health and disease. *Nat Rev Nephrol*. (2020) 16:77–98. doi: 10.1038/s41581-019-0197-5

Batchelor EK, Kapitsinou P, Pergola PE, Kovesdy CP, Jalal DI. Iron deficiency in chronic kidney disease: updates on pathophysiology, diagnosis, and treatment. *J Am Soc Nephrol*. (2020) 31:456–68. doi: 10.1681/ASN.2019020213

Kautz L, Jung G, Valore EV, Rivella S, Nemeth E, Ganz T. Identification of erythroferrone as an erythroid regulator of iron metabolism. *Nat Genet*. (2014) 46:678–84. doi: 10.1038/ng.2996

Peyssonnaux C, Zinkernagel AS, Schuepbach RA, Rankin E, Vaulont S, Haase VH, et al. Regulation of iron homeostasis by the hypoxia- inducible transcription factors (HIFs). *J Clin Invest*. (2007) 117:1926–32. doi: 10.1172/JCI31370

Frazer DM, Andreson GJ. The regulation of iron transport. *Biofactors*. (2014) 40:206–14. doi: 10.1002/biof.1148

Wong MMY, Tu C, Li Y, Perlman RL, Pecoits-Filho R, Lopes AA, et al. Anemia and iron deficiency among chronic kidney disease Stages 3-5ND patients in the chronic kidney disease outcomes and practice patterns study: often unmeasured, variably treated. *Clin Kidney J*. (2019) 13:613–24. doi: 10.1093/ckj/sfz091

Lopes MB, Tu C, Zee J, Guedes M, Pisoni RL, Robinson BM, et al. A real- world longitudinal study of anemia management in non-dialysis-dependent chronic kidney disease patients: a multinational analysis of CKDopps. *Sci Rep*. (2021) 11:1784. doi: 10.1038/s41598-020-79254-6

Locatelli F, Covic A, Eckardt K, Wiecek A, Vanholder R. Anaemia management in patients with chronic kidney disease: a position statement by the Anaemia Working Group of European Renal Best Practice (ERBP). *Nephrol Dial Transplant*. (2009) 24:348–54. doi: 10.1093/ndt/gfn653

(NICE) NI for H and CE. *Chronic Kidney Disease: Managing Anaemia*. (2015). Available online at: nice.org.uk/guidance/ng8 (accessed March 11, 2021).

Bock HA, Hirt-Minkowski P, Brünisholz M, Keusch G, Rey S, Von Albertini Darbepoetin alpha in lower-than-equimolar doses maintains haemoglobin levels in stable haemodialysis patients converting from epoetin alpha/beta. *Nephrol Dial Transplant*. (2008) 23:301–8. doi: 10.1093/ndt/gfm579

Palmer SC, Salanti G, Craig JC, Mavridis D, Salanti G. Erythropoiesis-stimulating agents for anaemia in adults with chronic kidney disease: a network meta-analysis (Review). *Cochrane Database Syst Rev*. (2014) 2013:CD010590. doi: 10.1002/14651858.CD010590

Hahn D, Ci E, Elserafy N, Ac W, Em H. Short-acting erythropoiesis-stimulating agents for anaemia in predialysis patients. *Cochrane Database Syst Rev*. (2017) 1:CD011690. doi: 10.1002/14651858.CD011690.pub2

Sakaguchi Y, Hamano T, Wada A, Masakane I. Types of erythropoietin-stimulating agents and mortality among patients undergoing hemodialysis. *J Am Soc Nephrol*. (2019) 30:1037–48. doi: 10.1681/ASN.2018101007

Minutolo R, Garofalo C, Chiodini P, Aucella F, Del Vecchio L, Locatelli F, et al. Types of erythropoiesisstimulating agents and risk of ESKD and death

in patients with non-dialysis chronic kidney disease. *NDT*. (2021) 26:267–74. doi: 10.1093/ndt/gfaa088

Locatelli F, Hannedouche T, Fishbane S, Zoe Morgan DO, White WB. Cardiovascular safety and all-cause mortality of methoxy polyethylene glycol-epoetin beta and other erythropoiesis-stimulating agents in anemia of CKD a randomized noninferiority trial. *CJASN*. (2019) 14:1701–10. doi: 10.2215/CJN.01380219

Gandra SR, Finkelstein FO, Bennett AV, Lewis EF, Brazg T, Martin ML. Impact of erythropoiesis- stimulating agents on energy and physical function in nondialysis CKD patients with anemia: a systematic review. *Am J Kidney Dis*. (2010) 55:519–34. doi: 10.1053/j.ajkd.2009.09.019

Johansen KL, Finkelstein FO, Revicki DA, Evans C, Wan S, Gitlin M, et al. Systematic review of the impact of erythropoiesis-stimulating agents on fatigue in dialysis patients. *Nephrol Dial TransplantDialTransplant*. (2012) 27:2418–25. doi: 10.1093/ndt/gfr697

Besarab A, Bolton WK, Browne JK, Egrie JC, Nissenson AR, Okamoto DM, et al. The effects of normal as compared with low hematocrit values in patients with cardiac disease who are receiving hemodialysis and epoetin. *N Engl J Med*. (1998) 339:584–90. doi: 10.1056/NEJM199808273390903

Drüeke TB, Locatelli F, Clyne N, Eckardt K-U, Macdougall IC, Tsakiris D, et al. Normalization of hemoglobin level in patients with chronic kidney disease and anemia. *NEJM*. (2006) 335:2071–84. doi: 10.1056/NEJMoa062276

Singh AK, Szczech L, Tang KL, Barnhart H, Sapp S, Wolfson M, et al. Correction of anemia with epoetin alfa in chronic kidney disease. *N Engl J Med*. (2006) 355:2085–98. doi: 10.1056/NEJMoa065485

Pfeffer MA, Burdmann EA, Chen C-Y, Cooper ME, de Zeeuw D, Eckardt K-U, et al. A trial of darbepoetin alfa in type 2 diabetes and chronic kidney disease. *NEJM*. (2009) 361:2019–32. doi: 10.1056/NEJMoa0907845

Vaziri ND, Zhou XJ. Potential mechanisms of adverse outcomes in trials of anemia correction with erythropoietin in chronic kidney disease. *Nephrol Dial Transplant*. (2009) 24:1082–8. doi: 10.1093/ndt/gfn601

Parfrey PS, Foley RN, Wittreich BH, Sullivan DJ, Zagari MJ, Frei D. Double-blind comparison of full and partial anemia correction in incident hemodialysis patients without symptomatic heart disease. *J Am Soc Nephrol*. (2005) 16:2180–9. doi: 10.1681/ASN.2004121039

Umanath K, Jalal DI, Greco BA, Umeukeje EM, Reisin E, Manley J, et al. Ferric citrate reduces intravenous iron and erythropoiesis- stimulating agent use in ESRD. *J Am Soc Nephrol*. (2015) 26:2578–87. doi: 10.1681/ASN.2014080842

Fishbane S, Block GA, Loram L, Neylan J, Pergola PE, Uhlig K, et al. Effects of ferric citrate in patients with nondialysis-dependent CKD and iron deficiency anemia. *J Am Soc Nephrol*. (2017) 28:1851–8. doi: 10.1681/ASN.2016101053

Rottembourg J, Kadri A, Leonard E, Dansaert A, Lafuma A. Do two intravenous iron sucrose preparations have the same efficacy? *Nephrol Dial Transplant*. (2011) 26:3262–7. doi: 10.1093/ndt/gfr024

Kortman GAM, Reijnders D, Swinkels DW. Oral iron supplementation: potential implications for the gut microbiome and metabolome in patients with CKD. *Hemodial Int*. (2017) 21(Suppl. 1):S28–36. doi: 10.1111/hdi.12553

Cigarran Guldris S, González Parra E, Cases Amenós A. Microbiota intestinal en la enfermedad renal crónica. *Nefrologia*. (2017) 37:9–19. doi: 10.1016/j.nefro.2016.05.008

Lewis GD, Malhotra R, Hernandez AF, McNulty SE, Smith A, Felker GM, et al. Effect of oral iron repletion on exercise capacity in patients with heart failure with reduced ejection fraction and iron deficiency: the IRONOUT HF randomized clinical trial. *JAMA*. (2017) 317:1958–66. doi: 10.1001/jama.2017.5427

Anker SD, Colet JC, Filippatos G, Willenheimer R, Dickstein K, Drexler H, et al. Ferric carboxymaltose in patients with heart failure and iron deficiency. *N Engl J Med*. (2009) 361:2436–48. doi: 10.1056/NEJMoa0908355

Ponikowski P, Van Veldhuisen DJ, Comin-Colet J, Ertl G, Komajda M, Mareev V, et al. Beneficial effects of long-term intravenous iron therapy with ferric carboxymaltose in patients with symptomatic heart failure and iron deficiency. *Eur Heart J*. (2015) 36:657–68. doi: 10.1093/eurheartj/ehu385

Van Veldhuisen DJ, Ponikowski P, van der Meer P, Metra M, Böhm M, Doletsky A, et al. Effect of ferric carboxymaltose on exercise capacity in patients with chronic heart failure and iron deficiency. *Circulation*. (2017) 136:1374–83. doi: 10.1161/CIRCULATIONAHA.117.027497

Ponikowski P, Kirwan B, Anker SD, Mcdonagh T, Dorobantu M, Drozdz J, et al. Ferric carboxymaltose for iron deficiency at discharge after acute heart failure: a multicentre, double-blind, randomised, controlled trial. *Lancet.* (2020) 396:1895–904. doi: 10.1016/S0140-6736(20)32339-4

Filippatos G, Farmakis D, Colet JC, Dickstein K, Lüscher TF, Willenheimer R, et al. Intravenous ferric carboxymaltose in iron-deficient chronic heart failure patients with and without anaemia: a subanalysis of the FAIR-HF trial. *Eur J Hear Fail.* (2013) 15:1267–76. doi: 10.1093/eurjhf/hft099

Toblli JE, Di Gennaro F, Rivas C. Changes in echocardiographic parameters in iron deficiency patients with heart failure and chronic kidney disease treated with intravenous iron. *Hear Lung Circ.* (2015) 24:686–95. doi: 10.1016/j.hlc.2014.12.161

Núñez J, Monmeneu JV, Mollar A, Núñez E, Bodí V, Miñana G, et al. Left ventricular ejection fraction recovery in patients with heart failure treated with intravenous iron: a pilot study. *ESC Hear Fail.* (2016) 3:293–8. doi: 10.1002/ehf2.12101

Klip IT, Jankowska EA, Enjuanes C, Voors AA, Banasiak W, Bruguera J, et al. The additive burden of iron deficiency in the cardiorenal-anaemia axis: scope of a problem and its consequences. *Eur J Hear Fail.* (2014) 16:655–62. doi: 10.1002/ejhf.84

Ahmed A, Campbell R. Epidemiology of chronic kidney disease in heart failure. *Hear Fail Clin.* (2008) 4:387–99. doi: 10.1016/j.hfc.2008.03.008

Cases Amenós A, Ojeda López R, Portolés Pérez J. Heart failure in patients with kidney disease and iron deficiency: the role of iron therapy. *Nefrologia.* (2017) 37:587–91. doi: 10.1016/j.nefroe.2017.11.009

Cases A, Puchades MJ, de Sequera P, Quiroga B, Martin-Rodriguez L, Gorriz JL, et al. Iron replacement therapy in the management of anaemia in non- dialysis chronic renal failure patients: perspective of the Spanish Nephrology Society Anaemia Group. *Nefrologia.* (2021). doi: 10.1016/j.nefro.2020.11.003. [Epub ahead of print].

Neiser S, Rentsch D, Dippon U, Kappler A, Weidler PG, Göttlicher J, et al. Physico-chemical properties of the new generation IV iron preparations ferumoxytol, iron isomaltoside 1000 and ferric carboxymaltose. *Biometals.* (2015) 28:615–35. doi: 10.1007/s10534-015-9845-9

Jahn MR, Andreasen HB, Fütterer S, Nawroth T, Schünemann V, Kolb U, et al. A comparative study of the physicochemical properties of iron isomaltoside 1000 (Monofer), a new intravenous iron preparation and its clinical implications. *Eur J Pharm Biopharm.* (2011) 78:480–91. doi: 10.1016/j.ejpb.2011.03.016

Macdougall IC, White C, Anker SD, Bhandari S, Farrington K, Kalra PA, et al. Intravenous iron in patients undergoing maintenance hemodialysis. *N Engl J Med.* (2019) 380:447–58. doi: 10.1056/NEJMoa1810742

Rostoker G, Loridon C, Griuncelli M, Rabaté C, Lepeytre F, Ureña-Torres P, et al. Liver iron load influences hepatic fat fraction in end-stage renal disease patients on dialysis: a proof of concept study. *EBioMedicine.* (2019) 39:461–71. doi: 10.1016/j.ebiom.2018.11.020

Rostoker G, Griuncelli M, Loridon C, Couprie R, Benmaadi A, Bounhiol C, et al. Hemodialysis associated hemosiderosis in the era of erythropoiesis-stimulating agents: a MRI study. *Am J Med.* (2012) 125:991–9.e1. doi: 10.1016/j.amjmed.2012.01.015

Tolouian R, Mulla ZD, Diaz J, Aguila J, Ramos-Duran L. Liver and cardiac iron deposition in patients on maintenance hemodialysis by magnetic resonance imaging T2. *Iran J Kidney Dis.* (2016) 10:68–74.

Holman R, Olynyk JK, Kulkarni H, Ferrari P. Characterisation of hepatic and cardiac iron deposition during standard treatment of anaemia in haemodialysis. *Nephrol (Carlton).* (2017) 22:114–7. doi: 10.1111/nep.12735

Hougen I, Collister D, Bourrier M, Ferguson T, Hochheim L, Komenda P, et al. Safety of intravenous iron in dialysis a systematic review and meta-analysis. *Clin J Am Soc Nephrol.* (2018) 13:457–67. doi: 10.2215/CJN.05390517

Macdougall IC, Bhandari S, White C, Anker SD, Farrington K, Kalra PA, et al. Intravenous iron dosing and infection risk in patients on hemodialysis: a prespecified secondary analysis of the PIVOTAL trial. *JASN.* (2020) 31:1118– 27. doi: 10.1681/ASN.2019090972

Watts ER, Walmsley SR. Inflammation and hypoxia: HIF and PHD isoform selectivity. *Trends Mol Med.* (2019) 25:33–46. doi: 10.1016/j.molmed.2018.10.006

Chen N, Hao C, Peng X, Lin H, Yin A, Hao L, et al. Roxadustat for anemia in patients with kidney disease not receiving dialysis. *N Engl J Med.* (2019) 381:1001–10. doi: 10.1056/NEJMoa1813599

Chen N, Hao C, Liu BC, Lin H, Wang C, Xing C, et al. Roxadustat treatment for anemia in patients undergoing long-term dialysis. *N Engl J Med.* (2019) 381:1011–22. doi: 10.1056/NEJMoa1901713

Akizawa T, Iwasaki M, Yamaguchi Y, Majikawa Y, Reusch M. Phase 3, randomized, double-blind, active-comparator (Darbepoetin Alfa) study

of oral roxadustat in CKD patients with anemia on hemodialysis in Japan. *J Am Soc Nephrol.* (2020) 31:1628–39. doi: 10.1681/ASN.2019 060623

Akizawa T, Otsuka T, Reusch M, Ueno M. Intermittent oral dosing of roxadustat in peritoneal dialysis chronic kidney disease patients with anemia: a randomized, phase 3, multicenter, open-label study. *Ther Apher Dial.* (2020) 24:115–25. doi: 10.1111/1744-9987.12888

Fishbane S, Pollock CA, El-Shahawy MA, Escudero ET, Rastogi A, Van BP, et al. ROCKIES: an international, phase 3, randomized, open-label, active-controlled study of roxadustat for anemia in dialysis-dependent CKD patients. Abstract TH-OR022. *JASN.* (2019) 30:6.

Esposito C, Csiky B, Tataradze A, Reusch M, Han C, Sulowicz W. Two phase 3, multicenter, randomized studies of intermittent oral roxadustat in anemic CKD patients on (PYRENEES) and not on (ALPS) dialysis. Abstract SA-PO225. *J Am Soc Nephrol.* (2019) 30:822.

Charytan C, Manllo-Karim R, Martin ER, Steer D, Bernardo M, Dua SL, et al. SIERRAS: a phase 3, open-label, randomized, active-controlled study of the efficacy and safety of roxadustat in the maintenance treatment of anemia in subjects with ESRD on stable dialysis. Abstract SA-PO227 P. *JASN.* (2019) 30:822.

Provenzano R, Evgeny S, Liubov E, Korneyeva S, Kathresal AA, Poole L, et al. HIMALAYAS: a phase 3, randomized, open-label, active-controlled study of the efficacy and safety of roxadustat in the treatment of anemia in incident- dialysis patients. Abstract TH-OR021 Washington, DC: American Society of Nephrology. *JASN.* (2019) 30:5.

Provenzano R, Fishbane S, Wei LJ, Szczech L, Leong R, Saikali KG, et al. *Pooled Efficacy and Cardiovascular (CV) Analyses of Roxadustat in the Treatment of Anemia in CKD Patients on and Not on Dialysis.* Abstract FR-OR13. Washington, DC: American Society of Nephrology (2019).

Fishbane S, El-Shahawy MA, Pecoits-Filho R, Van BP, Houser MT, Frison L, et al. OLYMPUS: a phase 3, randomized, double-blind, placebo- controlled, international study of roxadustat efficacy in patients with non- dialysis-dependent (NDD) CKD and anemia. Abstract TH-OR023 O. *JASN.* (2019) 30:6.

Coyne DW, Roger SD, Shin SK, KimSG, Cadena AA, Moustafa MA, et al. ANDES: a phase 3, randomized, double-blind, placebo controlled study of the efficacy and safety of roxadustat for the treatment of anemia in CKD patients not on dialysis. Abatract SA-PO228. *JASN.* (2019) 30:822.

Barratt J, Andric′ B, Tataradze A, Schömig M, Reusch M, Udaya Valluri CM. Roxadustat for the treatment of anaemia in chronic kidney disease patients not on dialysis: a phase 3, randomised, open-label, active- controlled study. *Nephrol Dial Transplant.* (2020) 35:gfaa140.MO001. doi: 10.1093/ndt/gfaa140.MO001

Barratt J, Andric B, Tataradze A, Schömig M, Reusch M, Valluri U, et al. Roxadustat for the Treatment of Anemia in CKD Patients Not on Dialysis (NDD): A Phase 3, Randomized, Open-Label, Active-Controlled Study. [Abstract TH-OR02]. *J Am Soc Nephrol.* (2020) 31:1.

Nangaku M, Kondo K, Kokado Y, Ueta K, Kaneko G, Shiosaka M, et al. Randomized, open-label, active-controlled (darbepoetin alfa), phase 3 study of vadadustat for treating anemia in non-dialysis-dependent CKD patients in Japan. Abstract SA-PO229 P. *JASN.* (2019) 30:823.

Nangaku M, Kondo K, Ueta K, Kokado Y, Kaneko G, Matsuda H, et al. Randomized, double-blinded, active-controlled (Darbepoetin Alfa), phase 3 study of vadadustat in CKD patients with anemia on hemodialysis in Japan. Abstract TH-OR024 O. *JASN.* (2019) 30:6.

Akizawa T, Macdougall IC, Berns JS, Bernhardt T, Staedtler G, Taguchi M, et al. Long-term efficacy and safety of molidustat for anemia in chronic kidney disease: DIALOGUE extension studies. *Am J Nephrol.* (2019) 49:271–80. doi: 10.1159/000499111

Natale P, Palmer SC, Tong A, Ruospo M, Hodson EM, Cooper TE, et al. Hypoxia-inducible factor stabilisers for the anaemia of chronic kidney disease. *Cochrane Database Syst Rev.* (2020) CD013751. doi: 10.1002/14651858.CD013751

Provenzano R, Besarab A, Wright S, Dua S, Zeig S, Nguyen P, et al. Roxadustat (FG-4592) versus epoetin alfa for anemia in patients receiving maintenance hemodialysis: a phase 2, randomized, 6- to 19-week, open-label, active-comparator, dose-ranging, safety and exploratory efficacy study. *Am J Kidney Dis.* (2016) 67:912–24. doi: 10.1053/j.ajkd.2015.12.020

Richardson S, Hirsch JS, Narasimhan M, Crawford JM, McGinn T, Davidson KW, et al. Presenting characteristics, comorbidities, and outcomes among 5700 patients hospitalized with COVID-19 in the New York City Area. *JAMA.* (2020) 323.2052–9. doi: 10.1001/jama.2020.6775

Fishbane S, Hirsch JS. Erythropoiesis-stimulating agent treatment in patients with COVID-19. *Am J Kidney Dis.* (2020) 6:303–5. doi:

10.1053/j.ajkd.2020.05.002

Serebrovska ZO, Chong EY, Serebrovska TV, Tumanovska LV, Lei X. Hypoxia, HIF-1α, and COVID-19: from pathogenic factors to potential therapeutic targets. *Acta Pharmacol Sin.* (2020) 41:1539–46. doi: 10.1038/s41401-020-00554-8

Khodour Y, Kaguni LS, Stiban J. Iron-sulfur clusters in nucleic acid metabolism: varying roles of ancient cofactors. *Enzymes.* (2019) 45:225256. doi: 10.1016/bs.enz.2019. 08.003

Liu W, Zhang S, Nekhai S, Liu S. Depriving iron supply to the virus represents a promising adjuvant therapeutic against viral survival. *Curr Clin Microbiol Reports.* (2020) 143:110173. doi: 10.1007/s40588-020-00140-w

20

Iron Deficiency Anemia in Inflammatory Bowel Disease: What do we Know?

Tamás Resál, Klaudia Farkas and Tamás Molnár*

Gastroenterology Unit, Department of Medicine, University of Szeged, Szeged, Hungary

*Correspondence:
Tamás Molnár
molnaribd@hotmail.com

One of the most common extraintestinal manifestations of inflammatory bowel disease is iron deficiency anemia. It is often an untreated condition that significantly impairs patients' quality of life and elevates mortality and morbidity. Although it is often accompanied by mild symptoms (e.g., fatigue, lethargy), it can provoke severe health conditions, such as dyspnea, palpitation, angina, and mental disorders, and increases hospitalization and mortality rate as well. As anemia develops through several pathomechanisms, such as occult bleeding, chronic inflammation, and medicines (e.g., methotrexate), treating anemia effectively requires to manage the underlying pathological changes as well. Based on international publications and data, it is a frequent condition and more frequent in pediatrics. According to Goodhand et al., iron deficiency is present in more than 60% of children, whereas only 14% of them received oral iron therapy. Compared to adult patients, 22% have iron deficiency, and 48% of them received oral and 41% intravenous iron therapy. Miller et al. also highlighted that among young patients iron deficiency anemia is a frequent condition, as almost 50% of the patients were anemic in their cohort. European Crohn's and Colitis Organisation's statements are clear regarding the diagnosis of iron deficiency anemia, and the iron supplementation as well. Third-generation parenteral iron supplementations seem to be safer and more effective than oral iron pills. Oral iron in many cases cannot replace the iron homeostasis as well; furthermore, it can provoke dysbiosis, which can potentially lead to relapse. As a result, we claim that both oral and parenteral should be used more frequently; furthermore, intravenous iron could replace oral medicines as well in certain cases. Despite the fact that iron deficiency anemia is examined by many aspects, further questions can be raised. Can it imply underlying pathological lesions? Are both oral and intravenous iron therapy safe and effective? When and how are they used? We demand that more studies should be conducted regarding these issues.

Keywords: inflammatory bowel disease, iron deficiency anemia, iron supplementation, anemia, parenteral iron supplementation, oral iron supplementation

INTRODUCTION

Inflammatory bowel disease [IBD: Crohn disease (CD), ulcerative colitis (UC)] is a chronic, immune-mediated disease that impairs patients' quality of life (QoL), and it is associated with many comorbidities. One of the most common concomitant diseases is iron deficiency anemia (IDA), which also worsens the condition of patients and mostly remains untreated (1). It can occur at any stage of IBD and can be the first symptom of the disease as well. It is often associated with frequent chronic activity, but can also be encountered without clinical signs of activity. In such cases, the IDA diagnosis raises the possibility of asymptomatic, subclinically occurring inflammation and mucosal damage in the presence of long-term chronic activity that damages the condition and function of the intestine (1).

Frequency of IDA

At the time of the diagnosis, the prevalence of IDA in patients younger than 18 years is approximately 41–75% (2), whereas in adult patients it is also high; however, it varies with wide ranges, from 6 to 74% (3). According to a Swedish study, conducted by Sjöberg et al., the prevalence of IDA is almost twice as high in children (55%) as in adult patients (27%) at the time of the diagnosis. Furthermore, they found significant difference as well in the prevalence of IDA among patients with CD, compared to UC, following the first year after the diagnosis. They also found that anemia in CD was more common in colonic engagement, and in UC, extensive inflammation increased the prevalence (4). Eriksson et al. conducted a study to assess the incidence, prevalence, and clinical outcome of anemia in IBD, comparing CD and UC, and they found as well that CD is associated with higher prevalence and a worse outcome regarding the resolution of anemia (5).

Symptoms and Clinical Role

Generally speaking, it should be highlighted that patients with IDA claim to have decreased QoL. In a Spanish study, conducted by García-López et al., it was found that treating IDA improves the QoL, regardless of the symptoms of IBD (6).

As iron plays key role in the function of many cells (e.g., erythrocyte, macrophage), cellular proteins, and enzymes (e.g., cytochromes, myoglobin), the symptoms of IDA vary over a wide range (7, 8). Key symptoms, such as shortness of breath, palpitation, tachycardia, and even angina, occur because of the hypoxemia. As a result of the decreased blood oxygen level, there is a compensatory decrease in intestinal blood flow, which may cause motility disorder, malabsorption, nausea, weight loss, and abdominal pain. Central hypoxia may lead to headache, vertigo, and lethargy, as well as cognitive impairment, and several studies proved that normalizing anemia improves cognitive functions (9–12) (Table 1).

Michailidou et al. compared the risk of postoperative complications between anemic and nonanemic patients. In their study consisting of more than 15,000 people, it was found that patients with anemia were more likely to have postoperative complications (e.g., morbidity and mortality rate; undesirable cardiovascular, renal, pulmonary, and wound healing complications; postoperative sepsis and shock) (13).

Etiology of Anemia in IBD

The most common causes of anemia in IBD are IDA, chronic inflammation, and anemia of mixed origins, whereas B_{12} deficiency and folic acid deficiency (mostly due to medications) belong to the less common causes. In addition, it may also occur

TABLE 1 | Symptoms of iron deficiency anemia.

Nervous system	Headache, lethargy, vertigo, syncope, cognitive impairment, depression
Cardiovascular system	Palpitation, tachycardia, hypotension, angina, ischemic electrocardiographic signs, cardiac failure
Respiratory system	Shortness of breath
Skin	Paleness, alopecia, cold intolerance
Gastrointestinal symptoms	Anorexia, nausea, motility disturbances, angular stomatitis, glossitis (Plummer–Vinson syndrome)
Immune system	Disorder of the innate and adaptive immune system
Urogenital symptoms	Decreased libido, menstrual disorders
General symptoms	Decreased quality of life, lower physical activity

TABLE 2 | Ethiology of anemia in IBD.

Most common causea of anemia in IBD	- Iron deficiency anemia - Anemia of chronic inflammation - Anemia of mixed origins
Less common causes	- Folic acid/B_{12} deficiency
Rare causes	- Hemolysis - Myelodysplastic syndrome - Aplasia - Protein starvation - Liver disease

because of hemolysis, myelodysplastic syndrome/medication-induced aplasia, protein starvation, and liver disease (e.g., primary sclerosing cholangitis) (14, 15) (Table 2).

Pathophysiology of IDA

In IBD, the IDA can develop through several pathomechanisms (16):

I. Intestinal mucosal damage resulting in occult, chronic blood loss

II. Chronic inflammation

a) Reduced iron-absorbing capacity of enterocytes
b) Iron is trapped in macrophages
c) Inhibition of the erythropoietin and the differentiation/proliferation of the erythroid progenitor cells

Cytokines and acute-phase proteins cause changes in iron homeostasis during inflammation. Hepcidin plays the central role in the regulatory process. It is an antimicrobial protein, produced by the liver in case of iron surplus and in inflammation, triggered by interleukin 6 and lipopolysaccharides. Hepcidin binds to the iron-transporting ferroportin receptor and degrades it, which results in decreased iron transport from the enterocytes to the circulation, and causes retention of the iron in the monocytes/macrophages; these processes are enhanced by anti–tumor necrosis factor α. In addition, hepcidin reduces the absorption of the Fe^{2+} from the duodenum, through the inhibition of the DMT1 (divalent metal transporter 1) (17).

Transferrin is the main iron carrier protein, and during inflammation, acute-phase proteins (e.g., α-1 antitrypsin) bind

TABLE 3 | Pathomechanisms of different type of anemias in IBD.

Iron deficiency anemia	Chronic blood loss Reduced absorption of Fe^{2+} (bowel resection, inflammation) Anorexia
Anemia of chronic disease	Iron retention in monocytes/macrophages Reduced absorption of Fe^{2+} (inflammation) Reduced biological half-life of erythrocytes (e.g., erythrophagocytosis) Inhibition of erythropoiesis
Other origin	Vitamin deficiency (B12, folic acid) Drug-induced bone marrow suppression (methotrexate, azathioprine)

TABLE 4 | World Health Organization's anemia criteria.

	Hemoglobin (g/dL)	Hematocrit(%)
Children between 6 months and 5 years	11	33
Children between 5 and 11 years	11.5	34
Children between 12 and 13 years	12	36
Pregnant women	11	36
Women	12	33
Men	13	39

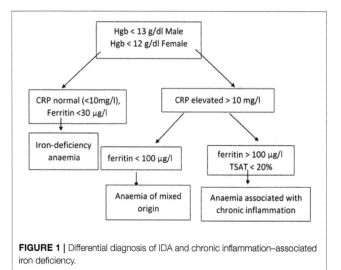

FIGURE 1 | Differential diagnosis of IDA and chronic inflammation–associated iron deficiency.

to transferrin receptors and inhibit the iron uptake in the erythroid progenitors cells, resulting in reduced differentiation and proliferation (18).

Diagnosis/Differential Diagnosis in Anemia

Anemia and iron homeostasis should be monitored regularly in IBD (depending on activity and the type of the treatment):

- At the time of diagnosis
- During activity—every 3 months
- In remission—every 6 to 12 months

Vitamin B_{12} and folic acid should be monitored every year, in case of presence of risk factors (e.g., resection, pouch, extensive ileal disease) every 3–6 months.

The diagnosis of anemia is assessed by the World Health Organization (WHO) diagnostic criteria, depending on the gender and age of the patients (**Table 3**).

Differential Diagnosis in Anemia

According to the European Crohn's and Colitis Organization (ECCO) recommendations, the following parameters should be monitored if hemoglobin is below normal (**Table 4**): erythrocyte count, serum ferritin, C-reactive protein (CRP) concentration, transferrin saturation, reticulocyte count, erythrocyte width distribution, and mean corpuscular volume. Ferritin is an acute-phase protein produced by the liver, and it is responsible for binding and storing iron in the liver, spleen, and reticuloendothelial system. It is reduced in case of iron deficiency and elevated in inflammation. Hence, in determining the cause of anemia in IBD, it is important to assess disease activity based on disease scoring systems (Crohn's Disease Activity Index and Mayo score) and serum CRP and fecal calprotectin levels. In case of inflammation, transferrin saturation helps in differential diagnosis. Transferrin saturation (accepted normal range = 20–45%) is lower in inflammation, liver disease, malignancy, nephrotic syndrome, and anorexia, whereas it is elevated in iron deficiency and pregnancy (19).

IDA (19):

a) Anemia based on WHO criteria (low hemoglobin and hematocrit). Clinically and endoscopically, no inflammation

can be found, CRP level is normal, and serum ferritin is <30 µg/L.

b) Anemia based on WHO criteria. Clinically and/or endoscopically, inflammation can be found, CRP is elevated, and ferritin is <100 µg/L.

Anemia associated with chronic inflammation:

- Anemia based on WHO criteria. Clinically and/or endoscopically, inflammation can be found, CRP is elevated, ferritin is >100 µg/L, and transferrin saturation is <20%.

Anemia of mixed origin:

- Anemia based on WHO criteria. Clinically and/or endoscopically, inflammation can be found, CRP is elevated, and ferritin is between 30 and 100 µg/L (**Figure 1**).

Iron Supplementation

Goodhand et al. pointed out how undertreated the IDA is in IBD. In children (88%) and adolescents (83%), the incidence of IDA is much higher compared to that in adults (55%), and only a small proportion of patients received oral (children 13%, adolescents 30%, adults 48%) or parenteral iron supplementation (children 0%, adolescents 30%, adults 41%) (20).

In addition to improving the QoL, the goal of iron supplementation is to normalize hemoglobin, serum ferritin, and transferrin saturation and to refill iron stores (ferritin >100 g/L).

TABLE 5 | Administration of parenteral iron replacement.

Hemoglobin (g/dL)	Body weight <70 kg	Body weight ≥70 kg
10–12 (Female) 10–13 (Male)	1,000 mg	1,500 mg
7–10	1,500 mg	2,000 mg

Based on the recommendation of the ECCO (19):

Iron supplementation is recommended to all patients with anemia associated with iron disorder. If iron deficiency exists without anemia, iron supplementation requires consideration of the patient's individual clinical status, as there is no evidence in IBD regarding the efficacy of the treatment (19).

Oral iron supplementation is recommended to every patient with IDA with hemoglobin >10 g/dL in case of remission (no clinical/endoscopic activity, normal CRP level). The recommended oral iron intake is 100 mg/day for adults (higher doses are not recommended), and 2–3 mg/kg body weight per day in children. An acceptable therapeutic response is an increase of 2 g/dL in hemoglobin over 4 weeks. If there is intolerance, adverse effects or unsatisfactory therapeutic response is present, intravenous iron therapy is recommended (19).

Parenteral iron supplementation is recommended as a first choice in IDA in case of active IBD (elevated CRP levels and/or clinically active IBD), or hemoglobin level <10 g/dL, or previous intolerance to iron supplementation is present. If the elevation is <2 g/dL in hemoglobin level after 4 weeks' therapy, it is recommended to complete the treatment with Erythropoietin (EPO) stimulant. The required iron intake is estimated based on the body weight and the hemoglobin, as it is more effective in patients with IBD suffering from iron deficiency than the traditional Ganzoni formula (19) (**Table 5**).

Following the resolution of IDA with parenteral iron supplementation, ferritin level is recommended to be maintained above 400 μg/L to prevent short-term recurrence. After successful iron supplementation, patients should be monitored every 3 months in the first year following the correction and every 6–12 months thereafter (including hemoglobin, ferritin, transferrin saturation, CRP). Recurrent anemia may indicate underlying inflammation despite clinical and biochemical remission. The goal of preventive treatment is to keep ferritin and hemoglobin at normal levels. Reinitiation of intravenous iron supplementation is recommended in cases where the ferritin level falls below 100 μg/L or the hemoglobin level is <12–13 g/dL (female/male) (19).

When considering between oral and intravenous iron therapy, the advantages and disadvantages of the therapeutic approaches should be considered as well (21–23).

Oral Iron Supplementation

a.   Advantages
    Low cost
    Easier to implement in daily practice
    More accessible
    Effective in good intestinal absorption

b.   Disadvantages
    Compliance issues
    Certain foods reduce iron absorption (e.g., tea, coffee, dairy products, fiber)
    Certain medications reduce iron absorption

    i.   Multivitamin/dietary supplements (Ca^{2+}, Zn^{2+}, Cu^{2+})
    ii.   Antacids, H_2 blockers, PPI
    iii. Quinolones, tetracyclines

    Dysbiosis
    Dysbiosis induced relapse
    Side effects are more common compared to parenteral iron suppl.

    i.   Nausea
    ii.   Abdominal pain
    iii. Diarrhea
    iv.   Constipation

Parenteral Iron Supplementation

a.   Advantages
    More effective
    Fast correction of iron homeostasis
    Safe and well tolerated
    Fewer side effects
    Effective in inflammation
    The condition of the mucosa does not influence the efficacy

b.   Disadvantages
    Higher cost
    Harder to implement in daily practice
    Potential risk of iron overload
    Potential risk of anaphylaxis
    Possibility of hypophosphatemia

Parenteral Iron Supplementation

Intravenous iron supplementations consist of an Fe^{3+} core and a carbohydrate layer. The side effect profile, clearance, tolerable dose, and duration of the infusion are dependent on the magnitude of the core and quality of the carbohydrate layer. The different generations of intravenous iron supplementation comprised different carbohydrate layers (24).

- First generation—high-molecular-weight iron dextran
- Second generation—low-molecular-weight iron dextran

    a. Ferrous gluconate
    b. Iron sucrose

- Third generation

    a. Ferumoxytol
    b. Iron carboxymaltose
    c. Iron isomaltoside

The disadvantage of the HMWID is the higher probability of anaphylactic reaction/side effects; because of that, it is advised to use higher-generation products. The representatives of the second generation are more efficient with fewer side effects; however, they are not as stable complexes as the representatives of the third-generation preparations; consequently, they can only be administered in low doses, and so they require frequents visits. Third-generation preparations are much more efficient, with minimal side effect profile; furthermore, they can be implemented easier in the daily practice. These formulations are more stable, so they can be administered in higher doses, resulting in faster correction of the iron homeostasis, and the duration of the infusion is lesser (23, 25).

DISCUSSION

Anemia and IDA are common consequences of IBD in the developed world. Despite that we know how frequent it is, physicians tend to pay less attention to treat it, even though it affects the course of the disease and heavily reduces the patients' QoL. Although modern medicine knows many facts about the pathophysiology of anemia and IDA, and there are many efficient agents in the therapeutic arsenal, it still raises relevant questions. However, the ECCO's recommendations are clear; we would like to highlight that it should be still a matter of individual judgment, and in certain cases, parenteral iron supplementation should be the choice, instead of oral, because of the side effects. Based on international publications and data, as intravenous iron supplementation tends to be more efficient and safe in IBD, we claim that more studies should be conducted regarding third-generation agents and clarify the boundary line in the recommendations. However, to sum up, we demand that both oral and intravenous iron treatments should be more widespread.

AUTHOR CONTRIBUTIONS

All authors listed have made a substantial, direct and intellectual contribution to the work, and approved it for publication.

FUNDING

This work was supported by the research grants of the National Research, Development and Innovation Office (Grant ID: 125377, 129266, and 134863), by the National Excellence Programme (20391-3/2018/FEKUSTRAT to KF), by the New National Excellence Program of the Ministry of Human Capacities (UNKP-19-4-SZTE-44, UNKP-20-5-SZTE-161 to KF), Janos Bolyai Research Grant (BO/00598/19/5) and the Géza Hetényi Research Grant (to KF) by the Faculty of Medicine, University of Szeged.

ACKNOWLEDGMENTS

The authors would like to take this opportunity to thank Mariann Rutka MD. Ph.D. and Anita Bálint MD. Ph.D., for suggesting we publish this article in Frontiers in Medicine.

REFERENCES

Jimenez KM, Gasche C. Management of Iron Deficiency Anaemia in Inflammatory Bowel Disease. *Acta Haematol.* (2019) 142:30–6. doi: 10.1159/000496728

Wiskin AE, Fleming BJ, Wootton SA, Beattie RM. Anaemia and iron deficiency in children with inflammatory bowel disease. *J Crohns Colitis.* (2012) 6:687–91. doi: 10.1016/j.crohns.2011.12.001

Bergamaschi G, Di Sabatino A, Albertini R, Ardizzone S, Biancheri P, Bonetti E, et al. Prevalence and pathogenesis of anemia in inflammatory bowel disease. Influence of anti-tumor necrosis factor-alpha treatment. *Haematologica.* (2010). 95:199–205. doi: 10.3324/haematol.2009.009985

Sjöberg D, Holmström T, Larsson M, Nielsen AL, Holmquist L, Rönnblom Anemia in a population-based IBD cohort (ICURE): still high prevalence after 1 year, especially among pediatric patients. *Inflamm Bowel Dis.* (2014) 20:2266–70. doi: 10.1097/MIB.0000000000000191

Eriksson C, Henriksson I, Brus O, Zhulina Y, Nyhlin N, Tysk C et al. Incidence, prevalence and clinical outcome of anaemia in inflammatory bowel disease: a population-based cohort study. *Aliment Pharmacol Ther.* (2018) 48:638–45. doi: 10.1111/apt.14920

García-López S, Bocos JM, Gisbert JP, Bajador E, Chaparro M, Castaño C, et al. High-dose intravenous treatment in iron deficiency anaemia in inflammatory bowel disease: early efficacy and impact on quality of life. *Blood Transfus.* (2016) 14:199–205. doi: 10.2450/2016.0246-15

Kaitha S, Bashir M, Ali T. Iron deficiency anemia in inflammatory bowel disease. *World J Gastrointest Pathophysiol.* (2015) 6:62–72. doi: 10.4291/wjgp.v6.i3.62

Pickett JL, Theberge DC, Brown WS, Schweitzer SU, Nissenson AR. Normalizing hematocrit in dialysis patients improves brain function. *Am J Kidney Dis.* (1999) 33:1122–30. doi: 10.1016/S0272-6386(99)70150-2

Cappellini MD, Musallam KM, Taher AT. Iron deficiency anaemia revisited. *J Intern Med.* (2020) 287:153–70. doi: 10.1111/joim.13004

DeLoughery TG. Iron deficiency anemia. *Med Clin North Am.* (2017) 101:319–32. doi: 10.1016/j.mcna.2016.09.004

Çekiç C, Ipek S, Aslan F, Akpinar Z, Arabul M, Topal F et al. The effect of intravenous iron treatment on quality of life in inflammatory bowel disease patients with nonanemic iron deficiency. *Gastroenterol Res Pract.* (2015) 2015:582163. doi:10.1155/2015/582163

Ebner N, Jankowska EA, Ponikowski P, Lainscak M, Elsner S, Sliziuk V, et al. The impact of iron deficiency and anaemia on exercise capacity and outcomes in patients with chronic heart failure. Results from the Studies Investigating Co-morbidities Aggravating Heart Failure. *Int J Cardiol.* (2016) 205:6–12. doi: 10.1016/j.ijcard.2015.11.178

Michailidou M, Nfonsam VN. Preoperative anemia and outcomes in patients undergoing surgery for inflammatory bowel disease. *Am J Surg.* (2018). 215:78–81. doi: 10.1016/j.amjsurg.2017.02.016

Gomollón F, Gisbert JP. Anemia and inflammatory bowel diseases. *World J Gastroenterol.* (2009) 15:4659–65. doi: 10.3748/wjg.15.4659

Semrin G, Fishman DS, Bousvaros A, Zholudev A, Saunders AC, Correia CE, et al. Impaired intestinal iron absorption in Crohn's disease correlates with disease activity and markers of inflammation. *Inflamm Bowel Dis.* (2006) 12:1101–6. doi: 10.1097/01.mib.0000235097.86360.04

Weiss G, Gasche C. Pathogenesis and treatment of anemia in inflammatory bowel disease. *Haematologica.* (2010) 95:175–8. doi: 10.3324/haematol.2009.017046

Przybyszewska J, Zekanowska E. The role of hepcidin, ferroportin, HCP1, and DMT1 protein in iron absorption in the human digestive tract. *Prz Gastroenterol.* (2014) 9:208–13. doi: 10.5114/pg.2014. 45102

Weiss G, Goodnough LT. Anemia of chronic disease. *N Engl J Med.* (2005) 352:1011–23 doi: 10.1056/NEJMra041809

Dignass AU, Gasche C, Bettenworth D, Birgegård G, Danese S, Gisbert JP, et al. European consensus on the diagnosis and management of iron deficiency and anaemia in inflammatory bowel diseases. *J Crohns Colitis.* (2015) 9:211–222. doi:10.1093/ecco-jcc/jju009

Goodhand JR, Kamperidis N, Rao A, Laskaratos F, McDermott A, Wahed M, et al. Prevalence and management of anemia in children, adolescents, and adults with inflammatory bowel disease. *Inflamm Bowel Dis.* (2012) 18:513–19. doi: 10.1002/ibd.21740

Nielsen OH, Soendergaard C, Vikner ME, Weiss G. Rational management of iron-deficiency anaemia in inflammatory bowel disease. *Nutrients.* (2018) 10:82 doi: 10.3390/nu10010082

Bou-Fakhredin R, Halawi R, Roumi J, Taher A. Insights into the diagnosis and management of iron deficiency in inflammatory bowel disease. *Exp Rev*

Hematol. (2017) 10:801–8. doi: 10.1080/17474086.2017.13 55233

Lee T, Clavel T, Smirnov K, Schmidt A, Lagkouvardos I, Walker A, et al. Oral versus intravenous iron replacement therapy distinctly alters the gut microbiota and metabolome in patients with IBD. *Gut.* (2017) 66:863–71. doi: 10.1136/gutjnl-2015-309940

Biggar P, Hahn KM. Bedeutung der verschiedenen i.v.-Eisengenerationen für den medizinischen alltag [Importance of the different i.v. iron generations for everyday medical practice]. *MMW Fortschr Med.* (2013) 155(Suppl. 1):18–24. doi: 10.1007/s15006-013-0732-4

Silverstein SB, Rodgers GM. Parenteral iron therapy options. *Am J Hematol.* (2004) 76:74–8. doi: 10.1002/ajh.2 0056

Anemia Increases Oxygen Extraction Fraction in Deep Brain Structures but not in the Cerebral Cortex

Jian Shen[1], Xin Miao[2], Chau Vu[1], Botian Xu[1], Clio González-Zacarías[3], Aart J. Nederveen[4] and John C. Wood[1,5]*

[1]Biomedical Engineering, University of Southern California, Los Angeles, Los Angeles, CA, United States, [2]Siemens, Boston, MA, United States, [3]Neuroscience Graduate Program, University of Southern California, Los Angeles, Los Angeles, CA, United States, [4]Amsterdam UMC, Radiology and Nuclear Medicine, University of Amsterdam, Amsterdam, Netherlands, [5]Department of Pediatrics and Radiology, Children's Hospital Los Angeles, Los Angeles, CA, United States

*Correspondence:
John C. Wood
JWood@chla.usc.edu

Sickle cell disease (SCD) is caused by a single amino acid mutation in hemoglobin, causing chronic anemia and neurovascular complications. However, the effects of chronic anemia on oxygen extraction fraction (OEF), especially in deep brain structures, are less well understood. Conflicting OEF values have been reported in SCD patients, but have largely attributed to different measurement techniques, faulty calibration, and different locations of measurement. Thus, in this study, we investigated the reliability and agreement of two susceptibility-based methods, quantitative susceptibility mapping (QSM) and complex image summation around a spherical or a cylindrical object (CISSCO), for OEF measurements in internal cerebral vein (ICV), reflecting oxygen saturation in deep brain structures. Both methods revealed that SCD patients and non-sickle anemia patients (ACTL) have increased OEF in ICV (42.6% ± 5.6% and 30.5% ± 3.6% in SCD by CISSCO and QSM respectively, 37.0% ± 4.1% and 28.5% ± 2.3% in ACTL) compared with controls (33.0% ± 2.3% and 26.8% ± 1.8%). OEF in ICV varied reciprocally with hematocrit (r^2 = 0.92, 0.53) and oxygen content (r^2 = 0.86, 0.53) respectively. However, an opposite relationship was observed for OEF measurements in sagittal sinus (SS) with the widely used T_2-based oximetry, T_2-Relaxation-Under-Spin-Tagging (TRUST), in the same cohorts (31.2% ± 6.6% in SCD, 33.3% ± 5.9% in ACTL and 36.8% ± 5.6% in CTL). Importantly, we demonstrated that hemoglobin F and other fast moving hemoglobins decreased OEF by TRUST and explained group differences in sagittal sinus OEF between anemic and control subjects. These data demonstrate that anemia causes deep brain hypoxia in anemia subjects with concomitant preservation of cortical oxygenation, as well as the key interaction of the hemoglobin dissociation curve and cortical oxygen extraction.

Keywords: sickle cell anemia, oxygen extraction fraction, internal cerebral vein, susceptibility, QSM, CISSCO, trust

INTRODUCTION

Sickle Cell Disease (SCD) is a genetic disorder characterized by a single base pair mutation in the beta subunit of hemoglobin that causes the abnormal hemoglobin S (HbS) to polymerize after deoxygenation leading to chronic hemolytic anemia and neurovascular complications (Ohene-Frempong et al., 1998). SCD patients have an abnormally high and early risk for stroke (Hassell, 2010). The incidence of primary overt stroke has been significantly reduced by Transcranial

Ultrasound (TCD) screening and chronic transfusion therapy (Adams, 2005). However, silent cerebral infarction (SCI) is even more common and there is lack of established relationship between SCI presence and TCD measurements (Wang et al., 2000). Imaging of brain oxygenation could be a powerful tool to assess the risk of stroke and aid in its prevention. The oxygen extraction fraction (OEF) has been recognized as an accurate and specific marker for tissue viability and a predictor of misery perfusion in carotid artery disease (Tanaka et al., 2008; Muroi et al., 2011). However, compared with other markers such as cerebral blood flow (CBF), studies on the oxygenation estimation in SCD, especially in deep brain structures, are scarce and results have been conflicting (Jordan et al., 2016; Bush et al., 2017; Fields et al., 2018; Guilliams et al., 2018; Juttukonda et al., 2019). The gold standard for oxygen metabolism is Positron Emission Tomography (PET) imaging (Mintun et al., 1984; Diringer et al., 2007). However, PET is limited by its high cost, invasiveness, long scan time, poor availability, and high exposure to radiation. Therefore, noninvasive estimates of global and regional brain oxygenation are strongly needed.

Currently, T_2-Relaxation-Under-Spin-Tagging (TRUST) is a widely used MRI technique to quantitatively estimate global brain blood oxygenation via the measurement of pure blood T_2 (Lu and Ge, 2008; Lu et al., 2012). Unfortunately, TRUST can only provide global saturation for the whole brain without offering oxygenation information in deep brain structures. Furthermore, there exists uncertainty in the proper calibration between T_2 and oxygen saturation in SCD patients because red blood cell (RBC) morphology and permeability are deranged in these patients (Bush et al., 2021). Unlike T_2 oximetry, susceptibility-based oximetry (SBO) methods are based on the paramagnetic susceptibility of venous blood. These methods usually measure magnetic susceptibility shift of a vein and there is a linear relationship between magnetic susceptibility shift of blood and concentration of deoxyhemoglobin. Quantitative Susceptibility Mapping (QSM) is a widely used technique to derive a pixel-wise susceptibility map from its induced magnetic field based on the 3D dipole convolution model (Wang and Liu, 2015). Through multiple image processing steps, QSM allows quantification of susceptibility for tissue with arbitrary geometry and orientation, which can be used to estimate oxygen saturation in deep brain structures. An alternative susceptibility-based method called CISSCO (Complex Image Summation around a Spherical or a Cylindrical Object) was introduced to quantify the susceptibility of any narrow cylindrical object at any orientation using a typical multi-echo gradient echo sequence (Cheng et al., 2009; Hsieh et al., 2015a, 2015b). The CISSCO method is based on the complex MR signal whereas QSM calculation is based on the phase signal, and they can be both generated from a typical multi-echo gradient echo scan. Despite the increasing applications of QSM and CISSCO, neither has been used in patients with chronic anemia and *in vivo* validation of these two techniques remains lacking.

The primary purpose of this study was to compare oxygen utilization in deep cerebral structures compared to oxygen saturation from the cerebral cortex. To accomplish this, we performed compared QSM and CISSCO measurements of oxygen saturation in the internal cerebral vein (ICV) with oxygen values derived from TRUST in the sagittal sinus in healthy subjects (CTL), sickle cell anemia patients (SCD) and anemia patients with normal hemoglobin (ACTL). The secondary objective was to cross-validate QSM and CISSCO measurements in the ICV.

MATERIALS AND METHODS

Study Design

This study was approved by our Institutional Review Board (CCI#11-00083) at Children's Hospital Los Angeles, and all subjects provided written informed consent prior to participation. Data from 28 SCD patients, 18 ACTL patients and 27 healthy control subjects were acquired. Complete blood count, metabolic panel, and hemoglobin electrophoresis were measured at the same day of their MRI scan. Four of the SCD and seven of the ACTL patients were receiving chronic transfusion therapy; these patients were studied on the morning of their transfusion visit prior to transfusion. Genotypes for the SCD patients were SS 25, Sβ+ 1, and SC 3. ACTL patients consisted of thalassemia major 6, hemoglobin H constant spring 3, hemoglobin H disease 2, hereditary spherocytosis 3, Eβ thalassemia major 1, aplastic anemia 1, and autoimmune hemolytic anemia 1. Control subjects were age and ethnicity matched to the SCD population. Eight of these subjects had sickle trait, but prior work from our laboratory has demonstrated indistinguishable cerebral blood flow and brain oxygenation patterns between hemoglobin AA and AS subjects (Vu et al., 2021). The exclusion criteria for all subjects included: 1) pregnancy; 2) hypertension; 3) diabetes; 4) stroke or other known neurologic insult; 5) seizures; 6) known developmental delay or learning disability; and 7) hospitalization within the month prior to the study visit.

Images were acquired on a clinical 3 T Philips Achieva system (Philips Healthcare, Best, Netherlands) with a 32-channel RF coil and a digital receiver chain. The 3D gradient echo sequence had parameters: TR = 30 ms; α = 25°; 2 echoes: TE1 = 4.94 ms, ΔTE = 5.2 ms; FOV = 210 * 190 * 120 mm^3; spatial resolution: 0.6 * 0.6 * 1.3 mm^3; SENSE acceleration rate = 2 in the phase-encoding direction; BW = 289 Hz/pix and total acquisition time = 6 min 50 s. Flow-compensation was added in the readout direction only, which was the anterior-posterior (AP) direction.

T_2-Relaxation-under-Spin-Tagging (TRUST) images were acquired from the sagittal sinus as previously described (Lu and Ge, 2008; Miao et al., 2019). Sequence parameters were as follows: TR = 3,000 ms; four effective echoes (eTE) at 0, 40, 80, 160 ms; CPMG τ = 10 m; voxel size = 3.44 * 3.44 mm^2; FOV = 220 * 220 mm^2; matrix size = 64 * 64; inversion time (TI) = 1,022 ms and total scan time = 1 min 12 s.

QSM Processing

For each subject, phase images were fitted to generate a B_0 field map. Brain extraction and phase unwrapping was performed using FSL (v6.0) (Jenkinson et al., 2012). Background field was removed using projection onto dipole fields (PDF) (Liu et al.,

2011). Unreliable phase voxels were identified using the condition of spatiotemporal smoothness of the GRE phase data and removed from the brain mask for subsequent processing (Schweser et al., 2011). L1-regularized field-to-susceptibility inversion was performed to derive the susceptibility map and a weighting parameter $\lambda = 4 \times 10^{-4}$ was applied (Bilgic et al., 2012). Venous oxygen saturation (S_vO_2) was computed based on:

$$\chi = (1 - S_vO_2)\chi_{d-o}Hct + \chi_{o-w}Hct, \qquad (1)$$

where χ is the susceptibility measurement of the internal cerebral vein, χ_{d-o} is the susceptibility shift per unit hematocrit between fully oxygenated and fully deoxygenated erythrocytes, and χ_{o-w} is the susceptibility shift between oxygenated blood cells and water. Values of 0.27 ppm and -0.03 ppm were used for χ_{d-o} and χ_{o-w} (Spees et al., 2001; Langham et al., 2009).

The ROI mask of the internal cerebral vein was manually selected based on the susceptibility map that was threshold at 0.1 ppm to avoid partial-volume effect. The angle between ROI and AP axis was calculated manually from the 3D dataset based on the coordinates of the two end points of the cylinder. Only the segment that had an angle below 30° was included. The purpose was to exclude regions that were susceptible to flow artifact.

CISSCO Processing

A more detailed description of CISSCO method for susceptibility quantification of a cylindrical object has been presented in (Hsieh et al., 2015a). Here we summarized with the major points and equations. CISSCO integrates the complex MR signals in three annuli around the cylinder of interest. The complex sums were cast into equations containing three unknown parameters, the susceptibility and radius of the vessel, and the proton spin density. The overall MR complex signal S within a coaxial cylinder with radius R was:

$$S = \pi l \rho_0 \vartheta \int_{\vartheta/R^2}^{g'} \frac{dx}{x^2} J_0(x) + \pi l a^2 \rho_{0,c} e^{i\varphi_{in}}, \qquad (2)$$

where a is the vessel radius, the phase value inside the cylinder $\phi_{in} = -\gamma\Delta\chi/6(3cos^2\theta - 1)B_0T_E$, $\Delta\chi$ is the susceptibility difference between tissues inside and outside, l is the slice thickness of the image, ρ_0 and $\rho_{0,c}$ are the effective spin densities of the tissue outside and inside the object, ϑ is the effective magnetic moment, $g' = (0.5 \gamma B_0\Delta\chi T_E)*sin^2\theta$ is the extremum phase value on the surface of the cylinder, θ is the orientation of the cylinder, and J_0 is the zeroth order Bessel function.

Equation 2 can be applied to all three annuli, allowing us to solve for the three unknown variables; complex signal differences between any two annuli eliminate the second term, eliminating two variables. First, the magnitude and phase images in coronal view were cropped to 64*64 and a 16*16 Gaussian high pass filter was applied to remove background phase. Next, θ was estimated based on the coordinates of the two endpoints of the innermost annuli. The calculated θ was 82.3 ± 5.6°, revealing that the internal cerebral vein is nearly perpendicular to the direction of B_0.

Finally, after applying the equation to three coaxial cylinders, the effective magnetic moment, the effective spin densities, and the susceptibility difference can be solved sequentially.

The resulting $\Delta\chi$ was converted to oxygen saturation using **Eq. 1**, the same as for QSM.

TRUST Processing

Control–label difference images for each echo time were averaged and fit to a simple mono-exponential function. In control and ACTL patients, the decay time constant was corrected for T_1 using an estimated calculated from hematocrit, assuming deoxygenated blood (Lu et al., 2004). In non-transfused SCD patients, venous T_1 was estimated to be 1818 ms (Václavuu et al., 2016), and for transfused SCD patients T_1 was estimated using a simple mixture assumption based upon the fraction of circulating hemoglobin S. In control subjects, the resulting T_2-apparent was converted to oxygen saturation using a calibration derived from human blood (Bush et al., 2018; Li et al., 2020). In SCD patients, a consensus calibration model (Bush et al., 2021) was used to convert T_2-apparent to oxygen saturation. Separate equations were used for transfused and non-transfused subjects, taking care to correct T_2-apparent for imperfections in the 180° pulse (Bush et al., 2021).

Physiological Background

To gain physiological insight into predictors of oxygen saturation in the ICV compared with the sagittal sinus, oxygen extraction fraction (OEF) was calculated separately for the two venous locations (OEF$_{ICV}$, OEF$_{SS}$) as follows:

$$OEF = \frac{(S_aO_2 - SvO_2)}{S_aO_2}, \qquad (3)$$

where S_aO_2 is the arterial saturation measured by pulse oximetry. We compared OEF$_{ICV}$ and OEF$_{SS}$ to O_2 content using linear regression, with variable transformation when appropriate. O_2 content was derived as follows, neglecting the impact of dyshemoglobins (Wasserman and Whipp, 1975):

$$O_2 \ content = 1.34*Hb*S_aO_2. \qquad (4)$$

To provide some physiological background, the equation between O_2 content, cerebral blood flow (CBF) and cerebral metabolic rate of oxygen (CMRO$_2$) is also shown here:

$$CMRO_2 = OEF*CBF*O_2 \ content. \qquad (5)$$

Alternatively, **Eq. 5** can be recast as follows:

$$OEF = \frac{CMRO_2}{(CBF*O_2 \ content)}. \qquad (6)$$

Thus, OEF is expected to vary reciprocally with the product of CBF and O_2 content, which is also referred to as cerebral oxygen delivery.

Statistical Analysis

Statistical analysis was performed in JMP (SAS, Cary, NC). Demographic and laboratory variables were compared using Analysis of Variance (ANOVA) with Dunnett's post hoc

TABLE 1 | Subject demographics. Group averages and standard deviations are given.

	Healthy controls	ACTL patients	SCD patients
N	24	17	25
Age	27.3 ± 8.2	21.6 ± 5.6	24.1 ± 6.8
Sex	11F, 13M	10F, 7M	11F, 14M
Hematocrit (%)	40.8 ± 4.1	35.2 ± 5.9*	26.8 ± 4.3*δ
Hemoglobin (g/dl)	13.6 ± 1.4	11.5 ± 2.8*	9.5 ± 1.7*δ
HbS (%)	12.4 ± 17.5	2.5 ± 10.2	67.8 ± 25.2*δ
HbF (%)	0	4.5 ± 6.0*	12.1 ± 10.5*δ
Systolic blood pressure (mmHg)	114.7 ± 9.0	115.2 ± 11.5	114.0 ± 10.0
Diastolic blood pressure (mmHg)	69.0 ± 7.5	62.1 ± 8.1*	61 ± 6.3*
Oxygen Saturation (%)	99.1 ± 1.2	99.2 ± 1.0	98.6 ± 1.4
O$_2$ content (ml O$_2$/ml blood)	18.5 ± 1.9	15.6 ± 3.8*	12.9 ± 2.4*δ
Lactose dehydrogenase (LDH)	548.2 ± 86.4	635.2 ± 250.0	863.0 ± 432.2*δ
MCV (cubic um/red cell)	85.5 ± 7.4	79.5 ± 9.7	96.1 ± 16.6*δ
MCH (pg/cell)	28.8 ± 2.6	25.8 ± 5.3*	34.0 ± 6.7*δ
MCHC (g Hgb/dl)	33.4 ± 1.3	31.7 ± 4.1	35.2 ± 1.6*δ
Reticulocytes (%)	1.5 ± 0.7	3.6 ± 3.4*	8.4 ± 4.9*δ
Transfused	0/24	7/17*	4/25

*Denotes p < 0.05 with respect to control, δ denotes p < 0.05 with respect to ACTL.

correction. OEF values derived by QSM and CISSCO (OEF-QSM, OEF-CISSCO) were compared across study groups using ANOVA with Dunnett's post-hoc correction. Inter-modality comparison was performed using Bland-Altman analysis, with bias assessed using a two-sided, one-sample t-Test. Shapiro-Wilks tests of normality were applied to each variable, with transformation, outlier exclusion, or nonparametric testing used when appropriate.

We examined predictors of OEF$_{ICV}$ and OEF$_{SS}$ using linear regression, with variable transformation when appropriate. Predictors included hemoglobin, hematocrit, oxygen saturation, oxygen content, hemoglobin S%, left shifted hemoglobin %, LDH, reticulocyte count, cell free hemoglobin, WBC, MCV, MCH, MCHC, WBC, platelets, and mean platelet volume. All variables with p values greater than 0.05 were retained for stepwise regression. Models were built iteratively (two variable models, followed by three variable models, etc), retaining variables yielding the highest combined r^2. No nonlinear variable interactions were considered.

Given the collinearity between the three strongest predictors (hemoglobin, hematocrit, and oxygen content), we also explored models where one of these three variables was "locked" in the model to inform us about potentially important covariates.

RESULTS

Demographics

Among the 73 volunteers participated in the experiment, data from seven subjects were discarded due to motion or low SNR. There were 25 SCD patients, 17 ACTL patients and 24 healthy controls in the final data processing, and the demographics were shown in **Table 1**. Controls were slightly older than either patient group, but the groups were well balanced for sex. Anemia, corresponding erythropoietic and hemolytic markers, hemoglobin F and total left shifted levels were increased in ACTL and SCD, but more severe in SCD. Oxygen saturation was not different across groups, but diastolic blood

TABLE 2 | Differences between hemoglobin F, hemoglobin S and OEF by three methods with or without hydroxyurea (HU) for non-transfused SCD patients.

	With HU	Without HU	p-value
Hb	9.5 ± 1.4	12.1 ± 2.7	**< 0.001**
Hb F (%)	18.4 ± 8.8	1.4 ± 3.3	**< 0.001**
Hb S (%)	78.2 ± 8.3	18.2 ± 27.9	**< 0.001**
OEF-TRUST (%)	28.2 ± 6.1	35.3 ± 5.7	**< 0.001**
OEF-CISSCO (%)	42.9 ± 5.5	36.2 ± 5.2	**< 0.001**
OEF-QSM (%)	30.1 ± 4.4	28.0 ± 2.7	0.1034

Bold text depicts a p-value < 0.05.

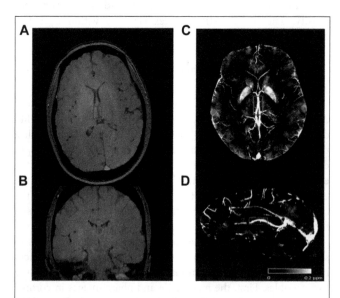

FIGURE 1 | Representative image and region of the internal cerebral vein (ICV, highlight by red rectangle). **(A)** Magnitude in axial view. **(B)** Magnitude in coronal view. **(C)** Axial view, and **(D)** Sagittal view of ROI in the max intensity projection of a representative susceptibility map.

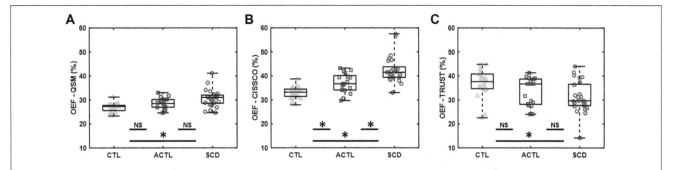

FIGURE 2 | Group differences for OEF measurements by CISSCO, QSM and TRUST. **(A)** Boxplot for OEF-QSM in internal cerebral vein for SCD, ACTL and CTL. **(B)** Boxplot for OEF-CISSCO in internal cerebral vein for SCD, ACTL and CTL. **(C)** Boxplot for OEF-TRUST in sagittal sinus for SCD, ACTL and CTL. (* denoted statistically significant $p < 0.05$; NS denoted no significant difference).

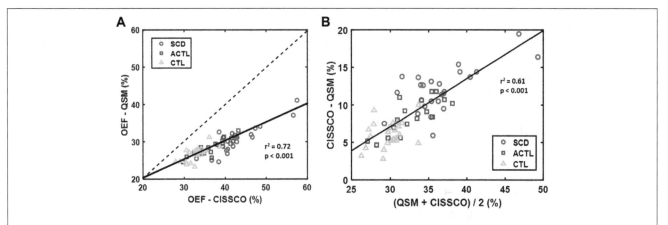

FIGURE 3 | **(A)** Scatter plot of OEF-CISSCO and OEF-QSM with linear correlation line (solid) and identity line (dashed) ($r^2 = 0.72$, $p < 0.001$). **(B)** Bland-Altman plot for OEF-CISSCO and OEF-QSM. The linear correlation line (solid) is shown ($r^2 = 0.61$, $p < 0.001$).

pressure was 10% lower in both anemic groups. Forty percent of the ACTL patients were transfused, compared with 16% of SCD, and none of the control subjects.

Table 2 summarizes the Hb, HbS%, HbF%, and OEF values in non-transfused SCD patients with and without hydroxyurea. Patients taking hydroxyurea had higher F%, higher OEF CISSCO, lower S%, and lower sagittal sinus OEF measurements than patients not on hydroxyurea. None of the controls or ACTL patients were taking hydroxyurea.

Figure 1A–C show representative magnitude and phase images in both axial and coronal views. The processed susceptibility map by QSM is shown in Figure 1D. ICV generally lies parallel to the axial plane and typically has a quantifiable length around 11 mm by QSM. By CISSCO, the calculated vessel radius, a, was 1.1 ± 0.5 mm and was independent of disease state and hemoglobin level.

Comparison of OEF Measurements in ICV (by QSM and CISSCO) and SS (by TRUST) for Different Groups

Figure 2A,B summarize the OEF measurements in the internal cerebral vein using QSM (OEF-QSM) and CISSCO (OEF-CISSCO), respectively. Mean OEF-QSM measurements were 30.1% in SCD, 28.5% in ACTL, and 26.6% in CTL ($p < 0.01$). On Dunnett's post hoc

correction, SCD was different from CTL ($p < 0.001$), but ACTL was not ($p = 0.1069$). Mean OEF-CISSCO measurements were 42.5% in SCD, 37.0% in ACTL, and 33.0% in CTL ($p < 0.01$), with both SCD ($p < 0.001$) and ACTL ($p = 0.007$) significantly different from control subjects. Figure 2C shows the OEF measurements in the sagittal sinus vein using TRUST (OEF-TRUST). Mean OEF-TRUST measurements were 31.2% in SCD, 33.4% in ACTL and 36.8% in CTL ($p < 0.01$). After Dunnett's analysis, we found that SCD was different from CTL ($p = 0.0034$) and ACTL was not ($p = 0.1291$).

Figure 3 characterizes the bias between the two OEF_{ICV} measurements using linear correlation (Figure 3A) and Bland-Altman analysis (Figure 3B). A strong linear relationship was observed between OEF-QSM and OEF-CISSCO ($r^2 = 0.72$, $p < 0.001$). The mean OEF-CISSCO is 9.3% higher than OEF-QSM ($p < 0.001$). In addition, the bias was proportional to the mean value ($r^2 = 0.61$, $p < 0.001$) and was larger in anemic subjects.

Relationships Between OEF Measurements and O₂ Content in ICV

The relationship between OEF measurements in the internal cerebral vein and O_2 content is shown in Figures 1A,B. Both methods demonstrate a reciprocal relationship with O_2 content,

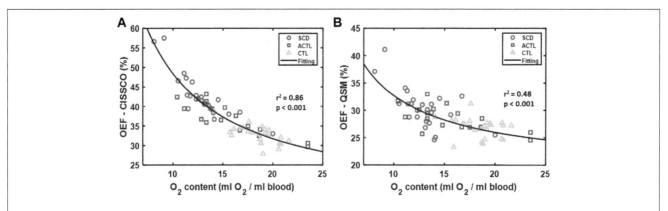

FIGURE 4 | Relationship between OEF and O_2 content in SCD, ACTL and CTL. **(A)** Scatterplot between OEF-CISSCO and O_2 content. The fitting reciprocal line is shown in black with $r^2 = 0.86$, $p < 0.001$. **(B)** Scatterplot between OEF-QSM and O_2 content. The fitting reciprocal line is shown in black with $r^2 = 0.48$, $p < 0.001$.

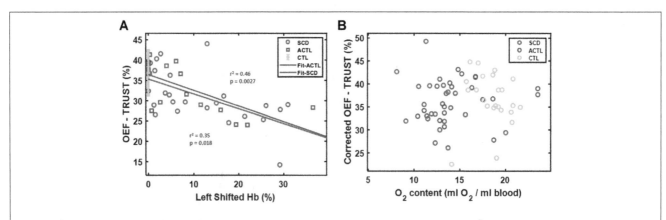

FIGURE 5 | **(A)** Relationship between OEF-TRUST with left shifted hemoglobin. Linear correlations are shown in blue line ($r^2 = 0.46$, $p = 0.0027$) for ACTL and red line ($r^2 = 0.35$, $p = 0.0018$) for SCD. The control group is shown as 36.8 ± 5.5 (mean ± std) in green. **(B)** Relationship between corrected OEF-TRUST with O_2 content.

but the variance is significantly less for OEF-CISSCO compared with OEF-QSM ($p < 0.01$ by F test). Importantly, when this relationship is removed, all group differences in OEF disappear for both techniques.

Relationships Between OEF, Left Shifted Hemoglobin and O_2 Content in SS.

Figure 5A demonstrates OEF-TRUST in the sagittal sinus as a function of left shifted hemoglobin concentration. The left shifted hemoglobin included hemoglobin F in SCD patients and fast moving hemoglobin in ACTL patients with alpha-thalassemia. It revealed that OEF-TRUST in the sagittal sinus declined with increasing left shifted hemoglobin for both SCD ($r^2 = 0.35$, $p = 0.018$) and ACTL ($r^2 = 0.46$, $p < 0.0027$). The slope was statistically identical in SCD and ACTL, as were the intercepts for all three groups. Thus, after controlling for inter-subject variability in the left shifted hemoglobin, the corrected OEF in the sagittal sinus was independent of group and O_2 content, as shown in **Figure 5B**.

Predictors for OEF in ICV and SS

Table 3 summarizes the primary and secondary predictors for OEF in the ICV and sagittal sinus. For OEF-CISSCO, there were two equivalent models predicting OEF in the ICV with a combined r^2 of 0.94 and 0.95 respectively. The dominant variable was either oxygen delivery ($r^2 = 0.86$), hemoglobin ($r^2 = 0.85$) or hematocrit ($r^2 = 0.92$), which are intrinsically co-linear ($r^2 = 0.90$). To explore what hematocrit reflected, beyond oxygen transport, we locked oxygen content (or hemoglobin alone) into the model, displacing hematocrit but introducing mean corpuscular hemoglobin concentration (MCHC) into the model. If hematocrit entered the model first, hemoglobin, oxygen content, and MCHC were displaced. With either the primary or the alternative model, oxygen saturation by pulse oximetry was positively associated with OEF-ICV.

After controlling OEF-TRUST for left shifted hemoglobin concentration, there was no residual relationship with patient group, Hb, Hct, RBC or O_2 content. There were also weak associations with systolic blood pressure (SBP), and the collinear variables MCV and MCH ($r^2 = 0.92$ with respect to each other). On stepwise analysis, left shifted hemoglobin, SBP and MCV persisted with a combined r^2 of 0.47.

TABLE 3 | OEF predictors by stepwise regression.

Residual OEF-CISSCO and O_2 Content			Residual OEF-TRUST and HbF%		
Parameter	r^2	p-value	Parameter	r^2	p-value
MCHC	0.34	<0.0001	MCH	0.16	0.008
Oxygen Saturation	0.19	0.0003	MCV	0.10	0.03
MCH	0.17	0.001	Height	0.10	0.03
HbS%	0.16	0.009	Weight	0.09	0.05
Weight	0.08	0.03	-		
RBC	0.07	0.04			
MCV	0.07	0.04			
Final Stepwise Model OEF-CISSCO			Final Stepwise Model OEF-TRUST		
$1/O_2$ content	0.85	<0.0001	HbF	0.34	0.0001
MCHC	+0.05	<0.0001	MCV	+0.13	0.004
Oxygen Saturation	+0.04	<0.0001	-	-	-
Total r^2	0.94	-	Total r^2	0.53	-
Alternative Model OEF-CISSCO			-		
1/Hematocrit	0.92	<0.0001			
Oxygen Saturation	+0.03	<0.0001			
Total r^2	0.95	-			

DISCUSSION

In this manuscript, we studied 66 subjects across a broad range of hemoglobin values and identified an increase in OEF in deep brain structures in patients with chronic anemia by two susceptibility-based methods. OEF in the ICV was reciprocally related to hematocrit, which reflected a combination of oxygen content and mean cellular hemoglobin concentration. OEF in the ICV was also directly proportional to peripheral oxygen saturation. In contrast, sagittal sinus OEF was decreased in anemic subjects, proportionally to hemoglobin, hematocrit, and oxygen content. However, after controlling for the impact of left shifted hemoglobin (hemoglobin F, hemoglobin H, hemoglobin Barts), OEF was independent of patient group and oxygen content. OEF by QSM and CISSCO were highly correlated, but QSM yielded systematically lower OEF estimates.

Previous work from our laboratory, and others, has suggested disparate oxygen extraction fraction estimates measured using sagittal sinus oximetry when compared to tissue oximetry performed in deep brain structures (Bush et al., 2018; Croal et al., 2019; Fields et al., 2018). In particular, tissue oximetry suggests profound deep brain hypoxia with worsening anemia (Fields et al., 2018; Guilliams et al., 2018), while sagittal sinus oximetry suggests normal or even decreased oxygen extraction (A. M. Bush et al., 2018; Li et al., 2020). We have previously postulated that a vascular steal phenomenon may exist, where oxygen delivery to brain cortex is preserved at the expense of deep brain structures (Chai et al., 2019). Arterial transit time is decreased in sickle cell disease patients (Afzali-Hashemi et al., 2021), leading to decreased exchange of labeled spins into the cerebrovasculature (A. Bush et al., 2018; Juttukonda et al., 2019). However, this manuscript is the first to document deep brain hypoxia in anemia subjects with concomitant preservation of sagittal sinus oxygen extraction.

The internal cerebral vein is one of the major deep cortical veins, and its oxygen saturation provides insight into the oxygenation of the basal ganglia, corpus callosum and

thalamus. OEF estimates using either QSM or CISSCO demonstrated an inverse relationship with O_2 content (**Figure 4**), similar to whole brain estimates of OEF by Asymmetric Spin Echo (ASE) (**Supplementary Figure S1**) (Fields et al., 2018). Although there is a bias between the two datasets, both demonstrate a comparable reciprocal relationship with O_2 content. The similarity should not be surprising, however, as ASE is dominated by tissue oxygenation in the white matter and deep gray structures; in ASE, much of the signal from cortex is contaminated by susceptibility artifacts from superficial veins and excluded from global OEF measurements. ASE oximetry measurements yield spatially averaged tissue oxygenation that weigh grey matter and white matter equally, despite their markedly disparate contribution to brain metabolism.

According to **Eq. 6**, OEF may be cast as the ratio of the cerebral metabolic rate of oxygen divided by the product of cerebral blood flow and oxygen content (i.e., O_2 delivery). On a whole-brain basis, CBF increases reciprocally with O_2 content in anemic subjects (Borzage et al., 2016; Bush et al., 2016), preserving global oxygen delivery. However, compensatory hyperemia is blunted or eliminated in deep watershed structures (Chai et al., 2019). By **Eq. 6**, OEF in the ICV (and by ASE) should vary inversely with oxygen content if deep brain blood flow does not augment appropriately.

The other two predictors of deep brain OEF also provide physiological insights. The positive relationship between ICV OEF and S_pO_2 arises organically from **Eq. 3**. The brain operates within a very narrow range of pO_2, which translates to a much broader range of S_vO_2 because of inter-subject variability in the hemoglobin dissociation curve (Wood, 2019). Powerful physiological compensation mechanisms limit declines in S_vO_2 under hypoxic conditions. Thus, inter-subject variability in S_aO_2, even within the normal range, introduces a positive relationship with OEF by providing more "headroom" for oxygen extraction. The positive association of MCHC and OEF in the ICV is more challenging to explain. MCHC contributes powerfully to RBC deformability and viscosity. We speculate that MCHC could be modulating capillary transit time through its impact on red cell rheology, however this would have to be independently confirmed.

In the sagittal sinus, oxygen saturation is dominated by cortical blood flow and supply-demand matching. Venous oximetry techniques follow Fick-principle (oxygen mass balance) and are inherently flow-weighted rather than spatially weighted. Since grey matter has 3–4 times the metabolic activity of white matter, venous oximetry techniques reflect grey matter oxygen balance. Whole brain CBF rises inversely to oxygen carrying capacity such that oxygen delivery is preserved in anemic subjects (Borzage et al., 2016; Bush et al., 2016). There are also multiple other publications confirming these observations (Prohovnik et al., 2009; Kosinski et al., 2017). Regional flow assessment using ASL demonstrates that cortical oxygen delivery is normal (Chai et al., 2019). Preservation of OEF in the sagittal sinus, with normal or even decreased OEF despite worsening anemia, is the natural consequence of compensatory hyperemia (Bush et al., 2018). The mechanisms behind this "cortical sparing" are unknown but work in mice suggests that chronic hypoxia stimulates cortical capillary proliferation (Harb et al., 2013). Duffin modeled compensatory hyperemia using a "fail-safe" mechanism and proposed potential biochemical mediators (Duffin, 2020). Regardless of the mechanism, observed patterns of brain volume loss (Choi et al., 2019, 2017) and silent infarction (Fields et al., 2018) are consistent with cortical sparing at the expense of the deep watershed areas.

A second striking finding of this study was the powerful effect of hemoglobin F and other high affinity hemoglobin molecules on OEF measured in the sagittal sinus. This undoubtedly represents left-shift of the hemoglobin dissociation curve and resulting higher oxygen affinity of hemoglobin. While this phenomenon is well known, the magnitude of the effect is striking, with OEF decreasing 20 saturation points over the physiologic range of left shifted hemoglobin fraction in anemic subjects. Importantly, all group differences in sagittal sinus OEF were eliminated once differences in high affinity hemoglobin fraction was controlled for. These findings highlight the critical physiologic principle that cerebral OEF is not a regulated variable. The brain varies vascular tone to preserve capillary pO_2 in a narrow range (Wood, 2019). When hemoglobin is left-shifted, less oxygen is delivered for any brain pO_2. In SCD patients with high hemoglobin F concentration, resting CBF increases to preserve tissue oxygen unloading in the cortex (Afzali-Hashemi et al., 2021). In contrast, the deep structures have decreased compensatory hyperemia and are forced to operate at lower pO_2 (increased OEF compounded by tighter oxygen affinity).

So are hydroxyurea or other dissociation curve modifiers placing the deep structures of the brain at risk? The left-shift of hemoglobin cannot be interpreted in isolation. With hydroxyurea, the impaired oxygen unloading is at least partially compensated by a 10%–15% rise in O_2 content; to date no study has systematically evaluated regional oxygen delivery and metabolism in patients prior to and following hydroxyurea initiation to evaluate that balance between improved oxygen capacity and impaired oxygen unloading.

Studies are currently ongoing to explore these endpoints in voxelotor (Vichinsky et al., 2019; Herity et al., 2021), an allosteric modifier of hemoglobin affinity. The present study emphasizes the need to examine both global and regional responses to such therapies.

The powerful impact of HbF and other modulators of the hemoglobin dissociation curve must also be considered when comparing OEF from modern hemoglobinopathy cohorts, with historical data prior to the widespread use of hydroxyurea (Herold et al., 1986; Vu et al., 2021). TRUST studies from modern SCD cohorts (Bush et al., 2017; Afzali-Hashemi et al., 2021; Vu et al., 2021) consistently observed lower OEF values that reported in historical cohorts (Heyman et al., 1952; Herold et al., 1986). Hydroxyurea did not achieve widespread use until the last one to 2 decades. Current recommendations favor introduction at 18 months of age, and dose escalation to maximum tolerated dose, leading to robust hemoglobin F% induction in many patients. In our cohort, OEF was 7% points lower in patients taking hydroxyurea which is consistent with OEF differences exhibited by current and historical cohorts.

It is important to consider whether our two principle findings, i.e. cortical sparing and the powerful effect of left shifted hemoglobin fraction, could be artifacts resulting from the two different oximetry techniques. MRI venous oximetry can be performed using magnetic susceptibility or by R2, R2*, or R2′ relaxometries. If the calibration curves for these methods are unbiased across the patient subgroups, then the techniques can be used interchangeably, and our observed results are valid. The susceptibility calibration is considered the most robust because it is independent of red cell integrity. The linear dependence of susceptibility on hematocrit and oxygen saturation is incontrovertible but estimates of the intrinsic susceptibility of deoxygenated hemoglobin vary from 0.18–0.27 (Weisskoff and Kiihne, 1992; Langham et al., 2009; Jain et al., 2012; Eldeniz et al., 2017; Fields et al., 2018). Errors in this parameter could introduce bias but not alter the direction of change observed. Hemoglobin S has the same intrinsic susceptibility as hemoglobin A (Eldeniz et al., 2017) and there is little biophysical reason to believe that other hemoglobins should be significantly different because the electron shells of the heme moiety are identical (it is just the supporting scaffolding that's different).

The TRUST calibration in normal subjects (so-called hemoglobin AA calibration) is also fairly incontrovertible. Two independent laboratories have yielded superimposable results over a very broad range of hematocrit values (Bush et al., 2021; Bush et al., 2018; Li et al., 2020). This observation is important because the red blood cells in the ACTL group, and all transfused patients, predominantly contains normal hemoglobin. Results from these patients yield identical findings compared to the SCD patients. Thus, cortical sparing and the effect of left shifted hemoglobin cannot be attributed simply to a faulty oximetry calibration.

The TRUST calibration has challenges in the SCD population that we have characterizing for years (Bush et al., 2021; Bush et al., 2018; Li et al., 2020). The variation in calibration arises from damage to the red cell membrane as well as changes in red cell density and shape (Bush et al., 2021; Bush et al., 2018; Li et al.,

2020), not from any intrinsic magnetic difference in sickle hemoglobin (Eldeniz et al., 2017). Since patients with sickle cell trait have normal appearing red blood cells, their blood follows the AA calibration curve, not the SCD curve (Bush et al., 2018). The sickle calibration curve used in this study represents a "consensus" calibration using data pooled from two laboratories to yield a more stable estimate of the hematocrit interaction and to derive a model that accounts for the dilution effect of transfusion (Bush et al., 2021). We believe that the absence of a group effect in **Figures 4, 5**, despite combining controls, transfused SCD, non-transfused SCD, transfused ACTL, and non-transfused ACTL, offers strong evidence that our TRUST calibrations not introducing systematic bias that could be misinterpreted as physiologic change.

It is also reasonable to wonder about the potential impact of hemoglobin F on the T2 calibration in those patients with excellent response to hydroxyurea (e.g. >15%). The published calibration curve for hemoglobin F cells is quite similar to the HbA calibration (Bush et al., 2017; Liu et al., 2011, p. 2). In SCD patients, hemoglobin F upregulation will cause some degree of hemoglobin F cells to circulate (like hemoglobin A)...this we could potentially compensate for using the mixture model (SS + FF is similar to SS + AA). To determine whether the increased HbF in some of the non-transfused SCD has an important "dilutional" effect, similar to transfusions, we reran all the TRUST data using the mixture model and did not observe any significant qualitative differences to our findings (see **Supplementary Figure S2A,B**).

In the extremes of hemoglobin F expression (for example after gene therapy or hereditary persistence of fetal hemoglobin), the sickling process is almost completely abrogated and the resulting red cells are morphologically normal. Under this extreme case (which does NOT reflect even the highest F induction in this study), the hemoglobin A calibration would be appropriate. As a result, we also compared the results using the hemoglobin A calibration for all subjects as a "worst case" simulation. When we did this, the two principle findings (cortical sparing, OEF negatively correlated with hemoglobin F) were maintained (**Supplementary Figure S2C, D**). However, OEF was systematically higher in SCD patients. This is nonsensical because it would imply that cerebral metabolic rate is increased in SCD compared with controls and other anemic subjects. Studies using gold standard techniques like Kety-Schmidt and PET have proven exactly the opposite (see supplemental data in Vu et al., 2021).

Both the CISSCO and QSM methods reveal group differences in venous saturation measurements and similar relationships with hemoglobin. However, there exists significant bias between the two techniques with QSM exhibiting higher saturation values. There might be several reasons for the underestimation of susceptibility for QSM. Firstly, the existence of streaking artifact may affect the measurement of susceptibility indirectly (Li et al., 2015). Secondly, partial-volume effect causes susceptibility to be underestimated, particularly in small vessels like the internal cerebral vein (Zhang et al., 2017). Lastly, QSM estimates of vein saturation are impacted by

nonlinear phase accrual in moving spins. This effect could worsen with anemia severity as blood viscosity lessens and blood flow increases. We postulate that the latter two effects are responsible for the systemic bias between QSM and CISSCO oximetry in these patients. CISSCO overcomes these limitations by avoiding unstable dipole inversion and by inferring vessel susceptibility from its effect on surrounding tissue rather than from the blood itself, similar to asymmetric spin echo (ASE).

The CISSCO method is not without its own limitations. CISSCO is most accurate for veins perpendicular to the main magnetic field, making it most effective for the straight sinus and internal cerebral vein. It cannot be used for superficial veins like the sagittal sinus because a complete annulus cannot be drawn across it. CISSCO requires high SNR inside the vessel (over 5:1) for accurate measurements, which limits the choice of echo times and can be impacted by Gibbs ringing (Hsieh et al., 2015a). In practice, we first quantify the magnetic moment from the second echo time as the uncertainty of measurement of magnetic moment at the longer echo time is smaller (Cheng et al., 2009). Then we solve the susceptibility at the first echo time for a higher SNR inside the internal cerebral vein, after scaling the calculated magnetic moment. In addition, improper choice of radius of three annuli might produce up to 15% uncertainty to the calculated susceptibility through error propagation (Hsieh et al., 2015a). However, despite these limitations, the tight relationship of OEF_{ICV} with O_2 content and the similarity of this relationship with OEF by ASE suggest that it may be a better choice than QSM for venous oximetry in select vessels.

Other alternatives exist to quantify saturation in the deep veins. A variation of TRUST, called TRU-PC (Krishnamurthy et al., 2014), uses complex differencing rather than arterial spin labeling to eliminate partial volume effects and has sufficient signal to quantify T_2 in deep draining veins. It would be instructive, in the future, to compare OEF estimates by TRU-PC and CISSCO in SCD patients as a mechanism to cross-validate T_2 and susceptibility-based oximetry in this patient population.

CONCLUSION

In summary, we have demonstrated that anemia worsens hypoxia in deep brain structures while cerebral cortex appears to be spared, replicating observations using tissue-based oximetry ASE. Our findings resolve the apparent paradox observed between TRUST and ASE measurements. We also demonstrate that hemoglobin F and other high affinity hemoglobin molecules appear to be powerful modulators of OEF by TRUST and explain group differences in OEF observed between anemic and control subjects. These observations were conserved across diverse study populations, robust with respect to choice of sickle cell calibration, and physiologically plausible.

Although CISSCO was ideal for the present context because is robust to partial volume effects, independent of blood flow velocity, and unaffected by red cell properties, it is only suitable for select cerebral veins, limiting its generalizability. QSM is more generalizable and saturation estimates were qualitatively similar to CISSCO, but troubled by large biases from partial volume and flow effects. Future oximetry in the deep brain may require techniques such as TRU-PC.

ETHICS STATEMENT

The studies involving human participants were reviewed and approved by Institutional Review Board at Children's Hospital Los Angeles. Written informed consent to participate in this study was provided by the participants' legal guardian/next of kin.

AUTHOR CONTRIBUTIONS

JS, XM, and JW designed the research study and wrote the manuscript. JS, XM, CV, BX, and CG-Z collected the data. JS and XM analyzed the data. AN and JW assisted with the interpretation of the data. All authors edited and approved this manuscript.

FUNDING

This work is supported by the National Heart Lung and Blood Institute (1RO1HL136484-A1, 1U01HL117718-01), the National Institute of Clinical Research Resources (UL1TR001855-02), the National Center for Research (5UL1-TR000130-05) through the Clinical Translational Science Institute at Children's Hospital Los Angeles, and by research support in kind from Philips Healthcare. Philips Healthcare was not involved in the study design, collection, analysis, interpretation of data, the writing of this article or the decision to submit it for publication.

ACKNOWLEDGMENTS

The authors would like to acknowledge Mr. Bertin Valdez and Mr. Obdulio Carreras for their efforts coordinating the patient study visits. We would like to thank Dr. Hanzhang Lu for supplying the TRUST patch and Philips Healthcare for providing In-Kind research support.

REFERENCES

Adams, R. J. (2005). TCD in Sickle Cell Disease: an Important and Useful Test. *Pediatr. Radiol.* 35, 229–234. doi:10.1007/s00247-005-1409-7

Afzali-Hashemi, L., Baas, K., Schrantee, A., Coolen, B. F., Van Osch, M. J., Spann, S. M., et al. (2021). Impairment of Cerebrovascular Hemodynamics in Patients with Severe and Milder Forms of Sickle Cell Disease. *Front. physiology* 12, 430. doi:10.3389/fphys.2021.645205

Baas, K. P. A., Coolen, B. F., Petersen, E. T., Biemond, B. J., Strijkers, G. J., and Nederveen, A. J. (2022). Comparative Analysis of Blood T_2 Values Measured by T_2-TRIR and TRUST. *J. Magn. Reson Imaging.* doi:10.1002/jmri.28066

Bilgic, B., Pfefferbaum, A., Rohlfing, T., Sullivan, E. V., and Adalsteinsson, E. (2012). MRI Estimates of Brain Iron Concentration in Normal Aging Using Quantitative Susceptibility Mapping. *Neuroimage* 59, 2625–2635. doi:10.1016/j.neuroimage.2011.08.077

Borzage, M. T., Bush, A. M., Choi, S., Nederveen, A. J., Václavů, L., Coates, T. D., et al. (2016). Predictors of Cerebral Blood Flow in Patients with and without Anemia. *J. Appl. Physiology* 120, 976–981. doi:10.1152/japplphysiol.00994.2015

Bush, A., Borzage, M., Detterich, J., Kato, R. M., Meiselman, H. J., Coates, T., et al. (2017). Empirical Model of Human Blood Transverse Relaxation at 3 T Improves MRI T2oximetry. *Magn. Reson. Med.* 77, 2364–2371. doi:10.1002/mrm.26311

Bush, A., Chai, Y., Choi, S. Y., Vaclavu, L., Holland, S., Nederveen, A., et al. (2018). Pseudo Continuous Arterial Spin Labeling Quantification in Anemic Subjects with Hyperemic Cerebral Blood Flow. *Magn. Reson. imaging* 47, 137–146. doi:10.1016/j.mri.2017.12.011

Bush, A. M., Borzage, M. T., Choi, S., Václavů, L., Tamrazi, B., Nederveen, A. J., et al. (2016). Determinants of Resting Cerebral Blood Flow in Sickle Cell Disease. *Am. J. Hematol.* 91, 912–917. doi:10.1002/ajh.24441

Bush, A. M., Coates, T. D., and Wood, J. C. (2018). Diminished Cerebral Oxygen Extraction and Metabolic Rate in Sickle Cell Disease Using T2 Relaxation under Spin Tagging MRI. *Magn. Reson. Med.* 80, 294–303. doi:10.1002/mrm.27015

Bush, A., Vu, C., Choi, S., Borzage, M., Miao, X., Li, W., et al. (2021). Calibration of T 2 Oximetry MRI for Subjects with Sickle Cell Disease. *Magn. Reson Med.* 86, 1019–1028. doi:10.1002/mrm.28757

Chai, Y., Bush, A. M., Coloigner, J., Nederveen, A. J., Tamrazi, B., Vu, C., et al. (2019). White Matter Has Impaired Resting Oxygen Delivery in Sickle Cell Patients. *Am. J. Hematol.* 94, 467–474. doi:10.1002/ajh.25423

Choi, S., Bush, A. M., Borzage, M. T., Joshi, A. A., Mack, W. J., Coates, T. D., et al. (2017). Hemoglobin and Mean Platelet Volume Predicts Diffuse T1-MRI White

Matter Volume Decrease in Sickle Cell Disease Patients. *NeuroImage Clin.* 15, 239–246. doi:10.1016/j.nicl.2017.04.023

Choi, S., O'Neil, S. H., Joshi, A. A., Li, J., Bush, A. M., Coates, T. D., et al. (2019). Anemia Predicts Lower White Matter Volume and Cognitive Performance in Sickle and Non-sickle Cell Anemia Syndrome. *Am. J. Hematol.* 94, 1055–1065. doi:10.1002/ajh.25570

Croal, P. L., Leung, J., Phillips, C. L., Serafin, M. G., and Kassner, A. (2019). Quantification of Pathophysiological Alterations in Venous Oxygen Saturation: a Comparison of Global MR Susceptometry Techniques. *Magn. Reson. Imaging* 58, 18–23. doi:10.1016/j.mri.2019.01.008

Diringer, M. N., Aiyagari, V., Zazulia, A. R., Videen, T. O., and Powers, W. J. (2007). Effect of Hyperoxia on Cerebral Metabolic Rate for Oxygen Measured Using Positron Emission Tomography in Patients with Acute Severe Head Injury. *J Neurosurg.* 106, 526–529. doi:10.3171/jns.2007.106.4.526

Duffin, J. (2020). Fail-safe Aspects of Oxygen Supply. *J. Physiol.* 598, 4859–4867. doi:10.1113/jp280301

Eldeniz, C., Binkley, M. M., Fields, M., Guilliams, K., Ragan, D. K., Chen, Y., et al. (2021). Bulk Volume Susceptibility Difference between Deoxyhemoglobin and Oxyhemoglobin for HbA and HbS: A Comparative Study. *Magn. Reson Med.* 85, 3383–3393. doi:10.1002/mrm.28668

Eldeniz, C., Binkley, M., Ragan, D., Fields, M., Guilliams, K., Comiskey, L., et al. (2017). Sickle Hemoglobin vs Normal Hemoglobin: Any Changes in Susceptibility," in Proceedings of the 25th Annual Meeting of International Society for Magnetic Resonance in Medicine. pp. 22

Fields, M. E., Guilliams, K. P., Ragan, D. K., Binkley, M. M., Eldeniz, C., Chen, Y., et al. (2018). Regional Oxygen Extraction Predicts Border Zone Vulnerability to Stroke in Sickle Cell Disease. *Neurology* 90, e1134–e1142. doi:10.1212/wnl.0000000000005194

Guilliams, K. P., Fields, M. E., Ragan, D. K., Eldeniz, C., Binkley, M. M., Chen, Y., et al. (2018). Red Cell Exchange Transfusions Lower Cerebral Blood Flow and Oxygen Extraction Fraction in Pediatric Sickle Cell Anemia. *Blood, J. Am. Soc. Hematol.* 131, 1012–1021. doi:10.1182/blood-2017-06-789842

Harb, R., Whiteus, C., Freitas, C., and Grutzendler, J. (2013). *In Vivo* imaging of Cerebral Microvascular Plasticity from Birth to Death. *J. Cereb. Blood Flow. Metab.* 33, 146–156. doi:10.1038/jcbfm.2012.152

Hassell, K. L. (2010). Population Estimates of Sickle Cell Disease in the U.S. *Am. J. Prev. Med.* 38, S512–S521. doi:10.1016/j.amepre.2009.12.022

Herity, L. B., Vaughan, D. M., Rodriguez, L. R., and Lowe, D. K. (2021). Voxelotor: a Novel Treatment for Sickle Cell Disease. *Ann. Pharmacother.* 55, 240–245. doi:10.1177/1060028020943059

Herold, S., Brozovic, M., Gibbs, J., Lammertsma, A. A., Leenders, K. L., Carr, D., et al. (1986). Measurement of Regional Cerebral Blood Flow, Blood Volume and Oxygen Metabolism in Patients with Sickle Cell Disease Using Positron Emission Tomography. *Stroke* 17, 692–698. doi:10.1161/01.str.17.4.692

Heyman, A., Patterson, J. L., and Duke, T. W. (1952). Cerebral Circulation and Metabolism in Sickle Cell and Other Chronic Anemias, with Observations on the Effects of Oxygen Inhalation 1. *J. Clin. Invest.* 31, 824–828. doi:10.1172/jci102668

Hsieh, C.-Y., Cheng, Y.-C. N., Neelavalli, J., Haacke, E. M., and Stafford, R. J. (2015a). An Improved Method for Susceptibility and Radius Quantification of Cylindrical Objects from MRI. *Magn. Reson. imaging* 33, 420–436. doi:10.1016/j.mri.2015.01.004

Hsieh, C.-Y., Cheng, Y.-C. N., Xie, H., Haacke, E. M., and Neelavalli, J. (2015b). Susceptibility and Size Quantification of Small Human Veins from an MRI Method. *Magn. Reson. imaging* 33, 1191–1204. doi:10.1016/j.mri.2015.07.008

Jain, V., Abdulmalik, O., Propert, K. J., and Wehrli, F. W. (2012). Investigating the Magnetic Susceptibility Properties of Fresh Human Blood for Noninvasive Oxygen Saturation Quantification. *Magn. Reson. Med.* 68, 863–867. doi:10.1002/mrm.23282

Jenkinson, M., Beckmann, C. F., Behrens, T. E. J., Woolrich, M. W., and Smith, S. M. (2012). FSL. *NeuroImage* 62, 782–790. doi:10.1016/j.neuroimage.2011.09.015

Jordan, L. C., Gindville, M. C., Scott, A. O., Juttukonda, M. R., Strother, M. K., Kassim, A. A., et al. (2016). Non-invasive Imaging of Oxygen Extraction Fraction in Adults with Sickle Cell Anaemia. *Brain* 139, 738–750. doi:10.1093/brain/awv397

Juttukonda, M. R., Donahue, M. J., Davis, L. T., Gindville, M. C., Lee, C. A., Patel, N. J., et al. (2019). Preliminary Evidence for Cerebral Capillary Shunting in Adults with Sickle Cell Anemia. *J. Cereb. Blood Flow. Metab.* 39, 1099–1110. doi:10.1177/0271678x17746808

Kosinski, P. D., Croal, P. L., Leung, J., Williams, S., Odame, I., Hare, G. M. T., et al. (2017). The Severity of Anaemia Depletes Cerebrovascular Dilatory Reserve in Children with Sickle Cell Disease: a Quantitative Magnetic Resonance Imaging Study. *Br. J. Haematol.* 176, 280–287. doi:10.1111/bjh.14424

Krishnamurthy, L. C., Liu, P., Ge, Y., and Lu, H. (2014). Vessel-specific Quantification of Blood Oxygenation with T2 -Relaxation-Under-Phase-Contrast MRI. *Magn. Reson. Med.* 71, 978–989. doi:10.1002/mrm.24750

Langham, M. C., Magland, J. F., Epstein, C. L., Floyd, T. F., and Wehrli, F. W. (2009). Accuracy and Precision of MR Blood Oximetry Based on the Long Paramagnetic Cylinder Approximation of Large Vessels. *Magn. Reson. Med.* 62, 333–340. doi:10.1002/mrm.21981

Li, W., Wang, N., Yu, F., Han, H., Cao, W., Romero, R., et al. (2015). A Method for Estimating and Removing Streaking Artifacts in Quantitative Susceptibility Mapping. *Neuroimage* 108, 111–122. doi:10.1016/j.neuroimage.2014.12.043

Li, W., Xu, X., Liu, P., Strouse, J. J., Casella, J. F., Lu, H., et al. (2020). Quantification of Whole-brain Oxygenation Extraction Fraction and Cerebral Metabolic Rate of Oxygen Consumption in Adults with Sickle Cell Anemia Using Individual T2 -based Oxygenation Calibrations. *Magn. Reson Med.* 83, 1066–1080. doi:10.1002/mrm.27972

Liu, T., Khalidov, I., de Rochefort, L., Spincemaille, P., Liu, J., Tsiouris, A. J., et al. (2011). A Novel Background Field Removal Method for MRI Using Projection onto Dipole Fields (PDF). *NMR Biomed.* 24, 1129–1136. doi:10.1002/nbm.1670

Lu, H., Clingman, C., Golay, X., and Van Zijl, P. C. M. (2004). Determining the Longitudinal Relaxation Time (T1) of Blood at 3.0 Tesla. *Magn. Reson. Med.* 52, 679–682. doi:10.1002/mrm.20178

Lu, H., and Ge, Y. (2008). Quantitative Evaluation of Oxygenation in Venous Vessels Using T2-Relaxation-Under-Spin-Tagging MRI. *Magn. Reson. Med.* 60, 357–363. doi:10.1002/mrm.21627

Lu, H., Xu, F., Grgac, K., Liu, P., Qin, Q., and Van Zijl, P. (2012). Calibration and Validation of TRUST MRI for the Estimation of Cerebral Blood Oxygenation. *Magn. Reson. Med.* 67, 42–49. doi:10.1002/mrm.22970

Miao, X., Nayak, K. S., and Wood, J. C. (2019). *In Vivo* validation of T2- and Susceptibility-based SᵥO2 Measurements with Jugular Vein Catheterization under Hypoxia and Hypercapnia. *Magn. Reson Med.* 82, 2188–2198. doi:10.1002/mrm.27871

Mintun, M. A., Raichle, M. E., Martin, W. R., and Herscovitch, P. (1984). Brain Oxygen Utilization Measured with O-15 Radiotracers and Positron Emission Tomography. *J. Nucl. Med.* 25, 177

Muroi, C., Khan, N., Bellut, D., Fujioka, M., and Yonekawa, Y. (2011). Extracranial-intracranial Bypass in Atherosclerotic Cerebrovascular Disease: Report of a Single Centre Experience. *Br. J. Neurosurg.* 25, 357–362. doi:10.3109/02688697.2010.551673

N Cheng, Y.-C., Hsieh, C.-Y., Neelavalli, J., and Haacke, E. M. (2009). Quantifying Effective Magnetic Moments of Narrow Cylindrical Objects in MRI. *Phys. Med. Biol.* 54, 7025–7044. doi:10.1088/0031-9155/54/22/018

Ohene-Frempong, K., Weiner, S. J., Sleeper, L. A., Miller, S. T., Embury, S., Moohr, J. W., et al. (1998). Sickle Cell Disease, the C.S. of Cerebrovascular Accidents in Sickle Cell Disease: Rates and Risk Factors. Blood. *J. Am. Soc. Hematol.* 91, 288

Prohovnik, I., Hurlet-Jensen, A., Adams, R., De Vivo, D., and Pavlakis, S. G. (2009). Hemodynamic Etiology of Elevated Flow Velocity and Stroke in Sickle-Cell Disease. *J. Cereb. Blood Flow. Metab.* 29, 803–810. doi:10.1038/jcbfm.2009.6

Schweser, F., Deistung, A., Lehr, B. W., and Reichenbach, J. R. (2011). Quantitative Imaging of Intrinsic Magnetic Tissue Properties Using MRI Signal Phase: an Approach to *In Vivo* Brain Iron Metabolism? *Neuroimage* 54, 2789–2807. doi:10.1016/j.neuroimage.2010.10.070

Spees, W. M., Yablonskiy, D. A., Oswood, M. C., and Ackerman, J. J. H. (2001). Water Proton MR Properties of Human Blood at 1.5 Tesla: Magnetic susceptibility,T1,T2,T2, and Non-lorentzian Signal Behavior. *Magn. Reson. Med.* 45, 533–542. doi:10.1002/mrm.1072

Tanaka, M., Shimosegawa, E., Kajimoto, K., Kimura, Y., Kato, H., Oku, N., et al. (2008). Chronic Middle Cerebral Artery Occlusion: a Hemodynamic and Metabolic Study with Positron-Emission Tomography. *AJNR Am. J. Neuroradiol.* 29, 1841–1846. doi:10.3174/ajnr.a1234

Václavů, L., van der Land, V., Heijtel, D. F., van Osch, M. J., Cnossen, M. H., Majoie, C. B., et al. (2016). *In Vivo* T1 of Blood Measurements in Children with Sickle Cell Disease Improve Cerebral Blood Flow Quantification from Arterial Spin-Labeling MRI. *AJNR Am. J. Neuroradiol.* 37, 1727–1732. doi:10.3174/ajnr.A4793

Vichinsky, E., Hoppe, C. C., Ataga, K. I., Ware, R. E., Nduba, V., El-Beshlawy, A., et al. (2019). A Phase 3 Randomized Trial of Voxelotor in Sickle Cell Disease. *N. Engl. J. Med.* 381, 509–519. doi:10.1056/nejmoa1903212

Vu, C., Bush, A., Choi, S., Borzage, M., Miao, X., Nederveen, A. J., et al. (2021). Reduced Global Cerebral Oxygen Metabolic Rate in Sickle Cell Disease and Chronic Anemias. *Am. J Hematol* 96, 901–913. doi:10.1002/ajh.26203

Wang, W. C., Gallagher, D. M., Pegelow, C. H., Wright, E. C., Vichinsky, E. P., Abboud, M. R., et al. (2000). Multicenter Comparison of Magnetic Resonance Imaging and Transcranial Doppler Ultrasonography in the Evaluation of the Central Nervous System in Children with Sickle Cell Disease. *J. Pediatr. hematology/oncology* 22, 335–339. doi:10.1097/00043426-200007000-00010

Wang, Y., and Liu, T. (2015). Quantitative Susceptibility Mapping (QSM): DecodingMRIdata for a Tissue Magnetic Biomarker. *Magn. Reson. Med.* 73, 82–101. doi:10.1002/mrm.25358

Wasserman, K., and Whipp, B. J. (1975). Excercise Physiology in Health and Disease. *Am. Rev. Respir. Dis.* 112, 219–249. doi:10.1164/arrd.1975.112.2.219

Weisskoff, R. M., and Kiihne, S. (1992). MRI Susceptometry: Image-Based Measurement of Absolute Susceptibility of MR Contrast Agents and Human Blood. *Magn. Reson. Med.* 24, 375–383. doi:10.1002/mrm.1910240219

Wood, J. C. (2019). Brain O2 Reserve in Sickle Cell Disease. *Blood, J. Am. Soc. Hematol.* 133, 2356–2358. doi:10.1182/blood-2019-04-901124

Zhang, J., Zhou, D., Nguyen, T. D., Spincemaille, P., Gupta, A., and Wang, Y. (2017). Cerebral Metabolic Rate of Oxygen (CMRO2) Mapping with Hyperventilation Challenge Using Quantitative Susceptibility Mapping (QSM). *Magn. Reson. Med.* 77, 1762–1773. doi:10.1002/mrm.26253

22

Magnitudes of Anemia and its Determinant Factors Among Lactating Mothers in East African Countries: Using the Generalized Mixed-Effect Model

Biruk Shalmeno Tusa[1]*, Adisu Birhanu Weldesenbet[1], Nebiyu Bahiru[2] and Daniel Berhanie Enyew[1]

[1] Epidemiology and Biostatistics Department, College of Health and Medical Sciences, Haramaya University, Haramaya, Ethiopia, [2] Department of Public Health and Health Policy, School of Public Health, College of Health and Medical Sciences, Haramaya University, Haramaya, Ethiopia

*Correspondence:
Biruk Shalmeno Tusa
birukshalmeno27@gmail.com

Background: The number of studies on the magnitude of anemia and its determinant factors among lactating mothers is limited in East African countries regardless of its multivariate consequences. Even though few studies were conducted on the magnitude of anemia and its determinants, most of them focused on the country level and different parts of countries. Therefore, the current study is aimed to determine the magnitude of anemia and determinant factors among lactating mothers in East African countries.

Methods: From nine East African countries, a total weighted sample of 25,425 lactating mothers was included in the study. Determinate factors of anemia were identified using generalized linear mixed models (GLMM). Variables with a $p < 0.05$ in the final GLMM model were stated to confirm significant association with anemia.

Result: The magnitude of anemia in East African countries was found to be 36.5% [95% confidence interval (CI): 35.55%, 36.75%]. Besides, as for the generalized linear mixed-effect model, age, educational status, working status, country of residence, wealth index, antenatal care service, place of delivery, history of using family planning in a health facility, current pregnancy, and visited by fieldworker in the last 12 months were factors that have a significant association with anemia in lactating mothers.

Conclusion: In East Africa, more than one-third of lactating mothers have anemia. The odds of anemia were significantly low among young mothers (15–34), who had primary education, were working, country of residence, and higher wealth index (middle and high). In addition, the likelihood of anemia was also low among lactating mothers who had antenatal care, used family planning, delivered at a health facility, were pregnant during the survey, and visited by fieldworkers. Therefore, promoting maternal care services (family planning, Antenatal Care (ANC), and delivery at health facilities) and a field visit by health extension workers are strongly recommended.

Keywords: anemia, lactating mother, Eastern Africa, demographic and health survey data, generalized mixed effect model

BACKGROUND

Anemia is a disorder defined as a reduced absolute number of circulating red blood cells, indicated by a low serum hemoglobin concentration (1). It occurs when a low number of red blood cells in the circulatory system leaves the oxygen-carrying capacity insufficient to meet physiological needs (2). Besides, it is one of the major health problems which is estimated to affect nearly 2 billion people all over the world (3, 4).

Anemia is widely spread and prevalent in developing countries than in developed countries (3–6) where Sub-Saharan Africa and Southeast Asia bear the highest- burden (7). Globally, 54.1% of anemia cases contribute to mild, 42.5% moderate, and 3.4% severe problems in all age groups of the population of the world (8, 9). The magnitude of anemia among lactating mothers is 52.5% in South Asia (4), 60.3% in Myanmar, 20% in Nepal, 63% in India, and 28.3% in Ethiopia (4, 6, 10, 11).

A wide variety of factors attribute to anemia and most of them are coincident. Iron deficiency is the most significant contributor to the occurrence of anemia, which accounts for 50% of the cases. Whereas vitamin deficiencies (folate and vitamin B12), infections, and hemoglobinopathies contribute to the rest of the cases of anemia worldwide (1–3, 5, 6). Lactating women, women of reproductive age, adolescent girls, pregnant women, newborn infants, and young children are the major risk groups for anemia (3, 12).

Lactating mothers commonly acquire anemia during their pregnancy (6). Lactating mothers are vulnerable to anemia morbidity due to their susceptibility to iron depletion during pregnancy and bad consequences of blood loss during their childbirth (13). Anemia in lactating women is also associated with a history of abortion, residence, history of malaria, and tea consumption (6, 12, 13). Prominently, lack of formal education, rural residency, higher parity, lower antenatal care visits, lack of family planning utilization, underweight, lower dietary diversity, food insecurity, and malaria infection were factors associated with higher odds of developing anemia while taking iron supplementation, being employed women and rich wealth quintile were significantly associated with lower risk of anemia (14).

Despite the high prevalence of anemia among lactating mothers particularly in developing countries, information on the magnitude of anemia and its determinant factors among lactating mothers remains unclear. In addition, few studies conducted were at the country level and different parts of countries. Therefore, the purpose of this study is to determine the magnitude of anemia among lactating mothers and its determinant factors in East Africa. As a result, the finding from this study will be helpful for health planners, decision-makers, and health professionals in understanding the burden of anemia among lactating mothers and in designing evidence-based interventions in the region.

Abbreviations: AIC, Akaike information criterion; AOR, adjusted odds ratio; BIC, Bayesian information criterion; CI, confidence interval; DHS, Demography and Health Surveys; GLMM, generalized linear mixed models; ICC, intra-cluster correlation coefficient; IR, individual record; UN, United Nation.

METHODS

Study Setting

According to the classification of the United Nations (UN), the African continent is subdivided into five regions. Among these regions, East Africa is one of the largest regions that includes 19 countries (Burundi, Comoros, Djibouti, Ethiopia, Eritrea, Kenya, Madagascar, Malawi, Mauritius, Mozambique, Reunion, Rwanda, Seychelles, Somalia, Somaliland, Tanzania, Uganda, Zambia, and Zimbabwe). The current study was conducted based on the Demographic and Health Surveys (DHS) data. From these 19 East African countries, six countries (Djibouti, Somalia, Somaliland, Seychelles, Mauritius, and Reunion) have no DHS data. Among the rest 13 countries that have DHS data, two countries have DHS data that was conducted before 2010 (Eritrea-2002 and Madagascar-2008) and two countries (Kenya and Comoros) did not assess anemia levels. Therefore, we included the nine countries that conducted DHS after 2010.

Data Source

The data of these nine East African countries were taken from the DHS program official database www.measuredhs.com after authorization was approved as a result of an online request made by clarifying the aim of this study. DHS is a nationally representative household survey that contains data from a wide variety of population, health, and nutrition tracking and effect assessment measures with face-to-face interviews of women aged 15–49. It also adopts standardized methods involving uniform questionnaires, manuals, and field procedures. Three types of sampling—stratified, multistage, and random—are used in the survey. In each country, information was obtained from qualified women aged 15–49 years. Detailed survey techniques and methods of sampling used to collect data have been reported elsewhere (13). Dependent and independent variables were extracted from the individual record (IR file) data set. From nine East African countries, a total weighted sample of 25,425 lactating mothers was included in the study.

Study Variables

The dependent variable of the present study was anemia status. The outcome variable was binary and it was coded as 1 if the lactating mother is anemic and 0 if the lactating mother is non-anemic. Based on different literatures, age, marital status, educational level, current work status, place of residence, wealth index, sex of head of household, age of head of household, cigarette smoking, media exposure, visited by fieldworker in the last 12 months, visited a health facility in the last 12 months, parity, antenatal care, place of delivery, current pregnancy, and use of family planning were considered as independent variables.

Data Processing and Statistical Analysis

Data processing and analysis were done using STATA 14 software. The data were weighted using sampling weight, primary sampling unit, and strata before any statistical analysis was made in an attempt to restore the representativeness of the survey and

TABLE 1 | Model comparison between fixed effect and mixed effect logistic regression.

Proposed model	AIC value	BIC value	ICC (95% CI)
Fixed effect logistic regression	30514.99	30847.19	Not applicable
Mixed effect logistic regression	30462.71	30803.01	0.17 (0.12, 0.24)

AIC, Akaike information criterion; BIC, Bayesian information criterion; CI, confidence interval; ICC, intra-cluster correlation coefficient.

to tell the STATA to take into account the sampling design when calculating SEs to get reliable statistical estimates. In addition, cross-tabulations and summary statistics were conducted to describe the study population.

Since the DHS data have a hierarchical nature, lactating mothers within a cluster may be more similar to each other than lactating mothers in the other clusters. Due to this, the assumption of independence of observations and equal variance across clusters might be violated. Therefore, an advanced statistical model is necessary to take into account the between cluster variability to get a reliable SE and unbiased estimate. Accordingly, both fixed and mixed effects were fitted. Model comparison was done based on the Akaike and Bayesian information criteria (AIC and BIC). The intra-cluster correlation coefficient (ICC) was also computed to measure the variation between clusters. A mixed-effect model [Generalized Linear Mixed Model (GLMM)] with the lowest Information Criteria (AIC and BIC) was selected (**Table 1**). Variables with a $p \leq 0.05$ were declared as significant determinants of anemia.

RESULTS

Sociodemographic Characteristics

In this study, a total weighted sample of 25,425 lactating mothers from nine East African countries was included in the analysis. The larger proportion (18.32%) of the participants were from Ethiopia. The majority of lactating mothers (24.99%) included in the study were in the age range of 20–24 years. Most (86.04%) of the study participants were married at the time of the survey. More than half (50.62%) of the study participants attended primary level of education, and 55.05% were working at the time of the survey.

More than three-fourth (81.03%) of the lactating mothers were from rural areas, and the majority (47.53%) of them were from households with the poor wealth quintile. Regarding the age and sex of the household head, about 18.05% and more than three-fourth (78.22%) of respondents were in the age range of 25–29 years and from male-headed households, respectively (**Table 2**).

Behavioral and Obstetric Factors

Almost all (99.38%) of the study participants were no-smokers, and more than half (59.44%) had media exposure. About 74.57% of the study participants visited health facilities, and only 17.07% were visited by fieldworkers in the past 12 months preceding the survey. More than three-fourth (77.45%) of the pregnant

TABLE 2 | Sociodemographic characteristics of respondents for the study on magnitudes of anemia and its determinant factors among lactating mothers in East African countries, 2021.

Variables	Anemia		Weighted frequency	Percent
	Yes	No		
Age				
15–19	1,093	1,551	2,644	10.40
20–24	2,252	4,103	6,355	24.99
25–29	2,147	4,186	6,333	24.91
30–34	1,761	3,236	4,997	19.66
35–39	1,241	2,084	3,325	13.08
40–44	547	882	1,429	5.62
45–49	150	192	342	1.34
Marital status				
Never married	603	971	1,574	6.19
Currently married	7,763	14,113	21,876	86.04
Formerly/ever married	825	1,150	1,975	7.77
Educational level				
Uneducated	3,129	4,421	7,550	29.70
Primary	4,569	8,302	12,871	50.62
Secondary	1,360	3,137	4,497	17.69
Higher	133	374	507	1.99
Currently working				
No	4,119	7,308	11,427	44.95
Yes	5,072	8,926	13,998	55.05
Place of residence				
Urban	1,637	3,185	4,822	18.97
Rural	7,554	13,049	20,603	81.03
Country				
Burundi	1,329	1,626	2,955	11.63
Ethiopia	1,316	3,341	4,657	18.32
Malawi	599	1,436	2,035	8.01
Mozambique	2,230	1,971	4,201	16.52
Rwanda	366	1,527	1,893	7.44
Tanzania	1,618	1,878	3,496	13.75
Uganda	522	1,023	1,545	6.08
Zambia	830	2,176	3,006	11.82
Zimbabwe	381	1,256	1,637	6.44
Wealth index				
Poor	4,761	7,323	12,084	47.53
Middle	1,815	3,311	5,126	20.16
Rich	2,615	5,600	8,215	32.31
Sex of head of household				
Male	7,011	12,877	19,888	78.22
Female	2,180	3,357	5,537	20.99
Age of head of household				
15–19	103	119	222	0.88
20–24	804	1,373	2,177	8.56
25–29	1,614	2,975	4,589	18.05
30–34	1,628	3,325	4,953	19.48
35–39	1,525	2,706	4,231	16.64
40–44	1,044	1,905	2,949	11.60
45–49	813	1,194	2,007	7.89
>49	1,660	2,637	4,297	16.90

TABLE 3 | Responses on behavioral and obstetric factors for the study on prevalence and associated factors of anemia among lactating mothers in East African countries, 2021.

Variables	Anemia		Weighted frequency	Percent
	Yes	No		
Cigarette smoking				
No	9,131	16,136	25,267	99.38
Yes	60	98	158	0.62
Media exposure				
No	3,820	6,493	10,313	40.56
Yes	5,371	9,741	15,112	59.44
Visited by field worker in last 12 months				
No	7,948	13,137	21,085	82.93
Yes	1,243	3,097	4,340	17.07
Visited health facility last 12 months				
No	2,292	4,173	6,465	25.43
Yes	6,899	12,061	18,960	74.57
Parity				
Prim-Para	2,081	3,653	5,734	22.55
Multipara	7,110	12,581	19,691	77.45
Antenatal care				
No	876	1,396	2,272	8.94
Yes	8,315	14,838	23,153	91.06
Place of delivery				
Home	3,098	4,425	7,523	29.59
Health facility	6,093	11,809	17,902	70.41
Currently pregnant				
No	16,003	9,073	25,076	98.63
Yes	118	231	349	1.37
Family planning used				
No	6,710	9,033	15,743	61.92
Yes	2,481	7,201	9,682	38.08

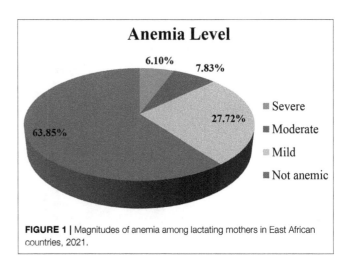

FIGURE 1 | Magnitudes of anemia among lactating mothers in East African countries, 2021.

women were multiparous and the majority (91.06%) had an ANC follow-up. Around 38.08% of the pregnant women reported that they used family planning and more than two-thirds (70.46%) delivered at health facilities (**Table 3**).

Magnitudes of Anemia Among Lactating Mothers

The overall prevalence of anemia among lactating mothers in East African countries was 36.15% [95% confidence interval (CI): 35.55, 36.75%]. Regarding the severity of anemia among lactating mothers, 6.10% had a severe form of anemia, and the majority (27.72%) and 7.83% had mild and moderate anemia, respectively (**Figure 1**). The highest prevalence of anemia was reported among lactating mothers from Mozambique (53.08%) followed by those from Tanzania (46.28%), whereas the lowest prevalence was from Rwanda (19.33%). The prevalence of anemia was highest (43.86%) among lactating mothers in the age group of 45–49 years and lowest (33.90%) in the age group of 25–29 years (**Table 2**).

Factors Associated With Anemia Among Lactating Mothers

Age of mother, educational status, working status, country of residence, wealth index, being visited by fieldworker within 12 months, ANC visit, being pregnant, place of delivery, and family planning usage were significant predictors of anemia among lactating mothers (**Table 4**).

The odds of having anemia decreased by 14% [adjusted odds ratio (AOR) = 0.86, 95% CI: 0.76, 0.97], 16% (AOR = 0.84, 95% CI: 0.73, 0.96), and 16% (AOR = 0.84, 95% CI: 0.73, 0.98) among lactating mothers aged 20–24, 25–29, and 30–34 years, respectively, as compared to those aged 15–19 years. The likelihood of being anemic was 13% (AOR = 0.87, 95% CI: 0.80, 0.94) lower among lactating mothers with a primary level of education compared to those who are uneducated. Anemia prevalence was lower by 13% (AOR = 0.87, 95% CI: 0.80, 0.94) among pregnant women who were working at the time of the survey as compared to those who were not working at the time of the survey.

The odds of having anemia were 2.02 (AOR = 2.02, 95% CI: 1.73, 2.36), 1.37 (AOR = 1.37, 95% CI: 1.16, 1.60), 2.47 (AOR = 2.47, 95% CI: 2.15, 2.84), 2.44 (AOR = 2.44, 95% CI: 2.10, 2.82), and 1.40 (AOR = 1.40, 95% CI: 1.18, 1.66) times higher among lactating mothers from Burundi, Malawi, Mozambique, Tanzania, and Uganda, respectively, as compared to those from Ethiopia. On the other hand, the likelihood of having anemia decreased by 32% (AOR = 0.68, 95% CI: 0.57, 0.82) among lactating mothers from Rwanda as compared to mothers in Ethiopia.

The odds of having anemia decreased by 13% (AOR = 0.87, 95% CI: 0.80, 0.95) and 20% (AOR = 0.80, 95% CI: 0.74, 0.88) among pregnant women from households in the middle and rich wealth quintiles, respectively, as compared to those in poor wealth quintiles. The likelihood of lactating mothers was anemic and lower by 9% (AOR = 0.91, 95% CI: 0.84, 0.99) among mothers who were visited by fieldworkers as compared to those not visited by a fieldworker.

Having an ANC visit decreased the odds of developing anemia among lactating mothers by 15% (AOR = 0.85,

TABLE 4 | Bi-variable and multi-variable mixed effect GLM analysis of anemia among lactating mothers in East African countries, 2021.

Variables	Anemia		Odds Ratio [95% CI]		P-value
	Yes	No	COR	AOR	
Age					
15–19	1,093	1,551	1	1	
20–24	2,252	4,103	0.79 [0.71, 0.88]	**0.86 [0.76, 0.97]**	**0.012**
25–29	2,147	4,186	0.77 [0.70, 0.86]	**0.84 [0.73, 0.96]**	**0.013**
30–34	1,761	3,236	0.78 [0.70, 0.87]	**0.84 [0.73, 0.98]**	**0.024**
35–39	1,241	2,084	0.90 [0.80, 1.01]	0.91 [0.74, 1.06]	0.213
40–44	547	882	0.90 [0.77, 1.05]	0.85 [0.70, 1.01]	0.071
45–49	150	192	1.06 [0.82, 1.39]	0.90 [0.68, 1.19]	0.464
Marital status					
Currently married	7,763	14,113	1	1	
Never married	603	971	1.22 [1.08, 1.37]	1.04 [0.91, 1.20]	0.506
Formerly/ever married	825	1,150	1.21 [1.08, 1.35]	1.03 [0.92, 1.16]	0.621
Educational level					
Uneducated	3,129	4,421	1	1	
Primary	4,569	8,302	0.75 [0.70, 0.80]	**0.87 [0.80, 0.94]**	**<0.001**
Secondary	1,360	3,137	0.64 [0.59, 0.71]	0.90 [0.80, 1.01]	0.055
Higher	133	374	0.60 [0.48, 0.75]	1.08 [0.86, 1.36]	0.483
Currently working					
No	4,119	7,308	1	1	
Yes	5,072	8,926	0.89 [0.83, 0.95]	**0.89 [0.83, 0.95]**	**0.001**
Place of residence					
Urban	1,637	3,185	1	1	
Rural	7,554	13,049	1.25 [1.14, 1.36]	1.03 [0.93, 1.13]	0.575
Country					
Ethiopia	1,316	3,341	1	1	1
Burundi	1,329	1,626	1.65 [1.44, 1.90]	**2.02 [1.73, 2.36]**	**<0.001**
Malawi	599	1,436	0.95 [0.82, 1.09]	**1.37 [1.16, 1.60]**	**<0.001**
Mozambique	2,230	1,971	2.44 [2.14, 2.78]	**2.47 [2.15, 2.84]**	**<0.001**
Rwanda	366	1,527	0.48 [0.40, 0.56]	**0.68 [0.57, 0.82]**	**<0.001**
Tanzania	1,618	1,878	1.97 [1.73, 2.25]	**2.44 [2.10, 2.82]**	**<0.001**
Uganda	522	1,023	1.13 [0.97, 1.32]	**1.40 [1.18, 1.66]**	**<0.001**
Zambia	830	2,176	0.84 [0.73, 0.97]	1.04 [0.89, 1.21]	0.616
Zimbabwe	381	1,256	0.68 [0.58, 0.81]	1.01 [0.84, 1.21]	0.943
Wealth index					
Poor	4,761	7,323	1	1	
Middle	1,815	3,311	0.87 [0.80, 0.94]	**0.87 [0.80, 0.95]**	**0.001**
Rich	2,615	5,600	0.75 [0.70, 0.81]	**0.80 [0.74, 0.88]**	**<0.001**
Sex of head of household					
Male	7,011	12,877	1	1	
Female	2,180	3,357	1.14 [1.06, 1.22]	1.06 [0.98, 1.14]	0.165
Age of head of household					
15–19	103	119	1	1	
20–24	804	1,373	0.77 [0.57, 1.05]	0.95 [0.70, 1.30]	0.756
25–29	1,614	2,975	0.74 [0.55, 1.01]	0.99 [0.73, 1.35]	0.958
30–34	1,628	3,325	0.71 [0.53, 0.96]	0.96 [0.71, 1.31]	0.812
35–39	1,525	2,706	0.79 [0.58, 1.06]	0.99 [0.72, 1.35]	0.941
40–44	1,044	1,905	0.78 [0.58, 1.06]	0.96 [0.71, 1.31]	0.806
45–49	813	1,194	0.98 [0.72, 1.33]	1.15 [0.83, 1.58]	0.400
>49	1,660	2,637	0.95 [0.70, 1.28]	1.10 [0.81, 1.50]	0.535

(Continued)

TABLE 4 | Continued

Variables	Anemia		Odds Ratio [95% CI]		P-value
	Yes	**No**	**COR**	**AOR**	
Cigarette smoking					
No	9,131	16,136	1	1	
Yes	60	98	1.173 [0.82, 1.67]	1.08 [0.76, 1.53]	0.668
Media exposure					
No	3,820	6,493	1	1	
Yes	5,371	9,741	0.85 [0.794, 0.90]	0.94 [0.89, 1.01]	0.106
Visited by fieldworker in last 12 months					
No	7,948	13,137	1	1	
Yes	1,243	3,097	0.75 [0.69, 0.82]	**0.91 [0.84, 0.99]**	**0.037**
Visited health facility last 12 months					
No	2,292	4,173	1	1	
Yes	6,899	12,061	0.97 [0.91, 1.04]	1.01 [0.93, 1.08]	0.929
Parity					
Prim-Para	2,081	3,653	1	1	
Multipara	7,110	12,581	0.99 [0.92, 1.06]	1.01 [0.92, 1.11]	0.772
Antenatal care					
No	876	1,396	1	1	
Yes	8,315	14,838	0.76 [0.67, 0.85]	**0.85 [0.75, 0.97]**	**0.017**
Place of delivery					
Home	3,098	4,425	1	1	
Health facility	6,093	11,809	0.72 [0.67, 0.78]	**0.90 [0.83, 0.98]**	**0.012**
Currently pregnant					
No	16,003	9,073	1	1	
Yes	118	231	0.87 [0.67, 1.12]	**0.77 [0.59, 0.99]**	**0.038**
Family planning used					
No	6,710	9,033			
Yes	2,481	7,201	0.49 [0.46, 0.52]	**0.60 [0.56, 0.65]**	**<0.001**

AOR, Adjusted Odd Ratio; CI, confidence interval; COR, Crude Odd Ratio. The bold values shows variables that have a significant association with anemia.

95% CI: 0.75, 0.97). Similarly, the odds of being anemic decreased by 10% (AOR = 0.90, 95% CI: 0.83, 0.98) among lactating mothers who delivered at the health facility as compared to those who delivered at home.

Lactating mothers who were pregnant at the time of the survey had 23% lower odds of developing anemia (AOR = 0.77, 95% CI: 0.59, 0.99) as compared to those who were not pregnant at the time of the survey. Likewise, family planning usage was associated with a 40% decrease in the odds of having anemia among lactating mothers as compared to mothers who did not use family planning (**Table 3**).

DISCUSSION

Anemia in lactating mothers is an overlooked public health issue that affects both the mother and the newborn (15). Thus, we examined the magnitude and determinant factors of anemia among lactating women in East Africa. Accordingly, the magnitude of anemia in East African countries was found to be 36.5%. In relation to the generalized linear mixed-effect model, age, educational

status, working status, country of residence, wealth index, antenatal care service, place of delivery, history of using family planning, delivery at a health facility, being pregnant, and visited by fieldworkers in the last 12 months were factors that have a significant association with anemia in lactating mothers.

In this study, the prevalence of anemia among lactating mothers in East African countries was 36.5%, which is comparable to the study done in India (15). In addition, the prevalence of anemia observed among lactating mothers in this study was lower than the prevalence in studies conducted in Vietnam and Myanmar (11, 16). This might be because the mothers near and after delivery get enough maternity leave and consume animal products based on the culture and custom of their countries. The highest prevalence of anemia among East African countries was observed in Mozambique (53.08%), whereas the lowest was in Rwanda.

In the present study, the odds of having anemia were low among lactating mothers aged 20-34 years as compared to those aged 15-19 years. This is in-line with different studies that indicate the risk of anemia is greater in the later age group (17). Furthermore, in this study, the risk of anemia is lower by 13% in lactating mothers with education which is in-line with the study done in India (2).

On the other hand, the odds of having anemia are decreased as the wealth quantile is increased. This is in-line with the study done in Myanmar (11), and this might be because those lactating mothers with better socioeconomic status may access a balanced diet and buy a variety of iron-containing foods that help decrease the anemia incidence. Likewise, the likelihood of having anemia decreased among the lactating mothers who were visited by a fieldworker. This may imply that strengthening the fieldworker visits might decrease the anemia prevalence.

Moreover, lactating mothers with ANC follow-up had a decreased odd of having anemia. This is comparable with the study done in India (2). This could be because iron supplementation during pregnancy was provided to those who had ANC visits and decreased the prevalence of anemia. Besides, the current study documented that the odds of anemia among lactating mothers who delivered at the health facility were low as compared to their counterparts. This finding is in agreement with studies done in India (2), and this might be because the risk of hemorrhage among those lactating mothers who delivered at health institutions is lower. If it is happening in the context of skilled delivery, it can be easily managed, and this may contribute to the decrement of anemia.

Additionally, lactating mothers who were pregnant at the time of the survey had lower odds of developing anemia, which contradicts the study done in Ethiopia (18). This might be due to the ever-increasing coverage of maternal health services for pregnant mothers.

Furthermore, the odds of anemia in lactating mothers decreased among those who used family planning. This finding is in-line with studies done in Ethiopia (19, 20). This might be explained by the rationale that those lactating mothers who use family planning may have frequent contact with the health professional and in the process they may get additional nutritional advice that may contribute to decreasing anemia.

The current study has its strengths and limitations. The first strength is attributed to the use of a large sample size and nationally representative data set of each included country. Second, by considering the clustered nature of the data, the advanced model was applied. On the other hand, coming to the limitations of the present study, the findings might not be representative of all the East African countries, for some

countries have no DHS program, some did not assess anemia level, and some have old DHS data.

CONCLUSION

In East Africa, more than one-third of lactating mothers have anemia. The odds of anemia were significantly low among mothers aged 15–34 years, who had primary education, were working, country of residence, and had higher wealth index (middle and high). In addition, the likelihood of anemia was also low among lactating mothers who had antenatal care, used family planning, delivered in the health facility, were pregnant during the survey, and visited by fieldworkers. Therefore, promoting maternal care services (family planning, ANC, and health facility delivery) and a field visit by health extension workers is strongly recommended.

ETHICS STATEMENT

We requested Demography and Health Surveys (DHS) Program, and permission to download and use the data for this study from http://www.dhsprogram.com was approved by the 152155 reference number. What is more, there are no individual identifiers reported in any part of this manuscript. All the data management and analysis strictly followed the standard indicated in the manuals of DHS.

AUTHOR CONTRIBUTIONS

The conception of the study, design of the study, acquisition of data, analysis, and interpretation of data were conducted by BT. Data curation, drafting the article, revising it critically for intellectual content, validation, and final approval of the version to be published were done by AW, NB, and DE. All authors have read and approved the final manuscript.

ACKNOWLEDGMENTS

We thank DHS for providing the data for this study.

REFERENCES

Zopfs D, Rinneburger M, Pinto dos Santos D, Reimer RP, Laukamp KR, Maintz D, et al. Evaluating anemia using contrast-enhanced spectral detector CT of the chest in a large cohort of 522 patients. *Eur Radiol.* (2020) 31:4350– 7. doi: 10.1007/s00330-020-07497-y

Siddiqui MZ, Goli S, Reja T, Doshi R, Chakravorty S, Tiwari C. et al.

Prevalence of anemia and its determinants among pregnant, lactating, and nonpregnant nonlactating women in India. *Matern Child Health J.* (2017) 7:2158244017725555. doi: 10.1177/2158244017725555

Milman N. Anemia—still a major health problem in many parts of the world! *Annals of Hematology.* (2011) 90:369–77. doi: 10.1007/s00277-010-1144-5

Sunuwar DR, Singh DR, Chaudhary NK, Pradhan PMS, Rai P, Tiwari K. Prevalence and factors associated with anemia among women of reproductive age in seven South and Southeast Asian countries: Evidence from nationally representative surveys. *PLoS ONE.* (2020) 15:e0236449. doi: 10.1371/journal.pone.0236449

Chaparro CM, Suchdev PS. Anemia epidemiology, pathophysiology, and etiology in low- and middle-income countries. *Ann N Y Acad Sci.* (2019) 1450:15–31. doi: 10.1111/nyas.14092

Liyew AM, Teshale AB. Individual and community level factors associated with anemia among lactating mothers in Ethiopia using data from Ethiopian demographic and health survey, 2016; a multilevel analysis. *BMC Public Health.* (2020) 20:775.

Kebede A, Gerensea H, Amare F, Tesfay Y, Teklay G. The magnitude of anemia and associated factors among pregnant women attending public institutions of Shire Town, Shire, Tigray, Northern Ethiopia, 2018. *BMC Res Notes.* (2018) 11:595. doi: 10.1186/s13104-018-3706-x

Gardner W, Kassebaum N. Global, regional, and national prevalence of anemia and its causes in 204 countries and territories, 1990–2019. *Curr Dev Nutr.* (2020) 4:830. doi: 10.1093/cdn/nzaa053_035

De Benoist B, Cogswell M, Egli I, McLean E. *Worldwide Prevalence of Anaemia 1993–2005.* WHO Global Database of Anaemia (2008).

Chandyo RK, Henjum S, Ulak M, Thorne-Lyman AL, Ulvik RJ, Shrestha PS. et al. The prevalence of anemia and iron deficiency is more common in breastfed infants than their mothers in Bhaktapur, Nepal. *Eur J Clin Nutr.* (2016) 70:456–62. doi: 10.1038/ejcn.2015.199

Zhao A, Zhang Y, Li B, Wang P, Li J, Xue Y. et al. Prevalence of anemia and its risk factors among lactating mothers in Myanmar. *Am J Trop Med Hyg.* (2014) 90:963–7. doi: 10.4269/ajtmh.13-0660

Feleke BE, Feleke TE. Pregnant mothers are more anemic than lactating mothers, a comparative cross-sectional study, Bahir Dar, Ethiopia. *BMC Hematology.* (2018) 18:2. doi: 10.1186/s12878-018-0096-1

Julla BW, Haile A, Ayana G, Eshetu S, Kuche D, Asefa T. Chronic energy deficiency and associated factors among lactating mothers (15-49 years old) in Offa Woreda, Wolayita Zone, SNNPRs, Ethiopia. *World Sci Res.* (2018) 5:13–23. doi: 10.20448/journal.510.2018.51.13.23

Seifu B, Yilma DJBRJ. Prevalence and associated factors of anemia among lactating women in ethiopia from 2010 to 2020: a systematic review and meta-analysis. 2020;5(2):327-42.

Zhao A, Zhang J, Wu W, Wang P. Zhang YJAPjocn. Postpartum anemia is a neglected public health issue in China: a cross-sectional study. *Asia Pac J Clin Nutr.* (2019) 28:793.

Trinh LTT, Dibley MJAPjocn. Anaemia in pregnant, postpartum and non pregnant women in Lak district, Daklak province of Vietnam. *Asia Pac J Clin Nutr.* (2007) 16:310-5.

Pinho-Pompeu M, Surita FG, Pastore DA, Paulino DSM. Pinto e Silva JLJTJoM-F, Medicine N. Anemia in pregnant adolescents: impact of treatment on perinatal outcomes. *J Matern Fetal Neonatal Med.* (2017) 30:1158– 62. doi: 10.1080/14767058.2016.1205032

Kibret KT, Chojenta C, D'Arcy E. Loxton DJBo. Spatial distribution and determinant factors of anaemia among women of reproductive age in Ethiopia: a multilevel and spatial analysis. *BMJ Open.* (2019) 9:e027276. doi: 10.1136/bmjopen-2018-027276

Liyew AM, Teshale ABJBPH. Individual and community level factors associated with anemia among lactating mothers in Ethiopia using data from Ethiopian demographic and health survey, 2016; a multilevel analysis. *BMC Public Health.* (2020) 20:1–11. doi: 10.1186/s12889-020- 08934-9

Lakew Y, Biadgilign S, Haile DJBo. Anaemia prevalence and associated factors among lactating mothers in Ethiopia: evidence from the 2005 and 2011 demographic and health surveys. *BMJ Open.* (2015) 5:e006001. doi: 10.1136/bmjopen-2014-006001

23

Reducing Anemia Among School-Aged Children in China by Eliminating the Geographic Disparity and Ameliorating Stunting: Evidence from a National Survey

Jun-Yi Wang[1], Pei-Jin Hu[1], Dong-Mei Luo[1], Bin Dong[1], Yinghua Ma[1], Jie Dai[1], Yi Song[1*], Jun Ma[1] and Patrick W. C. Lau[2]*

[1] Institute of Child and Adolescent Health, Peking University School of Public Health, National Health Commission Key Laboratory of Reproductive Health, Beijing, China, [2] Department of Sport and Physical Education, Hong Kong Baptist University, Kowloon Tong, China

Correspondence:
Yinghua Ma
yinghuama@bjmu.edu.cn
Yi Song
songyi@bjmu.edu.cn

Background: The aim of this study was to assess the geographic disparity in anemia and whether stunting was associated with anemia in different geographic groups among school-aged children in China.

Methods: 71,129 Han children aged 7, 9, 12, and 14 years old were extracted from the 2014 cycle of Chinese National Surveys on Children Constitution and Health. Anemia, anemia severity, and stunting were defined according to WHO definitions. Binary logistic regression models were used to estimate the association between anemia and stunting in different geographic groups.

Results: The prevalence of anemia was significantly higher in girls (10.8%) than boys (7.0%). The highest anemia prevalence was in Group VII (lower class/rural, 12.0%). A moderate/severe prevalence of anemia was concentrated in Group VII and Group VIII (western/lower class/rural) for both sexes. The prevalence of anemia was higher in stunting boys than non-stunting boys in Group IV (lower class/city, $\chi^2 = 12.78$, $P = 0.002$) and Group VII ($\chi^2 = 6.21$, $P = 0.018$), while for girls, it was higher in stunting girls than their non-stunting peers only in Group II (upper class/large city, $\chi^2 = 4.57$, $P = 0.046$). Logistic regression showed that the stunting children have 30% higher risk of anemia than non-stunting children after adjustment for age, sex and school (OR = 1.30, 95% CI: 1.05–1.60).

Conclusion: A significant geographic disparity and an association between anemia and stunting among specific groups of school-aged children in China was demonstrated. Consequently, eliminating the geographic disparity and ameliorating stunting might contribute to the improvement of Chinese children's anemia. Specific guidelines and interventions are needed, especially for adolescent girls and the groups with serious anemia burden.

Keywords: anemia, geographic disparity, stunting, children, China

INTRODUCTION

Anemia, or low concentrations of hemoglobin (Hb), adversely affects cognitive and motor development and study capacity, and increases susceptibility to infection, which also exerts a substantial economic burden on the government (1, 2). Globally, 1.62 billion people suffer with anemia and the prevalence among children was 25.4%, according to a World Health Organization (WHO) (3) report. Asia is the hardest hit, especially in South Asia (4, 5), where an improvement in children's hemoglobin status may lead to a modest global increase in mean hemoglobin and a reduction in anemia prevalence. Globally, anemia is affecting people in both developed and developing countries with different health risks, and almost all age groups and both sexes are susceptible. Even for developed countries, such as Sweden, France, Australia, Denmark, Belgium, and Ireland, anemia prevalence has changed little during past two decades (6). Although iron deficiency anemia is the true indicator of poor nutritional status, considering that 90–95% of anemia cases in China are due to iron deficiency (7), anemia remains useful as an indicator of undernutrition and is particularly relevant for adolescents in the context of rapid growth and menstruation. Compared with children under five and pregnant women, adolescents have not been paid much attention. In 2016, 333 million adolescents with anemia lived in multi-burden settings, of which 194 million lived in India and China according to GBD (Global Burden of Disease study) data (6). Although the prevalence of anemia in China has declined in the past two decades at the national level (8), it was as high as 14.8% in some rural regions like Shanxi (9, 10). Nationwide, more than 19.2 million Chinese children were anemic and 389,198 had severe anemia in 2010, based on a total number of children aged 7–18 years (194,599,052). Nevertheless, updated information of geographic disparity on anemia among Chinese children is unclear. This information is urgently needed as it may provide a solid foundation to alleviate the geographic disparity of anemia among Chinese children.

In China, most anemia is due to prolonged iron deficiency, which impairs hemoglobin production and limits the amount of oxygen that red blood cells carry throughout the body and to the brain (11). Stunting is also a big issue in China and warrants monitoring because it is an undervalued indicator which reflects the cumulative effect of undernutrition with socioeconomic and other factors. These factors may contribute to anemia. Studies in Haiti and Angola confirmed that stunting increased the risks of developing anemia (12, 13). The question is still uncertain as to whether stunting is associated with anemia in China, especially in school-aged children who have been largely under-investigated. Moreover, if the association exists, does it vary or remain similar in different settings and populations?

Hemoglobin data from children aged 7 to 14 of both sexes across China was collected in the 2014 Chinese National Surveys on Students' Constitution and Health (CNSSCH). It provided a valuable opportunity to update the available information on anemia among school-aged children who have been largely neglected in research in China, compared with numerous publications on children under five and pregnant women (14).

The objectives of the present study were to: (1) delineate the geographic disparity of anemia; (2) identify the most susceptible population with the heaviest burden of anemia; and (3) examine the association between anemia and stunting, and the relationships across different geographic groups.

MATERIALS AND METHODS

Data was extracted from the 2014 cycle of CNSSCH, which was a large-scale cross-sectional survey of school-aged children conducted by six relevant ministries including the Ministries of Education, Health, Science and Technology, the State Ethnic Affairs Commission, and the State Sports General Administration, China. It spanned 31 provinces, excluding Hong Kong, Macau, and Taiwan. The sampling procedure, as previously described in detail (14), was the same in all CNSSCH survey sites. In brief, this survey was to investigate children's health status in China and used a multistage stratified cluster sampling design (14). In the first stage of sampling, in order to achieve better representation within the 30 provinces, populations were stratified by three socioeconomic indicator groups or three sets of prefecture-level cities (i.e., upper, moderate, low) at the regional level, defined by regional gross domestic product, total yearly income per capita, average food consumption per capita, natural growth rate of the population, and the regional social welfare index. In each group of three sub-provincial levels, one city was selected randomly and remained constant from the first survey in 1985. Within these sub-province regions, populations were also stratified by urban and rural area of residence. Within these stratified areas, a random selection of schools, including primary school, middle school, and high school, was conducted according to the established procedures. In the second stage, sampling took place in classes (primary sampling units or clusters) selected randomly from each grade in these schools, and all students in the selected class were included and listed in the investigation after meeting the inclusion criteria and after obtaining verbally informed consent from both students and their parents. Finally, within the primary sampling units, namely every age from 7 to 18 years for boys and girls, at least 50 Han ethnicity students, the minimum sample size, were included in the survey and sampling yielded equal numbers of the three socioeconomic indicator groups. Thus, the sample weight remained consistent in each age, sex, region (urban/rural), city (three socioeconomic indicators' groups at sub-province level), and province for students aged 7–18 years in each survey year. The participants in this study were Han children aged 7, 9, 12, and 14 years old from 26 provinces and four municipalities, except for Tibet (where the Han ethnicity is a minority). The children were recruited in this study if their parents and themselves had lived in their local regions more than a year.

Participants underwent a medical examination prior to the national survey and were excluded if they had one or more of the following conditions: (1) serious organ disease (e.g., heart, lung, liver, kidney); (2) abnormal physical development (e.g., pygmyism, gigantism); (3) physical impairment or deformity (e.g., severe scoliosis, pectus carinatum, limp, genu valgum, and gunu varum); or (4) acute disease symptoms (e.g., diarrhea, fever) during the past month and not yet recovered. Consequently, 71,129 children with complete data records on age, sex, urban/rural groups, height, weight and hemoglobin concentration were included in the analysis. Moreover, the ratio of boys/girls or urban/rural groups was approximately equal to 1:1 of each sex- and age-specific subgroup. The project was approved by the Medical Research Ethics Committee of Peking University Health Science Center (IRB00001052-18002). With data collected from schools across China, the school principals were able to determine the process for gaining informed consent from children's parents or guardians. All participants' information was anonymized and de-identified prior to analysis to protect their privacy.

Measures

Participants were required to wear light clothing and stand straight, barefoot, and at ease when height was measured. The heel, humerus, and shoulders were contacted to form a "three-point, one-line" standing position. Measurements were conducted by a team of trained field professionals who were required to pass a training course in anthropometric measurements. Height was measured to the nearest 0.1 cm with a portable stadiometer. The stadiometers were calibrated before use. The measurements were carried out at the same time of the day during the survey (better to be specific, e.g., morning, afternoon, during school recess, etc.). Height-for-age Z-score (HAZ) was calculated by using WHO 2007 references with the fixed population. Stunting was defined using the growth references of HAZ: stunting: $<-2SD$ (15, 16).

Hemoglobin concentration was measured by laboratory technicians for the participants in the selected school. Hemoglobin concentration was measured by HemoCue201+ (Origin: Sweden, Model: HemoCue201$^+$, Manufacturer: HemoCue AB) (17). Data collection was supervised as follows by well-trained on-site investigators: (a) the capillary blood sample was collected from the fingertip after discarding the first drop, and a small amount of blood was pressed out onto the fingertips. The blood was taken continuously with a micro cuvette, (b) the micro cuvette was inserted into the cuvette tank and reacted for 15s to 60s, (c) the score was determined and recorded on site (18). Age specific cut-off values of hemoglobin concentration were used to define anemia. Hemoglobin concentration was defined by using WHO criteria (19, 20) and categorized as: (1) for children aged 5 to 11 year: $\geq$115 g/L normal, <115 g/L anemia, 110–114 g/L mild anemia, $\leq$109 moderate/severe prevalence anemia; (2) for children aged 12–14 year: $\geq$120 g/L normal, <120 g/L anemia, 110–119 g/L mild anemia, $\leq$109 g/L moderate/severe prevalence anemia.

In order to compare the prevalence of anemia in different geographic groups with different socioeconomic status (SES), all subgroups were further divided into eight categories (21): Group I (large coastal city), Group II (upper class/large city), Group III (middle class/city), Group IV (lower class/city), Group V (upper class/rural), Group VI (middle class/rural), Group VII (lower class/rural), and Group VIII (western/lower class/rural). Group I included the nine largest cities (Beijing, Shanghai, Tianjin, Shijiazhuang, Shenyang, Dalian, Jinan, Qingdao, and

Nanjing) and Group II represented the upper urban class. Group VIII constituted the other extreme: rural regions in western provinces, home to the lowest SES class (data was shown in **Figure 1**).

Statistical Analyses

The prevalence of anemia in the Han children was described by sex, age, and geographic groups. Chi-square test was used to assess the difference of the prevalence and categories of anemia among different subgroups, while the inspection level was adjusted by Bonferroni method [$\alpha' = 2\alpha/k(k-1)$, k = 7]. To assess the geographic difference of association between anemia and stunting, binary logistic regression analyses were conducted with adjustments for sex and age. The design effect of cluster sampling by school was also added in the model. All analyses were conducted using Stata 12.1 (Stata Corp, College Station, Texas). A 2-sided P-value of <0.05 was considered significant.

RESULTS

The Prevalence of Anemia in Different Geographic Groups

As shown in **Table S1**, the prevalence of anemia was significantly higher in girls (10.8%) than boys (7.0%). The highest anemia prevalence was in Group VII (12.0%). The lowest prevalence of anemia was observed in Group I (5.2%), Group V (6.0%), and Group II (7.6%). The prevalence of anemia in Group I was more than twice that of Group VII. **Table S2** demonstrates that the moderate/severe prevalence of anemia was concentrated in Group VII and Group VIII for both sexes. The prevalence of anemia at each age group was similar to the total sample and the highest prevalence of anemia was found in the age 7 group, followed by 12 years, and the lowest prevalence was the 14-year-old boys group. For girls, those aged 12 and 14 years had significantly higher anemia prevalence than those of 7 and 9 years (data was shown in **Table S3**).

The Prevalence of Anemia in Susceptible Population

Girls had a higher prevalence of anemia than boys across different groups. The prevalence of anemia among girls in Group VII was 4–5 times higher than boys in Group I (**Table S1**). **Table 1** and **Table S4** indicate that the prevalence of anemia among stunting children was higher than their non-stunting counterparts. When stratified by sex, the prevalence of anemia was higher in stunting boys than non-stunting boys in Group IV ($\chi^2 = 12.78$, $P = 0.002$) and Group VII ($\psi^2 = 6.21$, $P = 0.018$), while for girls, the anemia prevalence was higher in stunting girls than their non-stunting peers only in Group II ($\chi^2 = 4.57$, $P = 0.046$).

The Association Between Anemia and Stunting Stratified by Geographic Groups and Sex

As shown in **Table 2**, the stunting children have a 30% higher risk of anemia than non-stunting children (OR = 1.30, 95% CI: 1.05–1.60). When stratified by geographic group, the association strengths ranged from 1.41 to 2.34 in Group II, III, IV, VI, and

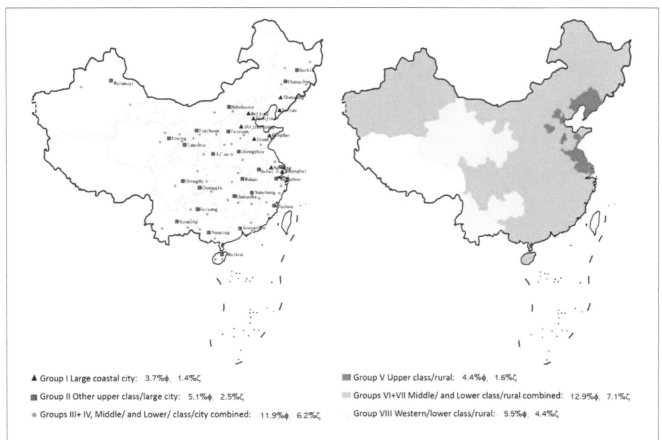

▲ Group I Large coastal city: 3.7%φ, 1.4%ζ

■ Group II Other upper class/large city: 5.1%φ, 2.5%ζ

● Groups III+ IV, Middle/ and Lower/ class/city combined: 11.9%φ, 6.2%ζ

Group V Upper class/rural: 4.4%φ, 1.6%ζ

Groups VI+VII Middle/ and Lower class/rural combined: 12.9%φ, 7.1%ζ

Group VIII Western/lower class/rural: 5.5%φ, 4.4%ζ

FIGURE 1 | The distribution of different geographic groups with different socioeconomic status (SES); note: φ the prevalence of mild anemia in 2014, ζ the prevalence of moderate/severe anemia in 2014.

VIII but with 95% CI overlap, while there was no significant association between anemia and stunting in Group I, V, and VII. After stratifying by sex, stunting boys were 1.74 times more likely to be anemic than non-stunting boys while there was no significant association between stunting and anemia among girls. The results of the associations by age stratification were consistent with total sample (data not shown).

DISCUSSION

In the present study, by using data from the 2014 CNSSCH covering 26 provinces and four municipalities in China, not only were the differences in the prevalence of anemia among school-aged children by geographic groups, sex, and stunting status documented, but also the major associations between anemia and stunting in school-aged children. On the whole, the prevalence of anemia was significantly higher in girls than in boys, and in addition there was low prevalence of anemia in areas with good economic conditions. However, some regions, such as the poorer rural setting of Group VII and middle-class cities of Group III might be overlooked.

Researchers have pointed out that geographic disparity was related inversely to SES, to wealth at a household level, and to income and education at an individual level (2, 22, 23).

Areas with SES were often geographically good, and also had better health care facilities and services (24). Compared to rural areas, individuals living in better SES have a greater availability of food and better housing, electricity, piped water, sanitation, and transportation. Moreover, these populations usually have a higher educational level, economic status, and employment opportunities. Studies in Indonesia have found child stunting to be associated with poor health care practices, inadequate sanitation and water supply, food insecurity, and low caregiver education (25). Sankar Goswmai's study used the wealth index to reflect the state of SES and the results indicated that, relatively, the poorest area had the highest prevalence of anemia (OR = 2.033, 95% CI:1.71-2.22), while the richer area had lowest prevalence of anemia (OR = 1.183, 95% CI:1.14-1.32) (26). In groups with these good economic development indicators, the prevalence of anemia was low; the study mentioned that a child living in a household in the lowest wealth quintile was 21% more likely to be anemic than were those in the highest wealth quintile (27), which is consistent with the present study. In Group I (large coastal city) and Group II (other upper class/large city), the economic development is relatively high and anemia prevalence is relatively lower than other groups. High quality living environments and facilities due to advanced economic development can contribute to anemia reduction among Chinese

TABLE 1 | The prevalence of anemia stratified by stunting status, geographic group, and sex among Chinese school-aged children.

Group[#]	Boys						Girls					
	Non-stunting		Stunting		χ^2	P	Non-stunting		Stunting		χ^2	P
	N	%	N	%			N	%	N	%		
I	98	3.3	1	5.0	13.39	0.066	207	6.9	0	0.0	0.67	1.000
II	299	6.6	4	14.8	2.92	0.100	388	8.5	6	19.4	4.57	0.046
III	374	7.6	8	13.8	3.06	0.084	619	12.7	13	18.6	2.10	0.150
IV	355	6.8	12	17.9	12.78	0.002	454	8.6	10	14.3	2.80	0.129
V	118	4.0	0	0.0	0.29	1.000	240	8.0	1	11.1	0.11	0.531
VI	295	6.7	8	8.6	0.51	0.408	397	9.1	15	15.0	4.04	0.053
VII	710	9.0	15	6.9	1.05	0.395	1201	15.2	29	12.0	1.92	0.202
VIII	161	8.1	22	13.8	6.21	0.018	225	11.3	19	11.6	0.01	0.898
Total	2,410	6.9	70	11.1	16.89	<0.001	3731	10.7	93	13.4	5.11	<0.001

[#]Group I (large coastal city), Group II (upper class/large city), Group III (middle class/city), Group IV (lower class/city), Group V (upper class/rural), Group VI (middle class/rural), Group VII (lower class/rural), and Group VIII (western/lower class/rural). Group I included the nine largest cities (Beijing, Shanghai, Tianjin, Shijiazhuang, Shenyang, Dalian, Jinan, Qingdao and Nanjing) and Group II, represented the upper urban class. Group VIII constituted the other extreme: rural regions in western provinces, home to the lowest SES class.

TABLE 2 | Association between anemia and stunting stratified by geographic group and sex among Chinese school-aged children.

Group[#]	Total[a]	Boys[b]	Girls[b]
I	1.17 (0.11–12.63)	29.20 (1.81–471.90)*	-
II	2.32 (1.24–4.36)*	2.78 (1.15–6.71)*	2.17 (0.85–5.55)
III	1.76 (1.12–2.77)*	2.13 (1.14–4.01)*	1.48 (0.88–2.50)
IV	2.34 (1.33–4.12)*	3.51 (1.72–7.15)*	1.72 (0.80–3.70)
V	0.99 (0.14–6.74)	-	1.38 (0.20–9.66)
VI	1.78 (1.16–2.72)*	1.89 (0.87–4.10)	1.79 (1.04–3.07)*
VII	0.77 (0.58–1.02)	0.86 (0.49–1.52)	0.73 (0.51–1.06)
VIII	1.41 (1.00–1.99)*	2.05 (1.30–3.22)*	1.03 (0.62–1.72)
Total	1.30 (1.05–1.60)[a]*	1.74 (1.30– 2.35)[a]*	1.09 (0.86–1.38)[b]

[a]Adjusted for age, sex, and group.
[b]Adjusted for age and group.
*Groups were significantly different by multivariate logistic regression analysis, P < 0.05.
(-):the sample size was too small to display the statistics results.
[#]Group I (large coastal city), Group II (upper class/large city), Group III (middle class/city), Group IV (lower class/city), Group V (upper class/rural), Group VI (middle class/rural), Group VII (lower class/rural), and Group VIII (western/lower class/rural). Group I included the nine largest cities (Beijing, Shanghai, Tianjin, Shijiazhuang, Shenyang, Dalian, Jinan, Qingdao and Nanjing) and Group II, represented the upper urban class. Group VIII constituted the other extreme: rural regions in western provinces, home to the lowest SES class.

children (2). A previous study conducted in 32 selected low-income and middle-income countries showed that a child living in a household in the lowest wealth quintile was 21% more likely to be anemic than those in the highest wealth quintile (2). However, the prevalence of anemia did not disappear in Group I and Group II, which indicated that improving the monitoring of anemia, scaling up coverage of prevention, and developing anemia prevention interventions were still needed in China (28, 29).

China has long been concerned about the imbalance of geographic disparity, thus, improving the health of children in rural western China remains a critical health priority (30). The national anemia prevention intervention policy was mainly implemented in the area of Group VIII, i.e., "National Nutrition Improvement Program for Rural Compulsory Education Students (NNIPRCES)" released by the general office of the State Council of China (2011) (31). Even though the prevalence of anemia in Group VIII has been significantly reduced after the implementation of the above policy (32), it is still serious due to its high baseline. Currently, Group VII has replaced Group VIII as the most serious burden of anemia because no extra attention has been given to this group. Other than continuing investment in anemia improvement in rural regions of western provinces, it is recommended that attention should be paid to other areas such as poorer rural settings in China. For example, nutritional education and improvement of diet quality should be included in the content of anemia intervention, to ensure the daily Recommended Dietary Allowance (RDA) of iron-containing foods (meat, milk, etc.) (33). These additional measures may play a more important role in decreasing anemia for vulnerable groups such as children living in western regions, boys with stunting issues, and adolescent girls (14).

Besides Group VII, Group III also had a surprisingly high prevalence of anemia. The higher prevalence of anemia in Group VII indicated that lower economic groups are susceptible and intervention needs to be focused here first, and as such it might be helpful to improve the anemic status by eliminating the geographic disparity. Considering the serious disparity, the government should reconsider the priorities around the anemic burden across the country and develop new strategies and interventions not only to the groups with serious burden, but also those at high risk like Group III.

In the present study, the association between anemia and stunting exists only in boys, but not in girls. Therefore, non-targeted anemia interventions, such as general nutrition improvement, may only work for boys. Ramachandran (34) pointed out that adolescent girls form a crucial segment of the population and constitute the vital "bridge" between the present generation and the next generation. The main reasons for this consequence among girls may be the menstrual bleeding during their puberty and weight loss (35, 36). In order to pursue a slim figure, adolescent girls deliberately lose their body weight by dieting, which may lead to insufficient iron intake (37). Iron deficiency may be a routine consequence of growth and skeletal development (38). Sex differences should be taken into account when implementing anemia interventions. Consequently, it is suggested that all children, especially adolescent girls, need health education due to their vulnerability to anemia (39). Furthermore, reliable measures on the causes of anemia are needed to guide interventions (40).

China, with its significant economic development in recent decades, has experienced epidemiological and demographic transitions which have affected its population's nutritional conditions and produced environments that have contributed to a change in anemia (41). Despite the nutritional transition and improved nutritional status, stunting and anemia remain a major public health problem in China (42). There were some common factors in the occurrence of anemia and stunting. As we all know, the main risk factor for anemia among children is low iron intake at a stage of life in which iron requirement is high. Iron, as an essential trace mineral, is necessary for linear growth and body tissue proliferation (43). Meanwhile, stunting is an indicator of long-term chronic malnutrition, which is primarily caused by insufficient nutrition supply (44). The supply of nutrients includes not only macro-nutrients, but also micronutrients, such as iron (45). One reason why stunting may be related to anemia is that stunting may pick up deficiencies in iron, which are also known to boost the risk of anemia through impaired erythropoiesis and oxidative stress pathways (44). Especially for children in groups with high prevalence of stunting, all age-groups of children were vulnerable groups for anemia (46). In addition, it is worth noting that school-aged children in Group III (middle class/city) in China have been facing the double burden of anemia and stunting. Therefore, "the child- and adolescent- specific dietary guidance" is able to guide children to a reasonable quality diet, which refers to the "recommended daily dietary allowances for children and adolescents" established by the Chinese Nutrition Society (47). WHO recommends that a diet containing adequate amounts of bioavailable iron could prevent and control anemia (48). In addition, community-based platforms for nutrition education and government commitment and focus on equity are also important factors that may lead to the implementation of interventions that prevent and treat child stunting (49–51).

There are limitations in the present study. Firstly, it was a cross-sectional study and it cannot infer causality between anemia and stunting. Secondly, samples of capillary blood from the fingertip of each child were collected after discarding the first drop. Capillary blood can't distinguish the type and cause of anemia. Thirdly, iron deficiency and other nutrient indicators were not assessed directly.

CONCLUSIONS

The present study demonstrated a large geographic disparity in anemia in China. Lower anemia is found in better SES groups, while the higher prevalence is shown in poorer SES groups. The prevalence of anemia in Group VIII was not only due to SES, but also stunting. In addition to focusing on the rural western regions, the government should also pay more attention and provide more resources to the population in middle class cities and lower-class rural areas. The present findings imply that previous measures aimed at improving anemia, regardless of sex and with a limited focus on school-aged children in poor groups, may not be comprehensive enough to tackle the anemia problem in China. Specific strategies and interventions should be developed for children in susceptible groups, and especially for girls.

ETHICS STATEMENT

The project was approved by the Medical Research Ethics Committee of Peking University Health Science Center (IRB00001052-18002).

AUTHOR CONTRIBUTIONS

J-YW and YS conceptualized and designed the study and completed the statistical analyses. J-YW drafted the initial manuscript and reviewed and revised the manuscript. YS and YM designed the study and collected the data. D-ML and YS assisted with the statistical analyses. YM, JM, PL, BD, P-JH, D-ML, JD, and YS critically reviewed and revised the manuscript. All authors were involved in writing the paper and had final approval of the submitted and published versions.

ACKNOWLEDGMENTS

We acknowledge the revision suggestions from Lain Kiloughery, and also appreciate the investigators and students who participated in the surveys.

REFERENCES

Stevens GA, Finucane MM, De-Regil LM, Paciorek CJ, Flaxman SR, Branca F, et al. Global, regional, and national trends in haemoglobin concentration and prevalence of total and severe anaemia in children and pregnant and non-pregnant women for 1995–2011: a systematic analysis of population-representative data. *Lancet Global Health.* (2013) 1:e16– 25. doi: 10.1016/S2214-109X(13)70001-9

Balarajan Y, Ramakrishnan U, Ozaltin E, Shankar AH, Subramanian SV. Anaemia in low-income and middle-income countries. *Lancet.* (2011) 378:2123–35. doi: 10.1016/S0140-6736(10)62304-5

Antwi-Bafour S, Hammond S, Adjei JK, Kyeremeh R, Martin- Odoom A, Ekem I. A case-control study of prevalence of anemia among patients with type 2 diabetes. *J Med Case Rep.* (2016) 10:110. doi: 10.1186/s13256-016-0889-4

Kojima S. Why is the incidence of aplastic anemia higher in Asia? *Exp Rev Hematol.* (2017) 10:277–79. doi: 10.1080/17474086.2017.1302797

WHO. *Worldwide Prevalence of Anaemia 1993-2005 - WHO Global Database on Anaemia.* Geneva: World Health Organization (2008). Available online at: http://www.who.int/iris/handle/10665/43894 (accessed May 2, 2019).

Azzopardi PS, Hearps SJC, Francis KL, Kennedy EC, Mokdad AH, Kassebaum NJ, et al. Progress in adolescent health and wellbeing: tracking 12 headline indicators for 195 countries and territories, 1990–2016. *Lancet.* (2019) 393:1101–18. doi: 10.1016/S0140-6736(18)32427-9

Cy J. *Modern Child and Adolescent Health.* 2nd ed. Beijing: People Health Press (2010).

China NBoSo. *Tabulation on the 2010 Population Census of the People's Republic of China.* (2011). Available online at: http://www.stats.gov.cn/tjsj/ pcsj/rkpc/6rp/indexch.htm (accessed May 5, 2019).

Zhan Y, Chen R, Zheng W, Guo C, Lu L, Ji X, et al. Association between serum magnesium and anemia: china health and nutrition survey. *Biol Trace Elem Res.* (2014) 159:39–45. doi: 10.1007/s12011-014- 9967-x

Gan QL, Chen J, Yang T, Li L, Xu P, Pan H, et al. Prevalence of anemia among students from National Improvement Program for Rural Compulsory Students in 2013. *Chin J Sch Health.* (2016) 37:674–75. doi: 10.16835/j.cnki.1000-9817.2016.05.011

Luo R K-WM, Rozelle S, Zhang L, Liu C, Sharbono B, Shi Y, et al. Anemia in Rural China's elementary schools- prevalence and correlates in Shaanxi Province's Poor Counties. *Ecol Food Nutr.* (2010) 49:357– 72. doi: 10.1080/03670244.2010.507437

Iannotti L, Delnatus JR, John ARO, Eaton JC, Griggs JJ, Brown S. Determinants of anemia and haemoglobin concentration in haitian school- aged children. *PLoS ONE.* (2015) 93:1092–98. doi: 10.4269/ajtmh.15-0073

Oliveira D, Ferreira FS, Atouguia J, Fortes F, Guerra A, Centeno- Lima S. Infection by intestinal parasites, stunting and anemia in school-aged children from Southern Angola. *PLoS ONE.* (2015) 10:e0137327. doi: 10.1371/journal.pone.0137327

Song Y, Wang HJ, Dong B, Wang Z, Ma J, Agardh A. National trends in haemoglobin concentration and prevalence of anemia among Chinese School-Aged Children, 1995-2010. *J Pediatr.* (2017) 183:164– 69.e2. doi: 10.1016/j.jpeds.2017.01.012

Organization WH. *WHO Reference 2007 SPSS Macro Package.* (2007). Available online at: http://www.who.int/entity/growthref/tools/readme_spss. pdf (accessed May 4, 2019).

Onis MD, Onyango AW, Borghi E, Siyam A, Nishida C, Siekmann J. Development of a WHO growth reference for school- aged children and adolescents. *Bull World Health Org.* (2007) 85:660–7. doi: 10.2471/BLT.07.043497

Nkrumah B, Nguah SB, Sarpong N, Dekker D, Idriss A, May J, et al. Haemoglobin estimation by the HemoCue(R) portable haemoglobin photometer in a resource poor setting. *BMC Clin Pathol.* (2011) 11:5. doi: 10.1186/1472-6890-11-5

World Health Organization (WHO). *Haemoglobin Concentrations for the Diagnosis of Anaemia and Assessment of Severity.* (2011). Available online at: http://apps.who.int/iris/bitstream/10665/85839/3/WHO_NMH_ NHD_MNM_11.1_eng.pdf (accessed May 4, 2019).

World Health Organization (WHO) U, UNU. *Iron Deficiency Anaemia Assessment, Prevention, and Control, A Guide for Programme Managers.* Geneva: World Health Organization (2001).

Chan M. *Haemoglobin Concentrations for the Diagnosis of Anaemia and Assessment of Severity.* China: World Health Organization (2011). p. 1–6.

Ji CY, Chen TJ, Working Group on Obesity in C. Empirical changes in the prevalence of overweight and obesity among Chinese students from 1985 to 2010 and corresponding preventive strategies. *Biomed Environ Sci.* (2013) 26:1–12.

Melku M, Addis Z, Alem M, Enawgaw B. Prevalence and predictors of maternal anemia during pregnancy in Gondar, Northwest Ethiopia: an Institutional Based Cross-Sectional Study. *Anemia.* (2014) 2014:108593. doi: 10.1155/2014/108593

Adamu AL, Crampin A, Kayuni N, Amberbir A, Koole O, Phiri A, et al. Prevalence and risk factors for anemia severity and type in Malawian men and women: urban and rural differences. *Popul Health Metr.* (2017) 15:12. doi: 10.1186/s12963-017-0128-2

Alexis J Comber CB, Robert Radburn. A spatial analysis of variations in health access- linking geography, socio-economic status and access perceptions. *Int J Health Geogr.* (2011) 10:1–11. doi: 10.1186/1476-072X-10-44

Beal T, Tumilowicz A, Sutrisna A, Izwardy D, Neufeld LM. A review of child stunting determinants in Indonesia. *Matern Child Nutr.* (2018) 14:e12617. doi: 10.1111/mcn.12617

World Health Organization (WHO). *Reducing Stunting in Children- Equity Considerations for Achieving the Global Targets 2025.* (2018). Available online at: https://apps.who.int/iris/handle/10665/260202 (accessed May 11, 2019).

Goswmai S, Das KK. Socio-economic and demographic determinants of childhood anemia. *J Pediatr.* (2015) 91:471–7. doi: 10.1016/j.jped.2014.09.009

Okumura MJ, Knauer HA, Calvin KE, Takayama JI. Caring for children with special health care needs: profiling pediatricians and their health care resources. *Matern Child Health J.* (2018) 22:1042–50. doi: 10.1007/s10995-018-2484-3

Dreshaj HNA. Global challenges for the environment, water clean and economic advantages. *Int J Eng Trends Technol.* (2013) 4:1–5. Available online at: https://ssrn.com/abstract=2835964

Huo YJ, Zhou H, Wang Y. Status of underweight and it's relative factors for children under 3 years old in 14 counties in the western areas of China. *Chin Journal Child Health Care.* (2017) 25:552–5. doi: 10.11852/zgetbjzz2017-25-06-04

Cardoso MA, Augusto RA, Bortolini GA, Oliveira CS, Tietzman DC, Sequeira LA, et al. Effect of providing multiple micronutrients in powder through primary healthcare on anemia in young Brazilian children: a multicentre pragmatic controlled trial. *PLoS ONE.* (2016) 11:e0151097. doi: 10.1371/journal.pone.0151097

Aonsfsl WT. *People's Republic of China: Health Industry Standard* (China). (1998).

de Souza Queiroz S, de A. Torres M. Iron deficiency anemia in children. *J Pediatr.* (2000) 76:298–304. doi: 10.2223/JPED.167

Ramachandran P. Health and nutrition in adolescents and young women: preparing for the next generation. *J Health Med Nurs.* (2017) 145:256–57. doi: 10.1016/j.ijhydene.2013.08.087

Choi JLMSS. Attempts to lose weight among US children- importance of weight perceptions from self, parents, and health professionals. *Obesity.* (2018) 26:597–605. doi: 10.1002/oby.22106

Powers J M, Stanek J R, Lakshmi S, Haamid FW, O'Brien SH. Hematologic considerations and management of adolescent girls with heavy menstrual bleeding and anemia in U.S. Children's Hospitals. *J Pediatr Adolesc Gynecol.* (2018) 31:446–50. doi: 10.1016/j.jpag.2018.06.008

Zhang CX, Chen YM, Chen WQ, Su YX, Wang CL, Wu JN. Food group intake among adolescents in guangzhou city compared with the Chinese Dietary Guidelines. *Asia Pac J Clin Nutr.* (2012) 21:450–6. doi: 10.6133/apjcn.2012.21.3.18

Verma A, Rawal VS, Kedia G, Kumar D, Chauhan J. Factors influencing anemia among girls of school going age (6–18 years) from the slums of Ahmedabad City. *Ind J Comm Med.* (2004) 29:25–6.

Thummakomma K, Meda P, Jayashankar T. Impact of change in dietary behavior and iron supplementation for reduction of iron deficiency anemia in rural adolescent girls. *Int J f Agric.* (2017) 7:525–28. doi: 10.24247/ijasraug201768

Patton GC, Sawyer SM, Santelli JS, Ross DA, Afifi R, Allen NB, et al. Our future: a Lancet commission on adolescent health and wellbeing. *Lancet.* (2016) 387:2423–78. doi: 10.1016/S0140-6736(16)00579-1

Mikki N, Abdul-Rahim HF, Awartani F, Holmboe-Ottesen G. Prevalence and sociodemographic correlates of stunting, underweight, and overweight among Palestinian school adolescents (13-15 years) in two major governorates in the West Bank. *BMC Public Health.* (2009) 9:485. doi: 10.1186/1471-2458-9-485

Zou Y, Zhang R-H, Xia S-C, Huang LC, Fang YQ, Meng J, et al. The rural- urban difference in BMI and anemia among children and adolescents. *Int J Environ Res Public Health.* (2016) 13:1020. doi: 10.3390/ijerph13101020

Bruce BR. Modern nutrition in health and disease (tenth edition). *Crit Care Med.* (2006) 34:529–32. doi: 10.1097/01.CCM.0000236502. 51400.9F

Fatimah APS. Iron intake and haemoglobin levels in stunting in adolescent. *Althea Med J.* (2016) 3:175–80. doi: 10.15850/amj.v3n2.782

Ramakrishnan U, Nguyen P, Martorell R. Effects of micronutrients on growth of children under 5 y of age: meta-analyses of single and multiple nutrient interventions. *Am J Clin Nutr.* (2008) 89:191– 203. doi: 10.3945/ajcn.2008.26862

Assefa S, Mossie A, Hamza L. Prevalence and severity of anemia among school children in Jimma Town, Southwest Ethiopia. *BMC Hematol.* (2014) 14:1–9. doi: 10.1186/2052-1839-14-3

Ge KY. *Chinese Nutrition Scientific Encyclopedia.* Beijing: People's Medical Publishing House (2004). p. 1521–44.

World Health Organization (WHO). *Global Nutrition Targets 2025: Anaemia Policy Brief.* (2014). Available online at: https://www.who.int/nutrition/ publications/ (accessed June 22, 2019)

Smith LC KF, Frankenberger TR, Wadud A. Admissible evidence in the court of development evaluation? The Impact of CARE's SHOUHARDO project on child stunting in Bangladesh. *IDS Working Papers.* (2011) 41:196– 216. doi: 10.1111/j.2040-0209.2011.00376_2.x

Bhutta ZA, Das JK, Rizvi A, Gaffey MF, Walker N, Horton S, et al. Evidence-based interventions for improvement of maternal and child nutrition: what can be done and at what cost? *Lancet.* (2013) 382:452– 77. doi: 10.1016/ S0140-6736(13)60996-4

Al Hassand N. The prevalence of iron deficiency anemia in a Saudi University female students. *J Microsc Ultrastruct.* (2015) 3:25. doi: 10.1016/j.jmau.2014.11.003

24

The Prognostic Significance of Anemia in Patients with Heart Failure

Haijiang Xia[1], Hongfeng Shen[1], Wei Cha[1] and Qiaoli Lu[2]*

[1] Department of Cardiology, Affiliated Hospital of Shaoxing University, Shaoxing, China, [2] Department of General Medicine, Zhuji People's Hospital of Zhejiang Province, Shaoxing, China

*Correspondence:
Qiaoli Lu
lql_dr@163.com

Background: Anemia is a commonly occurring comorbidity in patients with heart failure (HF). Although there are a few reports of a higher prevalence of mortality and hospitalization-related outcomes due to accompanying anemia, other studies suggest that anemia does not have an adverse impact on the prognostic outcomes of HF. Two meta-analyses in the past decade had reported the adverse impact of anemia on both mortality and hospitalization- related outcomes. However, only one of these studies had evaluated the outcome while using multivariable adjusted hazard ratios. Moreover, several studies since then reported the prognostic influence of anemia in HF. In this present study, we evaluate the prognostic impact of anemia on mortality and hospitalization outcomes in patients with HF.

Methods: We carried out a systematic search of the academic literature in the scientific databases EMBASE, CENTRAL, Scopus, PubMed, Cochrane, ISI Web of Science, clinicaltrial.gov, and MEDLINE based on the PRISMA guidelines. Meta-analysis was then performed to evaluate the effect (presented as risk ratio) of anemia on the overall mortality and hospitalization outcome in patients with HF.

Results: Out of 1,397 studies, 11 eligible studies were included with a total of 53,502 (20,615 Female, 32,887 Male) HF patients (mean age: 71.6 ± 8.3-years, Hemoglobin: 11.9 ± 1.5 g/dL). Among them, 19,794 patients suffered from anemia (Hb: 10.5 ± 1.6), and 33,708 patients did not have anemia (Hb: 13.2 ± 1.7 g/dL). A meta-analysis revealed a high-odds ratio (OR) for the overall mortality in patients with anemia (OR: 1.43, 95% CI: 1.29–1.84). A high-risk ratio was also reported for hospitalization as the outcome in patients with anemia (1.22, 1.0–1.58).

Conclusion: This systematic review and meta-analysis provide evidence of the high risk of mortality and hospitalization-related outcomes in patients with HF and anemia. The study confirms the findings of previously published meta-analyses suggesting anemia as an important and independent risk factor delineating the prognostic outcome of chronic HF.

Keywords: anemia, hemoglobin, heart failure, mortality, hospitalization

INTRODUCTION

Heart failure (HF) is one of the most common types of cardiovascular disorders in the world (1, 2). According to the American Heart Association, HF is a complex cardiac syndrome that occurs as a result of a structural or functional dysfunction resulting in an impaired blood ejection across the body (3). Mentz and O'Connor (4) suggested a range of dysfunctions in the endothelial, renal system, and venous pathways that could eventually result in the remodeling of the myocardial structure leading to HF. Based on the statistics from the Global Burden of Disease Studies, HF is categorized as a rising global epidemic that accounts for more than 17 million deaths worldwide each year (5–7).

The patients with HF also exhibit a range of comorbidities that have a substantial impact on the prognostic outcome of the disease (8, 9), and the patient's quality of life (10). Studies have suggested that anemia is one of the most common comorbidities associated with HF (11–13). Recent studies have reported a high prevalence rate of anemia (28 to 58%) in patients with HF (14–16). The inception of anemia in patients with HF is largely associated with multifactorial reasons including deficits in iron metabolism, renal function, bone marrow function, and synthesis/response of erythropoietin (14, 15). Anand (17) suggested that the dysfunctional blunted response of erythropoietin due to the disruption in renal function as a result of HF could be one of the most critical factors contributing to the development of anemia. A substantial reduction in the renal flow of blood, in combination with dysfunctions in changes in the glomerular filtration rate, could influence the PO_2 levels which ultimately has a detrimental effect on the structure of erythropoietin eventually leading to anemia.

Evidence also suggests that the adjunct medication-induced iron deficiency could explain the prevalence of anemia in patients with HF (18–20). Sirbu et al. (20) suggested that conventional drugs administered to patients with HF i.e., beta blockers, calcium channel blockers, Angiotensin converting enzyme inhibitor, and aspirin can substantially impair iron metabolism resulting in anemia.

In retrospect, anemia, accompanying HF, has an overall adverse impact on the prognostic outcome of patients. Nagatomo et al. (18) reported that anemia leads to an elevated hyper-hemodynamic in patients with HF. Moreover, increased cardiac workload by the means of stroke volume could also influence the sympathetic nervous activity which eventually can contribute to cardiac remodeling especially in the left ventricle, eventually promoting morbidity and mortality in HF patients (21, 22). Despite having an overall influence on the morbidity and mortality in the adult population, there is still no consensus regarding the prognostic influence of anemia on the mortality and hospitalization-related outcomes in patients with HF. Only a few high-quality studies have addressed the predominant impact of anemia on the prognostic outcome of HF patients in terms of mortality (23–26). However, only a few studies also report that anemia has no prognostic effect on the mortality and hospitalization-related outcomes in patients with HF (27, 28).

To date, only two systematic reviews and meta-analyses have reported the prognostic impact of anemia on the mortality and hospitalization-related outcomes in patients with HF (12, 29). Both of these studies reported a high relative risk ratio of mortality, hospitalization- related outcome in patients with HF, and anemia. However, several high-quality randomized controlled trials (23, 24), observation studies (25, 26), and retrospective cohort studies (30–32), that evaluate the prognostic influence of anemia on mortality and hospitalization outcomes in patients with HF, have been published recently. Therefore, there is a need for an updated systematic review and meta-analysis of the data.

This systematic review and meta-analysis provide an update on the current state of evidence regarding the prognostic influence of anemia in patients with HF, and risk ratios associated with the mortality and hospitalization-related outcomes in HF patients with anemia. The findings from the present study may provide cardiologists with a better understanding of the prognostic influence of anemia in patients with HF.

MATERIALS AND METHODS

A systematic review and meta-analysis was carried out based on the PRISMA (Preferred Reporting Items for Systematic Reviews and Meta-Analyses) guidelines (33).

Data Search Strategy

Scientific databases (EMBASE, MEDLINE, CENTRAL, PubMed, Cochrane, ISI Web of Science, and clinicaltrial.gov, and Scopus) were searched from inception until September 2020. The following MeSH keywords: "heart failure," "HF," "Chronic heart failure," "anemia," "Hemoglobin," and "Hb" were used in different combinations during the search across the academic databases. Manual screening of the bibliography section of the included studies were performed to identify further relevant studies. The inclusion criteria for the study were as follows:

- Studies that evaluated the prevalence of HF patients with anemia.
- Studies performed in the human population.
- Studies that evaluated the influence of anemia on the outcomes of short-, long-term mortality, and hospitalization outcomes.
- Studies published after 2008.
- Studies reporting the outcomes of mortality and hospitalization with the adjusted hazard ratio.
- Randomized-quasi-randomized and controlled clinical trials, observational prospective or retrospective studies.
- Studies published in peer-reviewed scientific journals or presented at conferences.
- English language studies.

The screening of the studies was independently performed by two reviewers. Cases of disagreements were resolved by discussions with a third independent reviewer. The following data were extracted from the included studies: author information, descriptive data, sample distribution, hemoglobin values, events of mortality, and events of hospitalizations. In cases of missing quantitative data, attempts were made to contact the corresponding authors of the publication.

Quality Assessment

Quality (risk of bias) of each study was assessed by ROBINS-I, a Cochrane risk of bias assessment tool for RCTs randomized controlled trials and non-RCTs randomized controlled trials i.e., ROBINS-I (34, 35) and Cochrane risk of bias assessment tool for the randomized controlled trials (36). The ROBINS-I tool considers inadequate randomization, selective reporting, concealed allocation, classification, and missing data as major threats for instigating bias. The Cochrane tool for assessing randomized controlled trials assesses biases such as concealment of allocation, generation of random sequence, selective reporting, and blinding of outcome. The evaluation of methodological quality was done independently by two reviewers. Cases of disagreements were resolved by discussion with the third reviewer.

Data Analysis

Meta-analysis of the included studies was done using the Comprehensive Meta-analysis software version 2.0 (37). The within group meta-analysis was performed using a random effects model (38). We estimated the pooled odds ratio from the included studies. Heterogeneity among the studies was assessed by I^2 statistics, with the threshold for interpreting heterogeneity as follows: I^2 statistics between 0 and 25%, negligible heterogeneity; 25–75%, moderate heterogeneity; and ≥75%, substantial heterogeneity (39). We distributed the

data and performed the analysis for the overall mortality and hospitalization outcome, reporting odds ratio, confidence intervals (CI) of 95% level of significance, and heterogeneity. We also carried out separated sub-group analyses to evaluate the comparative influence of mortality between HF patients with a reduced and preserved ejection fraction. Publication bias was estimated using the Duval and Tweedy's trim and fill procedure (40). This non-parametric method tests for publication bias and adjusts the estimated overall effect size. Briefly an iterative method is used in which some of the extreme values remaining are removed, and a new mean effect is calculated. The alpha level of significance was set at 95%.

RESULTS

A systematic search resulted in 1,370 studies. Additional 27 studies were identified after screening the bibliography of articles (**Figure 1**). A total of 11 studies fulfilled the inclusion criteria. Three of the included studies were retrospective cohort studies (30–32), three were prospective cohort studies (41–43), two were randomized controlled trials (23, 24), two were observation studies (25, 26), and one was a retrospective observational study (44). The characteristics of the included studies are summarized in **Table 1** and the clinical features of the patients are summarized in **Table 2**.

Participant Information

A total of 57,386 patients with HF were included in the 11 studies, among them, 20,615 were females and 35,944 were males. In

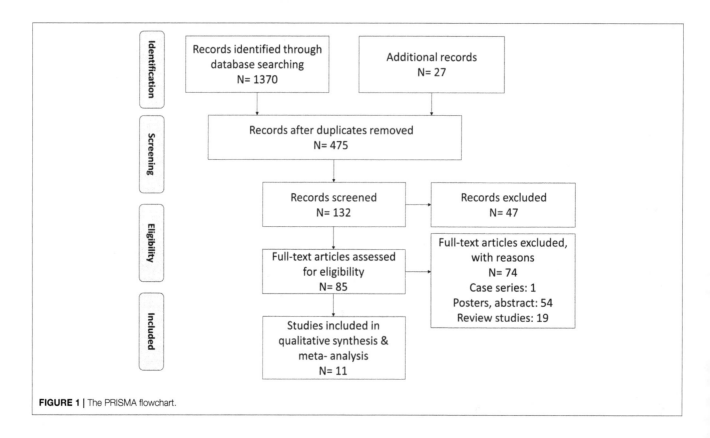

FIGURE 1 | The PRISMA flowchart.

TABLE 1 | Details of the included studies.

Study	Country	Study design	Sample size (female, male)	Overall age (M ± SD) years	Mean overall Hb (g/dl) (Mean ± SD)	Patients sample distribution size (female, male)	Distributed sample age (Mean ± SD) years	Mean Hemoglobin (g/dl) (Mean ± SD)	Mortality (n)	Hospitalization (n)
Ye et al. (32)	China	Retrospective cohort	3,279 (1,539 F, 1,740 M)	71	12.6	Anemia: 1,490 (742 F, 748 M) No anemia: 1,789 (797 F, 992 M)	Anemia: 74 No anemia: 67	Anemia: 10.7 No anemia: 14.1	Overall: 122 Anemia: 69 No anemia: 53	Overall: 1,817 Anemia: 801 No anemia: 1,016
Cherat et al. (30)	Thailand	Retrospective cohort	414 (228F, 186M)	62.6 ± 14.7	Male: 11.9 Female: 10.7	Anemia: 259 (153 F, 106M) No anemia: 155 (75 F, 80M)	Anemia: 64 No anemia: 58	Anemia: 10.0 No anemia: 13.6	Anemia: 52 No anemia: 19	Anemia: 79 No anemia: 47
Savarese et al (25)	Sweden	Observational study	42,985 (15,926 F, 27,059 M)	75	12.7	Anemia: 14,779 (4,957 F, 9,822 M) No anemia: 28,206 (10,969 F, 17,237 M)	Anemia: 77 No anemia: 73	Anemia: 11.5 No anemia: 13.9	Anemia: 23,711 No anemia: 16,865	Anemia: 4,209 No anemia: 8,933
Gupta et al (23)	USA	Randomized controlled trial	1,748 (872F, 876M)	72	12.8	Anemia: 716 (326 F, 390 M) No anemia: 1,032 (546 F, 486 M)	Anemia: 73 No anemia: 72	Anemia: 11.5 No anemia: 13.8	Anemia: - No anemia: -	Anemia: 451 No anemia: 516
Parcia et al. (24)	USA	Randomized controlled trial	215 (104 F, 111 M)	69	12.5	Anemia: 76 (27 F, 49 M) No anemia: 139 (77 F, 62 M)	Anemia: 71 No anemia: 67	Anemia: 11.5 No anemia: 13.5	Anemia: - No anemia: -	Anemia: 36 No anemia: 42
Kim et al. (44)	Korea	Retrospective observation study	384 (191 F, 193 M)	66.8	12.9	Anemia: 270 (139 F, 131 M) No anemia: 114 (52 F, 62 M)	Anemia: 71.3 ± 11.8 No anemia: 62.4 ±	Anemia: 11.3 ± 1.8 No anemia: 14.5 ± 1.5	Anemia: 48 No anemia: 12	Anemia: - No anemia: -
Jin et al. (42)	China	Prospective cohort study	1,604 (752 F, 852M)	74.3 ± 11.3	12.4 ± 2.0	Anemia: 818 (393 F, 425 M) No anemia: 786 (359 F, 427 M)	Anemia: 76.9 ± 10.2 No anemia: 71.6 ± 11.8	Anemia: 10.9 ± 1.4 No anemia: 13.9 ± 1.3	Anemia: 143 No anemia: 83	Anemia: 367 No anemia: 296
Wienbergen et al. (26)	Germany	Observational study	949 (240F, 709M)	69.5	13.0	Anemia: 409 No anemia: 540	Anemia: - No anemia: -	Anemia: - No anemia: -	Anemia: - No anemia: -	Anemia: - No anemia: -
Formiga et al. (31)	Spain	Retrospective cohort study	155 (119F, 36M)	92.4 ± 2	11.7 ± 2.0	Anemia: 127 No anemia: 28	Anemia: - No anemia: -	Anemia: - No anemia: -	Anemia: 7 No anemia: 2	Anemia: 80 No anemia: 8
van den Berge et al. (13)	Netherlands	Prospective cohort study	1,769 (644F, 1,125M)	63.6	7.8	Anemia: 850 (285F, 565M) No anemia: 919 (359 F, 560M)	Anemia: 63.1 ± 14.5 No anemia: 64.1 ± 15.0	Anemia: 6.7 ± 0.9 No anemia: 9.0 ± 0.8	Anemia: 365 No anemia: 257	Anemia: - No anemia: -
Goh et al. (41)	Singapore	Prospective cohort study	3,884 (827F, 3,057M)	60 ± 13	13.1 ± 2.1	Anemia: 1,606 (371F, 1,235M) No anemia: 2,278 (456F, 1,822M)	Anemia: 64 ± 13 No anemia: 58 ± 13	Anemia: 11.1 ± 1.2 No anemia: 14.5 ± 1.3	Anemia: - No anemia: -	Anemia: - No anemia: -

M, Male; F, Female; n, number; SD, Standard deviation.

TABLE 2 | Clinical characteristics of the patients.

Study	Cause of anemia	Diabetes (%)	Hypertension (%)	Chronic kidney disease (%)	Ejection fraction (%)
Ye et al. (32)	Nd	A: 25 NA: 36.2	A: 39.1 NA: 45.6	A: 26.4 NA: 7.2	A: 50 NA: 40
Chairat et al. (30)	Nd	A: 31 NA: 15	A: 55 NA: 41	A: 24 NA: 1	Preserved: A: 64.2 NA: 62.2 Reduced: A: 29.6 NA: 28.3
Savarese et al. (25)	Nd	A: 33.1 NA: 24.9	A: 71.9 NA: 70.1	A: 50.3 NA: 43.1	–
Gupta et al. (23)	Nd	A: 57.1 NA: 36	A: 90.6 NA: 89.5	–	A: 51 NA: 51
Parcha et al. (24)	Nd	A: 39 NA: 53	A: 68 NA: 114	–	–
Kim et al. (44)	Nd	A: 44.8 NA: 18.4	A: 59.6 NA: 54.4	A: 9.6 NA: 1.8	–
Jin et al. (42)	Nd	A: 29.5 NA: 25.2	A: 74.7 NA: 72.9	A: 45.5 NA: 24.2	A: 61.6 NA: 61.4
Wienbergen et al. (26)	Iron deficiency	A: 37.6 NA: 35.1	–	A: 54.7 NA: 52.9	–
Formiga et al. (31)	Nd	–	–	–	–
van den Berge et al. (43)	Nd	A: 23 NA: 20	A: 32 NA: 34	–	–
Goh et al. (41)	Nd	A: 53 NA: 34	A: 59 NA: 51	A: 58 NA: 36	A: 29 NA: 27

Nd, Not defined; A, Anemic; NA, Non-anemic.

the included studies, three studies defined that their patients suffered from acute HF (31, 32, 44) and one had reported that they included cases with both acute and chronic HF (26). The rest of the seven studies did not provide details concerning the nature of the HF cases they included (23–26, 30, 41, 42). Besides, five of the included studies had also reported the ejection fraction values for their sample (23, 30, 32, 41, 42). The average ejection fraction for all the included studies was found to be $47.5 \pm 15.2\%$ for the HF patients with anemia, and $44.9 \pm 15.6\%$ for the HF patients without anemia. Moreover, the HF was defined by seven of the included studies with echocardiography (23, 24, 30, 32, 41, 42, 44), one study used the NT-proB-type Natriuretic Peptide blood test (25), and three studies did not define their measures for identifying HF (26, 31, 43).

Furthermore, the average age of the patients was 70.5 ± 8.6-years. All the included 11 studies had followed the World Health Organization classification to define anemia i.e., hemoglobin levels <13.0 g/dl for males and <12.0 g/dl for females. Moreover, among the anemic patients, mild anemia was defined as $Hb \geq 9.1$ g/dl, moderate anemia was defined as 6.1 g/dl $\leq Hb < 9$ g/dl, and severe anemia was defined as $Hb < 6$ g/dl. In our study, the average hemoglobin level was 12 ± 1.5 g/dL. In the subgroup distribution for the patients with/without anemia, a total of 21,400 patients have anemia, whereas 35,986 patients do not have anemia. Two studies did not report the gender distribution for this sub-sample of the patients with/without anemia (26, 31). From the studies that reported the gender distribution, a total of 2,931 females and 17,933 males have anemia, whereas 13,690

females and 21,728 males do not have anemia. The average age of the sub sample with and without anemia was 70.4 ± 5.4 and 65.9 ± 5.7-years, respectively. The average hemoglobin levels in the sub sample with and without anemia was reported to be 10.5 ± 1.5 and 13.4 ± 1.6 g/dL, respectively.

Publication Bias

The Duval and Tweedy's trim and fill method was used to identify any missing studies based on the random effect models on both sides of the funnel plot. The overall random effect models determined the point estimates and the 95% confidence intervals for all the combined studies as 1.42 (1.23–1.64). The results of the trim and fill method indicated that one study was missing on the left side of the funnel plot. The trim and fill method reported the imputed estimate of 1.37 (1.18–1.60). The publication bias is reported in **Figure 2**.

Quality Assessment for Non-randomized Controlled Trials

We analyzed the risk of bias in the methodology of the non-randomized controlled trials with the ROBINS-I tool (summarized in **Table 3**). The overall risk was found to be low in the included studies. We observed that the methodological risk of bias was highest for the selection of reported results and deviation from intended intervention. The overall risk of bias is summarized in **Figure 3**.

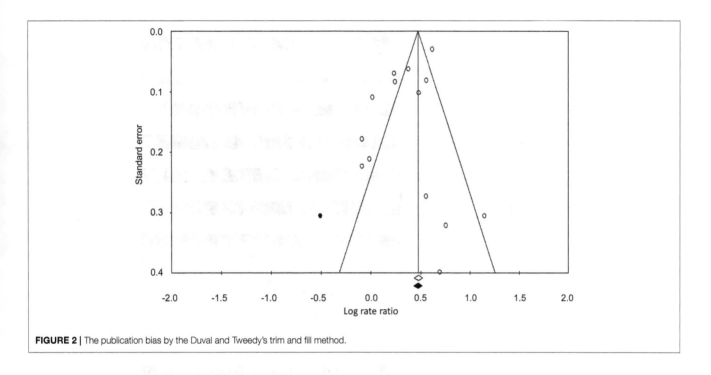

FIGURE 2 | The publication bias by the Duval and Tweedy's trim and fill method.

TABLE 3 | Risk of bias within studies according to the ROBINS-I scale.

Study	Confounding bias	Selection bias	Deviation from intended intervention	Missing data	Measurement in outcome	Selection of reported result	Classification of intervention
Ye et al. (32)	+	+	+	+	+	+	+
Chairat et al. (30)	+	+	+	+	+	+	+
Savarese et al. (25)	+	+	+	+	+	+	+
Kim et al. (44)	+	+	+	+	+	−	+
Jin et al. (42)	+	?	?	+	+	?	+
Wienbergen et al. (26)	+	+	?	+	+	−	+
Formiga et al. (31)	+	+	?	+	+	−	+
van den Berge et al. (43)	+	+	+	+	+	−	+
Goh et al. (41)	+	+	+	?	−	−	+

Quality Assessment for Randomized Controlled Trials

We analyzed the risk of bias for the randomized controlled studies using the Cochrane risk of bias assessment tool. Results are summarized in **Table 4**. The overall risk was low in the included studies. We observed an unclear risk of bias for the selective reporting section (**Figure 4**).

Meta-Analysis Report
Mortality Outcome

The overall mortality rate was reported by 10 studies (25, 26, 31, 41–47). The outcome was reported by all the studies for a 1-year duration. The estimated pooled odds ratio was 1.43 (95%

CI: 1.25–1.63, $p < 0.001$) (**Figure 5**), with moderate heterogeneity (I^2: 56.1%).

Sub-group analysis for the overall mortality rate with a reduced ejection fraction was reported by two studies (30, 41). The estimated pooled odds ratio was 1.25 (95% CI: 1.09–1.45, $p < 0.01$) (**Figure 6**), with no heterogeneity (I^2: 0%). Likewise, sub-group analysis for overall mortality rate with a preserved ejection fraction was reported by four studies (23, 30, 32, 42). The estimated pooled odds ratio was 1.38 (95% CI: 1.06–1.79, $p < 0.02$) (**Figure 7**), with moderate heterogeneity (I^2: 48.5%).

Hospitalization Outcome

The overall hospitalization outcome was reported by four studies (23, 24, 42, 44), with two studies reporting the outcome at

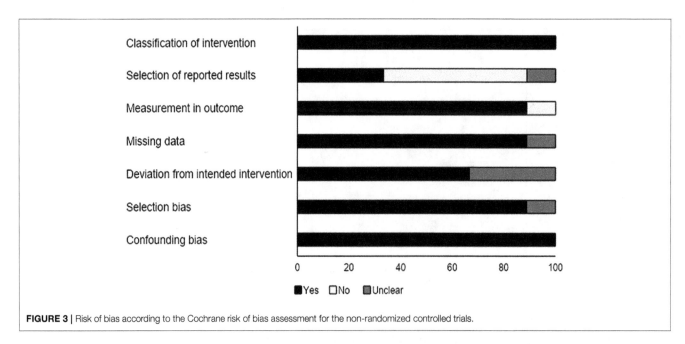

FIGURE 3 | Risk of bias according to the Cochrane risk of bias assessment for the non-randomized controlled trials.

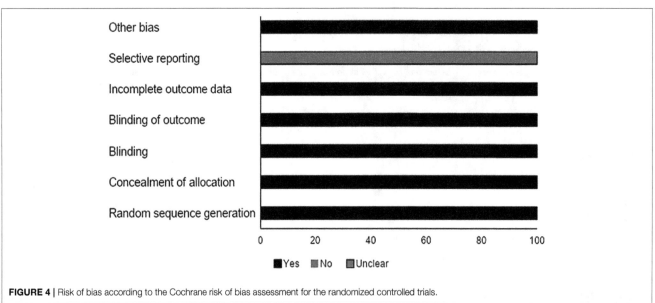

FIGURE 4 | Risk of bias according to the Cochrane risk of bias assessment for the randomized controlled trials.

TABLE 4 | Risk of bias within studies according to the Cochrane risk of bias assessment tool for randomized controlled trials.

Study	Random sequence generation	Concealment of allocation	Blinding	Blinding of outcome	Incomplete outcome data	Selective reporting	Other bias
Gupta et al. (23)	+	+	+	+	+	?	+
Parcha et al. (24)	+	+	+	+	+	?	+

a 1-year follow up (23, 42), one at a 1.5-year follow up (44), and one after 24-weeks (24). The pooled rate ratio was 1.22 (95% CI: 1.0–1.58, p: 0.04) (**Figure 8**), with no heterogeneity (I^2: 0%).

Sub-group analysis on only long-term (1–1.5-years) hospitalization outcomes showed a pooled risk ratio of 1.15 (95% CI: 0.84–1.56, p: 0.36) (**Figure 9**), with no heterogeneity (I^2: 0%).

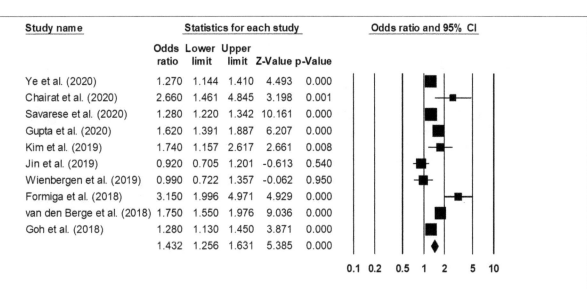

Study name	Odds ratio	Lower limit	Upper limit	Z-Value	p-Value
Ye et al. (2020)	1.270	1.144	1.410	4.493	0.000
Chairat et al. (2020)	2.660	1.461	4.845	3.198	0.001
Savarese et al. (2020)	1.280	1.220	1.342	10.161	0.000
Gupta et al. (2020)	1.620	1.391	1.887	6.207	0.000
Kim et al. (2019)	1.740	1.157	2.617	2.661	0.008
Jin et al. (2019)	0.920	0.705	1.201	-0.613	0.540
Wienbergen et al. (2019)	0.990	0.722	1.357	-0.062	0.950
Formiga et al. (2018)	3.150	1.996	4.971	4.929	0.000
van den Berge et al. (2018)	1.750	1.550	1.976	9.036	0.000
Goh et al. (2018)	1.280	1.130	1.450	3.871	0.000
	1.432	1.256	1.631	5.385	0.000

FIGURE 5 | Forest plot for studies evaluating the overall 1-year overall mortality outcome. The adjusted odds ratios are presented as black boxes, whereas 95% confidence intervals are presented as whiskers. A negative odds ratio represents a reduction in the risk of mortality in heart failure patients with anemia, whereas the positive odds ratio represents an increase in the risk of mortality in heart failure patients with anemia.

Study name	Odds ratio	Lower limit	Upper limit	Z-Value	p-Value
Chairat et al. (2020)	0.900	0.461	1.758	-0.308	0.758
Goh et al. (2018) low	1.280	1.130	1.450	3.871	0.000
	1.259	1.090	1.456	3.121	0.002

FIGURE 6 | Forest plot for studies evaluating the overall 1-year overall mortality outcome for HF patients with reduced ejection fraction. The adjusted odds ratios are presented as black boxes, whereas 95% confidence intervals are presented as whiskers. A negative odds ratio represents a reduction in the risk of mortality in heart failure patients with anemia, whereas the positive odds ratio represents an increase in the risk of mortality in heart failure patients with anemia.

Study name	Odds ratio	Lower limit	Upper limit	Z-Value	p-Value
Ye et al. (2020)	1.270	1.144	1.410	4.493	0.000
Chairat et al. (2020)	2.660	1.461	4.845	3.198	0.001
Gupta et al. (2020)	1.620	1.391	1.887	6.207	0.000
Jin et al. (2019)	0.920	0.705	1.201	-0.613	0.540
	1.380	1.063	1.793	2.416	0.016

FIGURE 7 | Forest plot for studies evaluating the overall 1-year overall mortality outcome for HF patients with preserved ejection fraction. The adjusted odds ratios are presented as black boxes, whereas 95% confidence intervals are presented as whiskers. A negative odds ratio represents a reduction in the risk of mortality in heart failure patients with anemia, whereas the positive odds ratio represents an increase in the risk of mortality in heart failure patients with anemia.

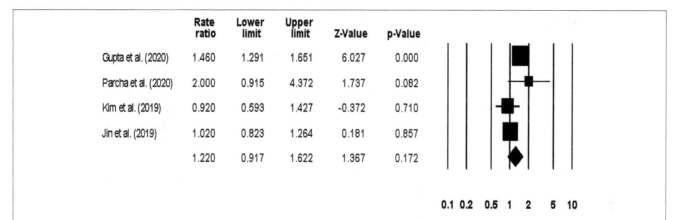

FIGURE 8 | Forest plot for studies evaluating the overall hospitalization outcome. The adjusted odds ratios are presented as black boxes, whereas 95% confidence intervals are presented as whiskers. A negative odds ratio represents a reduction in the risk of mortality in heart failure patients with anemia, whereas the positive odds ratio represents an increase in the risk of mortality in heart failure patients with anemia.

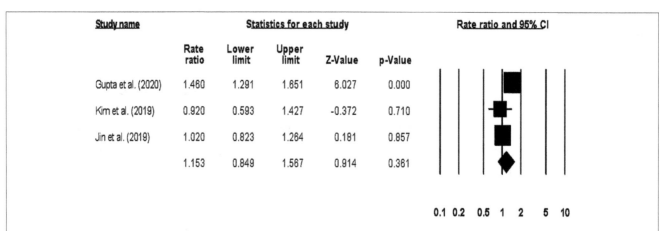

FIGURE 9 | Forest plot for studies evaluating the overall long-term hospitalization outcome. The adjusted odds ratios are presented as black boxes whereas 95% confidence intervals are presented as whiskers. A negative odds ratio represents a reduction in the risk of mortality in heart failure patients with anemia, whereas the positive odds ratio represents an increase in the risk of mortality in heart failure patients with anemia.

DISCUSSION

This systematic review and meta-analysis provide a comprehensive state of evidence regarding the prognostic influence of anemia in patients with HF. We observed high overall risk ratios associated with the overall mortality and hospitalization-related outcomes in HF patients with anemia.

The management of HF is one of the most challenging aspects for cardiologists worldwide due to its atypical pathophysiological mechanism, coexisting morbidities, and manifestations (48–50). Presence of comorbidities, such as anemia, makes it even more challenging for clinicians to evaluate the cardiovascular condition of the patient, thus potentially contributing to an increased morbidity and mortality-related outcomes (12, 51, 52). Recent literature has increasingly recognized the rising prevalence of anemia in patients with HF (53–55). Several mechanisms are linked with the aggravation of anemia in patients with HF (14, 17–19). The study by Anand and Gupta (14) suggests that the absolute/functional nutritional deficiency of iron, response/synthesis of erythropoietin, and adverse effects of medications are the most significant factors aggravating the

onset of anemia. Moreover, the increase in pro-inflammatory markers in patients with HF could also contribute to anemia by activating the GATA-binding proteins and nuclear factor kappa light chain enhancer, eventually inhibiting the production of renal erythropoietin or resulting in a blunted-erythropoietin response (56–58). In addition to these inflammatory changes, deficiency and/or mutation of genes that regulate hematopoiesis have also been reported to eventually worsen cardiac remodeling i.e., hypertrophy in the left ventricle (59, 60). These changes eventually promote the increased risks of morbidities that can lead to re-hospitalizations and eventually to an increased mortality (12).

In our present review, we analyzed a range of studies that reported a predominant influence of anemia on all-cause 1-year mortality related outcomes in patients with HF. Ye et al. (32) evaluated the overall all-cause mortality in 3,279 patients and reported a significant (*p*: 0.01) increase in the mortality-related events in HF patients with anemia as compared to patients without anemia. This relationship between anemia and mortality was proportional to the severity of the anemia i.e., the more severe the anemia, the higher the mortality rates. Similarly, Jin et al. (42) reported higher mortality related outcomes for the anemic group (14.6%) as compared to the non-anemic group (8.7%) in a Chinese cohort of 1,604 patients. The authors further showed that the mortality rates in anemic patients further increased in patients with renal dysfunction (21%). This increase in mortality-related events in HF patients with anemia may be due to several mechanisms, such as enhancement in oxidative stress, fluid-retention, cardiac-hypoxia, sympathetic nervous activity, and renin-angiotensin-aldosterone activity (61, 62). Sanderson (63) further suggested that a decrease in the neuro-hormonal activation as a result of a reduced vascular-resistance and decreased blood viscosity could further reduce the glomerular filtration rate and enhance the overall retention of water and salt content leading to an expanded extracellular plasma volume, eventually increasing the morbidity and mortality related outcomes in patients with HF. In our present meta-analysis, we confirm these findings and report a high-odds ratio (OR: 1.43, 95% CI: 1.25–1.63) associated with the overall mortality-related factors in patients with HF. Besides, in a further subgroup comparative analysis of mortality between HF patients with a reduced and preserved ejection fraction, we observed differences in terms of mortality between the two groups.

We also assessed the risk of hospitalization-related outcomes associated with anemia in patients with HF. We observed that all the studies included in our systematic review had reported an overall increase in the hospitalization-related outcomes for HF patients with anemia. Kim et al. (44) showed a high rate of re-hospitalization in anemic patients (Hazard ratio: 0.92, 0.59–1.42) as compared to non-anemic patients with HF. The authors also suggest that the anemia diagnosis at discharge could serve as a predictor not only for the morbidity-but also for the mortality-related outcomes, thus emphasizing the importance of managing anemia during hospitalization to reduce the adverse events in patients with HF. RELAX randomized controlled trial by Parcha et al. (24) reported a higher incidence of hospitalization in anemic patients primarily due to cardiac or renal problems even at the end of a 24-week period (24). The authors suggest that the timely recognition and management of anemia could be crucial for stemming the deterioration of the symptomatic manifestations in patients with HF.

Our meta-analysis is in agreement with these reports. We showed high risk ratios of re-hospitalizations in anemic patients with HF (1.22, 1.27–1.78). Subgroup analysis of long term (>1-year) hospitalization-related outcome also revealed a high-risk hospitalization ratio in anemic patients with HF (1.15, 0.84–1.56).

Our systematic review and meta-analysis have a few limitations. First and foremost, this systematic review and meta-analysis was not registered in a review repository such as PROSPERO. Although the lack of registration might raise concerns regarding the validity of this present review (64), we would like to assure our reader that we made attempts to register our review at these repositories, but because of the current pandemic crisis, the waiting time at the PROSPERO repository was >1-year. Secondly, we did not evaluate the gender differences

in terms of the risks of hospitalization and mortality associated with anemia in patients with heart failure. We understand the importance of evaluating the gender differences in terms of the prognostic significance it possesses for clinicians. Therefore, we strongly recommend future studies to address this limitation by conducting gender sub-group analysis to outline the gender differences in terms of the prognostic outcome of anemia in HF. Thirdly, our understanding of the short- and long-term hospitalization related outcomes in HF patients with anemia may be biased due to an insufficient data in the eligible included studies. In our included pool of four studies that had reported the hospitalization related outcomes in HF patients with anemia, only one study had evaluated the outcome during a 24-week follow-up (24), whereas the other three studies had evaluated the long-term (1–1.5-years) outcomes (23, 42, 44). Therefore, the outcomes of risk ratio overall hospitalization could be biased, and we would suggest our reader to evaluate this statistic with caution. Additionally, short- and long-term prognostic influences of anemia on mortality were not evaluated in this review and meta-analysis, since all the included studies had reported a 1-year mortality outcome. Previous studies have stressed upon the high risks of mortality-related outcomes especially during the short-term periods (43). Therefore, future studies are needed to address these limitations by conducting more high-quality studies and sharing their descriptive data in open access data repositories. The evaluation of these outcomes would be highly beneficial for medical practitioners to predict the prognostic outcomes regarding mortality and re-hospitalization in HF patients with anemia. Lastly, we would like to mention that usually an important limitation in the literature involving patients with heart failure is that the researchers do not report the definitions of anemia they adopted. In this present study, however, we found that all the included studies had adopted the World Health Organization's classification to define anemia i.e., Hb < 13.0 g/dl for males and Hb < 12.0 g/dl for females.

In conclusion, in this present systematic review and meta-analysis, we provide a confirmatory evidence regarding the high prognostic influence of anemia in patients with HF. We provide statistical evidence of the high mortality and hospitalization-related risks associated with anemia in patients with HF. The findings from the present study can further contribute in developing clinical awareness of the widespread prevalence of anemia in patients with chronic HF. This may help cardiologists to develop the best practice guidelines for determining the appropriate treatment approach for controlling adverse outcomes in HF patients with anemia.

AUTHOR CONTRIBUTIONS

HX conceived and designed the study and was involved in the writing of the manuscript. HS, WC, and QL collected the data and performed the literature search. All authors have read and approved the final manuscript.

REFERENCES

Cardiovascular Diseases (CVDs). Available online at: https://www.who. int/news-room/fact-sheets/detail/cardiovascular-diseases-(cvds) (accessed November 14, 2020).

Ziaeian B, Fonarow GC. Epidemiology and aetiology of heart failure. *Nat Rev Cardiol*. (2016) 13:368–78. doi: 10.1038/nrcardio.2016.25

Yancy CW, Jessup M, Bozkurt B, Butler J, Casey DE, Drazner MH, et al. 2013 ACCF/AHA guideline for the management of heart failure: a report of the American College of Cardiology Foundation/American Heart Association Task Force on Practice Guidelines. *J Am Coll Cardiol*. (2013) 62:e147– 239. doi: 10.1161/CIR.0b013e31829e8776

Mentz RJ, O'Connor CM. Pathophysiology and clinical evaluation of acute heart failure. *Nat Rev Cardiol*. (2016) 13:28–35. doi: 10.1038/nrcardio.2015.134

GBD 2013 Mortality and Causes of Death Collaborators. Global, regional, and national age-sex specific all-cause and cause-specific mortality for 240 causes of death, 1990-2013: a systematic analysis for the Global Burden of Disease Study 2013. *Lancet*. (2015) 385:117–71. doi: 10.1016/S0140-6736(14)61682-2

Savarese G, Lund LH. Global public health burden of heart failure. *Card Fail Rev*. (2017) 3:7–11. doi: 10.15420/cfr.2016:25:2

Zannad F. Rising incidence of heart failure demands action. *Lancet*. (2018) 391:518–9. doi: 10.1016/S0140-6736(17)32873-8

Sharma M, Nayanisri K, Jain R, Ranjan R. *Predictive Value of Fasting Plasma Glucose on First Antenatal Visit before 20 Weeks of Gestation to Diagnose Gestational Diabetes Mellitus*. JCDR (2018). Available online at: http://jcdr.n et/article_fulltext.asp?issn = 0973-709x&year = 2018&volume = 12&issue = 2&page = QC01&issn = 0973-709x&id = 11177 (accessed March 11, 2020).

Wong CY, Chaudhry SI, Desai MM, Krumholz HM. Trends in comorbidity, disability, and polypharmacy in heart failure. *Am J Med*. (2011) 124:136– 43. doi: 10.1016/j.amjmed.2010.08.017

Macabasco-O'Connell A, DeWalt DA, Broucksou KA, Hawk V, Baker DW, Schillinger D, et al. Relationship between literacy, knowledge, self-care behaviors, and heart failure-related quality of life among patients with heart failure. *J Gen Intern Med*. (2011) 26:979–86. doi: 10.1007/s11606-011- 1668-y

Grote Beverborg N, van Veldhuisen DJ, van der Meer P. Anemia in heart failure: still relevant? *JACC Heart Fail*. (2018) 6:201–8. doi: 10.1016/j.jchf.2017.08.023

Groenveld HF, Januzzi JL, Damman K, van Wijngaarden J, Hillege HL, van Veldhuisen DJ, et al. Anemia and mortality in heart failure patients a systematic review and meta-analysis. *J Am Coll Cardiol*. (2008) 52:818– 27. doi: 10.1016/j.jacc.2008.04.061

Nanas JN, Matsouka C, Karageorgopoulos D, Leonti A, Tsolakis E, Drakos SG, et al. Etiology of anemia in patients with advanced heart failure. *J Am Coll Cardiol*. (2006) 48:2485–9. doi: 10.1016/j.jacc.2006.08.034

Anand IS, Gupta P. Anemia and iron deficiency in heart failure: current concepts and emerging therapies. *Circulation*. (2018) 138:80– 98. doi: 10.1161/CIRCULATIONAHA.118.030099

Cleland JGF, Zhang J, Pellicori P, Dicken B, Dierckx R, Shoaib A, et al. Prevalence and outcomes of anemia and hematinic deficiencies in patients with chronic heart failure. *JAMA Cardiol*. (2016) 1:539– 47. doi: 10.1001/jamacardio.2016.1161

von Haehling S, Gremmler U, Krumm M, Mibach F, Schön N, Taggeselle J, et al. Prevalence and clinical impact of iron deficiency and anaemia among outpatients with chronic heart failure: the PrEP Registry. *Clin Res Cardiol*. (2017) 106:436–43. doi: 10.1007/s00392-016-1073-y

Anand IS. Anemia and chronic heart failure implications and treatment options. *J Am Coll Cardiol*. (2008) 52:501–11. doi: 10.1016/j.jacc.2008. 04.044

Nagatomo Y, Yoshikawa T, Okamoto H, Kitabatake A, Hori M, J-CHF Investigators. Anemia is associated with blunted response to β-blocker therapy using carvedilol - insights from Japanese Chronic Heart Failure (J-CHF) study. *Circ J*. (2018) 82:691–8. doi: 10.1253/circj.CJ-17-0442

Okonko DO, Anker SD. Anemia in chronic heart failure: pathogenetic mechanisms. *J Card Fail*. (2004) 10(Suppl. 1):S5– 9. doi: 10.1016/j.cardfail.2004.01.004

Sirbu O, Sorodoc V, Jaba IM, Floria M, Stoica A, Profire L, et al. The influence of cardiovascular medications on iron metabolism in patients with heart failure. *Medicina*. (2019) 55:329. doi: 10.3390/medicina55070329

Vaisman N, Silverberg DS, Wexler D, Niv E, Blum M, Keren G, et al. Correction of anemia in patients with congestive heart failure increases resting energy expenditure. *Clin Nutr*. (2004) 23:355–61. doi: 10.1016/j.clnu.2003.08.005

Varat MA, Adolph RJ, Fowler NO. Cardiovascular effects of anemia. *Am Heart J*. (1972) 83:415–26. doi: 10.1016/0002-8703(72)90445-0

Gupta K, Kalra R, Rajapreyar I, Joly JM, Pate M, Cribbs MG, et al. Anemia, mortality, and hospitalizations in heart failure with a preserved ejection fraction (from the TOPCAT Trial). *Am J Cardiol*. (2020) 125:1347– 54. doi: 10.1016/j.amjcard.2020.01.046

Parcha V, Patel N, Kalra R, Bhargava A, Prabhu SD, Arora G, et al. Clinical, demographic, and imaging correlates of anemia in heart failure with preserved ejection fraction (from the RELAX Trial). *Am J Cardiol*. (2020) 125:1870– 8. doi: 10.1016/j.amjcard.2020.03.006

Savarese G, Jonsson Å, Hallberg A-C, Dahlström U, Edner M, Lund LH. Prevalence of, associations with, and prognostic role of anemia in heart failure across the ejection fraction spectrum. *Int J Cardiol*. (2020) 298:59– 65. doi: 10.1016/j.ijcard.2019.08.049

Wienbergen H, Pfister O, Hochadel M, Fach A, Backhaus T, Bruder O, et al. Long-term effects of iron deficiency in patients with heart failure with or without anemia: the RAID-HF follow-up study. *Clin Res Cardiol*. (2019) 108:93–100. doi: 10.1007/s00392-018-1327-y

Kosiborod M, Curtis JP, Wang Y, Smith GL, Masoudi FA, Foody JM, et al. Anemia and outcomes in patients with heart failure: a study from the National Heart Care Project. *Arch Intern Med*. (2005) 165:2237– 44. doi: 10.1001/archinte.165.19.2237

Tymin´ska A, Kapłon-Cie´slicka A, Ozieran´ski K, Peller M, Balsam P, Marchel M, et al. Anemia at hospital admission and its relation to outcomes in patients with heart failure (from the Polish Cohort of 2 European Society of Cardiology Heart Failure Registries). *Am J Cardiol*. (2017) 119:2021– 9. doi: 10.1016/j.amjcard.2017.03.035

He S-W, Wang L-X. The impact of anemia on the prognosis of chronic heart failure: a meta-analysis and systemic review. *Congest Heart Fail*. (2009) 15:123–30. doi: 10.1111/j.1751-7133.2008.00030.x

Chairat K, Rattanavipanon W, Tanyasaensook K, Chindavijak B, Chulavatnatol S, Nathisuwan S. Relationship of anemia and clinical outcome in heart failure patients with preserved versus reduced ejection fraction in a rural area of Thailand. *Int J Cardiol Heart Vasc*. (2020) 30:100597. doi: 10.1016/j.ijcha.2020.100597

Formiga F, Chivite D, Ariza-Solé A, Corbella X. Mild anemia and mortality in very old adults hospitalized for acute heart failure. *J Am Geriatr Soc*. (2018) 66:2432– 4. doi: 10.1111/jgs.15562

Ye S-D, Wang S-J, Wang G-G, Li L, Huang Z-W, Qin J, et al. Association between anemia and outcome in patients hospitalized for acute heart failure syndromes: findings from Beijing Acute Heart Failure Registry (Beijing AHF Registry). *Intern Emerg Med*. (2020) 16:183– 92. doi: 10.1007/s11739-020-02343-x

Moher D, Liberati A, Tetzlaff J, Altman DG, PRISMA Group. Preferred reporting items for systematic reviews and meta-analyses: the PRISMA statement. *PLoS Med*. (2009) 6:e1000097. doi: 10.1371/journal.pmed.1000097

Jørgensen L, Paludan-Müller AS, Laursen DRT, Savovic´ J, Boutron I, Sterne JAC, et al. Evaluation of the Cochrane tool for assessing risk of bias in randomized clinical trials: overview of published comments and analysis of user practice in Cochrane and non-Cochrane reviews. *Syst Rev*. (2016) 5:80. doi: 10.1186/s13643-016-0259-8

Sterne JA, Hernán MA, Reeves BC, Savovic´ J, Berkman ND, Viswanathan M, et al. ROBINS-I: a tool for assessing risk of bias in non-randomised studies of interventions. *BMJ*. (2016) 355:i4919. doi: 10.1136/bmj.i4919

Savovic´ J, Weeks L, Sterne JAC, Turner L, Altman DG, Moher D, et al. Evaluation of the Cochrane Collaboration's tool for assessing the risk of bias in randomized trials: focus groups, online survey, proposed recommendations and their implementation. *Syst Rev*. (2014) 3:37. doi: 10.1186/2046-4053-3-37

Bax L, Yu L-M, Ikeda N, Moons KG. A systematic comparison of software dedicated to meta-analysis of causal studies. *BMC Med Res Methodol*. (2007) 7:40. doi: 10.1186/1471-2288-7-40

Higgins JPT, Thompson SG, Spiegelhalter DJ. A re-evaluation of random- effects meta-analysis. *J R Stat Soc Ser A Stat Soc*. (2009) 172:137– 59. doi: 10.1111/j.1467-985X.2008.00552.x

Higgins JPT, Thompson SG. Quantifying heterogeneity in a meta-analysis. *Stat Med*. (2002) 21:1539–58. doi: 10.1002/sim.1186

Duval S, Tweedie R. Trim and fill: a simple funnel-plot-based method of testing and adjusting for publication bias in meta-analysis. *Biometrics*. (2000) 56:455–63. doi: 10.1111/j.0006-341X.2000.00455.x

Goh VJ, Tromp J, Teng T-HK, Tay WT, Van Der Meer P, Ling LH, et al. Prevalence, clinical correlates, and outcomes of anaemia in multi-ethnic Asian patients with heart failure with reduced ejection fraction. *ESC Heart Fail*. (2018) 5:570–8. doi: 10.1002/ehf2.12279

Jin X, Cao J, Zhou J, Wang Y, Han X, Song Y, et al. Outcomes of patients with anemia and renal dysfunction in hospitalized heart failure with preserved ejection fraction (from the CN-HF registry). Int J Cardiol Heart Vasc. (2019) 25:100415. doi: 10.1016/j.ijcha.2019.100415

van den Berge JC, Constantinescu AA, van Domburg RT, Brankovic M, Deckers JW, Akkerhuis KM. Renal function and anemia in relation to short- and long-term prognosis of patients with acute heart failure in the period 1985-2008: a clinical cohort study. PLoS ONE. (2018) 13:e0201714. doi: 10.1371/journal.pone.0201714

Kim MC, Kim KH, Cho JY, Lee KH, Sim DS, Yoon HJ, et al. Pre- discharge anemia as a predictor of adverse clinical outcomes in patients with acute decompensated heart failure. Korean J Intern Med. (2019) 34:549- 58. doi: 10.3904/kjim.2017.337

Negi PC, Dev M, Paul P, Pal Singh D, Rathoure S, Kumar R, et al. Prevalence, risk factors, and significance of iron deficiency and anemia in nonischemic heart failure patients with reduced ejection fraction from a Himachal Pradesh heart failure registry. Indian Heart J. (2018) 70(Suppl. 3):S182-8. doi: 10.1016/j.ihj.2018.10.032

Parrish JB, Weinstock-Guttman B, Smerbeck A, Benedict RHB, Yeh EA. Fatigue and depression in children with demyelinating disorders. J Child Neurol. (2013) 28:713-8. doi: 10.1177/0883073812450750

Simone M, Viterbo RG, Margari L, Iaffaldano P. Computer-assisted rehabilitation of attention in pediatric multiple sclerosis and ADHD patients: a pilot trial. BMC Neurol. (2018) 18:82. doi: 10.1186/s12883-018-1087-3

Braunwald E. The war against heart failure: the Lancet lecture. Lancet. (2015) 385:812-24. doi: 10.1016/S0140-6736(14)61889-4

Gutierrez C, Blanchard DG. Diastolic heart failure: challenges of diagnosis and treatment. Am Fam Phys. (2004) 69:2609-16. Available online at: https://www.aafp.org/afp/2004/0601/p2609.html

McLean RC, Jessup M. The challenge of treating heart failure: a diverse disease affecting diverse populations. JAMA. (2013) 310:2033- 4. doi: 10.1001/jama.2013.282773

Beale AL, Warren JL, Roberts N, Meyer P, Townsend NP, Kaye D. Iron deficiency in heart failure with preserved ejection fraction: a systematic review and meta-analysis. Open Heart. (2019) 6:e001012. doi: 10.1136/openhrt-2019-001012

Jacob C, Altevers J, Barck I, Hardt T, Braun S, Greiner W. Retrospective analysis into differences in heart failure patients with and without iron deficiency or anaemia. ESC Heart Fail. (2019) 6:840-55. doi: 10.1002/ehf2.12485

Ezekowitz JA, McAlister FA, Armstrong PW. Anemia is common in heart failure and is associated with poor outcomes: insights from a cohort of 12 065 patients with new-onset heart failure. Circulation. (2003) 107:223- 5. doi: 10.1161/01.CIR.0000052622.51963.FC

Ikama MS, Nsitou BM, Kocko I, Mongo NS, Kimbally-Kaky G, Nkoua JL. Prevalence of anaemia among patients with heart failure at the Brazzaville University Hospital. Cardiovasc J Afr. (2015) 26:140-2. doi: 10.5830/CVJA-2015-021

Tang Y-D, Katz SD. Anemia in chronic heart failure: prevalence, etiology, clinical correlates, and treatment options. Circulation. (2006) 113:2454- 61. doi: 10.1161/CIRCULATIONAHA.105.583666

Dabek J, Kułach A, Gasior Z. Nuclear factor kappa-light-chain-enhancer of activated B cells (NF-κB): a new potential therapeutic target in atherosclerosis? Pharmacol Rep. (2010) 62:778-83. doi: 10.1016/S1734-1140(10)70338-8

Dec GW. Anemia and iron deficiency–new therapeutic targets in heart failure? N Engl J Med. (2009) 361:2475-7. doi: 10.1056/NEJMe0910313

van der Meer P, Voors AA, Lipsic E, Smilde TDJ, van Gilst WH, van Veldhuisen DJ. Prognostic value of plasma erythropoietin on mortality in patients with chronic heart failure. J Am Coll Cardiol. (2004) 44:63- 7. doi: 10.1016/j.jacc.2004.03.052

Jaiswal S, Natarajan P, Silver AJ, Gibson CJ, Bick AG, Shvartz E, et al. Clonal hematopoiesis and risk of atherosclerotic cardiovascular disease. N Engl J Med. (2017) 377:111-21. doi: 10.1056/NEJMoa1701719

Sano S, Oshima K, Wang Y, MacLauchlan S, Katanasaka Y, Sano M, et al. Tet2-mediated clonal hematopoiesis accelerates heart failure through a mechanism involving the IL-1β/NLRP3 inflammasome. J Am Coll Cardiol. (2018) 71:875-86. doi: 10.1016/j.jacc.2017.12.037

Silverberg D, Wexler D, Blum M, Wollman Y, Iaina A. The cardio-renal anaemia syndrome: does it exist? Nephrol Dial Transplant. (2003) 18(Suppl. 8):viii7-12. doi: 10.1093/ndt/gfg1084

Bock JS, Gottlieb SS. Cardiorenal syndrome: new perspectives. Circulation. (2010) 121:2592-600. doi: 10.1161/CIRCULATIONAHA.109.886473

Sanderson JE. Pathogenesis of oedema in chronic severe anaemia: studies of body water and sodium, renal function, haemodynamic variables and plasma hormones. Br Heart J. (1994) 71:490. doi: 10.1136/hrt.71.5.490-b

Editors. Best practice in systematic reviews: the importance of protocols and registration. PLoS Med, (2011) 8:e1001009.

Permissions

The contributors of this book come from diverse backgrounds, making this book a truly international effort. This book will bring forth new frontiers with its revolutionizing research information and detailed analysis of the nascent developments around the world.

We would like to thank all the contributing authors for lending their expertise to make the book truly unique. They have played a crucial role in the development of this book. Without their invaluable contributions this book wouldn't have been possible. They have made vital efforts to compile up to date information on the varied aspects of this subject to make this book a valuable addition to the collection of many professionals and students.

This book was conceptualized with the vision of imparting up-to-date information and advanced data in this field. To ensure the same, a matchless editorial board was set up. Every individual on the board went through rigorous rounds of assessment to prove their worth. After which they invested a large part of their time researching and compiling the most relevant data for our readers.

The editorial board has been involved in producing this book since its inception. They have spent rigorous hours researching and exploring the diverse topics which have resulted in the successful publishing of this book. They have passed on their knowledge of decades through this book. To expedite this challenging task, the publisher supported the team at every step. A small team of assistant editors was also appointed to further simplify the editing procedure and attain best results for the readers.

Apart from the editorial board, the designing team has also invested a significant amount of their time in understanding the subject and creating the most relevant covers. They scrutinized every image to scout for the most suitable representation of the subject and create an appropriate cover for the book.

The publishing team has been an ardent support to the editorial, designing and production team. Their endless efforts to recruit the best for this project, has resulted in the accomplishment of this book. They are a veteran in the field of academics and their pool of knowledge is as vast as their experience in printing. Their expertise and guidance has proved useful at every step. Their uncompromising quality standards have made this book an exceptional effort. Their encouragement from time to time has been an inspiration for everyone.

The publisher and the editorial board hope that this book will prove to be a valuable piece of knowledge for researchers, students, practitioners and scholars across the globe.

List of Contributors

Joames K. Freitas Leal, Roland Brock, Merel Adjobo-Hermans and Giel Bosman
Department of Biochemistry, Radboud University Medical Center, Nijmegen, Netherlands

Frank Preijers
Laboratory for Hematology, Department of Laboratory Medicine, Radboud University Medical Center, Nijmegen, Netherlands

Satheesh Chonat
Department of Pediatrics, Emory University School of Medicine, Atlanta, GA, United States
Aflac Cancer and Blood Disorders Center, Children's Healthcare of Atlanta, Atlanta, GA, United States

Mary Risinger
College of Nursing, University of Cincinnati, Cincinnati, OH, United States

Haripriya Sakthivel, Tamara Maghathe and Katie G. Seu
Cancer and Blood Diseases Institute, Cincinnati Children's Hospital Medical Center, Cincinnati, OH, United States

Omar Niss and Theodosia A. Kalfa
Cancer and Blood Diseases Institute, Cincinnati Children's Hospital Medical Center, Cincinnati, OH, United States
Department of Pediatrics, University of Cincinnati College of Medicine, Cincinnati, OH, United States

Jennifer A. Rothman
Duke University Medical Center, Durham, NC, United States

Loan Hsieh
Division of Hematology, CHOC Children's Hospital and UC Irvine Medical Center, Orange, CA, United States

Stella T. Chou, Janet L. Kwiatkowski and Eugene Khandros
Division of Hematology, Children's Hospital of Philadelphia, Philadelphia, PA, United States
Department of Pediatrics, Perelman School of Medicine, University of Pennsylvania, Philadelphia, PA, United States

Matthew F. Gorman
Kaiser Permanente Santa Clara Medical Center, Santa Clara, CA, United States

Donald T. Wells
Dell Children's Medical Center, Austin, TX, United States

Neha Dagaonkar
Genomics Analysis Facility, Institute for Genomic Medicine, Columbia University, New York, NY, United States

Kejian Zhang
Coyote Bioscience Co., Ltd., San Jose, CA, United States

Wenying Zhang
Department of Pediatrics, University of Cincinnati College of Medicine, Cincinnati, OH, United States
Laboratory of Genetics and Genomics, Division of Human Genetics, Cincinnati Children's Hospital Medical Center, Cincinnati, OH, United States

Ahmar Urooj Zaidi
Children's Hospital of Michigan, Detroit, MI, United States

Steven Buck and Yaddanapudi Ravindranath
Children's Hospital of Michigan, Detroit, MI, United States
Wayne State University School of Medicine, Detroit, MI, United States

Manisha Gadgeel, Miguel Herrera-Martinez, Araathi Mohan, Kenya Johnson, Shruti Bagla and Robert M. Johnson
Wayne State University School of Medicine, Detroit, MI, United States

Gloria Barbarani, Cristina Fugazza and Antonella E. Ronchi
Dipartimento di Biotecnologie e Bioscienze, Università degli Studi Milano-Bicocca, Milan, Italy,

John Strouboulis
School of Cancer & Pharmaceutical Sciences, Faculty of Life Sciences & Medicine, King's College London, London, United Kingdom

Maddalena Raia
CEINGE Biotecnologie Avanzate, Naples, Italy

Sule Unal
Division of Pediatric Hematology, Hacettepe University, Ankara, Turkey

Susanna Barella
SSD Talassemie, Anemie Rare e Dismetabolismi del Ferro, Ospedale Pediatrico Microcitemico Antonio Cao, Azienda Ospedaliera Brotzu, Cagliari, Italy

Cristian Tornador
BloodGenetics S.L., Barcelona, Spain
Teresa Moreto Foundation, Barcelona, Spain

Edgar Sánchez-Prados
Bioinformatics for Health Sciences Master Programme, Universitat Pompeu Fabra, Barcelona, Spain

Beatriz Cadenas
Whole Genix SL., Barcelona, Spain
Universitat de Vic-Universitat Central de Catalunya, Vic, Spain
Iron Metabolism: Regulation and Diseases Group, Josep Carreras Leukaemia Research Institute, Campus Can Ruti, Barcelona, Spain

Veronica Venturi
Iron Metabolism: Regulation and Diseases Group, Department of Basic Sciences, Faculty of Medicine and Health Sciences, Universitat Internacional de Catalunya, Barcelona, Spain

Mayka Sánchez
BloodGenetics S.L., Barcelona, Spain
Iron Metabolism: Regulation and Diseases Group, Department of Basic Sciences, Faculty of Medicine and Health Sciences, Universitat Internacional de Catalunya, Barcelona, Spain

Ines Hernández-Rodriguez
Haematology Service, Hospital Germans Trias i Pujol University Hospital, Oncology Catalan Institute, Barcelona, Spain

Annelies J. van Vuren and Eduard J. van Beers
Van Creveldkliniek, Department of Internal Medicine and Dermatology, University Medical Center Utrecht, Utrecht University, Utrecht, Netherlands

Carlo A. J. M. Gaillard
Department of Internal Medicine and Dermatology, University Medical Center Utrecht, Utrecht University, Utrecht, Netherlands

Michele F. Eisenga
Department of Internal Medicine, Division of Nephrology, University Medical Center Groningen, University of Groningen, Groningen, Netherlands

Elisa Fermo, Cristina Vercellati, Anna Paola Marcello, Anna Zaninoni, Alberto Zanella, Wilma Barcellini and Paola Bianchi
UOC Ematologia, UOS Fisiopatologia delle Anemie, Fondazione IRCCS Ca' Granda Ospedale Maggiore Policlinico di Milano, Milan, Italy

Selin Aytac and Mualla Cetin
Department of Pediatric Hematology, Faculty of Medicine, Hacettepe University, Ankara, Turkey

Ilaria Capolsini
Pediatric Oncohematology Section with BMT, Santa Maria della Misericordia Hospital, Perugia, Italy

Maddalena Casale
Department of Woman, Child and General and Special Surgery, University of Campania "Luigi Vanvitelli", Naples, Italy

Sabrina Paci
Dipartmento di Pediatria, ASST Santi Paolo e Carlo, Presidio Ospedale San Paolo Universita' di Milano, Milan, Italy

Emmanuelle Charrin, Camille Faes, Amandine Sotiaux, Sarah Skinner and Cyril Martin
Interuniversity Laboratory of Human Movement Biology, University Claude Bernard Lyon 1, University of Lyon, Lyon, France
Laboratory of Excellence "GR-Ex", Paris, France

Vincent Pialoux and Philippe Connes
Interuniversity Laboratory of Human Movement Biology, University Claude Bernard Lyon 1, University of Lyon, Lyon, France
Laboratory of Excellence "GR-Ex", Paris, France
Institut Universitaire de France, Paris, France

Philippe Joly
Interuniversity Laboratory of Human Movement Biology, University Claude Bernard Lyon 1, University of Lyon, Lyon, France
Laboratory of Excellence "GR-Ex", Paris, France
Groupement Hospitalier Est, UF "Biochimie des Pathologies érythrocytaires" Centre de Biologie Est, CHU de Lyon, Lyon, France

Asena Abay
Dynamics of Fluids, Department of Experimental Physics, Saarland University, Saarbrücken, Germany
Landsteiner Laboratory, Sanquin, Amsterdam, Netherlands

Emile van den Akker and Marieke von Lindern
Landsteiner Laboratory, Sanquin, Amsterdam, Netherlands

Greta Simionato, Laura Hertz and Lars Kaestner
Dynamics of Fluids, Department of Experimental Physics, Saarland University, Saarbrücken, Germany
Theoretical Medicine and Biosciences, Saarland University, Homburg, Germany

Revaz Chachanidze
Dynamics of Fluids, Department of Experimental Physics, Saarland University, Saarbrücken, Germany
Université Grenoble Alpes, CNRS, Grenoble INP, LRP, Grenoble, France

Marc Leonetti
Université Grenoble Alpes, CNRS, Grenoble INP, LRP, Grenoble, France

Giampaolo Minetti
Laboratory of Biochemistry, Department of Biology and Biotechnology, University of Pavia, Pavia, Italy

Christian Wagner
Dynamics of Fluids, Department of Experimental Physics, Saarland University, Saarbrücken, Germany
Physics and Materials Science Research Unit, University of Luxembourg, Luxembourg City, Luxembourg

Gianluca De Rosa, Francesco Manna, Barbara Eleni Rosato, Antonella Gambale, Roberta Russo, Roberta Marra, Immacolata Andolfo and Achille Iolascon
Department of Molecular Medicine and Medical Biotechnologies, University of Naples Federico II, Naples, Italy
CEINGE, Biotecnologie Avanzate, Naples, Italy

Edoardo Errichiello and Orsetta Zuffardi
Department of Molecular Medicine, University of Pavia, Pavia, Italy

Annalisa Vetro
Pediatric Neurology, Neurogenetics and Neurobiology Unit and Laboratories, Department of Neuroscience, A. Meyer Children's Hospital, University of Florence, Florence, Italy

Valeria Calcaterra
Pediatric Unit, Department of Maternal and Children's Health, Fondazione IRCCS Policlinico San Matteo, University of Pavia, Pavia, Italy

Gloria Pelizzo
Department of Pediatric Surgery, Children's Hospital "G. Di Cristina", ARNAS Civico-Di Cristina-Benfretelli, Palermo, Italy

Lucia De Franceschi
Department of Medicine, University of Verona, Verona, Italy

Polina Petkova-Kirova
Institute of Molecular Cell Biology, Saarland University, Homburg, Germany

Jens Danielczok
Theoretical Medicine and Biosciences, Saarland University, Homburg, Germany

Rick Huisjes and Richard van Wijk
Department of Clinical Chemistry & Haematology, University Medical Center Utrecht, Utrecht, Netherlands

Asya Makhro and Anna Bogdanova
Red Blood Cell Research Group, Institute of Veterinary Physiology, Vetsuisse Faculty, Zurich Center for Integrative Human Physiology (ZIHP), University of Zürich, Zurich, Switzerland

Maria del Mar Mañú-Pereira
Vall d'Hebron Research Institute, Vall d'Hebron University Hospital, Barcelona, Spain

Joan-Lluis Vives Corrons
Red Blood Cell Defects and Hematopoietic Disorders Unit, Josep Carreras Leukaemia Research Institute, Barcelona, Spain

Catherine Qiu Hua Chan
Department of Family Medicine and Continuing Care, Singapore General Hospital, Singapore

Lian Leng Low and Kheng Hock Lee
Department of Family Medicine and Continuing Care, Singapore General Hospital, Singapore
Family Medicine, Duke-NUS Medical School, Singapore

Xisheng Weng
Department of Orthopaedic Surgery, Peking Union Medical College Hospital, Chinese Academy of Medical Sciences & Peking Union Medical College, Beijing, China

Chang Han
Department of Orthopaedic Surgery, Peking Union Medical College Hospital, Chinese Academy of Medical Sciences & Peking Union Medical College, Beijing, China
Peking Union Medical College, Eight-year MD program, Chinese Academy of Medical Sciences, Beijing, China

Yimin Dai
Peking Union Medical College, Eight-year MD program, Chinese Academy of Medical Sciences, Beijing, China

Karima Landelouci and Geneviève Pépin
Département de Biologie Médicale, Université du Québec à Trois-Rivières, Trois-Rivières, QC, Canada Groupe de Recherche en Signalisation Cellulaire, Université du Québec à Trois-Rivières, Trois-Rivières, QC, Canada

Shruti Sinha
Department of Biotechnology, GITAM Institute of Technology, GITAM deemed to be University, Visakhapatnam, India

Qinrui Li, Furong Liang, Weilan Liang, Wanjun Shi and Ying Han
Department of Pediatrics, Peking University First Hospital, Beijing, China

Guan-ying Nie, Peng Liu, Ming Li and Dian-jun Sun
Key Lab of Etiology and Epidemiology, National Health Commission & Education Bureau of Heilongjiang Province (23618504), Key Laboratory of Trace Elements and Human Health, Center for Endemic Disease Control, Chinese Center for Disease Control and Prevention, Harbin Medical University, Harbin, China

Rui Wang
Examination Department, Central Hospital Affiliated to Shenyang Medical College, Shenyang, China

Alessia Pagani and Clara Camaschella
Division of Genetics and Cell Biology, San Raffaele Scientific Institute, Milan, Italy

Antonella Nai and Laura Silvestri
Division of Genetics and Cell Biology, San Raffaele Scientific Institute, Milan, Italy
Vita-Salute San Raffaele University, Milan, Italy

Jose Portolés and Leyre Martín
Department of Nephrology, Puerta de Hierro Majadahonda University Hospital, Madrid, Spain
Anemia Working Group Spanish Society of Nephrology, Madrid, Spain

Aleix Cases
Anemia Working Group Spanish Society of Nephrology, Madrid, Spain
Instituto de Investigaciones Biomédicas August Pi i Sunyer (IDIBAPS), Universitat de Barcelona, Barcelona, Spain

José Jesús Broseta
Instituto de Investigaciones Biomédicas August Pi i Sunyer (IDIBAPS), Universitat de Barcelona, Barcelona, Spain

Tamás Resál, Klaudia Farkas and Tamás Molnár
Gastroenterology Unit, Department of Medicine, University of Szeged, Szeged, Hungary

Jian Shen, Chau Vu and Botian Xu
Biomedical Engineering, University of Southern California, Los Angeles, Los Angeles, CA, United States

Xin Miao
Siemens, Boston, MA, United States

Clio González-Zacarías
Neuroscience Graduate Program, University of Southern California, Los Angeles, Los Angeles, CA, United States

Aart J. Nederveen
Amsterdam UMC, Radiology and Nuclear Medicine, University of Amsterdam, Amsterdam, Netherlands

John C. Wood
Biomedical Engineering, University of Southern California, Los Angeles, Los Angeles, CA, United States
Department of Pediatrics and Radiology, Children's Hospital Los Angeles, Los Angeles, CA, United States

Adisu Birhanu Weldesenbet and Daniel Berhanie Enyew
Epidemiology and Biostatistics Department, College of Health and Medical Sciences, Haramaya University, Haramaya, Ethiopia

Nebiyu Bahiru
Department of Public Health and Health Policy, School of Public Health, College of Health and Medical Sciences, Haramaya University, Haramaya, Ethiopia

Mei Luo, Bin Dong, Yinghua Ma, Jie Dai, Yi Song and Jun Ma
Institute of Child and Adolescent Health, Peking University School of Public Health, National Health Commission Key Laboratory of Reproductive Health, Beijing, China

Patrick W. C. Lau
Department of Sport and Physical Education, Hong Kong Baptist University, Kowloon Tong, China

Hongfeng Shen and Wei Cha
Department of Cardiology, Affiliated Hospital of Shaoxing University, Shaoxing, China

Qiaoli Lu
Department of General Medicine, Zhuji People's Hospital of Zhejiang Province, Shaoxing, China

Index

Printed in the USA
CPSIA information can be obtained
at www.ICGtesting.com
JSHW051411091023
49903JS00006B/376